Neurogenic Disorders of Language

Theory Driven Clinical Practice

D1384961

Dedication

To my late husband, Dennis—you are sadly missed, but your memories are happily cherished.—Laura Murray

To Carla Hess, Wayne Swisher, and Kevin Fire—your boundless enthusiasm and relentless confidence inspired a future beyond my imagination.—Heather Clark

Neurogenic Disorders of Language

Theory Driven Clinical Practice

Laura L. Murray, PhD, CCC-SLP

Associate Professor

Department of Speech and Hearing Sciences

Indiana University

Heather M. Clark, PhD, CCC-SLP

Associate Professor

Communication Disorders Program

Appalachian State University

North Carolina

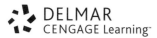
DELMAR
CENGAGE Learning

Australia • Brazil • Japan • Korea • Mexico • Singapore • Spain • United Kingdom • United States

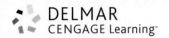

DELMAR
CENGAGE Learning™

Neurogenic Disorders of Language:
Theory Driven Clinical Practice
Laura L. Murray, Heather M. Clark

Vice President, Health Care Business Unit:
  William Brottmiller

Editorial Director: Cathy L. Esperri

Acquisitions Editor: Kalen Conerly

Development Editor: Juliet Steiner

Editorial Assistant: Molly Belmont

Marketing Director: Jennifer McAvey

Marketing Coordinator: Chris Manion

Production Editor: John Mickelbank

Art and Design Coordinator: Christi DiNinni

For product information and technology assistance, contact us at
Cengage Learning Customer & Sales Support, 1-800-354-9706
For permission to use material from this text or product,
submit all requests online at **www.cengage.com/permissions**
Further permissions questions can be emailed to
permissionrequest@cengage.com

Library of Congress Control Number: 2005014066

ISBN-13: 978-1-56593-703-1

ISBN-10: 1-56593-703-1

Delmar
Executive Woods
5 Maxwell Drive
Clifton Park, NY 12065
USA

Cengage Learning is a leading provider of customized learning solutions with
office locations around the globe, including Singapore, the United Kingdom,
Australia, Mexico, Brazil, and Japan. Locate your local office at
international.cengage.com/region

Cengage Learning products are represented in Canada by
Nelson Education, Ltd.

To learn more about Delmar, visit **www.cengage.com/delmar**

Purchase any of our products at your local bookstore or at our preferred
online store **www.ichapters.com**

Printed in Canada
5 6 7 11 10 09

Contents

Acknowledgments

This book represents a major accomplishment for us, but could not have come to fruition without the assistance and support of numerous colleagues, friends, and family members. First, we acknowledge with great gratitude William Irwin for his chapter contribution and timely work effort that assured the completion of this book. Second, we thank Katy Taylor for her tireless assistance compiling the glossary and reference list, Laura Karcher and Jamie Mayer for their reviewing expertise, and Hye-Young Kim for her contributions to the glossary. Third, we are indebted to our past and current mentors and colleagues, whose support and research not only have influenced the contents of this book, but also have inspired our own research and teaching endeavors. And finally, and most importantly, we are most grateful to our families, especially Dylan, Norman, Kehvon, and Ashlyn, for their encouragement and patience. They are no doubt as relieved as we are that this book is finally finished!

About the Authors

Laura L. Murray, Ph.D., CCC-SLP is an associate professor in speech and hearing sciences, a core faculty member in cognitive science and neural science programs at Indiana University, and an affiliated scientist for the Indiana University Center for Aging Research. Prior to her academic position, she worked as a speech-language pathologist in both school and hospital settings in Manitoba, Canada. As a professor, Dr. Murray has received several awards for her teaching efforts at both the graduate and undergraduate levels. Her research focuses on expanding traditional conceptualizations of acquired language disorders by extending theoretical and clinical examination and management of these disorders to cognitive domains beyond language. She has published approximately 40 research papers in refereed journals, and has contributed more than 70 invited and refereed papers to conferences at the national and international levels in the fields of aphasia, right hemisphere disorders, dementia, traumatic brain injury, and normal aging.

Heather M. Clark, Ph.D., CCC-SLP is an associate professor of communication disorders at Appalachian State University in North Carolina. After receiving her clinical training at the University of North Dakota, she pursued doctoral study at the University of Iowa. As a speech-language pathologist in an acute care setting, she developed a passion for serving adults with neurogenic communication disorders, and has thus focused her research efforts on better understanding the cognitive, linguistic, and motor processes that underlie normal communication in individuals both with and without neurologic injury or disease. She currently serves on the steering committee for ASHA Special Interest Division 2, Neurophysiology and Neurogenic Speech and Language Disorders, and was awarded the 2003 American Journal of Speech-Language Pathology Editor's Award.

Preface

In the United States and worldwide, brain damage due to stroke, traumatic brain injury (TBI), progressive neurological disease, and other etiologies is extremely common. Each year in the United States, approximately 1.4 million adults will suffer a TBI (Centers for Disease Control and Prevention, 2003), 41,000 will be diagnosed with a brain tumor (Central Brain Tumor Registry of the United States, 2005), 750,000 will have a stroke (National Stroke Association, 2002), and more than 500,000 will be diagnosed with a progressive disorder such as Alzheimer's disease, Parkinson's disease, or multiple sclerosis (National Institute of Aging, 2003; National Institute of Neurological Disorders and Stroke, 2001; 2003). Neurogenic language disorders are common consequences of these forms of brain damage and disease.

The purpose of this book is to provide a thorough review of neurogenic language disorders for speech-language pathology students, clinicians, and researchers, as well as those in related health care disciplines, such as occupational therapy, neuropsychology, physiatry, and nursing, who provide services to the above patient populations. Several features of this book, in terms of both content and organization, make it a valuable resource, regardless of the reader's degree of experience with neurogenic language disorders. First, a number of neurogenic language disorders are systematically described, including aphasia and cognitive-communicative disorders associated with right hemisphere brain damage, TBI, and dementing diseases such as Alzheimer's or Parkinson's disease. Second, traditional descriptions of these neurogenic language disorders are expanded upon by discussing both the linguistic and cognitive bases of these disorders, and by including a thorough review of cognitive assessment and treatment approaches. Third, as indicated by the title of our book, both theoretical and applied clinical issues are highlighted throughout, with a special emphasis on the World Health Organization's International Classification of Functioning, Disability, and Health (ICF) as a guiding framework for understanding and managing neurogenic language disorders (WHO; 2001). Accordingly, this book will serve not only as a comprehensive textbook for university courses that must cover a range of neurogenic language disorders, but also as an up-to-date reference for both researchers and clinicians looking to expand their knowledge base.

On an editorial note, readers will see that throughout the book we use the term *patients* to refer to individuals who have been diagnosed with a neurogenic language disorder. We acknowledge that there is a move in both research and clinical practice to replace terms that denote impairment with more neutral ones (e.g., *individuals* or *adults* vs. *patients*); however, in those sections of the book in which discussions focus on patients and caregivers, the text became too cumbersome and confusing when trying to use only neutral terminology. Therefore, for clarity purposes, we elected to use the term *patients*.

ORGANIZATION OF THIS TEXT

Several frameworks have been adopted to organize the contents of this book. First, the ICF classification system is used throughout the text to highlight the importance of addressing neurogenic language disorders in terms of not only linguistic and cognitive symptoms (i.e., ICF levels of body structure and function), but also the effects of these symptoms on the daily personal, social, education, and/or vocational endeavors (i.e., ICF levels of activity and participation) of the patients and, in at least some cases, caregivers as well. Second, a language processing model is followed to allow systematic and in-depth description of procedures for evaluating and remedying linguistic aspects of neurogenic language disorders. Last, because all neurogenic language disorders are associated with both linguistic and cognitive symptoms, rather than including separate discussions for each neurogenic language disorder (e.g., aphasia, dementia), management approaches are examined in terms of those appropriate for addressing linguistic problems and those appropriate for addressing cognitive problems.

The first three chapters of this book review constructs and conditions essential to managing neurogenic language disorders. Chapter 1 introduces and explains concepts fundamental to the book's organizational frameworks (e.g., ICF classification system). In Chapter 2, readers are familiarized with impairments and activity limitations associated with neurogenic language disorders, including those associated with aphasia, right hemisphere brain damage, TBI, or dementia, and in Chapter 3, common etiologies of these disorders are described.

The next four chapters pertain to diagnostic issues. Chapter 4 provides an overview of the assessment process. Chapters 5, 6, and 7, respectively, review procedures for quantifying and qualifying linguistic abilities, cognitive status, and daily communication activity and participation of patients with neurogenic language disorders.

The remaining book chapters primarily focus on treatment issues, beginning with Chapter 8, which offers an overview of evidence-based practice concepts. Chapter 9 describes and evaluates numerous behavioral methods for treating impaired linguistic and cognitive functions, Chapter 10 reviews pharmacological approaches, and Chapter 11 covers techniques designed to effect change at the ICF levels of activity and participation. In Chapter 12, the current health care system and its policies are discussed with respect to their impact on evaluating and treating neurogenic language disorders. This chapter, and thus the book, concludes with a brief consideration of possible ways in which the management of neurogenic language disorders may advance in the future.

FEATURES

Within each chapter, the reader will find a number of special features. These features were designed to augment the reader's experience and to help the reader successfully navigate the content. Special features include:

- *Learning Objectives*—Each chapter begins with a carefully constructed list of its main concepts. These can be used as a framework for what to expect as well as a review and study aid.
- *Key Terms*—Also setting the tone for each chapter is a list of its key terms. Definitions for each of these terms can be found in the Glossary. Readers can scan the terms as an orientation to the chapter's terminology as well as use them as review and study aids.
- *Sidebars*—Throughout the book, sidebars are included to place information in the context of real-life clinical practice. Directly related to the chapter, sidebars provide models for applying the theoretical concepts in clinical settings with clients.
- *Summary*—Each chapter concludes with a summary that pulls everything together and provides solid footing for moving on to subsequent chapters.
- *Comprehensive References*—The book provides a comprehensive, up-to-date, relevant list of references for readers looking for further information on the topics covered.

Given their prevalence, there is an ongoing need to identify effective and efficient means by which to manage neurogenic language disorders. By reviewing the current literature and highlighting areas in need of additional investigation, it is our hope that this book spurs further theoretical and clinical interest in understanding, assessing, and treating neurogenic language disorders, and, in turn, will result in improved outcomes for those patients and caregivers directly affected by neurogenic language disorders.

Chapter 1

Introduction: Models and Concepts

LEARNING OBJECTIVES

After reading this chapter you should be able to:

- Discuss the International Classification of Function and its application to the study and management of neurogenic language disorders.

- Identify and describe the linguistic processes (body functions) that support language comprehension and production.

- Identify and describe components of attention, memory, and executive functioning (body functioning) and their contribution to communication.

- Identify the neuroanatomy (body structures) that support language, attention, memory, and executive functioning.

KEY TERMS

activities and participation
attention
body function
body structure
cognition
cognitive flexibility
communication
environmental factors

executive functioning
inhibition
International Classification of Functioning, Disability, and Health (ICF)

language
memory
organization
planning
problem solving
repetition
self-monitoring

INTRODUCTION

As adults, most of us have progressed through our lives giving only passing notice to our ability to communicate. We listen, speak, read, and write, often without effort, and we expect other adults to experience similar ease in their communication with us. We know, however, that even otherwise healthy adults can experience illnesses or accidents that suddenly impact their communication in both subtle and dramatic ways. Likewise, as we age, we become more susceptible to a number of chronic diseases that may progressively and irreversibly limit our communication abilities as well as our thinking or cognitive skills. Adult neurogenic language disorders arise when these illnesses, accidents, or progressive diseases cause brain damage, and, in turn, that brain damage negatively impacts the communicative and possibly cognitive well-being of

1

the affected individual. Accordingly, speech-language pathologists serving adults must be familiar with the variety of medical conditions that can produce adult neurogenic language disorders. Additionally, they must possess the knowledge and skills necessary not only to evaluate how these accidents or diseases are affecting the communicative and cognitive functioning of their patients, but also to design and implement treatments that will remediate or stabilize the negative effects of these conditions. This book provides students as well as practicing clinicians with a comprehensive review of the concepts and procedures germane to managing adult neurogenic language disorders.

GUIDING FRAMEWORK

Throughout this text, a number of theoretical models addressing the characterization, assessment, and treatment of neurogenic language disorders will be presented. These models often explain relationships among areas of impairment, inform differential diagnosis, and direct selection of treatment targets and strategies. Consistent with the American Speech-Language-Hearing Association (2001) Scope of Practice for Speech-Language Pathology, we have chosen the World Health Organization (WHO, 2001) **International Classification of Functioning, Disability, and Health (ICF)** as a guiding framework for this text. Although the specific terms adopted by the ICF differ from those introduced in the original International Classification of Impairment, Disability, and Handicap (ICIDH; WHO, 1980), the key concepts of the ICIDH have been maintained in the revised ICF.

The ICF includes a system for describing the impact of disease or injury on the body and its functions, as well as patients' ability to complete tasks or activities relevant to their personal, social, educational, and/or vocational pursuits. The ICF constructs of **body structure** and **body function** are closely related, describing the integrity of tissues and organs along with the functions they perform. This level of description parallels the construct of **impairment** described in the ICIDH, and traditionally has been a primary focus of medical assessment as well as medical/surgical interventions. The categories of body structure particularly relevant to communication are *structures of the nervous system, structures of the eye, ear, and related structures, structures involved in voice and speech,* and *additional musculoskeletal structures related to movement* (e.g., muscles). Similarly, the body functions of *mental functions, sensory functions, voice and speech functions,* and *neuromusculoskeletal and movement-related functions* contribute to communication behaviors. With respect to language and neurogenic language disorders specifically, *the structures of the nervous system* and a number of the *specific mental functions* (e.g., attention, memory, mental functions of language) are of primary interest.

The ICF also incorporates the construct of **activities and participation,** which highlights the ability of the individual to use language to communicate in a variety of contexts. Although the ICF combines activities and participation in a single classification construct, the ICIDH terms of **disability** and **handicap** are roughly synonymous with activities and participation, respectively. Within the area of activities and participation, the primary construct of interest to the discussion of neurogenic language disorders is *communication,* which involves receiving and producing spoken, nonverbal, formal sign language, and/or written messages. Within this category the ICF also includes descriptions of conversation and the use of communication devices. Additional categories potentially influenced by the presence of neurogenic language disorders are *learning and applying knowledge, general tasks and demands, domestic life, interpersonal interactions and relationships, major life areas* (e.g., education, work, and employment), and *community, social, and civic life.*

The final primary construct of the ICF is **environmental factors,** which emphasizes the contribution of *products of technology* (e.g., assistive mobility devices), *environmental characteristics* (e.g., physical geography, lighting), *support and relationships* (e.g., family, care providers), *attitudes* of the individual as well as family members and care providers, and *services, systems, and policies* relating to the individual's ability to participate fully in desired activities.

Side Bar

The ICF Applied

The value of the ICF descriptors may be better appreciated through illustration. Consider Dick and Melvin, both men in their early sixties who have experienced strokes with resulting mild language disorders. With respect to underlying *body structure and function*, they demonstrate similar structural impairments of the central nervous system and disruption in the mental functions of receptive and expressive language, potentially leading to the prediction that each would be similarly impacted by their impairments.

A number of *environmental factors*, however, influence the effects of these functional impairments on each man's communicative *activity*. Dick is well educated and, as a vice president for a national banking corporation, has considerable experience communicating in a variety of settings using flexible linguistic styles. Thus, he easily, in fact nearly automatically, compensates for his new language disorder, and his communication impairment is judged to be quite mild by his friends and family.

Melvin, on the other hand, is a farmer in a rural community and did not complete education beyond his GED. His communication partners are limited to family and community members. Although his impairment is equal to Dick's, Melvin does not spontaneously compensate, and his communication impairments are notable during conversation and other interactions.

The ICF also provides a way to characterize the impact of a neurogenic language disorder on Dick's and Melvin's lives (*participation*). Considering again environmental factors, Melvin has a generally patient, laid-back personality, and does not express great frustration

(continued)

with his language symptoms (*individual attitude*). Because Melvin's communication partners are quite familiar with his typical conversation topics, communication is often successful in spite of linguistic errors. Moreover, the dialect in Melvin's geographic region is characterized by a relatively slow speech rate and precise articulation, which facilitate Melvin's comprehension. Ultimately, Melvin's neurogenic language disorder has little impact on his participation in activities he enjoyed prior to his stroke.

In contrast, both Dick's professional and leisure activities (e.g., leading group Bible studies, traveling) involve diverse communication contexts, most of which are demanding and relatively unaccommodating to reduced communicative efficiency (*attitudes of colleagues, strangers*). Thus, Dick expresses greater concern that his language disorder will significantly impact his participation in desired activities. Fortunately, a number of additional environmental factors will facilitate Dick's participation: Electronic communication options (*products and technology*) are available to Dick, and he is willing to utilize them (*individual attitude*). He lives in a metropolitan area with a wealth of community resources, and he has already made contact with an appropriate support group (*support and relationships*). Finally, Dick has access to sufficient economic resources and quality health care (*services, systems, and policies*) to assist with necessary adaptations to maximize participation.

It is clear that the nature of the neurogenic language disorder, which is the same for both men, does not tell the whole story. Only by considering the impact of the neurogenic language disorder on communicative effectiveness in real-life contexts, the implications on life participation, and the environmental factors influencing the impact of the disorder can we gain a more complete understanding of the patient's needs.

Readers familiar with the ICF may note that the overview provided here differs slightly from most descriptions included in other speech-language pathology (SLP) literature. Specifically, it is most common for SLP literature to discuss body structure and body function as a single construct (i.e., impairment) and to separate the construct of activities and participation into two distinct constructs of (1) activity and (2) participation. When the concepts are separated in this way, the term **activity** relates to the patient's ability to complete specific tasks (e.g., speak, write, comprehend gestures), whereas **participation** addresses the impact of impairments and activity limitations on the patient's ability to participate in desired life activities. This minimal modification of the published ICF framework is useful to clinicians managing communication disorders because it underscores the value of considering the nature of underlying language impairments and the resulting communication limitations as well as the impact of these deficits on life participation and quality of life.

In their original or modified form, the ICF constructs provide a framework for describing the myriad of characteristics possible in neurogenic language disorders, planning assessment and treatment strategies, and measuring outcomes. The

ICF recognizes the importance of multidisciplinary involvement throughout the care process, and emphasizes the value of full participation by the patient and family members in the planning and implementing of care plans.

The organization of this text reflects the ICF framework. In the current chapter, the various body structures and functions contributing to language behaviors are reviewed. Chapter 2 expands the discussion of body structure and function with a thorough description of the nature of various neurogenic language disorders. The chapters addressing assessment and treatment are organized with respect to underlying impairments, functional communication (i.e., activity), participation, and quality of life. Similarly, the discussion of treatment is structured such that strategies addressing underlying impairments, functional communication, and quality of life are considered. Finally, issues surrounding environmental factors are incorporated throughout the discussion of both assessment and treatment.

LANGUAGE AND COGNITION (BODY FUNCTION)

Before reviewing specific diseases or language disorders, familiarity and understanding of fundamental concepts such as communication, language, and cognition are essential. Therefore, in this section we provide explicit definitions of each of these terms and discuss the relationships among communication, language, and cognition. Next, we present more detailed information about the myriad of linguistic and cognitive processes that support language comprehension and expression.

Communication, defined as an exchange of ideas, is a fundamental human behavior. Even infants communicate their needs (primarily via crying), and as children age and develop, communication is enhanced by the development of speech, language, and sophisticated nonverbal communication skills. For adults, a primary communication tool is **language.** Language may be defined as a shared code for representing concepts through the use of symbols and rule-based combinations of symbols (Owens, Metz, & Haas, 2003). Language can manifest in various modalities, including spoken (e.g., listening, speaking), written (e.g., reading, writing), or nonverbal/gestural (e.g., facial expressions, conventional gestures, formal sign language). Regardless of the modality used to convey linguistic messages, language involves symbols (e.g., sounds, letters, words, signs) that convey meanings that may vary according to how they are combined, sequenced, or both. For example, the word "can" in the phrases "the can held tomatoes" and "she will can the tomatoes" describes an object in the first phrase and an action in the second phrase. Moreover, the meaning of identical linguistic messages may be influenced by the communicative context, as is illustrated by idioms and other figures of speech (e.g., "We had better get on the ball and fix that leak.").

Although the term "language" is typically used as a noun, it may be more accurate to think about language as a verb, in the sense that using language to communicate involves the execution of complex mental processes. In effect, humans "do" language. The following sections will underscore the highly active nature of language functions by providing an overview of not only the specific processes comprising language but also the additional cognitive processes that support language.

LANGUAGE AND COGNITIVE PROCESSING

Cognition encompasses all processes by which we transform, condense, elaborate, store, retrieve, and exploit sensory information, and thus allows us to cope with and process incoming information so that we can understand and interact with our environment (Guilford & Hoepfner, 1971; Neisser, 1967). Accordingly, language is considered a part of cognition, and shares an intimate relationship with other cognitive functions such as attention, memory, and executive functioning. Language, attention, memory, and executive functioning also are similar in that all are considered multidimensional, and consist of various subcomponents. Additionally, language and other cognitive processes are linked in terms of not only function and architecture, but also neurophysiological circuitry. That is, language, attention, memory, and executive functioning are subserved by many overlapping neural structures and pathways, and thus, when damage to one of these neural structures or pathways results in a neurogenic language disorder, it also, in addition to affecting language, will typically compromise several other cognitive functions. Therefore, having a good understanding of these cognitive functions and their subcomponents is germane to appropriate management of neurogenic language disorders.

Components of Language

As illustrated in Figure 1-1, language is comprised of several linguistic representation stores and operations. Collectively, these various linguistic processes function to support language comprehension, production, or both in one or more language modalities. Because neurogenic language disorders may be a product of impaired access to or functioning of one or a combination of these language subcomponents, assessment and treatment of neurogenic language disorders will depend on clinicians' familiarity with each of these functions within the linguistic system.

Phonological and Orthographic Processing

Understanding of phonological and orthographic processes is essential to the management of neurogenic language disorders in which production, comprehension, or both of spoken or written language, respectively, has been compromised. The phonological system encompasses both the set of sounds (i.e., phonemes) in

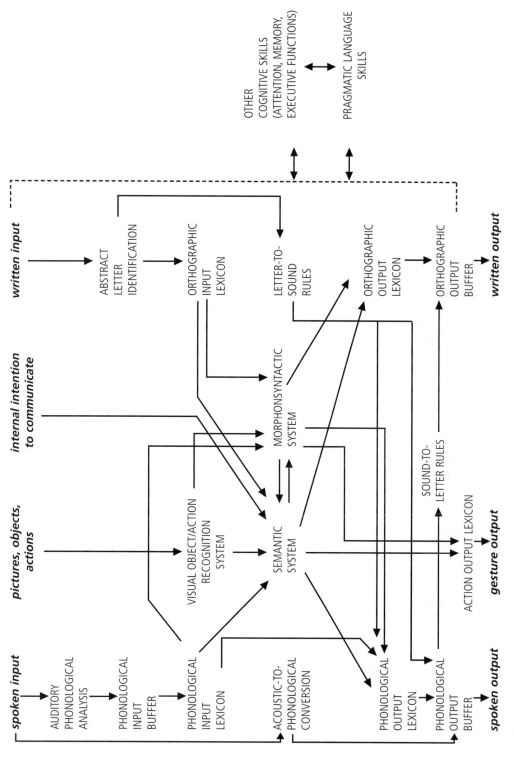

Figure 1-1. Model of linguistic processing (modified from Kay, Lesser, & Coltheart, 1996). Dashed line indicates that pragmatic language and other cognitive skills may exert an influence across most levels of linguistic processing.

one's language and the rules necessary to order and combine those sounds into words (Owens, 1984). It consists of two subsystems: (1) a segmental subsystem, which relates to our processing of distinctive sound elements or phonemes within syllables or words, and (2) a suprasegmental subsystem, which encompasses abilities such as processing of intonation (i.e., modulation of vocal pitch to indicate grammatical segmentation or complexity or emotional status), stress (i.e., accentuation of a certain sound or syllable to assist with determining word or utterance meaning), and pauses (Blumstein, 1998).

Phonological processes contribute at several levels to our understanding and production of spoken language (Goodglass, 1998; Hillis & Caramazza, 1994; Kay et al., 1996). For instance, the following processes depicted in Figure 1-1 involve manipulation and interpretation of phonological information: (1) auditory phonological analysis that allows discrimination of the incoming speech signal into words, syllables, and sounds, and determination of suprasegmental characteristics (e.g., stressed vs. unstressed syllables), despite different speech accents; (2) the phonological input buffer that provides temporary storage of spoken stimuli while they are being processed or prepared for processing; (3) the phonological input lexicon that represents our library of spoken words that have been previously heard; (4) acoustic-phonological conversion that allows translating what is heard directly into individual phonemes, a process needed to repeat aloud unfamiliar words; (5) the phonological output lexicon that represents our library of spoken words that have been previously produced; and (6) the phonological output buffer that temporarily stores the phonemes of a given word while the motor speech plans for producing that word are being instigated. Phonological processes also are interconnected with several orthographic processes, as described in the next paragraph.

The orthographic system functions to facilitate processing of graphemes, which are individual letters or letter clusters that represent a single phoneme (e.g., "c," "k," and "ck" are graphemes for the sound /k/) (Hillis & Caramazza, 1994; Kay et al., 1996). For reading, orthographic processes are engaged to convert graphemes into phonemes (i.e., letter-to-sound translation). Alternately, for writing, this aspect of the linguistic system functions to identify and arrange graphemes into words. In the model of linguistic processing represented in Figure 1-1, orthographic processing contributes to the following: (1) abstract letter identification that fosters visual recognition of letters written in various fonts or formats (e.g., cursive vs. printed letters, upper- vs. lowercase); (2) the orthographic input lexicon that stores the letter strings that correspond to our vocabulary of written words; (3) letter-to-sound rules that are used to translate graphemes into phonemes on a letter-by-letter basis, particularly when reading unfamiliar words; (4) sound-to-letter rules that are used to translate individual phonemes into graphemes, as when spelling unfamiliar words; (5) the orthographic output lexicon that stores spellings of written vocabulary we have previously used; and (6) the orthographic output buffer that temporarily holds word spellings while a word is being written or prepared to be written.

Lexical-Semantic Processing

Production and understanding of language content or meaning is a product of processing at the lexical-semantic level. The term "lexical" is typically used to refer to representations or processes related to word forms in the various language modalities (e.g., writing, spoken language), whereas "semantic" refers to the concepts that these word forms represent (Kay et al., 1996; Owens, 1984). In the model of linguistic processing shown in Figure 1-1, lexical-semantic processing relies upon the phonological input and output lexicons that store previously heard or produced spoken word forms, the orthographic input and output lexicons that store previously read or written word forms, and the semantic system that consists of the network of information we have acquired pertaining to objects, actions, people, attributes, experiences, and relationships, including superordinate, coordinate, and subordinate associations. Although most linguistic models (like the one depicted in Figure 1-1) propose an amodal semantic system in which one system provides meaning to all stimuli or ideas regardless of their input (e.g., picture, written word) or output (e.g., gesture, drawing, spoken word), contrasting models (e.g., Shallice, 1988) have been forwarded in which separate semantic stores are available for different input and/or output modalities.

Morphosyntactic Processing

Both morphological and syntactic language functions contribute to providing structure to linguistic input and output. More specifically, morphology encompasses the rule system that mediates assembling word forms from the basic elements of meaning (i.e., morphemes), and syntax consists of the set of rules that govern ordering words into sentences (Caplan, 1993; Owens, 1984). For example, in English, words can be formed by affixing derivational or inflectional morphemes. Derivational morphemes change words into different word classes (e.g., "slow," an adjective, into "slowly," an adverb), whereas inflectional morphemes provide information about syntactic relationships (e.g., subject-verb agreement of "talk" in the sentence "The child talks."). Our syntactic abilities allow us to produce and understand a variety of sentence types, including those with canonical (i.e., subject-verb-object order, as in active and conjoined sentences) or noncanonical word order (e.g., passive sentences with the less common object-verb-subject order).

Pragmatics and Discourse Processing

Pragmatics encompasses the system of rules and knowledge that direct our use and interpretation of language in social settings (Bates, 1976; Prutting, 1979). Therefore, our pragmatic abilities allow us to adjust our language to different communication partners (e.g., familiar vs. unfamiliar partner; person of authority vs. peer) and contexts or environments (e.g., at supper at home vs. during a church service; one-on-one vs. group setting; a happy vs. sad occasion). Pragmatics also includes our ability to use language for a variety of functions or intents (sometimes called speech acts), such as requesting, stating, greeting, asserting, and protesting (Dore, 1974; Lucas, 1980). These intents may be directly or indirectly expressed and comprehended through current, previous, and/or subsequent verbal output, as well as nonverbal cues such as facial expressions and gestures.

To be successful language users, we also must acquire a set of discourse rules that regulate our participation in conversation and other discourse genres (e.g., narration or story telling, procedural discourse) (Prutting & Kirchner, 1987; Stein & Glenn, 1979). For instance, conversational rules guide our turn-taking, topic selection, maintenance, and switching or termination, and use of repair or revision strategies (e.g., **repetition,** elaboration, simplification). Likewise, narrative rules govern how to construct (i.e., must include a setting, an initiating event, an action, and an outcome) and organize story episodes. Collectively, adherence to these rules should result in successful discourse, which according to Grice (1975) is achieved when: (1) a sufficient amount of information is provided by the message sender; (2) the information is truthful; (3) appropriate and relevant vocabulary are used; and (4) information is shared in a concise manner to prevent ambivalence and obscurity.

Components of Cognition

In addition to understanding of language, clinicians working with patients who have neurogenic language disorders must have appropriate insight into the structure and function of other cognitive skills, as these too may be compromised and contribute to their patients' communication difficulties. In fact, in certain patient populations (e.g., certain forms of dementia), the primary impairment is at the level of these cognitive functions, and communication problems are essentially a by-product of these cognitive versus linguistic deficits (Bayles, 2003; McDonald, 2000). Additionally, deficits in cognitive functions such as **attention,** memory, and executive functioning can also influence rehabilitation outcomes because of their effect on learning, whether related to the reacquisition of skills or the acquisition of compensatory strategies (Evans et al., 2003; Murray, 2004a). Accordingly, an understanding of the cognitive functions of attention, memory, and executive functioning and their subcomponents is essential to providing appropriate management of neurogenic language disorders.

Attention

Currently, it has yet to be resolved whether or not attention can be adequately defined by just one theoretical conceptualization. For example, many researchers describe attention as a capacity-limited system (e.g., Murray & Kean, 2004), whereas others view it as a cognitive bottleneck (e.g., Shuster, 2004). In capacity or resource models, attention is proposed to consist of (1) one or several finite pools (i.e., limited capacity) of attentional or processing resources, and (2) a governing system that manages distribution of these attentional resources to one or more activities (Kahneman, 1973; Norman & Shallice, 1986). According to capacity models, performance on a given task will suffer if an individual does not have access to a sufficient amount of attentional resources (i.e., capacity problem) and/or allots resources in an inefficient or inappropriate manner (i.e., allocation problem). For instance, if a lady was watching television and knitting at the same time, the quality of her knitting might suffer if she was very tired (i.e., had insufficient attention resources to split between watching television and knitting) or if she was paying more attention to the television program than to her knitting (i.e., inappropriate division of sufficient attention resources). In bottleneck or structural models of attention, an inescapable bottleneck is hypothesized to underlie limits on our attentional capabilities. That is, the time required to select a response is the restricting factor (i.e., bottleneck) that results in performance breakdowns, particularly when we attempt to complete two or more activities simultaneously (Pashler, 1994a, 1994b). In the previous example of the lady watching television and knitting, bottleneck theories would predict that the lady's knitting quality or her ability to follow her television program would primarily decline when she had to make a change in her knitting behavior (e.g., switch to a new type of knitting stitch, start a new row) because at that point she would need to select a new "knitting" response. Accordingly, her attention abilities at that point would switch from accomplishing two tasks at once (i.e., watching television and knitting) to completing just one task (i.e., hopefully, knitting) because of the bottleneck in our attentional system (i.e., in this example, the time needed to select a knitting behavior).

Although the debate over the adequacy of these two models of attention continues, researchers do agree that attention is multidimensional, and several attention functions have been identified (Kahneman, 1973; Van Zomeren & Brouwer, 1994). One of the more basic functions is **sustained attention,** sometimes also called vigilance, which refers to our ability to maintain attention and, thus, consistent performance over long periods of time. **Focused or selective attention** allows us to concentrate on and prioritize certain features of our external or internal environment in the presence of competing features or stimuli. **Divided attention** represents the more complex attentional skill of attending to and completing more than one task, or simultaneously attending to and processing multiple stimuli. **Attention switching** is also considered by several researchers to represent a separate attention function; this aspect of attention facilitates moving attentional focus from one task or stimulus to another. Examples of how these attention functions support our performance of daily activities are provided in Table 1-1.

Memory

The cognitive function of **memory** allows us to store, retain, and subsequently retrieve processed information (Guilford, 1967; Squire, 1987). Memory is viewed

Table 1-1. Activities that Exemplify Various Aspects of Attention

ACTIVITY	ATTENTION FUNCTION
Watching the ticker at the bottom of the television screen to determine if your child's school has been closed or delayed due to bad weather; Looking for whales on a whale watching boat trip	sustained attention/vigilance
Studying for a test in your dormitory room while your roommate is talking and laughing on the telephone with her boyfriend; Participating in a one-on-one conversation during your office's annual Christmas party	focused/selective attention
Driving and talking on your cell phone; Listening to a lecture and taking notes on that lecture	divided attention
Preparing two different dishes for a meal in which you alternate completing steps of each recipe; Switching between helping your child complete his homework and completing your own work	attention switching

as a multifaceted system consisting of various memory stores and processes that are essential to depositing and recovering information from these stores. A common framework used to conceptualize memory stores and functions divides memory into long-term memory and short-term or working memory capabilities, each of which can be further separated into different types of memory skills.

Long-Term Memory. Two forms of long-term memory, declarative and nondeclarative, have been identified. **Declarative memory** holds information that can be stored and accessed explicitly or consciously, and can be thought of as our "knowledge base" (Sohlberg & Mateer, 2001a, p. 168). It is often subdivided into **semantic** and **episodic** memory stores (Markowitsch, 1998; Squire, 1987). Whereas semantic memory holds context-independent, factual memories (e.g., state capitals, names of U.S. presidents, physics formulae, word definitions), episodic memory contains context-dependent memories and thus represents our autobiographical memory store (e.g., your first date, what you ate for breakfast this morning, where you were when you heard about the September 11, 2001 terrorist attacks). These two declarative memory subsystems are related in that many memories initially stored as episodic memories may over time be consolidated within semantic memory. For example, when you were first learning information pertaining to the United States Civil War, you might have tied that information to who taught you the information, what class covered the information, and what information was covered in which lecture. Over time, however, this contextual information can fade, and now you may just remember certain facts about this war.

In contrast to declarative memories, **nondeclarative memories** are implicit in that they can be evoked and, in some cases, stored unconsciously (Schacter, 1992). For example, **procedural memory** is a form of nondeclarative, long-term memory that holds your memory for motor (e.g., typing, fingering for a musical instrument) and cognitive (e.g., arithmetic operations) skills that are habitual and that require little effort to recall. Declarative and nondeclarative memory systems are not completely distinct in that some declarative memories, over time, may become procedural. For instance, when we first learn how to tie our shoes, the steps to complete this task may be stored in semantic or episodic memory; after a few months, however, this skill becomes automatic and may then become a procedural memory.

In patient populations, long-term memory (both declarative and nondeclarative forms) also may be subdivided into anterograde versus retrograde memory (Markowitsch, 1998; Squire, 1987). **Anterograde memories** are those long-term memories that are stored after brain damage has occurred, or after the onset of the neurological disease process. In contrast, **retrograde memories** are those that were acquired prior to brain damage or neurological disease onset. For example, in the case of a patient with dementia due to Alzheimer's disease, in the earlier stages of the disease, this patient may primarily have problems with anterograde memories such as where he left the car keys when he got home from work or the names of some new neighbors. As the disease progresses, this patient also experiences difficulties recalling retrograde memories such as what year he graduated from college, the capital city of the state in which he lives, or how to operate a power tool that he has owned for many years.

Short-Term and Working Memory. **Short-term memory** is our transient store of information, which for most people is limited to retaining seven, plus or minus two, pieces of information for a short time span of a few minutes (Baddeley, 1990; Markowitsch, 1998). In recent memory models, short-term memory has been replaced or encompassed by working memory. **Working memory** extends the function of short-term memory by not only temporarily storing information, but also by concurrently processing or manipulating that information (Baddeley, 2003; Kane, Bleckley, Conway, & Engle, 2001). Working memory is often conceptualized as consisting of several short-term buffers or stores, and an executive component that supervises information storage and manipulation within the buffers. Whereas the number and nature of short-term buffers vary across models (e.g., Crosson, 2000 vs. Baddeley, 2003), at least two storage systems are consistently proposed, a visuospatial sketchpad and a phonological buffer or loop dedicated to processing visuospatial and verbal-acoustic information, respectively. Working memory's executive system is domain-free and capacity limited, and therefore is similar to the governing system described in some attention models (e.g., Norman & Shallice,

1986). Furthermore, the executive component of working memory is proposed to manage sustaining target goals or information in a highly active state, particularly in the presence of distraction (Engle, 2002; Kane et al., 2001), and thus is also similar to inhibition, a cognitive function typically categorized as an executive function (see the following Executive Functioning section of this chapter).

Storage and Retrieval Memory Functions. Another important aspect of memory pertains to the functions responsible for helping keep information active in working memory, storing information into long-term memory, and subsequently retrieving information from long-term memory (Baddeley, 1990; Ellis & Hunt, 1993). **Encoding** functions such as association, rehearsal, categorization, chunking, and verbal mediation are used to maintain information in working memory as well as to transfer that information to long-term memory stores. More specifically, encoding refers to our ability to construct internal representations of incoming information or to associate that information with previously stored memories. For example, the encoding strategy of association might be used to help remember the name of a business associate, Lucy, because the business associate has red hair, like that of actress Lucille Ball.

Retrieval functions are essential to transferring information from long-term storage to consciousness. This transfer involves searching among activated memories for those that are most accurate and appropriate to the situation. Like encoding, a number of strategies can be used to facilitate memory retrieval; these include alphabet search (e.g., when trying to recall an individual's name, you start at the letter A to see if that helps cue recall of the correct name; if A does not work, you move to B and so on) and retracing or recreating the events or contexts in which the information was stored (e.g., retracing your trip to the mall to recall in what store you saw a product on sale, and what the sale price of that item was). Retrieval skills can be evaluated by comparing an individual's speed and accuracy of recall when completing recognition (e.g., multiple choice, true/false task) versus free recall (e.g., open-ended requests or questions such as "List the first 10 presidents of the United States." or "Whom did you visit with yesterday?") tasks. Because of the additional context information inherent in recognition tasks (i.e., the additional context will help activate the appropriate memories), it is normal for people to demonstrate superior recognition versus free recall performance.

Executive Functioning

Executive functioning refers to the set of high-level, interrelated cognitive abilities responsible for generating, selecting, planning, and monitoring goal-directed and adaptive responses that in turn sustain completion of independent, purposeful, and/or novel behavior (Dugbartey, Rosenbaum, Sanchez, & Townes, 1999; Ylvisaker et al., 1998). Because of the complex nature of these cognitive processes, theoretical models of executive functioning are not yet well specified, including how many or which cognitive functions should be considered "executive" (Murray & Ramage, 2000). Likewise there is variation in the nomenclature used to identify specific executive functions. Accordingly, the executive domains described below should not be considered the only possible set of executive functions, and differences are possible between the names we use to label these executive functions and those encountered in other textbooks or research articles.

There are several executive functions that we rely upon to succeed in completing our daily activities. Particularly important executive processes include: (1) **planning,** which allows us to devise strategies and sequence the steps of those strategies to achieve intended goals throughout our day; (2) **organization,** or the ability to structure or categorize incoming information as well as our own responses; (3) **inhibition,** which refers to our ability to regulate and repress automatic, routine, or extraneous processing or responding; (4) **cognitive flexibility,** which allows us to change or adapt our behavior in the event of failure; (5) **problem solving,** which includes problem identification, and generation, selection, and implementation of solutions; and (6) **self-monitoring,** or our ability to appraise and adjust our performance and behavior on the basis of environmental feedback, our knowledge of task difficulty, and our awareness of our own strengths and weaknesses. Again, it is important to keep in mind that additional domains of executive functioning may exist, and that cognitive processes within these domains may overlap.

Model of Linguistic Processing

There are several reasons for including and discussing the model shown in Figure 1-1. First, as previously mentioned, it depicts the multidimensional nature of linguistic processing by illustrating not only the various linguistic functions involved in comprehending and producing language across verbal, written, and gestural modalities, but also the relationships among these functions. Second, the model also demonstrates that other cognitive functions, such as attention, memory and executive functioning, and higher-level language skills that fall under the realm of pragmatics, not only influence each other, but also are interrelated with phonological, orthographic, action, semantic, and morphosyntactic processes. Third, this model can serve as a guide for assessing and treating neurogenic language disorders by helping clinicians identify which language behaviors or symptoms are dependent on which linguistic or cognitive processes. For example, a patient who has difficulty matching printed names of objects to pictures of those objects, but who has adequate visual abilities, good auditory comprehension (indicating that problems at the semantic level are unlikely), and can still read aloud (indicating that problems with abstract letter identification and use of letter-to-sound rules are unlikely) might be hypothesized to have a breakdown at the level of the orthographic input lexicon. Further examples of what language symptoms might occur following interruption at certain linguistic levels of this model are provided in our discussion of aphasia.

NEURAL BASES OF LANGUAGE AND COGNITION (BODY STRUCTURE)

It is commonly understood that the brain plays a critical role in the functioning of the entire body. Moreover, specific neural areas are proposed to be primarily responsible for specific functions or behaviors. The following section overviews our current understanding of the neural bases of linguistic and cognitive processes involved in communication. Although we have attempted to summarize the vast literature addressing relevant brain-behavior relationships, readers are cautioned that methods for investigating the function of various brain areas have not yet been perfected (see Side Bar), nor have all studies revealed the same findings.

Side Bar

Do we *really* know what the brain does?

The idea that specific parts of the brain are responsible for specific functions has been around only since the early 1800s, with the earliest theorists being ostracized for their radical speculations (see Roth & Heilman, 2000, for review). Fortunately, a number of scientists considered the notion worthy of study, and thus a number of methods for examining brain-behavior relationships have evolved, each with unique advantages and limitations. A general familiarity with these methods will be helpful to clinicians as they interpret studies examining brain-behavior relationships.

One of the earliest techniques for studying localization of brain function, and one that is still used today, is the **lesion method.** In this method, scientists note changes in behavior following brain injury and/or disease, and by deduction attribute the control of those behaviors to the injured neural area. In the early days of this science, identifying specific sites of brain injury was usually accomplished at autopsy, as no other means of visualizing the brain were possible except on the rare occasions when individuals survived a penetrating brain injury (Damasio, 1995). Presently, however, the lesion method capitalizes on imaging techniques such as **computerized tomography** (CT scans) and **magnetic resonance imaging** (MRI) (see Chapter 3), which allow scientists to identify brain lesions in live patients.

A criticism of many lesion studies is their failure to incorporate behavioral measures thorough or sensitive enough to characterize impaired behaviors (Caplan, 1981; Knopman & Rubens, 1986). Moreover, some authors (e.g., Caplan, 1981) have questioned whether it is appropriate to infer normal brain function from disruptions in function when the brain is damaged. That is, it may be that injury alters brain function to such an extent that examining brain-behavior relationships after brain injury does not provide an accurate picture of brain-behavior relationships typical of neurologically healthy individuals.

(continued)

These criticisms notwithstanding, a variation of the lesion method was developed in the late 1950s, when scientists discovered that temporary brain "lesions" could be produced by applying electrical stimulation to the brain. Applying **cortical stimulation** to patients undergoing brain surgery as a treatment for epilepsy, Penfield and Roberts (1959) were the first to describe its effects on behavior. More recently, studies using this method have "mapped" various communication functions such as naming (Ojemann & Whitaker, 1978), use of sign language (Mateer, Polen, Ojemann, & Wyler, 1982; Mateer, Rapport, & Kettrick, 1984), and memory, syntax, and phonology (Ojemann & Mateer, 1979). A related technology is **transcranial magnetic stimulation,** which alters the function of cortical neurons using magnetic fields (e.g., Floel et al., 2004; Kohler, Paus, Buckner, & Milner, 2004; Roux et al., 2004). Although both of these methods hold promise for advancing our understanding of brain functions, a key limitation is that stimulation results are not clearly interpretable. For example, studies often involve very small samples of behavior, frequently targeting only one stimulus type or response mode. Thus, a negative response (i.e., stimulation did not disrupt performance on a task) could indicate that the neural site was not active during the task, but does not rule out that the site would be active at different levels of task complexity or other variations of task parameters. Similarly, positive responses are difficult to interpret. First, a stimulated neural site may be relevant to processes targeted by the experimental task, but it may also be active for many other processes not targeted during the experiment. Further, due to the connectivity and conductivity of neurons, stimulation of one cortical site can elicit responses in neurons far from the stimulation site (Ojemann & Whitaker, 1978). Therefore it may be unclear if the task disruption was related to the directly or indirectly stimulated neurons.

Whereas both lesion and stimulation studies require inferring brain function based on *disruptions* of typical function, other methods instead attempt to measure the activity of specific brain areas during *normal* function. **Electroencephalography** (EEG), which measures electrical activity in the brain, and **magnetoencephalography** (MEG), which measures the magnetic fields generated by electrical activity of the brain, are closely related technologies and allow for gross localization of brain activity. **Functional magnetic resonance imaging (fMRI),** a variation of the more well-known imaging technique of MRI, provides images of changes in blood oxygenation within the brain. Because oxygenation changes are hypothesized to occur in response to neural activity, fMRI images have been used to identify brain areas that are active during specific cognitive and linguistic tasks (Krasuski, Horwitz, & Rumsey, 1996). Related imaging technologies, **positron emission tomography** (PET) and **single photon emission computed tomography** (SPECT), utilize injected radioactive isotopes to track blood flow in the brain, which, again, is thought to reflect neural activity.

A notable limitation is common to each of these methods of measuring brain activity. Because most tasks are proposed to involve a number of cognitive processes (e.g., reaching for a pencil involves the visual system, the attention system, the motor and sensory systems, etc.), it is anticipated that many areas of the brain are active during such tasks. Thus, even when neural activity is detected, it may be difficult to isolate the brain activity associated with discrete mental functions.

(continued)

In summary, although many technologies have been developed to study brain function, as of yet, no one tool reveals the whole story of brain-behavior relationships. When two or more tools are combined in a single experiment, however, (e.g., Dogil et al., 2004), or as a number of independent investigations report similar findings, the nature of brain-behavior relationships will become clearer. Nonetheless, given the limitations of the current methods, it is likely that our current understanding of how various brain areas contribute to language and cognition is at best incomplete and potentially even inaccurate. Thus, clinicians may wish to use lesion information to predict likely areas of impairment, but should not rule out the possibility of disruptions to other linguistic and cognitive functions.

NEURAL BASES OF LANGUAGE

It is widely accepted that the left, or dominant, hemisphere plays the primary role in language function for most individuals, even those who are left-handed. Within the left hemisphere, a number of specific brain areas have been associated with unique language functions (see Figure 1-2).

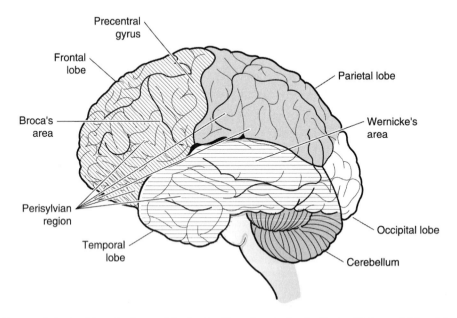

Figure 1-2. Left hemisphere of the brain. Broca's area in the frontal lobe and Wernicke's area in the temporal lobe are both located in the perisylvian region of the left hemisphere. Other areas important to language processing include the supramarginal and angular gyri. Dorsolateral prefrontal regions of both frontal lobes have been associated with high level cognitive abilities including executive functioning.

Broca's area, located in the inferior lateral frontal lobe, is generally proposed to play a primary role in language expression, regardless of output modality (e.g., speaking, writing, subvocalizing). With respect to specific linguistic processes, activation of Broca's area has been associated with maintenance of phonological representations (Hinke et al., 1993), production of speech sounds (Cuenod et al., 1995), and syntactic processing (Ni et al., 2000).

The area of the brain linked to language comprehension is **Wernicke's area,** which is located in the posterior aspects of the superior temporal lobe. Because comprehension involves processing of phonologic, semantic, and morphosyntactic structures, it is not surprising that activation of Wernicke's area is associated with these linguistic processes (see Gernsbacher & Kaschak, 2003, for review). The **supramarginal gyrus** and **angular gyrus** within the parietal lobe also have been found to contribute to comprehending written language. Activation in the cortical areas surrounding Broca's and Wernicke's areas, often termed **association areas** (e.g., temporal association area, parietal association area), is also common during language processing.

Side Bar

The naming power of discovery

Both Broca's and Wernicke's areas are named after the physician scientists who studied patients experiencing disruptions to their language abilities. Paul Broca and Carl Wernicke were pioneers in the thorough description of language impairments associated with damage to the left hemisphere.

In addition to these cortical areas (gray matter), bundles of axons (white matter) connecting cortical areas, known as association fibers, also function in language processing. The **superior longitudinal fasciculus** connects the frontal cortex with the parietal, temporal, and occipital cortices, and contains the **arcuate fasciculus,** which connects Wernicke's and Broca's areas. Accordingly, these fiber tracts play a critical role in the communication process by integrating receptive and expressive language processes.

Although the cerebral cortex is considered a primary contributor to our communication abilities, it is likely that select subcortical structures also function in language processing. Evidence for subcortical involvement comes primarily from studies describing patients with aphasia who demonstrated lesions in the **thalamus, basal ganglia,** and/or **internal capsule** (see Radanovic & Scaff, 2003, for review). The precise contribution of these subcortical structures (depicted in Figure 1-3) continues to be debated. The thalamus has been proposed to play a crucial role in verbal memory, and thus may influence both expressive and receptive language modalities

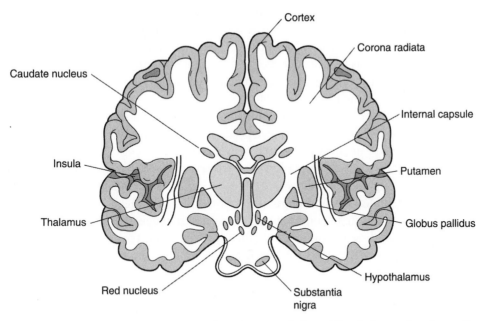

Figure 1-3. Subcortical structures viewed in the coronal plane. The thalamus, basal ganglia, and internal capsule may play a role in language processing. The thalamus and basal ganglia have also been associated with other cognitive functions, including certain attention, memory, and executive function abilities.

(Metter et al., 1983). Some researchers have theorized that the basal ganglia and surrounding white matter regulate the initiation of the motor production of language formulated by cortical structures (Crosson, 1985) or may serve to connect cortical structures (Alexander, Naeser, & Palumbo, 1987). More recent studies, however, have offered strong evidence that lesions involving the basal ganglia impact language functioning only when accompanied by reduced blood flow to cortical sites, (Hillis et al., 2004; Radanovic & Scaff, 2003), leading researchers to question the direct role of the basal ganglia in language processing.

Neural Bases of Cognition

Many of the neural structures and pathways upon which language functions rely also subserve one or more cognitive processes. Given that it is well beyond the scope of this book to examine all neural areas and circuits that support cognition, our review will highlight only those structures with well-established contributions to attention, memory, and/or executive functioning, and which are highly vulnerable to the forms of brain damage that result in neurogenic language disorders.

Neural Bases of Attention

Given that numerous neural structures and pathways located in a spectrum of cortical and subcortical regions have been found to support one or more attentional processes, it is not surprising that attention deficits are common among patients with neurogenic language disorders, even those with very little permanent brain damage (Penner, Rausch, Kappos, Opwis, & Radu, 2003; Van Zomeren & Brouwer, 1994). To help provide a framework by which to organize these various neural contributions, Filley (2002) has proposed two neural networks of attention, a diffuse network that supports primarily more basic attention functions (e.g., sustained and focused attention), and a right hemisphere network that mediates attention allocation to focal spatial stimuli. Important neural structures and pathways within the diffuse network include the thalamus, white matter connections between the thalamus and cortical areas of both cerebral hemispheres, and the lateral and medial aspects of both frontal lobes (Coull, 1998; Filley, 2002). There are some distinctions between right and left frontal lobes' contributions to this diffuse attention network: The right frontal lobe appears more dominant for sustained attention, whereas the left prefrontal cortex plays a fundamental role in functions such as attention-switching (Coull, 1998; Dreher & Grafman, 2003). Right posterior parietal cortex, prefrontal cortex, cingulate gyrus, and subcortical structures such as the thalamus and basal ganglia are important components of the right hemisphere attention network (Filley, 2002). Those structures that are more anteriorly located within the right hemisphere contribute to complex spatial attention functions, whereas more posteriorly located structures support more basic spatial attention abilities such as stimulus scanning and selection (Coull, 1998; Filley, 2002). Several of the neural structures that participate in attention functioning are depicted in Figures 1-3 and 1-4.

Neural Bases of Memory

Many neural regions help support the variety of memory stores and functions essential to our overall memory abilities. For example, several aspects of memory, including the application of encoding and retrieval memory strategies and working memory, rely on frontal lobe functioning (Crosson, 2000; Smith & Jonides, 1998; Squire, 1987). More specifically, research indicates that working memory's phonological buffer relies upon Broca's area, left supplemental motor, and premotor areas, the visuospatial buffer on right premotor cortex, and the executive

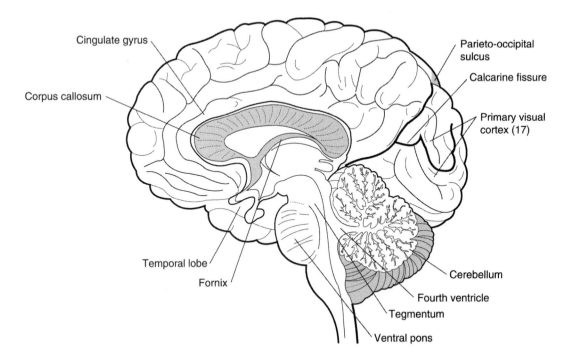

Figure 1-4. A sagital view of the right hemisphere. Attention functions have been related to the cingulate gyrus. Several deep structures, such as the fornix, may play a role in certain memory abilities.

component on the anterior cingulate gyrus and dorsolateral prefrontal areas of both hemispheres (see Figures 1-2 and 1-4). Additionally, subcortical structures such as the thalamus and basal ganglia, as well their connections with these frontal lobe regions, contribute to working memory, with a hypothesized specialization for preserving the temporal order of information being temporarily held in working memory buffers (Crosson, 2000; Kubat-Silman et al., 2002).

Long-term memory relies on both cortical regions and deeper brain structures (Nyberg, Forkstam, Petersson, Cabeza, & Ingvar, 2002; Squires, 1987). For instance, the hippocampus, located deep within the temporal lobe, and medial regions of the temporal lobe have been implicated in a number of memory functions, including declarative (particularly episodic memory) and anterograde memory (see Figure 1-3). In contrast, semantic memories appear to be stored in modality (e.g., auditory concepts within temporal cortex; visual concepts within parieto-occipital regions) and domain-specific regions (e.g., word meanings within temporoparietal cortex) of the cortex. Finally, subcortical areas such as the caudate nucleus and other basal ganglia structures illustrated in Figure 1-3 are germane to procedural memory. It is always important to keep in mind that these subcortical regions maintain communication with the many cortical structures that subserve memory, so that damage to the neural pathways that connect cortical and sub-cortical regions also can result in a variety of memory problems.

Neural Bases of Executive Functioning

Research consistently indicates that executive functioning is primarily achieved by frontal lobe areas (Filley, 2000 Stuss & Levine, 2002). Furthermore, within the frontal lobes, different regions have been found to support different executive functions. For example, inferior regions of the frontal lobes (i.e., orbitofrontal areas) have been associated with inhibition, superior regions (i.e., dorsolateral pre-frontal cortex) are more involved with problem solving and reasoning, and the frontal poles that encompass the most anterior portions of the frontal lobes appear to support some of the most complex executive functions, such as self-awareness (see Figure 1-2). Whereas the frontal lobes are clearly essential to executive functioning, other brain areas also appear to contribute. For example, imaging research indicates that the cerebellum is active during linguistic and nonlinguistic problem-solving tasks (Schatz, Hale, & Myerson, 1998). Likewise, pathways to and from the frontal lobes, in particular those connecting to subcortical structures such as the basal ganglia and thalamus, also participate in executive function abilities (Filley, 2000; Stuss & Levine, 2002).

○ SUMMARY AND LOOKING AHEAD

It is helpful to approach any area of study from a framework that will serve to high-light relationships among concepts and guide the development of clinical manage-ment strategies. In this beginning chapter, we have introduced the ICF classification system as the guiding framework for our examination of neurogenic language dis-orders. With the review of the body structures and functions supporting language and cognition as a foundation, Chapter 2 explores the nature of impairments and activity limitations resulting from damage to relevant body structures and/or dis-ruption of relevant body functions. The discussion of concepts foundational to managing neurogenic language disorders is continued in Chapter 3 as the etiolo-gies of these disorders are explored. The concepts explored in these introductory chapters inform both assessment and treatment of neurogenic language disorders, as will become clear in the remaining chapters.

An overview of the assessment process is provided in Chapter 4, followed by detailed descriptions of the strategies, methods, and tools employed in the assess-ment of linguistic and cognitive impairments in Chapters 5 and 6, respectively. Consistent with the ICF framework, Chapter 7 explores the assessment of func-tional communication (i.e., communication activity) and participation.

Chapter 8 introduces the discussion of treating adult neurogenic language disorders with a review of evidence-based practice concepts. Management strategies targeting underlying impairments in linguistic and cognitive processing are explored in Chapter 9, and pharmacological treatment approaches are summarized in Chapter 10. These chapters are followed by a discussion of procedures suitable for targeting functional communication and participation in Chapter 11.

Finally, in recognition that managing neurogenic language disorders does not take place in a vacuum but rather is framed within the larger health care culture and policies, Chapter 12 provides an overview of the United States health care system, exploring the influences of this system on our assessment and treatment of neurogenic language disorders. Chapter 12 concludes with an exploration of how our management of neurogenic language disorders may evolve in the coming decades.

So that this book may serve as a rich resource of clinical ideas, a comprehensive and diverse set of assessment procedures and treatment approaches are covered, some that can be applied to neurogenic language disorders in general and others that are specific to aphasia, cognitive-communicative disorders associated with right hemisphere brain damage or traumatic brain injury, or dementia. It is our hope that by reviewing the theoretical and applied material in this book, readers will acquire the conceptual background essential to managing adult neurogenic language disorders in a variety of health care settings.

Chapter 2

Overview of Neurogenic Language Disorders

LEARNING OBJECTIVES

After reading this chapter you should be able to:

- Define aphasia and describe the language impairments characteristic of aphasia.

- Identify and describe aphasia types based on the connectionist model of aphasia.

- Describe the nature of impairments in attention, memory, and executive functioning typical of RHD.

- Discuss the impact of the cognitive impairments in RHD on communication.

- Describe the nature of impairments in attention, memory, and executive functioning typical of TBI.

- Discuss the impact of the cognitive impairments in TBI on communication.

- Describe the nature of impairments in attention, memory, and executive functioning typical of dementia.

- Discuss the impact of the cognitive impairments in dementia on communication.

- Compare and contrast the language impairments of aphasia, RHD, TBI, and dementia.

KEY TERMS

agrammatism
agraphia
alexia
anomia
anomic aphasia
anosognosia
aphasia

coma
conduction aphasia
dementia
fluency
jargon
neglect syndrome
paragrammatism

paraphasias
primary progressive aphasia
post-traumatic amnesia
pure word deafness
subcortical aphasia

INTRODUCTION

This chapter describes a number of neurogenic language disorders with which patients in a variety of health care settings may present, highlighting how disruptions to specific linguistic and cognitive processes affect these patients' communication abilities. Readers may find that the model of linguistic and cognitive processing included in Chapter 1 (see Figure 1-1) will aid their understanding of the various linguistic and cognitive symptoms associated with neurogenic language disorders such as aphasia, cognitive-communicative disorders subsequent to right hemisphere brain damage (RHD) or traumatic brain injury (TBI), and dementia.

○ APHASIA

Although the term **aphasia** literally means "without speech," a number of specific definitions have been developed to capture more accurately the nature and features of this neurogenic language disorder (see Rosenbek, LaPointe, & Wertz, 1989, for review). In general, aphasia refers to a disruption in using and understanding language following neurological injury or disease (Brookshire, 2003; Goodglass, 1993) that is not related to general intellectual decline or sensori-motor deficits (Darley, 1982). Accordingly, a diagnosis of aphasia is typically not applied to patients with communication disorders related to traumatic brain injury, nondominant, or right, hemisphere brain damage, or a dementing disease because in these cases deficits in cognitive domains other than language (i.e., attention, memory, and/or executive functioning) often are the primary bases of these patients' communicative difficulties.

SYMPTOMS OF APHASIA

Aphasia is frequently characterized by impairments in a number of linguistic processes. The types of behavioral deficits resulting from these impairments, however, are usually grouped into disruptions of comprehension, speech fluency, naming, and repetition. Examples of the various aphasic behaviors are provided in Table 2-1.

Comprehension

Disruption in language comprehension, both in spoken and written modalities, is common in aphasia, although the severity of comprehension deficits varies greatly across patients. Comprehension deficits can arise from impairments to any of the linguistic processes contributing to assigning meaning to linguistic messages (e.g., phonological analysis, semantic processing, morphosyntactic parsing; see also Figure 1-1). Because the behavioral manifestations of auditory and reading comprehension deficits are often the same regardless of the underlying impairment (i.e., the patient fails to understand what is said or read), careful assessment is usually necessary to identify which specific linguistic impairment or combination of impairments are contributing to comprehension breakdowns (see Chapter 5).

Speech Fluency

The term "fluency" is often used to describe aspects of speech production affecting rate, rhythm, and ease of speech output. Disruptions to these features of speech fluency are called dysfluencies and are associated with speech disorders such as stuttering. With respect to the speech production of patients with aphasia, **fluency** refers primarily to phrase length (Rosenbek et al., 1989), but may also incorporate characteristics of melodic line, articulatory agility, speech rate, and grammatical

Table 2-1. **Examples of Speech Production Characteristics in Aphasia**

SPEECH BEHAVIOR	EXAMPLE	COMMON UNDERLYING IMPAIRMENT(S)
Anomic Pause	"Can you hand me the. . .er. . .remote?"	Semantic Representation Lexical Access Phonologic Representation Phonologic Processing
Semantic Paraphasia	"Can you hand me the TV?"	Semantic Representation Lexical Access
Phonemic Paraphasia	"Can you hand me the rebote?"	Phonologic Representation Phonologic Processing
Anomic Circumlocution	"Can you hand me the. . .other there. . .the clicker. . .for the TV?"	Semantic Representation Lexical Access Phonologic Representation Phonologic Processing
Neologism	"Can you hand me the jazzlepam?"	Semantic Representation Lexical Access Phonologic Representation Phonologic Processing
Jargon	"Griss me the jazzlepam."	Semantic Representation Lexical Access Phonologic Representation Phonologic Processing
Agrammatism	"You. . .uh. . .remote?"	Morphosyntactic Processing
Paragrammatism/Empty Speech	"Fast the jazzleman on the choose."	Semantic Representation Lexical Access Morphosyntactic Processing

form (Goodglass, Kaplan, & Barresi, 2001; Kertesz, 1982). Patients with aphasia-related fluency difficulties, referred to as nonfluent output, produce effortful, halting speech that is limited to short phrases and is often spoken at a slow rate with nominal melodic contour. In contrast, patients with fluent speech generally produce speech without apparent effort, even in the presence of sound, word, or grammatical errors, and sound "normal" in terms of their phrase length and intonation.

A phenomenon sometimes associated with nonfluent speech is **agrammatism** (also previously referred to as telegraphic speech), in which patients produce short utterances that consist primarily of content words such as nouns and verbs, lack function words such as articles and conjunctions, and have either simplified or incomplete grammatical structure. Agrammatism is hypothesized to reflect impairments in morphosyntactic processing and may also be characterized by morphologically simplified word forms (e.g., omitted plural endings and/or tense markers) (Caramazza & Berndt, 1985). Another speech characteristic proposed to reflect disrupted morphosyntactic processing is **paragrammatism,** which describes speech that incorporates atypical syntax (Goodglass, Kaplan, & Barresi, 2001). Whereas a patient exhibiting agrammatism may omit syntactic elements, a patient with paragrammatism may substitute inappropriate syntactic elements (e.g., using a verb where a noun should be). The concept of paragrammatism has been called into question (e.g., Davis, 2000), however, because careful study of paragrammatic speech has failed to reveal syntactic errors that vary significantly from those observed in agrammatic speech (see Heeschen & Kolk, 1988, for review). Additionally, because the presence of paragrammatism often results in a marked reduction or misuse of content words important for communicating meaning, the term "**empty speech**" may be appropriately used to describe fluent speech lacking in information content. It is important to note that patients' written output is often similar to their spoken output, and thus patients' written language might also be characterized as agrammatic or paragrammatic. For example, Figure 2-1 shows a writing sample from a patient with primary progressive aphasia that is an excellent example of agrammatic writing.

Naming

A common characteristic of aphasia is **anomia,** or difficulty recalling the names of people, objects, locations, and actions. Anomia may be manifest by a variety of behaviors, including delayed naming resulting in excessive pausing, errors in naming referred to as **paraphasias,** circumlocutions, and production of nonwords referred to as **neologisms.** Patients with severe anomia may produce entire sentences in which all content words and, in some cases, even functor words are replaced with neologisms, a phenomenon known as **jargon.** Impairments in several linguistic processes may produce anomia in patients' speech, writing, or both (see Figure 1-1). For example, degraded semantic representations may cause increased processing time as the appropriate concepts are accessed. Disrupted lexical access may result in pauses, circumlocutions, or word choice errors (i.e., semantic **paraphasias**). Finally, impairments to any of the various levels of phonological processing may result in anomic behaviors, particularly sound errors (i.e., phonemic **paraphasias**) (see Table 2-1 and Chapter 5 for further description and examples of paraphasic errors).

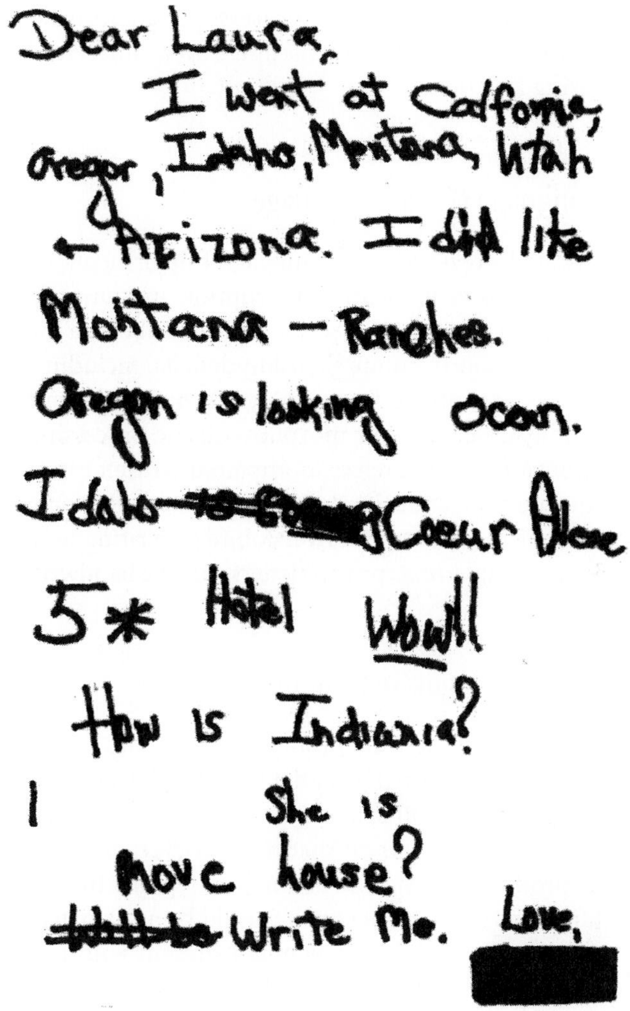

Figure 2-1. Example of agrammatic writing from a patient with primary progressive aphasia. See other Aphasia Types section of this chapter for a description of primary progressive aphasia.

Repetition

Another speech behavior impacted by aphasia is **repetition.** When asked to repeat words or phrases, some patients with aphasia will produce verbal output that is similar to their productions during spontaneous or elicited speech (e.g., agrammatic, paraphasic). Interestingly, other patients with aphasia will demonstrate repetition ability that is either much more or much less impaired than other spoken productions. Repetition without processing for meaning is proposed to involve a specific set of decoding and encoding processes (e.g., acoustic to phonologic conversion; see Figure 1-1) that may be disrupted to a different degree than other linguistic processing functions.

Disruptions in Written Language

As indicated previously, the language impairments of aphasia extend to written as well as spoken modalities. Disruption in comprehending written language is termed **alexia** or *acquired dyslexia*. As noted above, a number of underlying impairments may result in comprehension deficits, including difficulty decoding written forms (e.g., identifying letters or converting graphemes to phonemes), as well as disruptions in semantic or morphosyntactic processing (see Figure 1-1). **Agraphia** or *acquired dysgraphia* refers to impaired written expression, and may be manifest by the same characteristics described for spoken expression, as well as by difficulty in phoneme to grapheme conversion (e.g., writing to dictation) and production of specific allographs (e.g., printed letters, cursive handwriting) (Beeson & Hillis, 2001).

Concomitant Cognitive Symptoms

Although clearly linguistic problems are the most prominent symptoms observed in and typically reported by patients with aphasia, a growing body of research indicates that aphasia is often accompanied by deficits in cognition that extend beyond language processing. Given that there is overlap in the lesion locations that commonly produce aphasia and the neural regions that support nonlinguistic cognitive functions (see Chapter 1), it should be anticipated that patients with a variety of aphasia types and severities might present with impairments of one or several of these nonlinguistic cognitive abilities. Indeed, aphasia is commonly accompanied by problems of attention, memory, and executive functioning, and according to some researchers these latter cognitive problems may not only contribute to or exaggerate the language difficulties of patients with aphasia but also impede their recovery of language abilities, their acquisition of compensatory strategies, or both (McNeil, Odell, & Tseng, 1991; Murray, 2004a; Purdy, 2002; Van Mourik, Verschaeve, Boon, Paquier, & Van Harskamp, 1992).

Attention Problems

The results of previous investigations indicate that one, some, or all aspects of attention might be impaired in patients with aphasia (see Murray, 1999; 2002, for reviews). More specifically, compared to their healthy age-matched peers, patients with aphasia have been found to be less accurate, slower, or both on sustained attention (Gerritsen, Berg, Deelman, Visser-Keizer, & Meyboom-de Jong, 2003; Korda & Douglas, 1997), attention switching (Connor, Olber, Tocco, Fitzpatrick, & Albert, 2001; Ziegler, Kerkhoff, Cate, Artinger, & Zierdt, 2001), and focused and divided attention tasks (King & Hux, 1996; Murray, 2000). Furthermore, these performance differences between aphasic and non-aphasic adults are evident regardless of whether the attention tasks have relatively high or low linguistic demands.

Patients with aphasia also may display neglect, an attention deficit more frequently associated with right hemisphere brain damage (for a more detailed description of neglect, see the Right Hemisphere Disorders section of this chapter). It is estimated that between 15 and 65% of patients who suffer left hemisphere brain damage will present with right-sided neglect, or impaired attention to information presented on the right side of the body (Bartolomeo, Chokron, & Gainotti, 2001; Kerkhoff, 2001). Although symptoms of visual neglect are easiest to observe (e.g., failing to eat food on the right side of the plate; omitting words on the right side of the page when reading aloud), neglect can affect processing of and responding to information presented in other modalities as well (e.g., failing to attend to sounds presented to their right ear; failing to notice that their eyeglasses are not sitting properly on their right ear).

Memory Problems

As with attention, most if not all facets of memory appear vulnerable in patients with aphasia. For example, Visser-Keizer and colleagues (2002) interviewed stroke survivors and their caregivers about troublesome stroke-related symptoms and found that more than half of the left hemisphere stroke study participants (close to half of whom had aphasia) and their partners reported memory impairments following their stroke.

With respect to the various memory functions, short-term and working memory problems appear to coincide frequently with aphasia. These memory impairments have been identified when patients with aphasia complete tasks that involve the temporary storage and subsequent recall of verbal (Caspari, Parkinson, LaPointe, & Katz, 1998; Knott, Patterson, & Hodges, 2000; Tompkins, Bloise, Timko, & Baumgaertner 1994), episodic (Yasuda et al., 2000), auditory-nonverbal (Gordon, 1983), or visuospatial information (Bartha & Benke, 2003; Butters et al., 1970). Although only a limited number of studies have evaluated long-term memory subsequent to aphasia onset, initial findings suggest that getting verbal or visual information into or out of long-term memory stores is difficult for many patients with aphasia (Beeson et al., 1993; Burgio & Basso, 1997; Della Barba, Frasson, Mantovan, Gallo, & Denes, 1996). Further investigations are necessary, however, to determine which patients are at greatest risk for concomitant long-term memory deficits, as the current research has produced disparate findings with respect to the influence of lesion location and aphasia variables (i.e., aphasia type, severity) on long-term memory status.

Executive Function Problems

Researchers have been interested in evaluating the executive function abilities of patients with aphasia for many decades. Whereas initial studies (e.g., Kertesz & McCabe, 1975) were driven by the quest to determine if aphasia compromised intelligence, the impetus of more recent research (e.g., Purdy, 2002) has been to establish whether the influential negative relationship between the presence of executive function impairments and rehabilitation and functional outcomes observed in other neurogenic patient populations (e.g., Chen, Sultzer, Hinkin, Mahler, & Cummings, 1998) also applies to patients with aphasia. Findings from most aphasia studies indicate that these patients are at risk for deficits in a variety of executive domains, including problem solving and reasoning, planning, organization, inhibition, self-monitoring, and cognitive flexibility (Glosser & Goodglass, 1990; Keil & Kaszniak, 2002; Nehemkis & Lewinsohn, 1972; Purdy, 2002). There is little consensus, however, on whether a significant relationship exists between presence of executive function problems and aphasia type or severity, or lesion size or location (e.g., Kertesz & McCabe, 1975 vs. Gainotti et al., 1986). Accordingly, future research is needed to determine whether any language, medical, or demographic variables might help clinicians identify which patients with aphasia are at greatest risk for these high-level cognitive impairments.

EXPLANATIONS OF APHASIA

Although descriptions of the behavioral characteristics of aphasia are largely agreed upon, several differing views exist regarding the pattern of characteristics necessary to warrant the label of aphasia. One notion is that aphasia reflects a generalized impairment of all language functions, such that the term aphasia applies only to individuals who exhibit deficits across modalities and linguistic functions (Darley, 1982; Schuell & Jenkins, 1959). Other researchers have argued that the term aphasia can and should be additionally applied to selective impairments of specific language functions (e.g., naming, reading) (Caplan & Utman, 1992; Caramazza, Berndt, & Basili, 1983; Caramazza & Miceli, 1991; Caramazza, Papagno, & Ruml, 2000; Damasio, 1981; Goodglass & Kaplan, 1983; Ni et al., 2000). Contributing to the debate regarding behavioral criteria for the diagnosis of aphasia is a lack of consensus about the precise nature of the impairments underlying aphasia.

A first area of disagreement is whether underlying language skills, processes, or representations are lost as a result of the brain injury causing the aphasia (i.e., **loss of language competence**) (Goodglass, 1993; Grodzinsky, 1984; Lichtheim, 1885), or instead whether aphasia reflects disrupted access to or execution of intact language structures (i.e., disrupted **language performance**) (Friederici & Frazier, 1992; McNeil, 1982; Schuell, Jenkins, & Jimenese-Pabon, 1964). Evidence often cited to support viewing aphasia as disrupted language performance is the observation that patients with aphasia are often able to demonstrate specific language skills that are thought to be impaired (lost) when certain conditions are modified (e.g., change in response modality, enhanced contextual cues, reduced task complexity). Proponents argue that if a skill can be demonstrated under *any* circumstances, then underlying linguistic competence must exist (McNeil et al., 1991).

Theorists also disagree about which specific processes are disrupted in aphasia (see Chapey & Hallowell, 2001, for review). Early characterizations of aphasia suggested a *reduced ability to use language propositionally* (i.e., with the intent to communicate a specific meaning) (Jackson, 1878). This view accounts for the observation that many patients with aphasia may successfully use non-propositional language (e.g., rote recitation, automatic greetings). Subsequently, Goldstein and Scheerer (1948) suggested that aphasia results from an *impaired ability to form abstractions*, a skill required to manipulate linguistic symbols. More recently, a prominent explanation for aphasia has arisen out of the fields of psycholinguistic and cognitive neuropsychology, and specifies that *disruptions to specific linguistic processes*, either individually or in concert, result in predictable language performance breakdowns (Caplan & Utman, 1992; Caramazza et al., 1983; Caramazza & Miceli, 1991; Caramazza et al., 2000; Damasio, 1981). Finally, the language characteristics of aphasia also have been characterized as either a *disruption of the cognitive processes supporting language* (Chapey, 1986) or *reduced access to or inefficient allocation of cognitive resources to the mental processes relevant to language* (McNeil et al., 1991; Murray, 2000, 2004a).

CLASSIFICATION SYSTEMS FOR APHASIA

As indicated previously, patients with aphasia may demonstrate varying degrees of impairment in the areas of comprehension, speech fluency, naming, and repetition, as well as across modalities. Researchers who subscribe to a unidimensional view of aphasia (e.g., Darley, 1982; Schuell et al., 1964) consider these variations in behavioral manifestations as just that: *variations* in the presentation of a uniform disorder, and all patients with aphasia are diagnosed with aphasia (without adjectives, Rosenbek et al., 1989). Other researchers, and likewise clinicians, however, find it helpful to assign different designations for the various patterns of aphasic behaviors; thus a number of aphasia classification systems have evolved.

Dichotomous Classification Systems

One of the more common ways of classifying aphasia subtypes is by speech fluency. Patients with **nonfluent aphasia** typically exhibit speech characterized by utterances of four words or fewer, often produced haltingly and with great effort

(Rosenbek et al., 1989). In contrast, patients with **fluent aphasia** demonstrate an ease of speech production, with melodic line, rhythm, rate, and flow similar to non-aphasic speakers. This classification system does not, however, address other language characteristics, in that patients with either fluent or nonfluent aphasia may demonstrate impaired comprehension, naming, and/or repetition. These overlapping symptoms are no doubt responsible for the difficulty and unreliability that have been associated with attempting to classify most patients into one of these two aphasia categories (Gordon, 1998).

Patients with aphasia also have been classified according to degree of comprehension deficit. The term **receptive aphasia** has been used to describe the language characteristics of significantly impaired auditory and written comprehension, whereas **expressive aphasia** denotes relatively spared language comprehension but compromised language output abilities. Similar to the fluent/nonfluent dichotomy, however, the labels of expressive or receptive aphasia do not imply a specific level of impairment in speech fluency, naming, or repetition. Additionally, these terms are slight misnomers, given that patients who might be classified as having receptive aphasia typically have expressive deficits as well.

Although the two dichotomies described above are based solely on behavioral characteristics, researchers have proposed that each of these aphasia types can be associated with specific lesion sites (e.g., Goodglass, 1981). For example, both nonfluent and expressive forms of aphasia have historically been associated with relatively anterior lesions (e.g., damage to Broca's area or surrounding frontal association areas). In contrast, fluent and receptive forms of aphasia are traditionally associated with relatively posterior lesions (e.g., damage to Wernicke's area or surrounding temporal and parietal association areas). Lesion and imaging studies (e.g., Binder et al., 1997; Mazzocchi & Vignolo, 1979; Metter et al., 1989; Naeser, Palumbo, Helm-Estabrooks, Stiassny-Eder, & Albert, 1989), however, have revealed a number of exceptions to this lesion pattern, potentially reflecting, at least in part, that behavioral characteristics (e.g., severity, fluency) change over the course of recovery even when the lesion is static (Rosenbek et al., 1989).

Connectionist Classification System

The classification system adopted by commonly used aphasia diagnostic batteries, the *Boston Diagnostic Aphasia Examination–3* (Goodglass, Kaplan, & Barresi, 2001) and the *Western Aphasia Battery* (Kertesz, 1982) (see Chapter 5), and thus used most frequently by professionals serving patients with aphasia, is a system that incorporates both behavioral characteristics as well as neuroanatomical correlates of the observed behaviors. This system is often termed the connectionist model because of the inherent assumption that the various aphasic subtypes reflect disruption of specific brain centers or to the connections between these centers (see Table 2-2).

Table 2-2. Connectionist Aphasia Types

APHASIA TYPE	PREDICTED SITE OF LESION	COMPREHENSION	FLUENCY	NAMING	REPETITION
Broca's	Broca's Area	Mild to moderately impaired	Nonfluent	Impaired	Similar to spontaneous speech
Wernicke's	Wernicke's Area	Moderately to severely impaired	Fluent	Impaired	Similar to spontaneous speech
Global	Anterior and posterior left hemisphere	Moderately to severely impaired	Nonfluent	Impaired	Similar to spontaneous speech
Transcortical Motor	Anterior or superior to Broca's Area	Mild to moderately impaired	Nonfluent	Impaired	Less impaired than spontaneous speech
Transcortical Sensory	Posterior temporal lobe extending into the occipital lobe	Moderately to severely impaired	Fluent	Impaired	Less impaired than spontaneous speech
Transcortical Mixed (Isolation)	Anterior and posterior association areas in the left hemisphere	Moderately to severely impaired	Nonfluent	Impaired	Less impaired than spontaneous speech
Conduction	Left arcuate fasciculus and/or supramarginal gyrus in the inferior parietal lobe	Mild to moderately impaired	Fluent	Impaired	More impaired than spontaneous speech
Anomic	Anywhere in the left hemisphere	Normal to mildly impaired	Fluent	Impaired	Similar to spontaneous speech

Broca's aphasia, named for physician Paul Broca, who first described this behavior pattern and the brain lesion responsible for it, is characterized by nonfluent language output and relatively spared language comprehension compared to output fluency difficulties (i.e., these patients may have comprehension problems but they are not as prominent as their output difficulties). As might be deduced from the name, aphasias of this type are thought to result from damage to Broca's area, but also may be associated with lesions in surrounding frontal lobe areas and the white matter beneath the frontal cortex (Basso, Della Sala, & Farabola, 1987; Mazzocchi & Vignolo, 1979; Naeser et al., 1989).

Often considered the aphasia type in greatest contrast to Broca's aphasia is **Wernicke's aphasia,** which is characterized by marked comprehension, naming, and repetition impairments. Language output in Wernicke's aphasia, though fluent, typically contains many paraphasias, and is often described as "empty speech," reflecting the paucity of information that is communicated. Although exceptions are not uncommon (e.g., Binder et al., 1997; Mazzocchi & Vignolo, 1979), Wernicke's aphasia is usually associated with lesions to Wernicke's area and other regions within or near the posterior superior temporal lobe.

The aphasia type marked by significant impairments in all language modalities and functions (i.e., comprehension, speech fluency, naming, and repetition) is **global aphasia.** As might be expected from the breadth of impairments, global aphasia typically results from large lesions affecting both anterior and posterior language centers, although exceptions have been noted (Vignolo, Boccardi, & Caverni, 1986).

Each of the aphasias described above (i.e., Broca's, Wernicke's, and global) are characterized by repetition that is similar to spontaneous speech with respect to fluency, presence of paraphasic errors, morphosyntactic accuracy, and so forth. The following three aphasia types are similar to these hallmark aphasia types, with the exception that repetition is much less impaired than would be predicted from spontaneous speech. **Transcortical motor aphasia** is similar to Broca's aphasia with respect to speech fluency, comprehension, and naming. When patients with transcortical motor aphasia are asked to repeat phrases and sentences, however, their spoken output is generally more fluent and contains fewer errors than their spontaneous verbal output. Lesions resulting in transcortical motor aphasia are usually anterior or superior to Broca's area, and are hypothesized to reflect a disconnection between Broca's area and the supplemental motor area (Freedman, Alexander, & Naeser, 1984).

Similar to Wernicke's aphasia, **transcortical sensory aphasia** is characterized by poor comprehension and fluent speech. Repetition tends to be more preserved than spontaneous speech, which typically contains many paraphasias and neologisms. Lesions resulting from disrupted blood supply to the posterior cerebral artery that affect the inferior temporal lobe and parts of the occipital lobe are typically associated with transcortical sensory aphasia (Alexander, Hiltbrunner, & Fischer, 1989; Kertesz, Sheppard, & MacKenzie, 1982).

The final transcortical aphasia type is **transcortical mixed aphasia,** also known as **isolation aphasia.** Similar to global aphasia, patients with isolation aphasia exhibit notable impairments in comprehension, speech fluency, and naming, but retain the ability to repeat at a level not predicted by the severity of their other language deficits. As might be anticipated, isolation aphasia tends to be associated with large lesions involving both anterior and posterior language association areas (Maeshima et al., 2002).

In contrast to the aphasia types characterized by preserved repetition ability, **conduction aphasia** is notable for disproportionately severe deficits during repetition. Patients with conduction aphasia tend to have relatively good comprehension and fluent speech, with mild to moderate naming deficits. However, when they are asked to repeat, their speech may become more nonfluent, or paraphasias may become more prominent than is observed during their spontaneous speech. The lesion sites traditionally associated with conduction aphasia are the left arcuate fasciculus, the supramarginal gyrus in the inferior parietal lobe, or both (Anderson et al., 1999; Arnett, Rao, Hussain, Swanson, & Hammeke, 1996).

The final classic connectionist aphasia type is **anomic aphasia.** Patients with anomic aphasia exhibit a relatively isolated impairment of naming, with fluent speech and good comprehension. Although some patients may demonstrate anomic aphasia early post onset, other patients' impairments will evolve via spontaneous recovery and language treatment into anomic aphasia (Pedersen, Vinter, & Olsen, 2004). Unlike the other aphasia types, which have been associated with lesions to specific brain structures or pathways, anomic aphasia can result from brain damage to various cortical and subcortical regions.

Other Aphasia Types

Although not necessarily included in the traditional aphasia classification systems, additional aphasia types have been identified. **Subcortical aphasia,** referring to aphasia resulting from damage to non-cortical sites (e.g., thalamus, basal ganglia), has been reported by a number of researchers (Jodzio, Gasecki, Drumm, Lass, & Nyka, 2003; Metter et al., 1983; Naeser et al., 1982; Radanovic & Scaff, 2003; Robin & Scheinberg, 1990). The behavioral descriptions of subcortical aphasia are quite varied (see Hillis et al., 2004, for review) and may overlap with those for any other type of aphasia. As discussed in Chapter 1, the direct role of subcortical structures in language function and related aphasias has been called into question by recent studies demonstrating that language disruptions associated with subcortical lesions can be explained by reduced oxygenation to relevant cortical sites (e.g., Hillis et al., 2004). Nonetheless, clinicians should be aware that patients with subcortical lesions may demonstrate aphasia and that the nature of their aphasia may not be predictable from their lesion site.

Crossed aphasia describes aphasia resulting from lesions to the right hemisphere. Because even most left-handed individuals are left-hemisphere dominant for language, crossed aphasia is quite rare (Zangwill, 1967). Similar to subcortical aphasias, the pattern of language impairment in crossed aphasia is quite variable. Moreover, crossed aphasia may result from lesions to a number of right-hemisphere sites (Coppens, Hungerford, Yamaguchi, & Yamadori, 2002). Interestingly, the language characteristics of crossed aphasia may co-occur with the cognitive-communicative deficits (e.g., neglect) more commonly associated with right- hemisphere lesions (Paghera, Marien, & Vignolo, 2003).

Occasionally, the term **pure aphasia** is used to denote apparently isolated impairments of specific language functions. For example, patients who demonstrate reading difficulties in the absence of any other language impairment are said to demonstrate **pure alexia,** or word blindness (Barriere & Lorch, 2003; Buchman et al., 1986; Polster & Rose, 1998; Wee & Menard, 1999). Similarly, **pure agraphia** refers to isolated impairments of writing (Barriere & Lorch, 2003; Luzzi & Piccirilli, 2003; Nagaratnam, Plew, & Cooper, 1998), and **pure word deafness** describes profound auditory comprehension deficits without evidence of impairment in other language functions (e.g., speaking, reading) (Buchman, Garron, Trost-Cardamone, Wichter, & Schwartz, 1986; Polster & Rose, 1998; Wee & Menard, 1999). Such isolated linguistic impairments are uncommon, and as indicated previously, some authors would not consider isolated impairments indicative of aphasia. Nonetheless, such impairments are likely to be identified and managed in ways similar to those employed for the more typical aphasias.

The final aphasia type to be described is unique primarily with respect to etiology. Whereas aphasia most frequently results from acute neurological injury (e.g., strokes—see Chapter 3), it also may be a symptom of progressive disease. Aphasia of this type is called **primary progressive aphasia** (PPA) and is generally associated with left hemisphere pathology, although no single disease has yet been identified as the primary cause of PPA. Patients with PPA may demonstrate a range of impairments in comprehension, naming, speech fluency, and reading and writing skills (Duffy & Peterson, 1992). Unlike aphasia resulting from acute brain injury, which is generally expected to improve over time, the deficits associated with PPA continue to progress. In fact, one of the diagnostic criteria for PPA is that patients show a relatively isolated decline of language abilities for at least two years (Weintraub, Rubin, & Mesulam, 1990). Because of the gradual onset of PPA, it may be confused with early dementia, although careful assessment will generally reveal that broader intellect, including memory and executive functions, and the ability to complete daily activities independently are relatively spared, often for many, many years (Duffy & Peterson, 1992).

RIGHT HEMISPHERE DISORDERS

In contrast to the primarily linguistically based symptoms of patients with aphasia, the communication difficulties of patients who have suffered right hemisphere brain damage (RHD) are for the most part a product of concomitant cognitive deficits (Burrell, Linebaugh, & Cozens-Hoffman, 1996; Surian & Siegal, 2001; McDonald, 2000). For this reason, the term cognitive-communicative disorders is often used when referring to the types of communicative symptoms observed following RHD. An ever-increasing research literature indicates that patients with RHD can vary significantly in terms of the nature and severity of their cognitive-communicative disorder. This heterogeneity no doubt arises from the variety of deficits, including impairments of perception, attention, memory, executive functioning, and certain aspects of language, that may directly or indirectly influence these patients' communication abilities. Despite progress in understanding the types of cognitive-communicative disorders associated with RHD, limited data exist to help predict the frequency with which these disorders may occur. Whereas early estimates and small sample studies suggested that approximately 50% of RHD patients should be expected to present with some form of cognitive-communicative disorder (e.g., Benton & Bryan, 1996), Lehman Blake and colleagues (2002) more recently found that 96% of the RHD patients identified in their review of an inpatient hospital's medical charts had been diagnosed with at least one type of cognitive-communicative symptom. Accordingly, given that cognitive-communicative disorders may be a frequent consequence of RHD, clinicians must be aware of the range of deficits with which this patient population may present.

PERCEPTUAL PROBLEMS

Deficits in perceiving either visual or auditory information frequently occur following RHD (Cummings & Burns, 1996; Lehman Blake, Duffy, Meyers, & Tompkins, 2002; Vignolo, 2003). An understanding of these perceptual problems is necessary, given that they may be the underlying basis of some language symptoms (McDonald, 2000; Nicholson et al., 2003; Peper & Irle, 1997). For instance, problems with pitch discrimination may contribute to the prosody processing difficulties that are sometimes observed following RHD. Likewise, complex visuospatial discrimination and integration problems may result in a variety of communicative symptoms, such as a decreased ability to profit from nonverbal cues (e.g., patients are unable to discriminate the facial expressions of their communicative partners), inappropriate proxemics (e.g., patients with depth perception problems may get too close to their communicative partners), poor writing legibility, and illogical verbal output (e.g., a patient's narrative sample does not match with the picture stimulus because of his inability to perceive the items and events depicted in the picture). A list of possible perceptual problems associated with RHD is provided in Table 2-3, and further information about several of these deficits is provided later in this book (see Chapter 4).

COGNITIVE SYMPTOMS

Patients with RHD may experience a variety of cognitive problems subsequent to the onset of their brain damage. As will be summarized below, all major domains of cognition (i.e., attention, memory, and executive functioning) may be compromised. The specific symptoms with which a given patient presents will depend on

Table 2-3. Visual and Auditory Perceptual and Related Disorders Associated with RHD and Certain Dementing Diseases

VISUAL DISORDERS	AUDITORY DISORDERS
Visual integration deficits	Sound localization deficits
Topographical disorientation	Amusia/music perception problems
Impaired figure/ground perception	*Auditory agnosia
Impaired depth perception	Impaired pitch discrimination
Geographic disorientation	Impaired categorical processing of voice
*Prosopagnosia/facial recognition deficits	Impaired loudness discrimination
*Visual agnosia	
Achromatopsia/color perception deficits	
Impaired visual closure/perception of incomplete visual stimuli	
Simultanagnosia/poor integration of details	
Environmental agnosia	
Pallinopsia/abnormal persistence of visual images	

*Agnosias (i.e., problems applying meaning to what is being seen or heard) most frequently occur following bilateral brain damage, but also have been periodically reported following unilateral RHD.

which neural structures and pathways within the right hemisphere were compromised by the brain damage. Therefore, clinicians must keep in mind that it is unlikely that all RHD patients will display all of the following cognitive impairments. Instead, clinicians must utilize assessment procedures and findings to determine which of the following cognitive symptoms may be influencing the communication abilities of their right hemisphere patients.

Attention Problems

Attention is one of the most commonly impaired cognitive functions subsequent to RHD (Lehman Blake et al., 2002). All aspects of attention including sustained attention, focused attention, attention-switching, and divided attention may be compromised (Burrell et al., 1996; Hjaltason et al., 1996; Ruff et al., 1992). These attention problems are important to qualify and quantify as they may be the source of several communicative symptoms (Murray, 2000). For instance, pragmatic and discourse problems such as poor eye contact, understanding of lengthy conversations, and inadequate topic maintenance may be a by-product of decreased sustained attention abilities, rather than an impairment of higher-level language abilities.

Neglect Syndrome

Without question, the most frequently studied attention symptoms associated with RHD are collectively referred to as **neglect syndrome.** Generally, neglect refers to a set of attention problems in which patients are slow or inaccurate at reporting, reacting to, orienting to, or seeking out stimuli that are presented contralateral to the side of their brain damage (Cherney, 2002; Heilman, Watson, & Valenstein, 1985; Robertson & Halligan, 1999). Therefore, if patients with RHD present with neglect, they will have difficulty attending to information presented on their left side. Although neglect is most obvious when it affects patients' attention to visual information or stimulation, it also may negatively influence information processing in other modalities (e.g., auditory, tactile, olfactory). Whereas estimates of neglect prevalence following RHD vary, most suggest that over 50% of RHD patients will display one or more neglect symptoms (e.g., Lehman Blake et al., 2002). Research indicates that neglect also can occur in patients with left hemisphere brain damage, but that neglect associated with RHD is more severe and enduring (Heilman et al., 1985; Robertson & Halligan, 1999). Researchers have hypothesized that neglect is more debilitating following RHD because of the right hemisphere's relative dominance for allocating attention within both hemispaces (Mesulam, 1981); in contrast, the left hemisphere may contribute to distributing and directing attention within the right hemispace, but if it is damaged, the right hemisphere can compensate and continue to support attention to the right hemispace. Because of the frequency with which this cognitive deficit may occur, because it can be a persistent symptom, and because several studies have found neglect to be a particularly influential negative prognostic indicator of functional outcome (Cherney, Halper, Kwasnika, Harvey, & Zhang, 2001; Jehkonen et al., 2000b, 2001), understanding the variety of symptoms that may contribute to the syndrome of neglect is essential to managing patients with RHD.

One of the most overt neglect symptoms is **hemi-inattention,** which includes problems such as (1) poor response to or report of stimuli presented contralaterally in the absence of sensory impairments, or (2) poor performance of tasks or activities in the contralateral hemispace that cannot be attributed to motor impairments (Cherney, 2002; Heilman et al., 1985; Robertson & Halligan, 1999). When this symptom occurs in the visual modality, several other terms may be applied, including hemispatial neglect, visuospatial neglect, or unilateral spatial neglect. Symptoms such as omitting details from the left side of their drawings (see Figure 2-2), failing to brush teeth on the left side of their mouths, leaving their left shoe lace untied, and bumping into furniture that is on their left side are also considered a product of hemi-inattention. These behaviors are considered to have an attentional basis because neither sensory nor motor impairments can explain their occurrence (e.g., patients are not failing to brush teeth on the left side of their mouths because of hemiparesis or apraxia), and when you draw patients' attention to the information or task on their neglected side, they are able to process the information or complete the task.

Another obvious symptom of neglect is **hemiakinesia,** which is also sometimes referred to as hemihypokinesia or motor extinction, impersistence, or neglect. Patients with hemiakinesia underuse or in some cases never use the left side of their body, even in the absence of hemiparesis. Signs of hemiakinesia include poor balance because postural muscles on the left side of the body are not being fully exploited, failing to evade painful stimuli, difficulties completing bilateral tasks (e.g., problems buttoning a shirt or putting hair in a ponytail), and minimal exploration of the left hemispace with the left hand or limb when an activity necessitates this exploration.

Other neglect symptoms are not as obvious. For instance, sensory extinction to simultaneous stimulation refers to the phenomenon in which patients with neglect

Figure 2-2. Example of a free-hand drawing of a butterfly from a patient with left visuo-spatial neglect subsequent to a right hemisphere stroke.

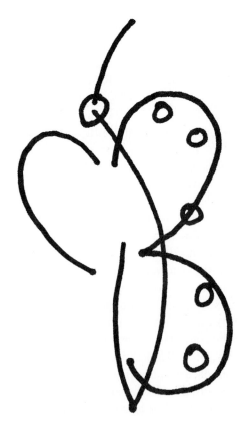

fail to report being stimulated on their left side when stimulation was presented bilaterally. For example, if the examiner touches the right and left sides of the RHD patient's back, the patient would report only being touched on the right side. Interestingly, this symptom often persists even after hemi-inattention has recovered. Another less noticeable symptom is **allesthesia.** This term is applied when RHD patients report being stimulated on their right side when they were actually stimulated on their left side. For instance, the clinician might enter an RHD patient's hospital room from the left side and then greet the patient from that left side. If the patient has allesthesia, she will look to her right to respond to the clinician.

The presence of neglect will have significant effects on RHD patients' language abilities. For example, patients with visual hemi-inattention may have reading difficulties related to not attending to the left side of words or the left side of the page. When these types of reading problems occur, patients may be diagnosed with **neglect dyslexia.** Similarly, **neglect dygraphia** refers to writing problems related to neglect. Signs that neglect is affecting writing include failing to cross or dot letters (e.g., "t," "f," "x," "i," "j"), leaving a large left side margin that increases in width as patients' writing progresses down the page, and displaying a right upward slant to their writing as they progress from the left to the right side of the page.

Memory Problems

RHD frequently produces a variety of memory impairments (Lehman Blake et al., 2002). Traditionally, RHD has been associated with impaired temporary as well as long-term recall of nonverbal more so than verbal material (Lange, Waked, Kirshblum, & DeLuca, 2000; Lewis-Jack, Campbell, Ridley, & Ocampo, 1997; Rausch, 1985). That is, patients with RHD might be expected to have difficulty encoding and remembering one or more of the following: (1) visual information such as complex designs, faces and facial expressions, and spatial locations and routes; (2) auditory information such as the rhythm or tune of a song; or (3) information presented in other sensory modalities such as olfaction (Rausch, Serafetinides, & Crandall, 1977). Additionally, RHD patients, particularly those with frontal lobe lesions, may display problems remembering the temporal order of the to-be-recalled nonverbal information (e.g., they forget what sequence in which a series of faces was shown), or under what circumstances they encoded the information (i.e., source memory deficit) (Buklina, 2003).

Although nonverbal memory problems have been traditionally associated with RHD and verbal memory problems with left hemisphere damage, researchers have more recently found that encoding and subsequent recall of verbal information may be additionally compromised following RHD (Culbertson et al., 1998; Halper et al., 1996; Murray, 2004b). For example, Tompkins and colleagues (1994) found that their study participants with RHD performed an auditory-verbal working memory task more poorly than their non-brain-damaged study participants.

Furthermore, the working memory performances of the RHD participants correlated with their performances of a discourse comprehension task that involved resolving contextual discrepancies or revising linguistic inferences. Accordingly, the memory problems of RHD patients need to be identified given their potential to interfere with discourse and other communicative abilities.

Executive Functioning Problems

Whereas currently only limited data are available regarding the nature and extent of executive functioning deficits following RHD, it is clear that executive skills such as planning, problem solving, cognitive flexibility, and inhibition will be compromised in at least some patients with RHD, particularly those with damage to their frontal lobe or to connections between their right frontal lobe and subcortical structures such as the thalamus (Annoni et al., 2003; Lehman Blake et al., 2002). A particularly problematic RHD symptom related to executive dysfunctioning is **anosognosia,** or an impaired awareness or denial of one's own deficits (Hartman-Maeir, Soroker, Ring, & Katz, 2002; Robertson & Halligan, 1999). Several forms of anosognosia are possible. The term verbal asomatognosia (also sometimes called somatognosia) is used when patients deny ownership of their limb or limbs contralateral to the side of their brain lesion. If patients admit they are experiencing symptoms subsequent to the onset of their brain damage, but appear unconcerned or show nominal emotional response about these symptoms, they may be diagnosed with anosodiaphoria.

Anosognosia in its various forms is common in RHD patients, particularly those with neglect (Ghika-Schmid, van Melle, Guex, & Bogousslavsky 1999; Hartman-Maeir et al., 2002; Jehkonen et al., 2000a). Patients may be unaware of just one symptom, several symptoms, or all of their symptoms, although it is more common for patients to have limited awareness of their cognitive rather than motor or sensory impairments. Like neglect, anosognosia is a negative prognostic indicator (Jehkonen et al., 2001). Accordingly, diagnosing anosognosia is imperative, as patients who are unaware of their deficits or who cannot appreciate the consequences of their deficits will not understand the need for treatment, will not be motivated to apply whatever strategies are suggested if they attend treatment, or may place themselves in physical or emotional jeopardy by attempting activities that are beyond their current ability level (Ghika-Schmid et al., 1999; Hartman-Maeir et al., 2002).

COMMUNICATIVE SYMPTOMS

Generally, the communicative problems of patients with RHD might be viewed as the inverse of those described for patients with aphasia: Whereas aphasia is associated with impaired phonological, lexical-semantic, and morphosyntactic processing, but relatively preserved pragmatic abilities, RHD is associated with relatively intact phonological, lexical-semantic, and morphosyntactic processing, but compromised pragmatic skills. That is, patients with RHD are typically capable of communicating on superficial levels but may experience breakdowns in more complex, less structured, abstract, and sophisticated communicative situations. This means that in acute care settings, the communicative problems of patients with RHD may not be obvious (Benton & Bryan, 1996). Instead, only when these patients return to their home, work, or other more demanding and unpredictable environments and communicative activities may their communicative difficulties be fully realized by the patients themselves or their caregivers.

Before describing the types of pragmatic and related discourse problems associated with RHD, it is important to evaluate research pertaining to lexical-semantic abilities following RHD. Some studies suggest deficits at this level of language processing, whereas others do not. More specifically, patients with RHD may display lexical-semantic comprehension and production difficulties, but often these difficulties reflect problems in perception or other areas of cognition rather than in lexical-semantic processes per se (Hough, DeMarco, & Schmitzer, 1997; Joanette, Goulet, & Hannequin, 1990; Fassbinder & Tompkins, 2001). For instance, problems with visuoperceptual discrimination may result in inaccurate completion of confrontation naming tasks. Attention problems also may contribute to apparent lexical-semantic breakdowns as several studies have indicated that patients with RHD display more difficulties with word finding under more complex attention conditions (e.g., Murray, 2000). Additionally, the patient's native language may influence whether deficits at the lexical-semantic level will be present following RHD. For example, patients with RHD who speak and write Chinese display similar levels of word-finding difficulties as their peers with left hemisphere damage because the neural representation of Chinese is more bilateral compared to other languages such as English (Cheung, Cheung, & Chan, 2004).

Clinicians are most likely to observe communicative problems at pragmatic and discourse levels of language processing in their patients with RHD. In terms of comprehension, difficulties with one or more of the following have been observed: (1) appreciating humor; (2) comprehending nonliteral language (e.g., indirect speech acts, idioms, sarcasm, proverbs, metaphors); (3) sensitivity to and interpretation of cues related to communicative context and partners, including extralinguistic aspects of communication (e.g., body gestures, facial expressions); (4) resolving lexical ambiguity based on previous world knowledge and/or current communicative content and context; (5) inferencing or revising of preliminary inferences; (6) differentiating between relevant versus irrelevant information; and (7) identifying the moral or theme of a story (Benton & Bryan, 1996; Bryan & Hale, 2001; Lehman Blake, 2003; Mackenzie, Begg, Lees, & Brady, 1999). In terms of language expression, the informativeness and efficiency of spoken and written output of patients with RHD may be negatively affected by deficits such as: (1) inefficient organization and summarization of information; (2) inclusion of tangential or irrelevant details; (3) problems with discourse cohesion (e.g., pronoun referencing, conjunctions) and coherence; (4) confabulation or inclusion of fabricated verbal material; and (5) inaccurate or incomplete discourse macrostructure (e.g., inappropriate turn-taking skills, incomplete or incorrect sequence of story episodes) (Benton & Bryan, 1996; Bryan & Hale, 2001; Kennedy, 2000; McDonald, 2000). All of the above comprehension and production symptoms are exacerbated as the cognitive demands of the communicative task or context increase. For example, for many patients with RHD, nominal discourse comprehension or production problems would be expected when they are conversing in a typical one-on-one situation with a familiar partner about a common and straightforward topic. In contrast, these same patients might be predicted to demonstrate conversational difficulties in a group discussion with unfamiliar communicative partners when the conversational topic is unusual and the communicative setting is novel.

Research has focused on determining processing deficits that might underlie pragmatic and discourse-level comprehension and production problems associated with RHD. For example, several investigators have suggested that other cognitive deficits (e.g., attention, working memory) cause or contribute to the pragmatic and discourse impairments of patients with RHD (Lehman Blake, 2003; Surian & Siegal, 2001). For instance, sustained and focused attention deficits may interfere with the ability of patients with RHD to process and select relevant contextual cues, which in turn may result in misinterpretation of their conversational partners' discourse output, inappropriate selection of their own conversational content or style, or both. Another hypothesis is that patients with RHD have difficulty suppressing word meanings or discourse interpretations that are irrelevant or incompatible with the communicative context (Fassbinder & Tompkins, 2001; Tompkins, Lehman Blake, Baumgaertner, & Fassbinder, 2001). Inefficient or inappropriate suppression may be particularly problematic in contexts in which patients must make revisions to their preliminary interpretations of the linguistic stimuli, as is necessary when understanding jokes or following complex story plots. Such deficits would affect not only their understanding of discordant or ambiguous information, but also their verbal output choices (Kennedy, 2000). For example, failure to suppress certain discourse or vocabulary options might result in including irrelevant information or inappropriate word selections. Further investigation of factors that contribute to the variety of pragmatic and discourse symptoms observed following RHD remains needed (McDonald, 2000; Tompkins et al., 2001); the findings of such research will be essential to helping clinicians identify and subsequently treat patients with RHD who are most at risk for these high level language difficulties that have the potential to severely restrict resumption of social and vocational activities.

TRAUMATIC BRAIN INJURY

Traumatic brain injury (TBI) results when external forces (e.g., sudden impact of striking one's head on a car dashboard in a car accident, or on the ground because of a fall) cause brain damage that leads to temporary or permanent physical, cognitive, emotional, and behavioral impairments (National Head Injury Foundation, 1989). Similar to RHD, communication problems following TBI are typically referred to as cognitive-communicative disorders to capture that for most TBI patients there is a stronger cognitive, rather than linguistic, basis to their communicative limitations. Typically, the type and severity of cognitive-communicative disorders displayed by a given patient with TBI will depend upon the patient's stage of TBI recovery, and the location and extent of his or her brain damage. Whereas Chapter 3 provides further description of the mechanisms of TBI, a summary of cognitive and communicative symptoms associated with TBI is presented in this chapter.

STAGES OF RECOVERY

As patients recover from a TBI, they may progress through one or more of the following stages: (1) coma or a period of unconsciousness, (2) post-traumatic amnesia or a phase of severe confusion and disorientation, (3) a rapid recovery phase of about three to six months in which they experience significant progress, and (4) a long-term plateau recovery phase in which they experience more gradual progress. Understanding these recovery phases is germane to providing families with appropriate education and counseling, particularly during the acute stages in which patients may have impaired consciousness or profound confusion. Accordingly, a more detailed description of disorders of consciousness and post-traumatic amnesia is provided below.

Coma

Patients who are in a **coma** exhibit no or minimal organized or purposeful response to external stimuli within their environment. That is, even following exposure to painful, tactile, auditory, olfactory, kinesthetic, or visual stimuli, these patients display no overt behavioral responses. Coma is more likely if the TBI was associated with rotational external forces, there is diffuse cortical and subcortical brain damage, and areas of the brain associated with arousal and awareness are compromised (e.g., brain stem regions such as the reticular formation) (Zeman, 1997).

In the acute stages, coma duration and depth are quantified and qualified because these variables can help guide predictions about survival and head injury severity (Formisano et al., 2004; Lieberman et al., 2003). Typically, a diagnosis of a severe TBI will be made if coma extends beyond 24 hours. To document coma depth, the Glasgow Coma Scale (GCS; Teasdale & Jennett, 1976) is most frequently used. For this scale, clinicians determine the patient's level of eye-opening (e.g., never opens eyes vs. will open eyes if asked to do so), and best verbal (e.g., only produces sounds and unintelligible word approximations vs. produces words but these words do not make sense) and motor response (e.g., displays abnormal extension posture vs. can complete simple motor tasks). GCS scores vary from a minimum of "3," indicating no response to external stimulation, to "15," indicating good orientation and alertness. When patients' scores rise above "8," they are no longer considered to be in a comatose state.

Vegetative State

Whereas most patients with TBI will progress from coma to a phase of post-traumatic amnesia, a small percentage will appear to awaken from coma (i.e., open their eyes) but will continue to demonstrate no willful interaction with their external or internal environment and no communication ability (Zeman, 1997). The term **vegetative state** may be used to describe patients with this type of consciousness disorder; if the vegetative state persists for longer than one month, the term persistent vegetative state may be applied. Although "vegetative" may be construed to have negative connotations, it is used to indicate that essential, "vegetative," life-sustaining abilities such as breathing, digestion, and sleep-wake cycles have recovered. In addition to eye opening, patients in this state also may display abnormal or spontaneous motor responses such as primitive reflexes (e.g., grasp reflex), teeth grinding, chewing, and even smiling or grunting. Vegetative state is most frequently seen in patients with TBI who suffer profound cortical damage but have relatively intact brain stem functioning (Beuthien-Baumann et al., 2003). The longer the duration of vegetative state, the less likely it is that patients will show improvements, and after one year in this state, it is unlikely that patients will recover even a rudimentary awareness of their environment (Zeman, 1997).

Post-Traumatic Amnesia

Fortunately, the majority of patients who emerge from coma will progress into a phase of **post-traumatic amnesia** (PTA) rather than vegetative state. PTA refers to an acute and commonly temporary recovery phase in which patients are extremely confused and disoriented. More specifically, patients in PTA are disoriented to person (e.g., their name, marital status, address, birthday), time, and place, have incoherent language output, impaired language comprehension, and emotional and behavioral disturbances such as marked agitation, **lability** (i.e., difficulty controlling one's emotions), impulsivity, and possible physical or verbal aggression. These symptoms are related to severe memory, attention, and executive function deficits that include problems remembering daily events and circumstances that transpired prior to and since their TBI, impaired sustained and focused attention (i.e., poor concentration), decreased processing speed, and impaired awareness of their cognitive, physical, and behavioral difficulties. Because of these widespread cognitive problems, patients do not typically remember their time in PTA. In fact, the criterion for emerging from PTA is the return of continuous, accurate, and reliable memory. Like coma duration, length of PTA can provide information pertaining to TBI severity in that the longer patients remain in PTA, the more likely they will have persistent symptoms and poorer functional recovery (Dikmen, Machamer, Winn, & Temkin, 1995; Formisano et al., 2004). Because of the significant confusion and agitation associated with this phase of recovery, formal assessment and active rehabilitation services do not begin until patients with TBI have emerged from PTA.

COGNITIVE SYMPTOMS

Regardless of head injury severity, deficits of attention, memory, and executive functioning are a frequent if not invariable consequence of TBI and, in many cases, are stronger predictors of functional outcome than physical status (Bush et al., 2003; Hoofien, Gilboa, Vakil, & Barak, 2004). The exact type and severity of these cognitive disorders will be dependent, at least in part, on the location and extent of neural structures and pathways that were compromised by the head injury. For instance, if a given patient with TBI suffered brain damage that was more prominent in the right hemisphere, that patient's attention, memory, and executive functioning deficits would most likely be similar to those previously described for patients with RHD. As will be reviewed in Chapter 3, however, certain brain regions are especially vulnerable in head trauma (e.g., frontal lobes, anterior portions of the temporal lobes), and thus certain cognitive symptoms are particularly common following TBI. Accordingly, what follows is a description of attention, memory, and executive functioning problems associated with TBI, with a special emphasis on those that occur most frequently.

Attention Problems

Attention impairments are widespread among patients with TBI, regardless of their head injury severity (Azouvi et al., 2004; Mathias, Beall, & Bigler, 2004), and are important to quantify and qualify because they can contribute to other cognitive deficits (e.g., memory and executive functioning), communication problems (e.g., difficulty with topic maintenance or switching due to sustained or alternating attention limitations, respectively), and, consequently, poor functional outcomes (Perbal, Couillet, Azouvi, & Pouthas, 2003; Rios, Perianez, & Munoz-Cespedes, 2004). Attention problems are typically most apparent acutely, particularly when patients are still in PTA. In the earlier stages of recovery it is not uncommon for most, if not all, attention functions (i.e., sustained, selective, alternating, and divided attention) to be severely compromised. Because of these often profound attention impairments, most patients are inappropriate candidates for formal assessment or direct treatment at this point in their recovery because they lack the fundamental attention skills necessary to attend to the clinician, process task stimuli, and plan and carry out task responses.

As patients emerge from PTA, deficits of more basic attention functions (i.e., attention orienting) tend to resolve rapidly while impairment of more complex attention skills persist (Ryan & Warden, 2003). Several case reports indicate that left or right neglect syndrome may be another long-term attention problem following TBI (e.g., Cocchini, Beschin, & Della Salla, 2002). More frequently, however, patients with TBI in the chronic stages of recovery, particularly those who have suffered mild injuries, will demonstrate relatively intact attention functioning during simple or more routine daily activities, but will continue to report or display enduring attention problems when completing cognitively demanding tasks or when exposed to highly distracting environments (Azouvi et al., 2004; Mathias et al., 2004; Park, Moscovitch, & Robertson, 1999).

Memory Problems

A variety of memory abilities are compromised by TBI and can lead to problems completing many everyday activities and, relatedly, to high levels of caregiver burden (Hart et al., 2003; Marsh et al., 1998; Schmitter-Edgecombe & Wright, 2004). Working memory appears to be particularly vulnerable following TBI, even in cases of mild TBI (Hart et al., 2003; McAllister, Flashman, Sparling, & Sayking, 2004; Perbal et al., 2003). Furthermore, working memory deficits appear to be strongly associated with a number of TBI language impairments, including poor auditory comprehension and discourse production problems such as inadequate use of pronoun antecedents (Hartley & Jensen, 1991; Moran & Gillon, 2004; Turkstra & Holland, 1998).

Whereas all aspects of long-term memory may be negatively affected by TBI, most frequently problems with episodic memory are reported (Perbal et al., 2003; Ward, Shum, Dick, McKinlay, & Baker-Tweney, 2004). Often these episodic memory deficits are part of **retrograde amnesia** in patients with TBI, which may be continuous or interrupted (i.e., intermittent "islands" of memories stored prior to the TBI are inaccessible) (Carlesimo et al., 1998; Leplow et al., 1997). Whereas over time, most patients experience a shrinkage in their amnesia (i.e., a reduction in the amount of their past declarative and/or nondeclarative memories that they cannot recall), they typically are never able to recall the circumstances of their accident, most likely because the sudden onset of their brain damage interfered with encoding the events that occurred immediately prior to and during their accident.

Anterograde amnesia is another common memory problem following TBI that relates to difficulties storing and retrieving new long-term memories or, more generally, new information (Mathias et al., 2004; Shum, Harris, & O'Gorman, 2000; Ward et al., 2004). In many cases, inadequate use of deliberate encoding (e.g., chunking, semantic associations) and retrieval strategies underlies anterograde memory problems. For instance, researchers have shown that the word list recall performances of patients with TBI can be significantly improved if they are given training in the use of encoding strategies (Richardson & Barry, 1985).

Even though many aspects of memory are susceptible to TBI, others are commonly spared, and it is these memory skills that are often exploited in cognitive rehabilitation programs (see Chapter 9). More specifically, procedural memory is often an area of relative strength for many patients with TBI, even those who have suffered severe injuries (Vakil, Biederman, Liran, Groswaser, & Aeurbuch, 1994; Ward et al., 2004; Watt, Shores, & Konishita, 1999). Indeed, recent investigations have identified positive outcomes when treatment involved the use of the patients' procedural memory skills to learn verbal, visual, and other forms of new information (Turkstra, 2001).

Executive Functioning Problems

Given that frontal lobe damage is a frequent consequence of TBI, it is not surprising that executive function deficits including disinhibition, anosognosia, concrete and/or inflexible problem solving and reasoning, and poor planning are pervasive among patients representing the spectrum of TBI severity levels (Hart et al., 2003; Mathias et al., 2004; McDonald, Flashman, & Saykin, 2002; Rath et al., 2004). These high-level cognitive problems may be due to impairments of the executive functions themselves or to deficits in one or more of the other cognitive domains (e.g., attention) that support executive functioning (Rath et al., 2004; Rios et al., 2004), and may underlie certain pragmatic and discourse-level communication symptoms (Turkstra & Flora, 2002). Executive function deficits that appear to be particularly influential negative outcome predictors include unawareness of deficits (Hoofien et al., 2004) and cognitive inflexibility (Hart et al., 2003). Thus, detection and treatment of these executive function impairments will be vital to success in rehabilitation and eventual social and vocational reintegration.

COMMUNICATIVE SYMPTOMS

Variable language profiles may result following TBI. For example, if patients suffer more discrete dominant hemisphere lesions subsequent to their TBI, they may present with language symptoms consistent with an aphasia diagnosis (e.g., Gil, Cohen, Korn, & Groswasser, 1996). More frequently, however, TBI is associated with more diffuse brain damage, and in these cases, pragmatic and discourse deficits beyond the lexical-semantic or morphosyntactic levels are most prominent (Coelho, 2002; Hartley & Jensen, 1991). Like cognitive-communicative disorders associated with RHD, pragmatic and discourse production and comprehension problems are proposed to be primarily a product of attention, memory, and/or executive function deficits rather than a disordered linguistic system (Bate, Mathias,

& Crawford, 2001; Coelho, 2002; Moran & Gillon, 2004), and accordingly are also often referred to as cognitive-communicative disorders.

Overall, there is much overlap in the types of cognitive-communicative symptoms associated with TBI and those associated with RHD (Martin & McDonald, 2003). For example, frequently reported pragmatic deficits following TBI include poor topic management skills (e.g., excessive or infrequent topic initiation, inappropriate topic choices), inadequate discourse cohesion (e.g., nonspecific use of pronouns), decreased discourse informativeness (e.g., inclusion of irrelevant details, confabulation), impaired macrostructure (e.g., failure to include or sequence correctly essential story episodes), and difficulties processing implied information or figurative language (e.g., problems identifying the moral of a story; concrete interpretation of indirect speech acts) (Coelho, 2002; Davis & Coelho, 2004; Hartley & Jensen, 1991; Martin & McDonald, 2003). Again, the types of cognitive-communicative problems exhibited by a given patient with TBI will be dependent upon, at least in part, the location of that patient's brain damage and what other cognitive abilities have been compromised. For instance, patients with TBI who suffer damage to orbitofrontal regions are often highly disinhibited; thus, their language output and input abilities reflect this disinhibition (e.g., excessive topic switching, inappropriate vocabulary choices). In contrast, patients with TBI with damage to the dorsolateral frontal cortex are frequently apathetic (i.e., impaired initiation) and, accordingly, are more likely to have more passive or impoverished language profiles (e.g., infrequent conversational initiation or turns). Because of the direct relationship between pragmatics and successful social interactions, appropriate management of pragmatic and discourse problems is essential to facilitating resumption of participation in previous or new social activities for patients with TBI.

◇ DEMENTIA

Dementia refers to a set of cognitive, communicative, and behavioral symptoms that are caused by a variety of progressive medical or neurological conditions (see Chapter 3 for a description of reversible and irreversible causes of dementia). More specifically, a diagnosis of dementia will be considered if patients demonstrate, in addition to memory problems, unremitting deterioration in one of more of the following areas: perception, language, executive functioning, or personality (American Psychiatric Association, 1994; Grabowski & Damasio, 1997); additionally, these symptoms must be sufficiently significant so that they negatively affect social and occupational functioning. The types, severity, and breadth of cognitive and communicative symptoms with which a patient with dementia presents will be dependent on: (1) what disease (e.g., Alzheimer's vs. Parkinson's vs. Lewy body disease) is causing the dementia, as different diseases will affect different brain regions, and (2) in which disease stage the patient currently is (e.g., subtle vs. profound changes during early vs. late stages, respectively). Accordingly, dementia is characterized by a diverse set of communicative and cognitive impairments, most of which have already been described in preceding aphasia, RHD, and TBI sections of this chapter. Because many of these specific symptoms have been previously reviewed, a more general summary of perceptual, cognitive, and communicative problems associated with dementia is provided below.

PERCEPTUAL PROBLEMS

Because auditory and visual perceptual problems are often a product of either right hemisphere damage or bilateral brain damage, and because many dementing diseases cause not only right hemisphere but also bilateral brain damage, perceptual disorders are common among patients with dementia (Caselli, 2000; Crucian & Okun, 2003; Noe et al., 2004) (see Table 2-3). For example, because Alzheimer's disease affects predominantly posterior regions of both hemispheres, patients with this disease often display problems with complex visuospatial discrimination, prosopagnosia (i.e., facial recognition deficits), achromatopsia (i.e., problems perceiving colors), or propopagnosia (i.e., a disorder in which patients do not recognize their own image in a mirror) (Simard, van Reekum, & Myran, 2003). In contrast, patients with frontotemporal dementia, which, as the name implies, affects predominately anterior brain regions, may be more likely to present with auditory perceptual deficits including auditory agnosia (Hodges, 2001; Kaga, Nakamura, Takayama, & Momose, 2004). Importantly, perceptual problems can have negative effects on language and the other cognitive abilities of patients with dementia and, consequently, on their completion of a variety of daily activities (Caselli, 2000; Glosser et al., 2002).

COGNITIVE SYMPTOMS

As with the other adult neurogenic language disorders we reviewed in this chapter, all cognitive domains may be compromised in dementia. The relative severity of these various cognitive symptoms will differ among patients depending on what disease is causing their dementia and how far their dementing disease has progressed. Despite the diversity of cognitive profiles that can be seen across patients with dementia, these cognitive problems are consistently associated with significant caregiver burden and decreased ability to complete and participate in daily social and vocational activities (Chiu et al., 2004; Rizzo, Reinach, McGehee, & Dawson, 1997). Thus, the presence and severity of cognitive problems are important to document in each and every patient with dementia.

Attention Problems

All attention functions may be compromised in dementia; in fact, attention problems are one of the earliest symptoms in many types of dementia (Ballard, 2004; Chiu et al., 2004; Foldi, LoBosco, & Schaefer, 2002; Sieroff et al., 2004; Zgaljardic, Borod, Foldi, & Mattis, 2003). Whereas in the early stages of most dementing diseases only more complex aspects of attention (e.g., attention switching, divided attention) are deficient, as these diseases progress, more basic attention functions (e.g., sustained attention) will also deteriorate. It should also be noted that neglect syndrome may occur in some forms of dementia (Ishiai et al., 2000; Liu, McDowd, & Lin, 2004). Although neglect does not appear to be a frequent problem, Foldi and colleagues (2002) have suggested that (1) other cognitive problems may mask neglect symptoms, (2) only a subset of patients with predominantly right hemisphere involvement may develop neglect, and/or (3) bilateral neural deterioration may nullify attentional bias effects and thus, patients have problems attending to both sides.

Memory Problems

Strikingly different memory profiles can be observed among patients with dementia, depending on the etiology of their dementia. For example, in **Alzheimer's disease** (AD), persistent memory decline is a hallmark symptom, even in the earliest stages of the disease (Bayles, 2003; Noe et al., 2004). Over time, patients with AD will deteriorate from initially mild working and episodic memory problems (e.g., disoriented to place, misplacing personal items) to profound anterograde and retrograde amnesia and thus impairment of most memory stores and functions (e.g., working memory, episodic memory, semantic memory, encoding and retrieval strategies). Interestingly, however, procedural memory remains an area of relative strength well into the disease process, a finding that has been capitalized on in many dementia treatment programs (see Chapter 9). In contrast to the pattern of memory decline associated with AD, less prominent memory problems are observed in the early stages of other forms of dementia, including dementia with Lewy bodies (Ballard, 2004) and frontotemporal dementia (Elderkin-Thompson, Boone, Hwang, & Kumar, 2004). Likewise, in dementias associated with primarily subcortical degeneration such as Parkinson's disease, procedural memory appears most vulnerable (Zagaljardic et al., 2003). Despite these different patterns of memory decline, the vast majority of patients in the final stages of dementia will experience significant impairment of most if not all aspects of memory.

Executive Functioning Problems

Patients with dementia, regardless of the etiology of their dementia, invariably present with some form of executive dysfunctioning (Cannata, Alberoni, Franceschi, &

Mariani, 2002; Chen et al., 1998; Chiu et al., 2004). As just discussed with respect to memory problems, however, the type and severity of executive dysfunctioning can vary dramatically across the many dementing diseases. For instance, in frontotemporal dementia, the most striking initial symptoms are typically executive function deficits such as disinhibition, perseveration, and cognitive inflexibility (Elderkin-Thompson et al., 2004; Slachevsky et al., 2004). In contrast, in AD, executive function problems such as impaired reasoning are less prominent compared to memory and language impairments, and, according to some research, are possibly a product of other cognitive deficits (Cannata et al., 2002; Slachevsky et al., 2004). In **Parkinson's disease,** early deterioration of executive functioning is also common, but at least some of these executive function deficits, such as initiation and planning problems, are infrequently observed in early frontotemporal dementia (Zagaljardic et al., 2003). Regardless of these differences, by the middle and late stages of most dementing diseases, executive function deficits are significant and typically result in complete patient dependence and, consequently, significant caregiver burden (Chen et al., 1998; Torti, Gwyther, Reed, Friedman, & Schulman, 2004).

COMMUNICATIVE SYMPTOMS

Communication problems are common in dementia, regardless of etiology (Bayles, 2003; Zgaljardic et al., 2003). Like other cognitive domains, however, the profile of language symptoms varies across dementia types. In the early stages of AD and many cases of vascular dementia, language problems such as anomia and impaired comprehension of complex or figurative linguistic material are prominent symptoms (Cannata et al., 2002; Groves-Wright, Neils-Strunjas, Burnett, & O'Neill, 2004). In contrast, in frontotemporal dementia, morphosyntactic and pragmatic deficits and nonfluent output are often noted prior to or in addition to lexical-semantic difficulties (Elderkin-Thompson et al., 2004; Cooke et al., 2003). Furthermore, in other forms of dementia, such as that associated with Parkinson's disease, only more subtle, high-level language abilities (e.g., processing of complex, infrequent syntactic forms) appear compromised (Murray & Stout, 1999; Zgaljardic et al., 2003). By the middle stages of AD, language problems are more diverse and severe in that patients' spoken and written output becomes vague, perseverative, and difficult to follow, their discourse skills begin to decline (e.g., impaired topic maintenance and shifting), and comprehension of both concrete and figurative spoken and written language is now difficult (Bayles, 2003; Groves-Wright et al., 2004). By the final stages of many forms of dementia, patients are often able to produce little meaningful output and often become completely mute. Their language comprehension abilities are similarly ravaged by whatever disease is causing their dementia. Because communication abilities are necessary for not only the completion of daily activities but also to maintain social interactions, research indicates that the communication breakdown associated with dementia can lead to significant caregiver burden, and social isolation and depression in both the patient and the caregiver (Small et al., 1998; 2000). Importantly, as will be reviewed in subsequent treatment chapters (i.e., Chapters 9 through 11), researchers are continuing to develop new approaches to helping patients with dementia maintain their communicative and cognitive abilities, despite the progressive nature of this adult neurogenic language disorder.

SUMMARY

The number, variety, and complexity of underlying linguistic and cognitive impairments characterizing neurogenic language disorders can seem overwhelming. By considering the impairments within the framework of the process model depicted in Figure 1-1, however, readers may gain a clearer understanding of the relationships among impairments associated with the various neurogenic language disorders. The review of etiologies commonly associated with neurogenic language disorders provided in Chapter 3 will reveal additional relationships among impairments in body structure and function and resulting communication limitations.

Chapter 3

Neuropathology of Neurogenic Language Disorders

LEARNING OBJECTIVES

After reading this chapter you should be able to:

- List the major arteries that provide blood flow to the brain.
- Describe the two major types of stroke.
- Identify different types of benign and malignant tumors.
- Describe two infections that may cause neurogenic language disorders.
- Contrast open head and closed injury.
- Differentiate primary and secondary forms of structural and physiological damage associated with traumatic head injury.
- Distinguish between reversible and irreversible causes of dementia.
- Describe at least two etiologies of irreversible dementia.

KEY TERMS

Alzheimer's disease
aneurysm
arteriovenous
    malformation
carotid arterial
    system
closed head injury
contra coup effect
diffuse axonal
    shearing

embolus
frontotemporal
    dementia
irreversible
    dementia
ischemic stroke
hemorrhagic stroke
multi-infarct
    dementia
open head injury

reversible dementia
stroke/brain attack
thrombosis
transient ischemic
    attack
traumatic brain
    injury
tumor/neoplasm
vertebrobasilar
    arterial system

INTRODUCTION

Neurogenic language disorders are caused by a variety of pathologies that affect the structure and function of the central nervous system. The severity, type, and eventual outcome of our patients' neurogenic language disorders will depend, at least in part, on the site and extent of their brain damage. Therefore, it is important that we, as clinicians, understand at least basic information about the nature, course, and medical treatment of these pathologies. This chapter provides a description of the major types of pathology that underlie the linguistic and cognitive deficits typical of neurogenic language disorders. Familiarity with these pathologies will not only enhance our competency in managing the neurogenic language disorders experienced by our patients, but will also improve our skill in communicating more effectively with the variety of other professionals with whom we may interact in educational or health care settings.

 ## STROKE

A **stroke** refers to any disruption in blood flow to the brain. Sometimes referred to as cerebrovascular accident or, more recently, **brain attack,** stroke is the third leading cause of death following heart disease and cancer, and the leading cause of adult disability in the United States. According to the National Stroke Association (NSA, 2002), the number of new stroke cases reported each year is on the rise, increasing from around 500,000 about 20 years ago to the current estimate of 750,000 new cases each year. Stroke also is the most common cause of aphasia (Tonkonogy, 1986) and right hemisphere cognitive-communicative disorders (Tompkins, 1995), and the second most frequent cause of dementia (Fratiglioni & Rocca, 2001). Despite these sobering statistics, several studies have documented inadequate public knowledge of stroke, including risk factors and symptoms (Fisher, 2003; Goldstein & Gradison, 1999). For example, a Gallup survey conducted by the NSA in 1996 found not only that almost 40% of adults were unaware that a stroke occurs in the brain, but also that many could not recognize frequent symptoms of stroke.

As clinicians, it is our job to treat the variety of communication and cognitive deficits that may result from stroke. Because an important aspect of treatment involves educating our patients and their caregivers about stroke as well as their communication problems, clinicians must be cognizant of the mechanisms, outcomes, and medical management of stroke. To better understand the causes and consequences of stroke, it is helpful first to review the normal pattern of blood supply to the brain.

BLOOD SUPPLY

Although the brain typically comprises only 2% of our body weight, it requires about 17% of the cardiac output, and expends about 20% of the oxygen used by the entire body. Because the brain is unable to store oxygen, glucose, or other nutritional substances, even a brief interruption of blood flow will affect its functioning. For example, obstruction of blood flow for about ten seconds will result in unconsciousness, and as little as two to three minutes of blood flow cessation may cause permanent brain damage. The body is able to meet the blood supply demands of the brain via two major arterial systems, the carotid and the vertebrobasilar systems. As depicted in Figure 3-1, both of these arterial systems arise from the aorta, the major artery from the heart. The innominate or brachiocephalic artery comes directly off the right side of the aortic arch. This artery then subdivides into the right common carotid and right subclavian arteries. On the left

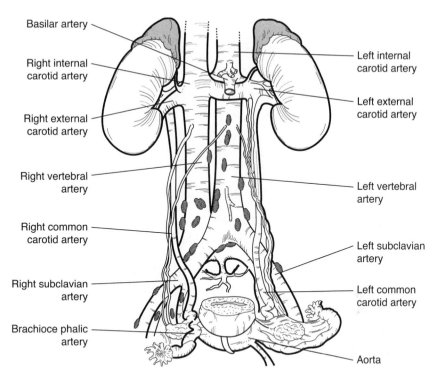

Figure 3-1. Carotid and vertebral basilar systems as they arise from the aorta. These two arterial systems are the basis of the cerebral vascular system.

side, the left common carotid comes off of the apex of the aortic arch, and then, in turn, sends off a branch, which is called the left subclavian artery.

The **carotid arterial system** begins at the left and right common carotid arteries. These two arteries ascend laterally to the trachea; at about the level of the larynx, each divides into external and internal carotid arteries. The internal carotid arteries are of particular importance because they enter the skull to provide the brain's anterior blood supply. Specifically, each internal carotid artery subdivides into an anterior and a middle cerebral artery. The anterior cerebral arteries supply the medial surfaces of the two cerebral hemispheres as well as the superior borders of the frontal and parietal lobes (Figure 3-2). The middle cerebral arteries travel along the lateral fissure to supply most of the lateral surface of the cerebral hemispheres, including superior and lateral portions of the temporal lobes and the lateral surfaces of the frontal lobes (Figure 3-2a). Consequently, the middle cerebral artery is of particular importance because it provides blood flow to the major speech and language brain areas (i.e., perisylvian language zone), including Broca's and Wernicke's areas. The middle cerebral artery also sends off smaller branches called the lenticulostriate arteries to supply deep structures such as the basal ganglia and internal capsule.

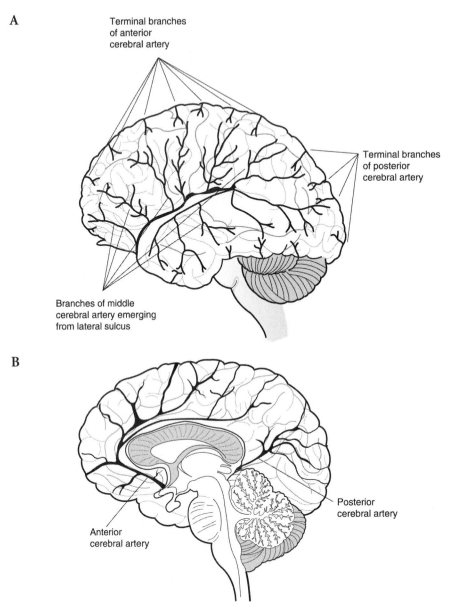

Figure 3-2. Cerebral vascular system. (a) Lateral view of the left side of the brain and the left middle cerebral artery that supplies most of the lateral aspects of the left hemisphere. Also shown are the terminal branches of the left anterior cerebral artery supplying superior aspects of the frontal and parietal lobes, and the terminal branches of the left posterior cerebral artery supplying inferior aspects of the temporal lobe and lateral aspects of the occipital lobe. (b) Medial view of the right side of the brain and the right anterior cerebral artery supplying medial aspects of the frontal and parietal lobes, and the right posterior cerebral artery supplying medial aspects of the occipital lobe.

The **vertebrobasilar arterial system** arises from the left and right subclavian arteries. Each of the subclavian arteries branches into a vertebral artery. These vertebral arteries ascend toward the brain via small holes in the upper vertebrae of the spine. They enter the skull through the foramen magna, and then at the level of the pons unite to form one basilar artery (Figure 3-3). The basilar artery then subdivides into the right and left posterior cerebral arteries. The posterior cerebral arteries provide blood to the occipital lobes as well as medial and inferior portions of temporal lobes. The posterior cerebral arteries also send arterial branches deep into the cerebral hemispheres to supply blood to important subcortical structures, such as the thalamus.

The carotid and vertebrobasilar artery systems are connected with each other through a ring of arteries referred to as the **Circle of Willis** (Figure 3-3). Located at the base of the brain, the Circle of Willis provides a collateral circulation system that can help compensate for a blockage in one of the major cerebral arteries. For example, if there is occlusion of the left internal carotid artery that in turn is

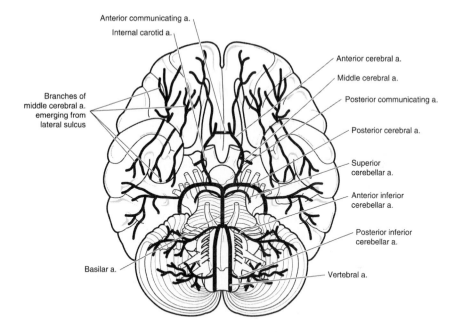

Figure 3-3. Inferior view of the brain and the cerebral vascular system. The posterior cerebral arteries are shown arising from vertebral basilar system. Also depicted is the Circle of Willis, the ring of arteries that connects carotid and vertebral basilar arterial systems and provides collateral cerebral circulation. The following arteries make up the Circle of Willis: posterior cerebral arteries, posterior communicating arteries, internal carotid arteries, middle cerebral arteries, anterior cerebral arteries and the anterior communicating artery.

reducing blood flow through the left middle and anterior cerebral arteries, the right carotid artery and the basilar artery can provide alternate sources of blood flow via the anterior communicating artery and the left posterior communicating artery, respectively. Unfortunately, with age, these communicating arteries often become less viable alternative blood flow routes due to narrowing associated with vascular disease.

Certain lateral areas of the hemispheres have some backup protection from blood flow occlusions because they are located where the distributions of major cerebral arteries overlap (Figure 3-2a). These areas are referred to as watershed areas or zones. The anterior watershed zone is found on the lateral surface of frontal and parietal lobes where the anterior and middle cerebral arteries meet, whereas the posterior watershed zone is found on the lateral surface of the occipital and temporal lobes where the middle and posterior cerebral arteries meet. Therefore, if blockage occurs in the posterior cerebral artery, there might be little damage to brain tissue within the posterior watershed area because this tissue is still receiving blood supply from the neighboring branches of the middle cerebral artery.

STROKE RISK FACTORS

Despite some built-in protective mechanisms within the cerebral circulatory system, every minute in the United States an individual suffers a stroke (NSA, 2002). Risk factors that increase an individual's likelihood of having a stroke include:

- age (e.g., whereas the incidence of stroke in the general population is approximately 2 per 1,000 individuals, this incidence increases to 1 per 100 individuals for adults over 70 years of age)
- hypertension or high blood pressure
- heart disease, including heart attacks or cardiac arrhythmias
- diabetes, which speeds up the process of atherosclerosis (i.e., hardening of the arteries) (Morley, 1999)
- smoking, which narrows blood vessels throughout the body
- obesity or, more accurately, high fat intake
- substance abuse (e.g., alcohol), which can lead to restriction of arteries, increased blood pressure, or both
- high cholesterol
- transient ischemic attacks (see below for description)

In terms of sex differences, 30% more men suffer strokes than women (NSA, 2002). This does not, however, translate into all good news for women. For example, each year in the United States more than twice as many women die from stroke than from breast cancer. Additionally, women over 30 years of age who take high-estrogen oral contraceptives and who smoke have a stroke risk rate that is 22 times higher than the average individual. There are also racial differences in terms of stroke occurrence; whereas strokes are more common among African-Americans than Caucasians, they are less common among other minority populations such as Hispanics and American Indians. Individuals who live in the southeast part of the United States also seem to be at a higher risk for suffering a stroke (Goldstein & Gradison, 1999). States such as Virginia, North Carolina, South Carolina, Georgia, Florida, Alabama, Arkansas, and Louisiana are often referred to as the "stroke belt" because of their high stroke incidence and mortality rates. Factors that may contribute to these rates include a higher than average population of African-Americans and elderly, and the traditional diet associated with these geographic areas.

TYPES OF STROKE

Although a number of diseases and complications of diseases cause strokes (Mlcoch & Metter, 2001; Reinmuth, 1997), there are only two major types of stroke, ischemic and hemorrhagic (Figure 3-4). Ischemic strokes are more common and account for about 85% of all strokes (NSA, 2002). In an **ischemic stroke,** there is a deficiency in blood flow to the brain due to blockage of an artery (Suarez, 2000). If the patient suffers a very small ischemic stroke, it may be called a lacunar stroke.

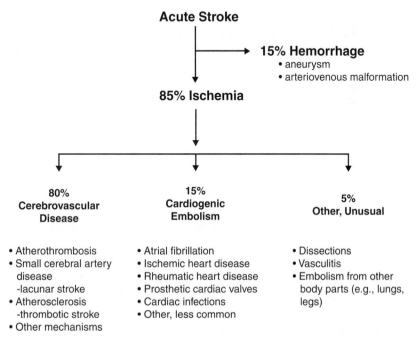

Figure 3-4. The two major types of stroke and their respective causes

Lacunar strokes typically involve small penetrating arteries that supply blood to structures deep within the brain (e.g., basal ganglia, internal capsule, thalamus) and result in a very small area of brain damage (i.e., 2 to 15 mm^2). The term **infarct** is used to describe the area of dead brain tissue that results from ischemia or blood flow deprivation. Two types of blockages may cause an ischemic stroke. One type is referred to as a **thrombosis.** In a thrombotic stroke, there is a buildup of atherosclerotic or fatty plaque on an artery that provides blood flow to the brain (Reinmuth, 1997). The process of forming the thrombosis or occlusion may take minutes or weeks, in part reflecting the size or number of affected arteries. The other type of ischemic stroke is due to an **embolus.** In an embolic stroke, a clot forms or a piece of fatty plaque breaks off from elsewhere in the circulatory system, and then travels to block off a smaller artery that supplies blood to the brain. The most common source of emboli is the heart, although clots may arise from disease or trauma to other parts of the body as well (e.g., lungs, legs, arms). In comparison to a thrombotic stroke, the clinical onset of an embolic stroke is typically faster, with maximal neurological symptoms manifesting themselves within seconds or minutes. For many patients, the exact mechanism of an ischemic stroke is never determined, so the medical charts of many patients indicate that they had a "thromboembolic" stroke.

A frequent precursor to an ischemic stroke is a **transient ischemic attack (TIA),** which is a small and temporary disruption of blood flow to the brain. During a TIA, an individual experiences the abrupt onset of stroke symptoms such as blurring or double vision, weakness or numbness of a limb or one side of the body, speech problems, aphasia, or dizziness (i.e., vertigo). Whereas these symptoms may persist up to 24 hours, most TIAs last only five to 30 minutes and cause no permanent brain damage or disability. It is vital that TIAs be taken seriously, as there is about a 10 to 20% chance of suffering a stroke during the first year after experiencing a TIA and a 30 to 60% chance within five years (Mlcoch & Metter, 2001). Medical treatment for a TIA focuses on either reducing the development of thrombi or the release of emboli. In the case of thrombosis, plaque buildup within the carotid artery may be removed by a surgical procedure called **endarterectomy.** Whereas endarterectomies may successfully reduce a patient's chance of suffering a stroke, in a small proportion of patients, they may induce an embolic stroke if a piece of plaque is dislodged during the arteriogram (i.e., the radiological procedure used to visualize the arteries; see also Chapter 4) or the surgical procedure itself (Hartmann et al., 1999). Another treatment option is to prescribe anticoagulants such as heparin or warfarin (e.g., Coumadin) to prevent thrombus formation and, consequently, the release of emboli. Antiplatelet medications such as aspirin or clopidogrel also may be used, as they help reduce the buildup of plaque on existing thrombotic areas (Gorelick et al., 1999). Taking one aspirin or fewer a day has been shown to reduce the risk of further TIAs, strokes, and even death, particularly in men (Albers & Tijssen, 1999).

The other major type of stroke, **hemorrhagic stroke,** occurs when an artery bursts and causes blood to escape and flood surrounding brain tissue. The buildup of blood is called a **hematoma,** and this pool of blood is dangerous because it can displace and compress adjacent brain tissue, arteries, or cranial nerves. Hemorrhagic strokes are most frequently associated with aneurysms, arteriovenous malformations, or a long medical history of hypertension. An **aneurysm** is a weak or thin spot on a blood vessel that causes the vessel to dilate or balloon (Figure 3-5). Aneurysms are often present from birth, and remain asymptomatic until they grow so large that they exert pressure and consequently affect the functioning of adjacent brain struc-

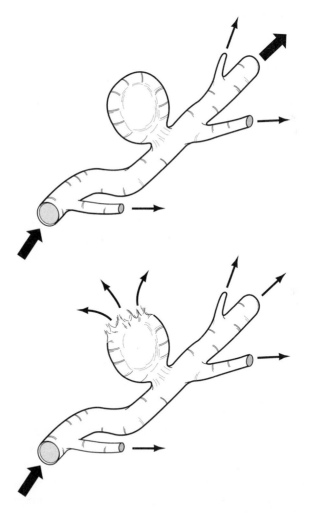

Figure 3-5. An illustration of an aneurysm on a cerebral artery. When an aneurysm bursts, as the lower drawings depicts, blood flow to structures supplied by the artery is reduced.

tures, or until they burst. If identified prior to a stroke, aneurysms may be treated by clipping the neck of the dilation or by spraying the dilation and adjacent vessels with plastics. An **arteriovenous malformation** (**AVM**) is a defect in the communication links between arteries and veins (i.e., regions in which oxygenated blood from arteries mixes with deoxygenated blood from veins), and consequently results in weakened arterial walls. Like aneurysms, AVMs are also present from birth and usually remain asymptomatic until early adulthood, when they can cause seizures or hemorrhages. When identified, AVMs may be removed with surgery or radiation, or embolized (filled with a material to prevent blood flow into the AVM) to prevent stroke.

Hemorrhagic strokes are often classified according to where they occur. For example, an intracerebral hemorrhage is one in which blood invades tissue within the brain. Whereas a severe headache is the most prominent early clinical symptom of an intracerebral hemorrhage, patients may also experience nausea, vomiting, and loss of consciousness. In a subarachnoid hemorrhage, blood spills into the pia-arachnoid space surrounding the brain. This type of hemorrhage is frequently caused by a ruptured aneurysm in the area of the Circle of Willis, or by a hemorrhaging AVM.

With respect to survival following a stroke, patients who suffer an ischemic stroke have the best chance of surviving, whereas those who suffer an intracerebral hemorrhagic stroke have the least chance of surviving. Although hemorrhagic strokes are associated with higher morbidity rates, patients who survive a hemorrhage often have a better recovery than survivors of ischemic stroke. That is because hemorrhagic strokes following successful acute medical treatment tend to produce less permanent brain damage compared to ischemic strokes (Reinmuth, 1997).

STROKE TREATMENT

Although strokes were previously referred to as cerebrovascular accidents, they have been more recently called **brain attacks.** This change in terminology has been instigated to emphasize that, like heart attacks, strokes should be treated as a medical emergency. That is, whereas in the past there was little that could be done to help a patient who was experiencing stroke symptoms, there are now medical treatments available that can be administered acutely to help prevent or reduce permanent brain damage and, consequently, the disability caused by strokes.

The first step to treating stroke is to recognize the symptoms (e.g., dizziness, confusion, severe headache, one-sided numbness or weakness, slurred speech) so that the patient can get immediate medical attention. Once at the hospital, the physicians will try to determine whether the patient is presenting with an ischemic or hemorrhagic stroke. If it is an ischemic stroke, the patient may be a candidate to receive one of several new drug treatments designed to reverse or minimize permanent brain damage. For example, thrombolytic drugs such as rtPA (recombinant tissue plasminigen activator) can be given within the first three hours of stroke onset to break up blood clots by speeding up the body's natural clot dissolving process (Hacke, Ringleb, & Stingele, 1999; Suarez, 2000). Unfortunately, the vast majority of stroke patients do not receive rtPA, primarily because they wait too long to seek medical treatment and thus miss the critical three-hour window in which rtPA has been shown to be effective (Katzan et al., 2000; O'Connor, McGraw, & Edelsohn, 1999). Another acute treatment option currently under development is the use of neuroprotective agents (Calabresi, Cupini, Centonze, Pisani, & Bernardi, 2003; Fisher, 2003; Lees, 1998). Drugs such as nimodipine (a calcium blocker), citicoline (an acetylcholine precursor), and antiepileptic medications can protect brain tissue directly adjacent to the infarct (i.e., penumbra) from the potentially fatal chemical changes that occur when its blood flow is reduced. Unfortunately, to date, clinical trials have been disappointing for many neuroprotective agents. Research, however, continues because neuroprotective agents have the potential to not only salvage brain tissue but also increase the three-hour treatment window of thrombolytic drugs to twenty-four hours (Clark & Lutsep, 1999; Fisher, 2003).

TUMOR

Although not as common as strokes, brain **tumors** or **neoplasms** also may cause neurogenic language disorders. It is estimated that each year, approximately 41,000 individuals in the United States will be diagnosed with a brain tumor (Central Brain Tumor Registry of the United States, 2005). Tumors are tissue masses that arise from an abnormally fast rate of cell reproduction. As the tumor grows, it progressively takes up more and more intracranial space, and consequently causes more and more compression or destruction of surrounding brain tissue, cranial nerves, and blood vessels. Onset of tumor symptoms reflects this progressive growth, and is characterized by the gradual appearance of problems with communication, cognition, or both; as the tumor continues to grow, communication and cognitive abilities continue to deteriorate. The specific symptoms that a patient may experience will depend on the location of the tumor.

Tumors may be benign or malignant. Benign brain tumors are noncancerous, and do not spread, or metastasize, to other parts of the body. Malignant brain tumors are cancerous and often recur despite treatment efforts; they may invade other parts of the body, or themselves be the product of cancer elsewhere in the body that has infiltrated the brain. There are many different types of intracranial tumors, each of which is named according to its tissue origin. A common tumor source within the brain is the supportive or glial cells. For example, one of the most common types of tumor in adults is a glioblastoma multiforme (also known as a high-grade astrocytoma) (Wen et al., 1995). Glioblastomas are malignant, and treatment may include chemotherapy, radiation, or surgical removal (i.e., resection).

Life expectancy following treatment for a glioblastoma varies from less than one year to about six years, depending on the size of the tumor and how fast the tumor is growing. The second most common type of brain tumor, a meningioma, arises from the arachnoid tissue that sheaths the brain. Meningiomas are benign and typically occur during adulthood. These tumors grow quite slowly, giving the brain time to accommodate, and thus cause few symptoms for a long time period. Prognosis is often favorable, as these tumors do not invade cortical tissue, tumor recurrence rates are low, and surgery is typically successful in removing the entire tumor.

Side Bar

How Big Tumors Can Cause "Little" Symptoms

Because some tumors have a very slow growth rate, patients may show nominal symptoms for some time. This phenomenon is sometimes referred to as the serial lesion effect and indicates that because of the slow, progressive nature of some tumors, the brain tissue and the neural circuits they support are able to adapt over time to the presence of the invading tumor. For example, I recently received a referral to assess a patient as part of a research study investigating attention and language abilities following right hemisphere brain damage. The patient's medical records indicated that she had recently undergone surgery to remove a large right frontal lobe meningioma. According to the patient's husband, the tumor had been the size of a golf ball. Based on this information about tumor size and location (note that the patient had not received any previous speech-language pathology or neuropsychology services), I was predicting that the patient would demonstrate significant difficulty on a number of the pragmatic and cognitive tests I had planned. During the assessment, however, I soon discovered my expectations were wrong, as the patient scored within and even above the normal range on most measures. I attributed the preservation of her linguistic and cognitive abilities not only to successful medical treatment of her tumor, but also to the serial lesion effect.

INFECTION

Certain bacterial and viral infections may invade the central nervous system to produce any number of neurogenic communication problems. In terms of bacterial infections, bacterial meningitis and brain abscesses are the most common. Bacterialmeningitis is associated with inflammation of the pia and arachnoid tissues that cover the brain. Symptoms include fever, fatigue, headache, a stiff neck, and, if severe, coma. Because this type of infection spreads rapidly, prompt medical treatment in the form of antibiotics is essential. In brain or intracerebral abscess, bacteria from another infection in the body attack a focal brain site. The inflammation caused by this infection leads to destruction of brain tissue, and may also exert pressure on adjacent brain structures and blood vessels. Brain abscesses are treated with both antibiotics and surgery to drain the abscess. Localized symptoms such as sensory loss or aphasia may occur prior to treatment, as well as persist following treatment if the abscess or its removal resulted in permanent brain damage.

The central nervous system also is vulnerable to viral infections such as herpes simplex encephalitis, viral meningitis, and syphilis. In acquired immune deficiency syndrome (AIDS), the human immunodeficiency virus (HIV) may invade the brain and cause widespread damage (particularly to white matter and subcortical brain structures) and, consequently, dementia (sometimes referred to as HIV encephalopathy). Recent research has indicated that approximately 10 to 30% of AIDS patients will develop dementia, usually in the later stages of this infection (Clifford, 2000; Heaton et al., 1995). Importantly, current HIV treatments appear to ameliorate or delay the onset the cognitive impairment, and consequently incidence rates of HIV dementia have declined as much as 50% since the early 1990s (Sacktor, 2002). For other viral infections, some antiviral medications are available, although treatment for many of these infections is palliative. That is, care focuses on making the patient as medically stable and comfortable as possible while waiting to see if the patient's own immune system can successfully eliminate the infection.

TRAUMATIC BRAIN INJURY

The National Head Injury Foundation (1989) defines **traumatic brain injury (TBI)** as an insult to the brain produced by external forces that may cause a variety of temporary or permanent physical, cognitive, emotional, and behavioral impairments. The external force may be created by projectiles striking the head (e.g., bullets, baseballs, clubs) or by the head suddenly striking a stationary object (e.g., a car windshield, a floor, a bathtub). When the skull is fractured or penetrated by an external force and the contents of the skull are exposed, the injury is referred to as an **open head injury.** In contrast, when the skull is not pierced by the external force and thus stays intact, the injury is referred to as a **closed head injury.** Individuals who have been shot or struck on the head by a sharp object typically suffer an open head injury, whereas individuals who have been involved in a car accident or who have fallen typically suffer a closed head injury. In open head injuries, brain damage is frequently focal or localized and the resulting functional impairments are likewise circumscribed. For example, if the focal brain damage affects the left hemisphere, the patient with TBI may present with aphasia. In closed head injuries, brain damage is typically more diffuse, affecting widespread areas of the brain, and consequently causes an array of cognitive and communicative deficits.

Currently in the U.S., someone receives a TBI every seven seconds, and every five minutes someone dies as a result of a TBI (Mackay, Chapman, & Morgan,

1997). The Centers for Disease Control and Prevention (CDC, 2003) have estimated that approximately 5.3 million or 2% of all Americans are presently living with disabilities caused by TBI. Additionally, TBI is the most common cause of death and disability among children in the U.S., resulting in an estimated 150,000 hospitalizations and more than 7,000 deaths each year. These statistics may represent an underestimation of the true occurrence rate of TBI, given that many individuals may not seek medical assistance for a head injury and individuals who are not hospitalized for their TBI are frequently not included in incidence or prevalence studies.

TRAUMATIC BRAIN INJURY RISK FACTORS AND CAUSES

There are a number of populations who are at greater risk for suffering a TBI. In terms of age, adolescents, young adults, and the elderly (i.e., 75 years or older) are more apt to sustain a TBI than other age groups, with individuals between 15 and 24 years of age having the highest TBI rates (Kraus & McArthur, 1999; Thurman, Alverson, Dunn, Guerrero, & Sniezek, 1999). Not only is TBI more common among the elderly than in the general population, but prognosis for recovery from TBI is poorer for elderly patients; for example, elderly patients with TBI have longer hospital stays and are more likely to die from their injuries compared to younger patients with TBI (Cifu et al., 1996; Pennings, Bachulis, Simons, & Slazinski, 1993). Generally, males are two to three times more likely to suffer a TBI compared to females (Kraus & McArthur, 1996; NIH Consensus Development Panel, 1999). This gender difference, however, inverses in patients over the age of 80 years, as in this age group, women are more likely to sustain a TBI (Goodman & Englander, 1992). Other risk factors for TBI include: (1) low socioeconomic level (Kraus & McArthur, 1996; Wagner, Sasser, Hammond, Wiercisiewski, & Alexander, 2000), (2) pre-traumatic psychiatric illness or family dysfunction (McGuire, Burright, Williams, & Donovick, 1998), (3) substance abuse—for example, 56% of patients have a positive blood alcohol concentration upon diagnosis of TBI (Bombardier & Thurber, 1998; NINDS, 2002; Wagner et al., 2000), and (4) previous TBI—that is, after suffering a TBI, a patient has a three times greater risk of suffering another TBI compared to the general population (CDC, 2003).

The most frequent cause of TBI in the general population is motor vehicle accidents (including when the victim is a vehicle occupant or a pedestrian/bicyclist), which account for approximately 50% of all TBI cases (Jagger, Levine, Jane, & Rimel, 1984; NIH Consensus Development Panel, 1999; NINDS, 2002). Among the elderly and young children, falls are the leading source of TBI. In fact, falls are responsible for more than 50% of all accidental deaths in adults aged 65 years or older. A number of medical factors may account for the high rates of falling among the elderly; these include medical conditions such as stroke, postural dizziness, hip disease, Parkinsonism, and diabetic neuropathy, which may affect the elderly adult's balance, coordination, or both (Isaacson & Rubin, 1999; Luukinen, Viramo, Koski, Laippala, & Kivela, 1999). Other common causes of TBI include assaults (e.g., gun wounds, physical abuse), suicide attempts, and sports and recreation accidents (CDC, 2003; Harrison et al., 1998; Matser, Kessels, Jordan, Lezak, & Troost, 1998; Wagner et al., 2000).

PATHOPHYSIOLOGICAL CONSEQUENCES OF TRAUMATIC BRAIN INJURY

There are a number of pathophysiological changes that take place within the brain subsequent to a TBI. These structural and physiological changes are often categorized according to whether they are the product of primary versus secondary damage (Graham, 1999). Primary damage refers to brain damage caused by the external or mechanical forces involved in the accident or trauma. In contrast, secondary damage refers to brain damage that is not mechanically generated and may develop hours to weeks following the head injury. Secondary damage is a product of complications arising from the primary damage or represents a pathophysiological process independent of the original, primary damage.

Type of primary damage depends, at least in part, on whether the patient suffered an open or closed head injury. In an open head injury, the primary damage is typically localized around the area of contact or the path of the penetrating object. Fragments of the skull, shattered pieces of the bullet, and debris from the penetrating object also may lacerate the brain. One type of primary damage associated with open head injuries is skull fractures, in which a bone or bones of the skull have been broken and consequently lacerate brain tissue. Contusions or bruises also form around the site of impact, as blood vessels also are typically lacerated by the injury. If the contusion is severe, resulting in an accumulation of blood that begins to displace brain mass, it may be diagnosed as a hematoma or blood clot (Table 3-1) (Graham, Adams, Nicoll, Maxwell, & Gennarelli, 1995; Mackay et al., 1997). Hematomas may form within brain tissue (i.e., intracerebral hematomas) or between the skull and brain tissue (i.e., epidural hematomas, subarachnoid hematomas, or subdural hematomas).

Contusions are a common form of primary damage following closed head injuries, and typically are found on the crests of gyri on the surface of the cerebral hemispheres. Contra coup effect or injury is the term used when contusions occur both at the site of impact (i.e., "coup") and at the opposite side of the brain (i.e., "contra"). That is, the force of the impact causes inward skull impression directly below the site of contact, and then also causes negative pressure changes (i.e., cavitation) to produce damage on the diametrically opposite side of the brain (Pang, 1985) (Figure 3-6). In addition to contra coup injury, certain brain regions are at great risk for contusions following closed head injury. For example, contusions often form on inferior and lateral surfaces of the frontal and temporal lobes because brain tissue and blood vessels can hit sharp, bony prominences located in

Table 3-1. Types of Hematomas or Blood Clots

TYPE	DESCRIPTION
Intracerebral Hematoma	Blood accumulation within brain tissue
	Commonly found within the frontal and temporal lobes following a closed or diffuse head injury
Epidural Hematoma	Blood accumulation between the skull and the dura
	Usually the result of arterial bleeding and thus enlarges rapidly
	Frequently associated with skull fractures
Subarachnoid Hematoma	Blood accumulation between the arachnoid and pia maters
	May cause compression of cerebral arteries or obstruction of the flow of cerebrospinal fluid
Subdural Hematoma	Blood accumulation underneath the dural membrane and above the arachnoid mater

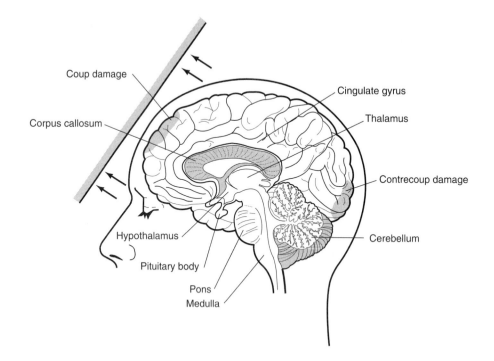

Figure 3-6. An illustration of coup (i.e., contusion and cavitation at the site of the external impact) and contre coup (i.e., contusion and cavitation at the side of the brain opposite to the external impact) brain damage.   [AU9]

those anterior areas of the skull. Contusions also are frequently found near the cor-
pus callosum, cerebral peduncles, and the cerebellar peduncles because these structures are located next to strong tentorial membranes against which they may strike
and bounce during a closed head injury. Diffuse axonal shearing or injury also
occurs following closed head injuries and is caused by high-velocity rotation of the
brain relative to the skull. As illustrated in Figure 3-7, this movement produces
microscopic damage, such as shearing axons from their myelin sheath or tearing of
the axons themselves (Maxwell, Watt, Graham, & Gennarelli, 1993; NINDS, 2002).
Diffuse axonal shearing frequently affects brain tissue at gray-white matter junctions, particularly in those cerebral areas already identified as vulnerable in terms
of contusions (e.g., inferior frontal lobe, cerebellar peduncles). Diffuse axonal
shearing has been identified as the major form of both focal and diffuse primary
damage following closed head injury, and is thought to be fundamental in causing
impairments of consciousness.

The thrust of medical management for both open and closed head injuries is
to prevent or minimize secondary forms of brain damage (Dearden, 1998; Graham
et al., 1995; Mackay et al., 1997). Of the various complications that may occur,
edema or swelling is quite common (particularly in pediatric patients with TBI)
and is the product of increased intra- and extracellular fluid in brain tissues.
Edema disrupts brain functioning because there is little room within the cranium
for the brain to expand. Consequently, edema tends to co-occur with increased

Figure 3-7. **Examples
of different forms of
diffuse axonal shearing
that may occur due to a
traumatic brain injury**

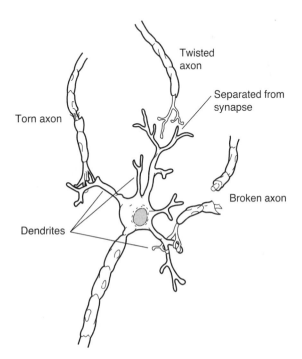

Twisted
axon

Separated from
synapse

Torn axon

Broken axon

Dendrites

intracranial pressure as brain tissue and blood vessels squeeze against the skull. Prolonged increased intracranial pressure (particularly when pressure exceeds 20 mmHg) is of concern because it can cause hypoxia (i.e., decreased oxygen in brain tissue), ischemic brain damage (i.e., cell death or infarction due to inadequate blood supply), or both. Hypoxia and ischemia also may be produced by decreased respiration (e.g., chest injuries that obstruct breathing) and low arterial blood pressure (e.g., excessive blood loss due to skeletal injuries). Medical treatments for edema and high intracranial pressure include drugs to decrease metabolic activity (e.g., sedatives or anti-seizure medications), fluid restriction to increase osmotic pressure to draw fluid off of the brain, and surgery to create a bone flap (i.e., cutting a hole in the skull to allow the brain more room to expand), to drain cerebrospinal fluid (i.e., ventriculostomy), or to insert a pressure transducer that allows continuous monitoring of intracranial pressure (Dearden, 1998; NINDS, 2002; Pentland & Whittle, 1999). Hypoxia may be prevented or treated by assuring that the patient has an adequate airway (e.g., inserting tracheostomy or endotracheal tubes) and by providing supplementary oxygen. Another possible form of secondary damage is infection (Landesman & Cooper, 1982). More specifically, meningitis and cerebral abscesses are common following open head injuries and skull fractures, and are treated with antibiotics to prevent outcomes that range from increased intracranial pressure to mortality.

Patients with TBI in both acute and chronic care facilities also typically suffer from a variety of other medical complications (Pentland & Whittle, 1999; NINDS, 2002). In some cases, these medical complications have direct effects on the patients' communication abilities. For example, prolonged intubation or use of endotracheal tubes may damage the vocal folds or nerves controlling phonation, leading to voice disorders. Other medical complications, such as contractures (i.e., decreases in joint range of motion due to shortening and other changes in muscles, tendons, and ligaments) and pressure sores can cause severe pain, which in turn can negatively affect a patient's ability and willingness to participate in speech-language assessment or treatment activities. Finally, any time the brain is injured, an individual is at risk for seizures. For patients with TBI, onset of seizures typically occurs within the first year or two post-trauma. It is estimated that approximately 5% of all patients with TBI will experience seizures, with more frequent incidence rates among pediatric patients and patients with open head injuries, regardless of age (Ludwig, 1993).

DEMENTING ILLNESSES

Dementia refers to a chronic, progressive deterioration in memory and at least one other area, such as personality, communication ability, or executive control functioning (American Psychiatric Association, 1994; see also Chapter 2). Currently, more than 50 causes of dementia have been identified (Table 3-2). It is imperative to determine what disease or condition is causing a patient's dementia

Table 3-2. **Some Reversible and Irreversible Causes of Dementia**

Reversible Causes	Depression (pseudodementia)
	Medications (e.g., side effects from certain anticholinergic or antihypertensive drugs)
	Infection (e.g., meningitis, encephalitis, urinary tract infection, West Nile Virus)
	Hearing loss
	Electrolyte imbalance
	Tumors
	Normal pressure hydrocephalus
	Mental and/or sensory deprivation
	Renal failure (dialysis dementia)
	Thyroid disease and other metabolic disorders
	Toxin exposure (e.g., lead poisoning)
	Vitamin deficiency (e.g., pellagra, Wernicke-Korsakoff syndrome)
Irreversible Causes	Alzheimer's disease
	Creutzfeld-Jakob disease
	Dementia with Lewy bodies
	Frontotemporal dementia or dementia of the frontal lobe type
	Human immunodeficiency virus encephalopathy
	Huntington's disease
	Korsakoff's disease
	Multi-infarct (i.e., multiple strokes) dementia
	Multiple sclerosis
	Parkinson's disease
	Pick's disease
	Progressive supranuclear palsy
	Traumatic brain injury (e.g., dementia pugilistica)
	Wilson's disease

because some etiologies are reversible and thus dementia symptoms may improve with the appropriate treatment. In contrast, other etiologies are irreversible and produce permanent cognitive impairments. Whereas it is not the responsibility of clinicians to diagnose dementia etiology, they must be cognizant of the numerous reversible and irreversible causes so as to treat and counsel their dementia patients appropriately.

REVERSIBLE CAUSES OF DEMENTIA

An estimated 10 to 30% of dementia cases are **reversible** in that they can improve with appropriate medical treatment. For example, depression can cause dementia and accounts for nearly 15% of all dementia cases (Rabins, 1983). Although depression does not always produce cognitive symptoms severe enough to qualify as dementia, approximately 10 to 20% of the depressed elderly will develop overt cognitive problems, sometimes referred to as **pseudodementia** (Beats, Sahakian, & Levy, 1996; Nussbaum, 1994). With respect to elderly patients, neither neuropsychological assessment nor biomedical methods (e.g., neuroimaging, neuroendocrine sampling) have proven sensitive or specific enough to permit timely, affordable, and confident diagnostic discrimination between pseudodementia and early or mild forms of irreversible dementia etiologies such as Alzheimer's disease (Christensen, Griffiths, MacKinnon & Jacomb, 1997; Nagaratnam & Lewis-Jones, 1998). Differential diagnosis is difficult because (1) pseudodementia has widespread cognitive symptoms (e.g., impaired memory and reasoning, visuospatial deficits) that are indistinguishable from those of early Alzheimer's disease (Jost & Grossberg, 1996); (2) presentation of depression in the elderly often is atypical in that their affective symptoms (e.g., depressed mood, feelings of worthlessness) may appear to be absent or secondary to their cognitive symptoms (Gallo et al., 1999); and (3) definitive diagnosis of Alzheimer's disease is possible only via autopsy to confirm Alzheimer-type neuropathology. Consequently, over 30% of elderly adults referred for a dementia evaluation are found to present with depression (Marin, Sewell, & Schlechter, 2002), and 5 to 20% of thoroughly evaluated patients who receive an initial diagnosis of irreversible dementia are rediagnosed with depression at a later date (Feinberg & Goodman, 1984).

Numerous medications and toxic substances may also produce reversible dementia. For example, dementia is a well-documented side effect of many anticholinergic drugs, including sedatives, antidepressants, and some antihypertensive medications (Stein & Strickland, 1998; Vogel, Carter & Carter, 2000). Exposure to toxins such as lead or mercury may also cause dementia. Notably, prolonged exposure to these toxins, particularly in children, may lead to an irreversible dementia.

A number of medical conditions, when left untreated, may also produce dementia. These include metabolic disorders (e.g., thyroid disease), hydrocephalus, vitamin deficiency (e.g., pellagra or B3 deficiency; Wernicke-Korsakoff syndrome or thiamine deficiency), renal failure (sometimes referred to as dialysis dementia), infection (e.g., meningitis, syphilis, encephalitis), and tumors (Kopelman, 1995; Mangino & Middlemiss, 1997). Whereas some of these medical disorders may eventually lead to permanent dementia, there is the potential to reverse the cognitive symptoms if the etiology is identified and treated early in the course of the disorder.

IRREVERSIBLE CAUSES OF DEMENTIA

In **irreversible dementia**, sometimes referred to as "primary degenerative dementia," cognitive symptoms are persistent and in many of these etiologies, progressive. The most common cause of irreversible dementia and dementia in general, particularly in North America, is **Alzheimer's disease** (**ADB**) (Canadian Study of Health and Aging Working Group, 1994; Ritchie & Lovestone, 2002). It is estimated that approximately 50 to 60% of the dementia population have AD. In terms of the general population, 10% of adults over the age of 65 and 40% to 60% of adults over the age of 85 are predicted to have the disease, and AD is identified as the fourth leading cause of death among the elderly (National Institute of Aging, 2003). Whereas the exact cause of AD has yet to be specified (see below), a variety of risk and protective factors have been identified (see Table 3-3) which may increase or decrease, respectively, an individual's chance of developing this dementing illness (O'Brien et al., 2003; Fratiglioni & Rocca, 2001).

Currently, the most accurate means of confirming a diagnosis of AD is the identification of neuropathological markers upon autopsy. For example, the pathologist will look for neurofibrillary tangles (i.e., unusual triangular and looped fibers

Table 3-3. Risk and Protective Factors Associated with Alzheimer's Disease

RISK FACTORS	PROTECTIVE FACTORS
old age	rich social network
Down syndrome or family history of Down syndrome	early diagnosis and treatment of vascular disorders
history of leukemia	possibly high education levels
advanced age of mother at birth	
family history of Alzheimer's disease	
presence of ApoE type 4 allele	
history of head trauma (particularly in presence of ApoE-4 allele)	
high blood pressure and high cholesterol	
smoking	
diabetes	

in the cytoplasm of neurons), which are typically most pronounced in the inferior temporal lobe, posterior association regions, and Wernicke's area, and neuritic or senile plaques (i.e., aggregations of degenerating neurons and the remains of degenerated nerve fibers), which are most pronounced in the medial temporal lobes. The brains of patients with AD also show widespread cortical atrophy and ventricular dilation. Importantly, bilateral areas of the brain are affected, although involvement may not necessarily be symmetrical (Cummings, 2000).

To help physicians and clinicians reliably diagnose AD in patients who are still living, a number of behavioral and medical criteria have been developed (McKhann et al., 1984). In particular, these criteria are aimed to help rule out other possible causes of dementia such as depression, stroke, alcoholism, malnutrition, or other diseases. For example, behavioral criteria include the presence of a deficit in memory and at least one other cognitive ability (i.e., attention, executive control functions, language, visuospatial skills) and that these cognitive deficits have been getting progressively worse. A medical criterion is that on CT, there should be the absence of focal lesions. Hypometabolism in posterior aspects of the temporal and parietal lobes is observed when positron emission tomography (PET) scans are completed on individuals with AD.

Finding the cause of AD has become the major thrust of much research. It is known that in approximately 5 to 10% of AD cases, the cause is genetic, due to an autosomal dominant inheritance pattern (Liddell, Lovestone, & Owen, 2001). These genetic cases tend to be associated with an early onset of AD (i.e., less than 65 years of age). So far, researchers have identified at least four genes that, when abnormal, may produce AD: (1) AD3, which is located on chromosome 14 and may be responsible for as many as 5% of AD cases; (2) AD4, which is not as common as AD3 and is found on chromosome 1; (3) AD1, which is located on chromosome 21 and has been associated with the high incidence of AD among individuals with Down syndrome; and (4) AD2, or apolipoprotein E (apoE), which is found on chromosome 19 and is described as a risk-modifying gene (i.e., the presence of this gene is not sufficient to produce AD). Another possible cause of AD revolves around abnormalities in neurotransmitters and neuromodulators (Ritchie & Lovestone, 2002). For example, patients with AD have decreased levels in choline acetyltransferase, a chemical responsible for making acetylcholine, a neurotransmitter known to be important for learning and memory. The mechanism responsible for these neurotransmitter deficiencies, however, has yet to be determined. Other possible causes of AD, which have so far received little empirical support, include exposure to toxins such as aluminum or silicon, immunologic disorders, and nutritional deficiency.

Pick's disease is another cause of irreversible dementia. This relatively rare disease typically occurs between the ages of 40 to 60 years and more frequently affects women than men (Rossor, 2001). Like AD, a diagnosis of Pick's disease can only be confirmed upon autopsy. At that time, the pathologist examines for the presence of neuropathological markers such as Pick bodies and atrophy in the anterior frontal and temporal cortices (Dickson, 2001). Behaviorally, Pick's disease can be distinguished from AD because in Pick's, personality changes (e.g., socially inappropriate behavior, disinhibition) are prominent early in the disease, whereas memory and visuospatial skills may be spared until later stages of the disease; the reverse behavioral profile is more common in AD. More recently, some researchers have proposed that Pick's disease may encompass or be a subtype of another form of irreversible dementia, **dementia of the frontal lobe type** (**DFT**) or **frontotemporal dementia,** which produces similar behavioral and cognitive symptoms (Grossman, 2002; Kertesz, Hillis, & Munoz, 2003; Razani, Boone, Miller, Lee, & Sherman, 2001). The name for this dementia type was coined when it was found that some patients with the behavioral symptoms of Pick's disease did not have the characteristic neuropathological markers of the disease (i.e., absence of Pick's bodies and AD pathology). Additionally, although both Pick's disease and DFT are associated with bilateral frontal lobe hypometabolism on PET scans, there are some reports of greater left hemisphere and anterior temporal lobe involvement in DFT cases. DFT tends to manifest after the age of 40 years and typically, patients with DFT are younger than patients with AD. It is estimated that DFT accounts for 5 to 20% of all dementia cases, and more frequently affects men than women (Bird et al., 2003). Currently, researchers are pursuing possible genetic (e.g., 25 to 40% of DFT cases are estimated to be familial) and neurochemical (i.e., deficits in serotonin) bases of DFT (Bird et al., 2003; Pasquier et al., 2003).

Side Bar

A Progressive Disorder with a Progressing Diagnosis

In many cases, the exact cause of patients' progressive communicative and cognitive deterioration is either only determined upon autopsy or, if an autopsy is not completed, never confirmed. For example, a couple of years ago a patient was referred to our clinic to receive treatment services for what his neurologist had diagnosed as primary progressive aphasia (see Chapter 2 for a more detailed description of this neurogenic language disorder). Indeed, this patient did initially report and present with relatively isolated progressive language decline in the form of increasing difficulty with word finding and sentence formulation. However, over the first few months that this patient attended individual and group therapy in our clinic, he began to demonstrate significant behavioral (e.g., inappropriate spending with his credit card) and motor symptoms (e.g., periodic falling, gait disturbance, dysarthria). The onset of these symptoms negated a diagnosis of primary progressive aphasia, which is typically only given when patients demonstrate isolated declines in their language for at least two years; in contrast, this patient was still within the first year of the onset of his language as well as other symptoms. Given the striking behavioral problems that this patient was developing, we hypothesized that he might be presenting with a variant of frontotemporal dementia, which is associated with both language and behavioral symptoms. The breadth and severity of motor symptoms with which this patient was presenting, however, were not consistent with frontotemporal dementia. We were aware, though, that his sister had recently passed away from amyotrophic lateral sclerosis (ALS or Lou Gerhig's disease), and consequently wondered if he might be presenting with more than one progressive disease.

(continued)

We continued to provide this patient and his wife with support for his deteriorating communication abilities that were soon confounded by the onset of additional cognitive impairments (e.g., memory and attention problems). For instance, although we quickly tried to identify an electronic augmentative communication system that would allow this patient to circumvent his rapidly escalating motor speech deficits, by the time his system arrived and we had begun training with the device, his cognitive and behavioral problems were interfering with successful device use (e.g., he could not remember how to access items not displayed on the main page of the device). Unfortunately, the patient's overall cognitive, communicative, behavioral, and motoric functioning deteriorated at very rapid rate, and about 18 months after his initial referral to our clinic, his wife was no longer able to care for him within their home. The patient was admitted to a nursing home, but within a few weeks passed away.

The patient's wife did seek an autopsy to determine the cause of her husband's neurological disease and subsequent death. She was particularly interested in finding out whether there might be a genetic component to whatever disease caused his demise, given that they had children and grandchildren. The results of the autopsy indicated that he did display some pathological changes consistent with Pick's disease or frontotemporal dementia. Other changes, however, suggested more widespread, nonspecific neural degeneration. Therefore, although the patient's wife never received a specific diagnosis, the autopsy findings did allay her fears somewhat, as ALS was ruled out. She also received comfort in knowing that the results of her husband's autopsy would be used to further research the understanding of frontotemporal dementia and other related, progressive neurological diseases.

Parkinson's disease (PD), which affects over half a million individuals in the U.S. (National Institute of Neurological Disorders and Stroke; NINDS, 2003), may cause irreversible dementia. PD is associated with deterioration of subcortical structures, such as the substantia nigra, and decreased levels of the neurotransmitter dopamine (Albin, Young & Penny, 1995; Rinne et al., 2000); disrupted functioning of other cortical (e.g., frontal lobe) and subcortical areas (e.g., putamen, globus pallidus) with which the substantia nigra connects also has been reported. It is not yet known what causes PD in the majority of patients, although in a small percentage of cases there appears to be a genetic origin, and twin studies indicate that environmental factors (e.g., herbicide and/or pesticide exposure) contribute to late-onset sporadic PD cases (Warner & Schapira, 2003). Symptoms of PD include dysarthria, bradykinesia or slowed movement, resting tremor, rigidity, gait and posture disturbances, micrographia (i.e., a mechanical disruption of writing that results in extreme reductions in letter size) (see Figure 3-8), and depression (Goldman, Baty, Buckles, Sahrmann, & Morris, 1998; Levin & Katzen, 1995). Currently, there is a lack of a consensus regarding how many patients with PD will develop irreversible dementia, with prevalence rates varying from around 10%

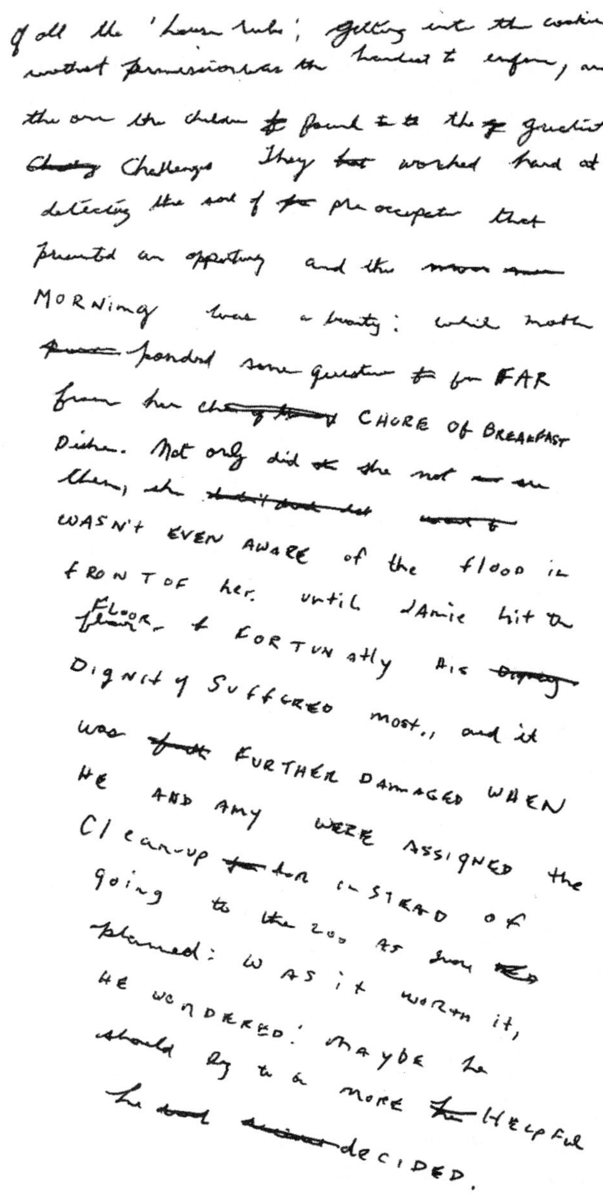

Figure 3-8. A sample of micrographia in the writing of a patient in the middle stages of Parkinson's disease. Note that the patient's strategy is to switch to printing when her writing becomes so small that even she can't read what she has written.

(Mayeux et al., 1988) to 40% (Cummings, 1988). Generally, patients with PD who develop dementia tend to be older, have had the disease for a shorter period of time, and display a faster rate of disease progression when compared to patients with PD who do not develop dementia. Although not all patients with PD develop dementia, over half of them will acquire mild cognitive deficits (Janvin, Aarsland, Larsen, & Hugdahl, 2003).

Another subcortical disease associated with irreversible dementia is Huntington's disease (HD). Approximately 30,000 individuals (with an additional 150,000 at a 50% chance of inheriting the disease) in the U.S. suffer from HD, with age of onset typically occurring somewhere between 35 and 50 years and death following 10 to 20 years after symptom onset (NINDS, 2001; Sutton-Brown & Suchowersky, 2003). In HD, the caudate nucleus undergoes gradual deterioration, which is eventually followed by cortical cell loss as well (Ho et al., 2001; Sutton-Brown & Suchowersky, 2003). HD is an autosomal dominant disease caused by a mutated gene on chromosome 4; autosomal dominant means that the mutated gene is located on a chromosome other than the sex-linked twenty-third chromosome, and that even if only one parent is carrying one copy of this mutated gene, that parent will develop the disease and there is a 50% chance of passing the disease on to all children born to that parent. In rare cases, chronic drug abuse may also lead to HD. Common symptoms of HD include chorea that affects speech (i.e., dysarthria), walking, swallowing (i.e., dysphagia), and other motor skills, bradykinesia, depression, and psychiatric problems such as social disinhibition (Berardelli et al., 1999; Kirkwood et al., 1999; Sutton-Brown & Suchowersky, 2003). Unlike PD, HD always is associated with a nonreversible dementia, which in some patients may actually precede motoric symptoms.

Chronic alcohol abuse can lead to a condition called Korsakoff's disease that is characterized by an irreversible dementia (Kopelman, 1995). Neuropathological changes associated with Korsakoff's disease include unilateral or bilateral damage to the thalamus, mammillary bodies, cerebellum, and diencephalic structures (e.g., hypothalamus, mammillary bodies); widespread cortical atrophy may also occur. Chronic abuse of other drugs such as cocaine also may cause permanent cognitive impairments that can progress in severity over time (Ardila, Rosselli, & Strumwasser, 1991).

The second most frequent cause of irreversible dementia in the elderly, accounting for about 20% of all dementia cases, is **multi-infarct dementia (MID)** (Fratiglioni & Rocca, 2001; O'Brien et al., 2003). MID refers to dementia caused by multiple strokes at both cortical and subcortical levels. The same factors that put individuals at risk for suffering one stroke also put them at risk for suffering multiple strokes (e.g., hypertension, cigarette smoking). In contrast to the previously described dementia etiologies, in which symptom onset is gradual and progressive, MID is associated with cognitive and physical symptoms that have an abrupt onset (co-occurring with stroke onset), and which over time tend to show a stepwise deterioration. Furthermore, unlike patients with one of the previously mentioned progressive diseases, patients with MID can have focal neurological symptoms and signs and may show an interim recovery of lost function (i.e., spontaneous recovery) following each of their strokes. Despite these differences, one form of MID, angular gyrus syndrome, is often confused with AD and pseudodementia (Benson, Cummings, & Tsai, 1982; Nagaratnam, Phan, Barnett, & Ibrahim, 2002). Angular gyrus syndrome is caused by multiple lesions to posterior and inferior parietal regions of the left hemisphere. It is difficult to discern from AD and pseudodementia because symptoms such as disorientation, anomia, and depression are characteristic of all three disorders, and because the lesions that produce angular gyrus syndrome are often so small they are not detected by CT scans.

DEMENTIA TYPES BASED ON LESION LOCATION

Dementia sometimes has been classified on the basis of what part of the brain is involved in the dementing disease or condition. The dementia associated with AD and Pick's disease is sometimes referred to as cortical dementia because the pathological changes associated with each of these diseases primarily affects cortical areas. In contrast, PD, HD, progressive supranuclear palsy, Wilson's disease, and multiple sclerosis are associated with subcortical dementia because each of these diseases produces alterations in primarily subcortical structures. This classification system also was designed to demarcate differences in the cognitive and behavioral profiles of patients with cortical versus subcortical dementia. For example, in subcortical dementia, initial symptoms are typically motoric in nature (e.g., dysarthria, gait disturbances), and language abilities remain intact. In contrast, in cortical dementia, initial symptoms are typically cognitive or behavioral in nature, and language is compromised. Recent research, however, indicates that patients with subcortical dementia may present with both language comprehension and production difficulties (Murray, 2000; Murray & Stout, 1999), and, in at least some cases, their initial symptoms may consist of cognitive or behavioral problems (e.g., Amann et al., 2000; Paulsen, Ready, Hamilton, Mega, & Cummings, 2001). In fact, not only is there overlap in terms of cognitive profiles, but also in terms of which areas of the brain are damaged in cortical and subcortical dementia (Ritchie & Lovestone, 2002). Consequently, clinicians would be well advised to avoid the terms cortical and subcortical dementia when describing their dementia patients.

SUMMARY

This chapter reviewed several diseases, medical conditions, and drugs that may produce neurogenic language disorders. Further information pertaining to many of these diseases and medical conditions is provided in the remaining chapters of this book; for example, in Chapter 11, a list of online information resources that are appropriate for clinicians as well as patients and their caregivers is provided (see Table 11-5). It is important to be aware that suffering from one of these diseases or conditions does not negate the possibility of acquiring another of these etiologies; thus, in many patients there are numerous reasons for their neurogenic language disorder (e.g., a patient with dementia who has a history of stroke and Parkinson's disease; a patient with Huntington's disease who suffers a fall and, consequently, a TBI). Accordingly, a comprehensive assessment, as will be reviewed in several subsequent chapters, is essential to identifying behaviors that can lead to the most accurate determination of the etiology or etiologies of each patient's neurogenic language disorder.

Chapter 4

A General Model of Assessment

LEARNING OBJECTIVES

After reading this chapter you should be able to:

- List four general goals of assessment.

- Describe factors that influence the determination of specific assessment goals.

- Describe the primary job responsibilities of the variety of health care professionals with whom speech language pathologists may interact.

- Identify pertinent information to collect for a case history.

- Describe sensory, motoric, perceptual, and psychiatric disorders that are important to identify prior to completing formal language testing.

- Define the psychometric properties of reliability, validity, and standardization.

- Differentiate the strengths and weaknesses of test bat-

teries versus tests of specific linguistic and cognitive functions.

- Describe the difference between qualitative and quantitative assessment information.

- Identify why a caregiver assessment might be needed.

- List important information that should be included in diagnostic reports.

KEY TERMS

agnosia
apraxia
bradykinesia
depression
dysarthria
hemianesthesia
hemianopia

hemiparesis
lability
neuropsychologists
occupational
    therapists
premorbid abilities
presbycusis

qualitative
    information
reliability
standardization
team approach
validity

INTRODUCTION

Clinicians who assess and treat adults with neurogenic language disorders may work in a variety of employment settings (e.g., acute care hospital, skilled nursing facility, home health) and with a variety of patient populations (e.g., varying in age, neurological disorder, time post-onset of the language disorder). Despite this variability, there are some generalities among the procedures used to quantify and qualify the acquired linguistic and cognitive impairments of their patients. Accordingly, the purpose of this chapter is to describe general assessment guidelines and procedures germane to planning an evaluation of a neurogenic language disorder, regardless of whether the patient presents with aphasia, right hemisphere damage (RHD), traumatic brain injury (TBI), and/or dementia. Specifically, this chapter defines what an assessment is and reviews both general and specific assessment goals. Next, general assessment procedures are described, followed by a brief review of assessment report writing.

ASSESSMENT: DEFINITION AND GOALS

An assessment represents an organized evaluation of the multiple factors (e.g., amount of environmental support) and abilities (e.g., linguistic and cognitive skills) that may influence a patient's language functioning. The general purposes of an assessment include (Murray & Chapey, 2001): (1) quantifying and qualifying communication strengths as well as weaknesses, (2) identifying the presence and possible influence of concomitant disorders, (3) establishing treatment goals, and (4) providing an informational basis from which to make predictions regarding recovery and treatment outcomes.

To satisfy these assessment goals, a clinician should ideally be completing an in-depth evaluation. Currently, however, there is a growing tendency for health care/insurance agencies to prescribe quick and cheap, versus comprehensive and, consequently, more costly language evaluations. Nevertheless, clinicians should, at the very least, attempt to obtain adequate time and financial support to complete the type of methodical assessment that is necessary to depict accurately their patients' linguistic and cognitive abilities, and thus plan appropriate treatment goals and procedures. Clinicians must be proactive and educate health care/insurance agencies about the subsequent time and financial savings associated with a thorough assessment. As Brookshire (1997) advised, it is clinicians' ethical responsibility "to ensure that gains in economy and efficiency do not come at the expense of their understanding of their patients' impairments and do not compromise their ability to provide the most efficacious treatment for those impairments" (p. 206).

SPECIFIC ASSESSMENT GOALS

Specific assessment goals define the nature and focus of the assessment (see Table 4-1). These goals are dictated by a variety of work-setting and patient-related factors. For example, the assessment provided to patients in temporary acute care units will differ from that provided to patients in rehabilitation units or facilities or skilled nursing facilities, or those receiving home health services. Whereas acute care assessment goals tend to focus more on immediate physical survival (e.g., presence and severity of dysphagia), basic communication needs (e.g., determining the reliability of yes/no responses; presence of motor speech vs. language dis-

Table 4-1. Examples of Specific Assessment Goals

INFLUENTIAL FACTOR		EXAMPLE GOAL
Work Setting	Acute Care	Determine caregivers' understanding of patient's current deficits.
		Determine presence or absence of dysphagia.
		Identify presence/absence of common right hemisphere cognitive-communicative deficits.
	Long-Term Care	Describe nature and severity of patient's neglect.
		Examine patient's productive discourse abilities in terms of macrolinguistic variables.
ICF Model	Functional Level	Describe nature and severity of patient's neglect.
		Examine patient's ability to understand spoken and written figurative language.
	Participation Level	Determine patient's current perception of his/her quality of life.
		Determine caregivers' current perception of the patient's quality of life.
Lesion Location	Right Hemisphere	Examine patient's productive discourse abilities in terms of macrolinguistic variables.
		Examine patient's ability to understand spoken and written figurative language.
	Left Hemisphere	Determine type and severity of aphasia.
		Examine patient's productive discourse abilities in terms of microlinguistic variables.

order), and the need for caregiver (family and medical staff) education and counseling, rehabilitation assessment goals are more comprehensive and should include detailed examination of specific linguistic and cognitive abilities.

Clinicians also should take into consideration the World Health Organization's (WHO; 2001) International Classification of Functioning, Disability, and Health (ICF) when deciding on specific assessment goals and procedures. Traditionally, the goal of assessment has been to evaluate the type and degree of language impairment (i.e., ICF level of Body Structure and Function). Consequently, the vast majority of standardized tests that are currently available assess linguistic (e.g., *Western Aphasia Battery, Boston Naming Test*) and/or cognitive (e.g., *Scales of Cognitive Ability for Traumatic Brain Injury, Wechsler Memory Scales–III*) impairments (see Chapters 5 and 6). More recently, however, there has been a trend in health care to determine how these impairments impact patients' daily activities and communication interactions (i.e., ICF level of Limitations of Personal Activities), as well as their ability to resume their premorbid social and vocational roles and activities (i.e., ICF level of Restrictions to Participation in Society). Accordingly, there is now a need to develop new or utilize existing tests (e.g., *ASHA Functional Assessment of Communication Skills for Adults*) that assess the extent to which patients' well-being and social and vocational lifestyle have been compromised by their neurogenic language disorder (see Chapter 7). It is particularly essential that test developers begin to design measures appropriate for patients with language deficits such as aphasia, as most existing tests for assessing problems at the ICF activity and society participation levels were created for patients with primarily physical deficits. Therefore, when using these tests with aphasic patients, clinicians must make guarded interpretations of the reliability and validity of their findings.

When setting specific assessment goals, particularly in rehabilitation, outpatient, and home health settings, clinicians should assure that their assessment protocols address each of the ICF levels (WHO; 2001) (i.e., Body Function and Structure, Activities, and Participation). It is important to incorporate assessment procedures specific to each of these levels, because research indicates there is no one-to-one correspondence among these levels (Frattali, 1998a, Ross & Wertz, 1999; Samsa & Matchar, 2004). That is, although clinicians might assume that patients who display severe impairments would also suffer severe activity and participation limitations, this is not necessarily the case.

Side Bar

Deficit Severity is in the Eye of the Beholder

Clinicians should never make assumptions about the impact of linguistic or cognitive impairments on their patients' participation in daily activities and social interactions. Take, for example, the following two patients who were receiving aphasia therapy in an outpatient rehabilitation clinic. Mr. McKibbin presented with a severe writing impairment following his stroke two months ago, and Ms. Ross presented with a mild reading deficit following her stroke four months ago. Whereas we might presume that Mr. McKibbin would also report greater daily activity and society participation setbacks compared to Ms. Ross, he does not; writing is not (and was not even prior to his stroke) an essential communication skill for Mr. McKibbin, a retired bricklayer who currently spends most of his days golfing with his wife (who records their golf scores). In contrast, Ms. Ross is currently completing a doctorate degree in education and, consequently, in addition to a mild reading impairment, presents with significant daily

(continued)

activity limitations and society participation restrictions. She is unable to complete reading assignments with the accuracy and speed with which she could prior to her stroke, and her success as a doctoral student and, subsequently, a professor is now being jeopardized.

In addition to the ICF levels of disease/disorder, clinicians should also consider other patient-related factors (e.g., lesion location, progressive vs. static brain damage, caregiver support) when developing specific assessment goals. For example, a request to evaluate a patient who has suffered a right hemisphere stroke would definitely suggest different specific assessment goals (e.g., analysis of visuospatial skills; analysis of high-level language comprehension abilities) than a request to evaluate a patient who has suffered a left hemisphere stroke (e.g., analysis of productive grammar skills; analysis of basic auditory comprehension abilities). Likewise, review of the patient's **premorbid abilities** (e.g., literacy skills, number and types of languages most frequently used) also is useful when setting specific assessment goals.

TEAM APPROACH CONSIDERATIONS

It is very important that, when planning assessments, clinicians take into consideration their role on the health care team. Throughout most countries in the world, the **team approach** to health care delivery is viewed as the optimal method for providing medical and rehabilitative services (Cifu & Steward, 1999; Golper, 2001; Langhorne & Duncan, 2001). Team organizational designs require establishing and maintaining collaboration among professionals from a variety of disciplines (Table 4-2). Because the precise composition of these health care teams may vary from work setting to work setting (e.g., rehabilitation ward vs. skilled nursing facility) and from patient to patient (e.g., comatose vs. mildly impaired traumatic brain injury patient), it is essential that speech-language pathologists first determine what professions are represented on the health care team to which they have been assigned. This is an important first step, as a number of team members may be capable of and interested in assessing the communication and cognition abilities of adults with neurogenic language disorders. Furthermore, depending on geographic location in the United States or Canada, by administering certain cognitive tests a speech-language pathologist may actually violate professional guidelines of that state or province. For example, frequently, only psychologists are licensed to purchase, administer, and/or interpret the results of certain tests of executive functioning (e.g., *Wisconsin Card Sorting Task*), as well as many cognitive test batteries (e.g., *Wechsler Adult Intelligence Scale–III*; *Wechsler Memory Scale–III*). Therefore, the health care team needs to determine who is responsible for assessing which communicative and cognitive abilities so as to avoid redundant testing procedures and, perhaps, breaching professional restrictions.

Table 4-2. **Professions Frequently Found on health Care Teams Serving Adults with Neurogenic Language Disorders**

PROFESSION	RESPONSIBILITIES
Audiology	Assess hearing abilities and balance/dizziness problems. Provide appropriate hearing devices and education/counseling.
Behavioral Psychology	Assess behavioral problems and develop and monitor implementation of behavioral modification programs.
Clinical/Rehabilitation Psychology	Assess psychosocial status (e.g., depression, grief, anxiety) and needs of patient and family. Provide counseling or make recommendations for other treatments (e.g., pharmacological treatment).
Neuropsychology	Assess cognitive abilities including perception, attention, memory, executive functions, and language. Infrequently directly involved in developing or providing communicative-cognitive treatment programs.
Nursing	Apply and monitor daily medical care as well as educate and train patient and family regarding ways to manage their own daily care. Essential to implementing behavioral treatments developed by other team members (e.g., encouraging patient use of a communication board; using appropriate behavioral modification techniques).
Nutrition	Assess nutritional (e.g., daily caloric intact) and hydration status and needs and develop dietary plans.
Occupational Therapy	Assess fine motor and sensorimotor abilities, skills involved in completing activities of daily living (e.g., grooming, cooking), and, in some settings, cognitive abilities such as perception, attention, and problem solving as they pertain to activities of daily living. Develop and provide treatment programs for deficits in those areas that they assess, including provision of and training with adaptive devices (e.g., switches, special eating utensils).
Physiatry	Determine the type of medical (e.g., laboratory tests) and rehabilitation (e.g., speech-language pathology, rehabilitation psychology) services needed and make requisitions for these services.

(continues)

Table 4-2. *Continued*

PROFESSION	RESPONSIBILITIES
Physical Therapy	Assess gross motor, balance, and postural abilities such as those involved in walking and transferring (e.g., moving from a wheelchair to a bed). Develop and provide treatment programs for deficits in those areas that they assess including provision of and training with adaptive devices (e.g., wheelchair, quad cane).
Speech-Language Pathology	Assess and provide treatment programs for motor speech, voice, language, cognitive, and swallowing disorders. Treatment includes not only individual services to patients, but also group therapy for patients, and education and counseling of patients and their caregivers.
Social Work	Assess social support status and needs, and make recommendations and assist in implementing patient discharges (e.g., arranging home health services; identifying financial concerns and possible funding sources). Sometimes provide patient and family counseling.
Therapeutic Recreation	Assess social interaction and leisure needs. Plan and implement recreational activities to improve social, emotional, behavioral, and communicative-cognitive functioning.
Vocational Rehabilitation	Determine appropriate vocational goals by identifying current work tolerance, past work history (to pinpoint transferable skills that are compatible with the patient's current physical, cognitive and behavioral limitations), and government or disability compensation funding.

Preferably, *all* team members should directly or indirectly contribute to the assessment of the communicative and cognitive abilities of patients with neurogenic language disorders. Team members who are typically best qualified for, and most frequently responsible for, the direct examination of abilities that speech-language pathologists commonly evaluate include **neuropsychologists** (or rehabilitation psychologists, clinical psychologist, etc.) and **occupational therapists.** Importantly, even when these other team members are in charge of directly assessing the linguistic and cognitive abilities of patients with neurogenic language disorders, speech-language pathologists must maintain as much active involvement as possible because of our unique expertise in examining and interacting with this patient population. Whereas these other team members often have had more training and experience in administering cognitive tests (i.e., attention, memory, and executive function assessment tools), speech-language pathologists typically are more educated about and proficient in accommodating test procedures for and interpreting the test results of patients with speech and language impairments. Likewise, when speech-language pathologists are responsible for the direct assessment of communication and cognition, it is very informative to interview other team members regarding their observations of a given patient's abilities. Their input will supplement direct assessment results by providing clinicians with a more comprehensive description of the patient's linguistic and cognitive abilities under varying communicative circumstances (i.e., different communicative partners, activities, and settings).

Lastly, clinicians must not overlook that the patients themselves, as well as their family or significant others are also integral members of the health care team. It is imperative that an assessment be driven by the needs voiced by patients (at least in those cases in which they are adequately cognizant of the type and extent of their impairments) and their families. Given the trend to incorporate ICF levels into current healthcare practice, inclusion of patients and their families in the assessment process is essential to quantifying and qualifying problems at the Body Function and Structure, and in particular at the Personal Activities and Participation in Society levels. Auditing bodies such as the Joint Commission of Accreditation of Healthcare Organizations (JCAHO) and the Commission on Accreditation of Rehabilitation Facilities (CARF) also require documented patient input. Finally, obtaining patient and family input is necessary because discrepancies among the perceptions of patients, families, and health care professionals regarding the nature of the problem and the types of medical and rehabilitation services required have been found (Code, Muller, & Herrmann, 1999; Herrmann, Johannsen-Horback & Wallesch, 1993). Consequently, a team approach to assessment should include procedures for identifying perceptual discrepancies among team members, and then assure that subsequent services resolve these discrepancies.

Side Bar

Community-Based Teams

All members of the health care team are not necessarily employees of the same facility. A small acute care hospital in rural Iowa employed only one speech-language pathologist, three physical therapists, and no occupational therapists. Therefore, some patients' health care team included occupational therapists as well as physician specialists (e.g., radiation oncologists) employed at the neighboring hospital. When a patient's care team extends beyond typical boundaries, special care must be taken to assure that communication among team members is accurate and efficient.

GETTING REFERRALS

One might expect that the presence of a neurogenic language disorder will be apparent to the patient, the patient's family, and the many health care professionals the patient encounters during a hospital stay. There is a variety of neurogenic communication disorders, however, that can go undetected while the patient is staying in structured health care settings. For example, patients with right hemisphere communication disorders (RHD) or with mild aphasia frequently demonstrate little difficulty in participating in the somewhat superficial and concrete conversations that occur throughout the day as their medical and physical problems are being addressed. Likewise, patients with executive function deficits are often able to act or function appropriately when staying in a health care facility because of the predictable and organized schedules of these institutions. That is, inherent to these facilities is the type of external structure and support that these patients need to compensate for their executive function problems (Dugbartey et al., 1999; Miyake, Emerson, & Friedman, 2000). Often it is only when these patients return to their homes, which tend to have less structured and controlled environments and routines, do the patients and/or their loved ones begin to observe the patients' higher-level or more subtle linguistic and cognitive deficits.

Consequently, in many medical settings, the clinician must educate other health care professionals and team members regarding possible high-level linguistic and cognitive problems associated with neurogenic disorders such as mild aphasia, mild TBI, and RHD. Information concerning general characteristics of the various neurogenic communication problems as well as strategies to compensate for these problems can be provided via in-service training, informal discussion, the provision of reading materials (e.g., handouts, pamphlets), or case presentations at clinical rounds. Such educational efforts will hopefully result in increases in the number of these at-risk patients who are referred for speech-language pathology services.

ASSESSMENT PROCEDURES

A variety of information-obtaining procedures should be used when completing an assessment (see Figure 4-1). Typically, the initial assessment procedures, such as obtaining a case history and completing informal observations, serve as a broad screen to identify the areas that will require more detailed and formal or structured assessment. The next step of the assessment process following collection of case history, observational, and formal test data is to integrate and interpret these findings to make decisions regarding the presence of a neurogenic language disorder, amount and type of treatment, and prognosis. Lastly, clinicians must keep in mind that assessment is an ongoing process: Following an initial evaluation, clinicians must continue to assess the accuracy and adequacy of their diagnostic and treatment decisions to ensure optimal provision of services to their patients.

CASE HISTORY

Case history information is essential to determining the patient's premorbid abilities, and consequently to identifying the presence of a neurogenic language disorder. This information is useful when planning subsequent assessment and treatment procedures

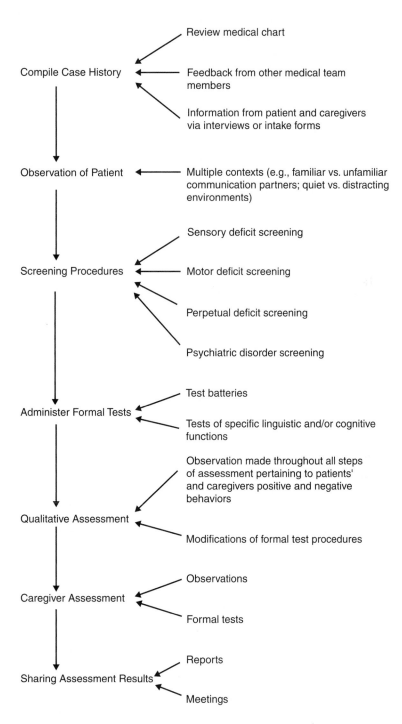

Figure 4-1. **General steps to completing an in-depth neurogenic language disorder evaluation.**

as well. For example, information pertaining to the patient's interests and hobbies can be used to develop motivating treatment stimuli and activities. To gather case history information, clinicians should not only review their patients' relevant medical records, but also interview the patients and their caregivers, including family and friends as well as other professionals on the health team.

Review of Previous and Current Medical Records

Medical charts and records contain the reports of all health care team members who have already assessed or treated the patient, and consequently provide a wealth of information about the patient's past and current level of functioning. With respect to developing assessment and treatment plans, identifying the following information will be of particular interest to speech-language clinicians:

1. personal information such as the patient's address, date and place of birth, educational background, occupation, ethnicity, and cultural background;

2. family and social history, including marital status, number of children, living situation (e.g., independent vs. assisted living), preferred social activities, and current level of family/social support;

3. past and present interests and hobbies;

4. premorbid speech and language abilities, including the languages that the patient uses, how frequently these languages are used, and competence and daily needs with respect to the various language modalities (e.g., pre-existing speech or language problems such as developmental stuttering or dyslexia; prior to his stroke, although the spoken language skills of a given bilingual patient were comparable, his written Spanish skills were stronger than his written English skills);

5. premorbid and present handedness; and

6. past and present medical, neurological, and psychiatric status, including current medications, description of physical, cognitive, and behavioral symptoms, symptom onset and duration, and type (e.g., focal vs. diffuse damage) and location of brain damage.

On the basis of this information, clinicians can begin to identify and implement appropriate assessment and treatment procedures. For example, information concerning the patient's age and education can be used to identify formal tests that have normative standards that are appropriate for that patient. Additionally, many formal linguistic and cognitive tests include questions pertaining to the above information; consequently, clinicians must know if their patients' responses to these test items are accurate.

With respect to reviewing patients' medical charts, speech-language clinicians also need to educate themselves regarding the assessment procedures, terminology, and abbreviations used by not only speech-language pathologists, but also other health care team members (see Table 4-3). This may be of particular importance

Table 4-3. Terms and Abbreviations Frequently Encountered in Medical Speech-Language Pathology

TERM OR ABBREVIATION	DEFINITION OR DESCRIPTION
AC	auditory comprehension
ADL	activities of daily living (e.g., bathing, teeth brushing, dressing)
A & O	alert and oriented
amb.	ambulatory
aq	water
ASHD	arteriosclerotic heart disease
Ba	barium, barium sulfate
bid	twice daily
biw	twice weekly
bp	blood pressure
bx	biopsy
c/o	complains of
CHF	congestive heart failure
COPD	chronic obstructive pulmonary disease
D/C	discontinue or discharge
DVT	deep vein thrombosis (i.e., blood clot that is often located in the leg)
ETOH	alcohol
F/U	follow-up
GERD	gastroesophagial reflux disease
h/a	headache
h/o	history of

(continues)

Table 4-3. *Continued*

TERM OR ABBREVIATION	DEFINITION OR DESCRIPTION
HTN	hypertension (i.e., high blood pressure)
IP	inpatient
LOC	loss of consciousness
LOS	length of stay
MVA	motor vehicle accident
NPO	nothing by mouth
NT	not tested
OP	outpatient
PNA	pneumonia
p.r.n.	as needed
p.o.	by mouth
q.d.	every day
RO	reality orientation (i.e., a form of cognitive stimulation often provided to patients with dementia or in post-traumatic amnesia following traumatic brain injury)
ROM	range of motion
SNF	skilled nursing facility
STG	short term goal
WFL	within functional limits

when trying to interpret the assessment findings of neurologists and radiologists. Table 4-4 describes some of the more frequently used procedures that clinicians may encounter in neurology reports, and Table 4-5 reviews the different structural and metabolic assessment techniques used to quantify and qualify brain damage in patients with neurogenic language disorders (Baylor, 2003; Silkes, 2003).

Table 4-4. Procedures Frequently Completed During a Neurological Examination to Identify the Presence and Possible Location of Nervous System Dysfunction

PROCEDURE	PURPOSE AND DESCRIPTION
Neck flexion	Checking for neck rigidity or stiffness, as these are indicative of a hemorrhage.
Auscultation	Applying a stethoscope over the carotid bifurcation (within the neck) to listen for evidence of bruits or abnormal pulsating sounds that indicate turbulent blood flow through an artery. Bruits are associated with artery stenosis or narrowing.
Palpation	Palpating the carotid arteries within the neck to feel for altered or unilateral pulsation that are indicative of arterial obstruction or occlusion.
Neuro-ophthalmologic exam	Inspecting the optic fundus or the vascular system at back of eye. Atherosclerosis, hypertension, diabetes, and other disorders produce recognizable retinal and vascular changes.
Motor function exam	Visually and manually inspecting muscular tone (e.g., spasticity vs. rigidity vs. flaccidity), bulk (e.g., wasting or hypertrophy), strength (e.g., hemiplegia or hemiparesis), and coordination, as well as for the presence of involuntary movements.
Sensory function exam	Assessing responses to primary sensory modalities (i.e., touch, pain, temperature, vibration, and position) and cortical sensations (e.g., two-point discrimination, stereognosis, graphesthesia).
Cranial nerve function exam	Examining for symptoms indicative of cranial nerve damage (e.g., lack of pupillary light reflex, impaired vertical and horizontal eye movements, presence of facial droop or asymmetry, asymmetrical soft palate movement, tongue deviation upon protrusion).
Reflex elicitation	Checking for the presence or absence of deep tendon reflexes (i.e., absence indicative of peripheral nerve damage, hyporeflexia indicative of lower motor neuron damage, hyperreflexia indicative of upper motor neuron) and pathological or release reflexes (i.e., reflexes that are normal in infants but that disappear over first to second year of life) such as the Babinski sign (i.e., when the lateral aspect of the sole of the foot is stroked the toes extend rather than flex), the snout reflex (i.e., tapping the upper lip causes an abnormal puckering response), the rooting reflex (i.e., when a cheek is tapped or stroked, there is an abnormal movement of the angle of the mouth toward the tap), or the grasp reflex (i.e., stroking the web between the thumb and first finger produces an abnormal involuntary grasp of the stroking fingers).
Exam of higher cognitive functions	Completing a brief screening of cognitive ability (e.g., orientation to person, place and time) and emotional-behavioral functioning (e.g., lability).

Table 4-5. Procedures for Assessing Structural and Metabolic Changes within the Brain

PROCEDURE	PURPOSE AND DESCRIPTION
Angiography	Injection of radiopaque material into an extracranial artery to obtain high resolution x-ray images of the cerebral vascular system (i.e., arterial supply and venous drainage). Used to identify structural abnormalities of intracranial blood vessels (e.g., arterial stenosis or occlusion, aneurysms, arteriovenous malformations, vasculitis) or alterations in the positions of these vessels (e.g., displacement may be indicative of a cerebral tumor). May also be used to confirm brain death. This technique is considered invasive with associated risks such as dislodging arterial plaque, producing emboli, and negative reaction to the contrast medium.
Ultrasonography	Noninvasive imaging of the carotid bifurcation or intracranial blood vessels using Doppler technology. Ultrasound exams are less sensitive than other vascular imaging techniques but can be conducted at bedside.
Computer assisted tomography/CT	X-ray cross-sectional images of the brain taken from various angles to identify the presence and location (within a few millimeters) of lesions. This technique is considered invasive because of x-ray/radiation exposure. Another risk is a negative reaction to the contrast medium. Whereas this is an affordable, rapid, and widely available assessment procedure, it does not allow immediate (e.g., within 24 hours) visualization of thrombotic or embolic infarctions and may fail to identify lacunae or tiny lesions.
Magnetic resonance imaging/MRI	Noninvasive images obtained by exposing the brain to a large magnetic field. Compared to CT scans, MRIs provide better visualization of gray versus white brain matter and small lesions, and quicker identification of infarction and edema (i.e., within 90 minutes). Relatively new MRI techniques include diffusion-weighted imaging (i.e., measures the average distance that water molecules move by diffusion in a fixed time) that can identify acute infarction within minutes of stroke onset, and perfusion-weighted imaging (i.e., involves injection of a contrast agent to provide information about blood flow or hemodynamics) that allows visualization of not only the infarction but also brain tissue at risk for infarction (i.e., penumbra). MRI also is useful for visualizing damage related to demyelinating diseases, tumors, infections, and degenerative diseases. Limitations of MRI include that it cannot be used with patients who have pacemakers or other metallic implants or prostheses because of the strong magnetic forces. Additionally patients with movement disorders or who are uncooperative will require sedation to avoid movement during the long scanning time.

(continues)

Table 4-5. *Continued*

PROCEDURE	PURPOSE AND DESCRIPTION
Magnetic resonance angiography/ MRA	Noninvasive imaging of extra- and intracranial blood vessels (e.g., identification of occlusions, aneurysms, arteriovenous malformations) based on MRI technology. MRA has fewer risks than angiography, but only allows imaging of the arterial or venous system during one examination unless scanning time is dramatically increased. Other limitations are similar to those mentioned for MRI.
Positron emission tomography/PET	Injection (or sometimes inhalation) of radioisotopes into an extracranial artery to visualize changes in regional cerebral blood flow (i.e., rCBF), cerebral glucose metabolism, or neurotransmitter levels. This technique is invasive because of the exposure to radioactive material, and is expensive and not widely available because the radioactive material must be generated in an on-site cyclotron.
Single photon emission-computed tomography/SPECT	Similar to PET, except the radioisotopes do not need to be generated by an on-site cyclotron. Although SPECT allows visualization of changes in cerebral blood flow (CBF), it is less precise than PET in terms of spatial resolution and identifying the etiology of CBF changes (e.g., tumor vs. stroke).

Patient and Caregiver Interviews

Information concerning patients' premorbid and current levels of functioning can also be obtained by interviewing patients and their caregivers (e.g., family members, friends, health care providers, or community members). Conducting an initial interview with patients and caregivers not only provides clinicians with much needed background information about their patients, but also gives clinicians an opportunity to establish rapport and mutual respect with patients and caregivers, qualities important to a therapeutic relationship. When an initial interview is not possible (usually due to time constraints), clinicians can obtain at least some of the same information by having patients and caregivers complete questionnaires.

One important question to ask during interviews pertains to what patients perceive to be their major problem or, perhaps more specifically, what they view to be their current, communicative and cognitive weaknesses and strengths. Patients' responses to this line of questioning not only can identify the patients' treatment priorities and expectations, which sometimes differ from those of the clinician (e.g., a patient might be much more concerned about an apparently mild auditory comprehension problem than his obviously severe reading deficit), but also can indicate if patients are unaware of (i.e., anosognostic) or in denial of their deficits. Patient interviews can also provide insight into patients' level of orientation (e.g., ability to answer correctly questions concerning personal background information), self-monitoring and correction skills (i.e., ability to determine whether they have made a mistake and, if so, to correct their error), and their pragmatic language abilities (e.g., ability to stay on topic, provide relevant vs. irrelevant information). Clinicians must, however, keep in mind that a number of factors may limit the amount of information that neurogenic patients can supply. For example, patients with aphasia may be unable to express this information or comprehend the interview questions due to their language problems, patients with RHI or TBI may have little insight into the presence or severity of their deficits due to cognitive impairments such as anosognosia, and the memory limitations of patients with dementia or TBI may reduce the amount or accuracy of the background information they share. Dysarthria or apraxia of speech, which limit speech production abilities, may further limit a patient's ability to respond to interview questions.

Consequently, it is equally important to interview family members and caregivers who have already assessed or treated the patient. The same questions should be posed to the patient's family and caregivers to identify any discrepancies in terms of perceptions of the patient's previous and current levels of functioning. Caregivers also should be asked to describe the communication style of the patient prior to the onset of neurological damage or disease. That is, the presence or severity of many communication disorders can only be determined with respect to the patient's premorbid abilities. For example, it would be inappropriate to diagnose a patient who has RHD with aprosodia if the family reported that the patient had always sounded monotone.

There are a number of tools available, both commercially and in the research literature, to help clinicians structure interviews with or collect information and observations from caregivers or patients. For example, clinicians working with aphasic patients might have caregivers (or perhaps the patients themselves) complete the *Communicative Effectiveness Index* (CETI; Lomas et al., 1989). On the CETI, individuals rate the current communicative performance of patients with aphasia in terms of "not at all able" to "as able as before the stroke" for a variety of daily communicative situations. Another example would be the *Neuropsychology Behavior and Affect Profile* (NBAP; Nelson et al., 1989, 1993), which caregivers complete twice: once rating the emotional-behavioral status of the patient prior to the onset of brain damage or neurological disease, and once rating the patient's current emotional-behavioral functioning. NBAP items pertain to areas such as indifference (e.g., anosognosia), inappropriate behavior, pragmatic problems, depression (e.g., apathy, sadness), and mania, and the tool has been validated to assess current level and type, and degree of change in affective functioning in patients with stroke or dementing illnesses.

In many assessment situations, the interview will be the primary, or only, means of evaluating the ICF level of participation. Chapter 7 discusses several ways to include formal and informal measures of participation and quality of life as part of the interview portion of the evaluation.

OBSERVATIONS AND INITIAL SCREENING PROCEDURES

Much information can be gleaned by a casual visit with patients and their family or caregivers. The main advantage of direct, informal observation is that it allows clinicians to examine the interaction between patients' behaviors and their environments, and thus may lead to identification of contextual factors (e.g., communication partners, ambient noise levels) that positively or negatively affect patients' communicative and cognitive abilities. Observational sessions also allow clinicians to identify positive (e.g., a spouse who always addresses his wife with left neglect on her right side, a patient with aphasia who uses gestures to augment her spoken output) and negative strategies (e.g., a caregiver who uses indirect requests with patients with RHD, a patient with dementia who avoids social situations) that enhance or hinder, respectively, the communication interactions of patients and caregivers (Holland, 1991).

Ideally, multiple informal observational samples should be completed to account for the variable behavior that is pervasive in adults with acquired neurogenic language disorders. For example, the language abilities of patients with aphasia have been found to vary not only across different communication contexts, topics, and activities (e.g., Glosser et al., 1988; Mayer & Murray, 2003), but also within identical communication situations (e.g., Freed, Marshall, & Chuhlantseff, 1996). Realistically, however, due to time and context limitations, most clinicians are able to complete only minimal amounts of observation and thus must acknowledge that they have a limited view of their patients' communicative behaviors in more naturalistic settings or circumstances. For instance, a clinician working in an outpatient clinic may be able to observe patients and caregivers/spouses interacting in the waiting room or during an occupational or physical therapy session, but have no opportunity to observe those patients' communication interactions in other, more frequently occurring settings such as their place of work, their home, or even their daily trip to the grocery store.

In addition to providing preliminary insight into patients' communicative and cognitive abilities, initial observations and screening procedures are useful for identifying complicating conditions that interfere with patients' current levels of functioning or future recovery. Failure to identify these complicating conditions prior to formal assessment of communicative and cognitive abilities can result in inaccurate diagnostic and prognostic conclusions. Complicating conditions with which patients with neurogenic language disorders frequently present and, consequently, of which clinicians must be cognizant include sensory deficits, motoric impairments, perceptual problems, and psychiatric disorders.

Screening for Sensory Deficits

Auditory, visual, and even tactile sensitivity problems may negatively influence a patient's performance on tests of communicative or cognitive abilities. Patients with neurogenic language disorders are at risk for hearing disorders because: (1) many of these patients are older and thus commonly present with age-related hearing problems (i.e., **presbycusis**), and (2) certain etiologies, such as traumatic brain injuries and infections (e.g., meningitis), frequently cause not only neurogenic language disorders, but also hearing loss (Cohn, 1999; Sakai & Mateer, 1984). Consequently, speech-language clinicians should assure that each of their patients has recently had, at a minimum, a hearing screening, and preferably a full audiological evaluation prior to administering any linguistic or cognitive tests. Determining the hearing acuity of patients with severe language impairments may be problematic if they have difficulty comprehending test instructions. With these patients, therefore, collaboration between the audiologist and speech-language clinician is imperative to ensure valid hearing assessment results. It also is important that for patients who require a hearing aid and/or other assistive listening devices, clinicians assure that the devices are in proper working condition (e.g., hearing aid battery is charged; device is free of cerumen buildup) before administering linguistic or cognitive assessment or treatment procedures.

Vision also is frequently compromised in adults with neurogenic language disorders. Patients might present with premorbid visual problems such as myopia, presbyopia (i.e., age-related visual problems), cataracts, or macular degeneration, with visual deficits caused by their brain damage or neurological disease such as visual field cuts (e.g., **left or right homonymous hemianopia**), nystagmus, diplopia (i.e., double vision), or optic neuritis (visual disorder found in multiple sclerosis and other medical conditions), or both (Campbell et al., 1999; Granadier, 2000; Rathore, Hinn, Cooper, Tyroler, & Rosamond, 2002). If an undiagnosed visual defect is suspected, clinicians should advocate for an ophthalmology or optometry referral. Likewise, clinicians should make sure that any visual assistive devices that their patients need are available and in suitable condition prior to completing their assessment. Clinicians also can help patients accommodate to visual field cuts by presenting visual stimuli in a vertical rather than horizontal display to reduce the possibility of inducing visual errors.

Many patients present with problems sensing temperature, pain, touch, or movement. In fact, it is estimated that 40 to 60% of stroke patients display some degree of somatosensory loss (Cary, 1995; Rathore et al., 2002). If these problems affect only one side of the body, the patient may be diagnosed with **hemianesthesia.** Clinician awareness of tactile deficits is important in terms of providing tactile cues or feedback. For example, a clinician getting a patient's attention by touching his hand would want to touch this patient's right hand if the patient had suffered a right hemisphere stroke and presented with left hemianesthesia.

Screening for Motoric Impairments

Adults with neurogenic language disorders may present with a variety of motoric impairments that may not only directly or indirectly affect their expressive communication abilities (e.g., motor speech, writing, gesturing, facial expressions), but also affect their ability to fulfill response requirements (e.g., speed and accuracy of a pointing response) of many frequently used linguistic and cognitive tests. Apraxia of speech and dysarthria are two common motoric problems that impact speech. Additionally, a number of motoric disorders may affect the limb and body movements of patients with neurogenic language disorders.

Apraxia of Speech

The diagnosis of **apraxia of speech** refers to difficulty with volitionally positioning muscles as well as planning and sequencing muscle movements for the production of phonemes and phoneme sequences (Croot, 2002; Yorkston, Beukelman, Strand, and Bell, 1999; Ziegler, 2002). Apraxia of speech is not a product of muscular weakness, slowness, or incoordination, particularly since patients are able to use the speech musculature without difficulty when completing reflexive or automatic motor acts. Frequently observed apraxia of speech symptoms include articulatory problems such as consistent or inconsistent articulatory substitutions, distortions, omissions, repetitions and additions, and prosodic disturbances such as a decreased speech rate, abnormal stress patterns, and excessive frequency or duration of pauses. The variability of these symptoms appears to be influenced, at least in part, by speech context variables such as the length and phonetic complexity of the word or utterance, word frequency, and type of speech activity (e.g., repetition task vs. reading aloud vs. spontaneous verbal output). Although apraxia of speech may occur following damage to many cortical and subcortical regions, it is most commonly associated with lesions to the premotor or parietal cortex, or insular regions of the left hemisphere, and consequently is frequently observed in patients with aphasia or TBI (Dronkers, 1996; Miller, 2002).

Because apraxia of speech and aphasia frequently co-occur, several aphasia batteries include subtests to assess for the co-existence of apraxia (e.g., *Boston Diagnostic Aphasia Examination–III*; Goodglass et al., 2001). There are also a number of tests designed to provide a more in-depth evaluation of the presence and severity of apraxia of speech, including the *Apraxia Battery for Adults–2* (Dabul, 2000) and the *Comprehensive Apraxia Test* (DiSimoni, 1989). Additionally, there are a few apraxia screening tools available, such as the *Quick Assessment for Apraxia of Speech* (Tanner & Culbertson, 1999c), that are designed to only establish the presence or absence of apraxia of speech. Despite the availability of these tools, trying to differentiate speech problems related to apraxia of speech from those related to certain types of aphasia (e.g., conduction aphasia, Broca's aphasia) remains difficult in many patients. Consequently, researchers continue to try to identify perceptual, acoustic, and/or physiological measures that might in the future help clinicians reliably distinguish the apraxic versus aphasic verbal output problems of their patients (Croot, 2002; Ziegler, 2002).

Dysarthria

When a motor speech disorder is caused by impairments of speech musculature (e.g., weakness or excessive tone) and/or control (i.e., incoordination, imprecise movements), the diagnosis of **dysarthria** applies (Darley, Aronson, & Brown, 1975; Kent, Kent, Duffy, & Weismer, 1998; Vogel & Cannito, 2001; Yorkston et al., 1999). In dysarthria, one or many of the basic components of motor speech may be compromised, including respiration, phonation, resonance, articulation, and prosody. In contrast to apraxia of speech, many symptoms of dysarthria tend to be more predictable and more consistent across speaking contexts. The frequency and types of motor speech symptoms, however, can vary significantly among patients with dysarthria depending on the location and etiology of their neurologic damage (Table 4-6). Because most muscle groups involved in speech have bilateral upper motor neuron innervation (i.e., are controlled by both cerebral hemispheres), typically only patients who have suffered bilateral brain damage will present with persistent and severe dysarthria. Consequently, in terms of neurogenic language disorder populations, patients with dementia and TBI are more apt to present with significant and enduring dysarthria than patients with aphasia or RHD, who often have suffered only unilateral brain damage and thus are more likely to present with a mild to moderate, mixed dysarthria if they have dysarthria (Kent et al., 1998). To identify the presence, type, and severity of dysarthria, clinicians can use one of the several commercially available tests, such as the *Assessment of Intelligibility of Dysarthric Speech* (Yorkston et al., 1984), the *Quick Assessment for Dysarthria* (Tanner & Culbertson, 1999b), the *Frenchay Dysarthria Assessment* (Enderby, 1983), and the *Dysarthria Examination Battery* (Drummond, 1993), or one of the research protocols described in the research literature (e.g., Kent et al., 1989). In addition to these tools that rely upon auditory-perceptual judgments, clinicians should also incorporate instrumental techniques (e.g., acoustic analyses, kinematic procedures) to provide further and, perhaps, more reliable quantification and qualification of their dysarthric patients' motor speech problems (Kent et al., 1998; Vogel & Cannito, 2001).

Other Motoric Disorders

In addition to motor speech impairments, patients with neurogenic language disorders often also present with motoric disturbances of other muscular systems that

Table 4-6. Types of Dysarthria

DYSARTHRIA TYPE	COMMON PERCEPTUAL FEATURES	ASSOCIATED NEUROLOGIC ETIOLOGIES (AND LOCATION)	POSSIBLE CO-EXISTING NEUROGENIC LANGUAGE DISORDER
Spastic	monopitch, monoloudness, reduced stress, slow speech rate, harsh and strained voice, imprecise articulation	Stroke, TBI, tumor (upper motor neuron, motor cortex, internal capsule, corona radiata)	Aphasia, RHD, TBI
Flaccid	*hypernasality, breathy voice, short phrases, imprecise articulation, slow speech rate	Stroke, TBI, tumor (lower motor neuron, brainstem, spinal nerves, cranial nerves)	TBI
Hyperkinetic	loudness variations, harsh and strained voice, irregular articulatory breakdowns, imprecise articulation, silent intervals	Stroke, TBI, tumor, Huntington's disease, dystonia (basal ganglia, putamen)	Dementia, TBI
Hypokinetic	monopitch, mono- and reduced loudness, breathy and rough voice, short rushes of speech, imprecise articulation	Parkinson's disease, progressive supranuclear palsy (basal ganglia)	Dementia, TBI
Ataxic	irregular articulatory breakdowns, imprecise articulation, excess and equal stress, monopitch or variable pitch changes, slow rate	Stroke, TBI, tumor, Friedreich's ataxia, multiple sclerosis (cerebellum)	Dementia, TBI
Mixed	varied and dependent on location of the multiple lesion sites	Strokes, TBI, multiple sclerosis, progressive supranuclear palsy, amyotrophic lateral sclerosis, olivo-pontine-cerebellar degeneration (diffuse brain damage/upper and lower motor neurons)	Dementia, TBI

*Variable depending on which cranial and/or spinal nerves were compromised by the brain damage.
Note. Table information synthesized from Kent et al. (1998), Darley et al. (1975), and Theodoros et al. (2001).

in turn can have a negative effect on their communication abilities, their ability to complete linguistic and cognitive tests, or both. One of the most frequent of these motor disturbances is **hemiparesis,** a muscular weakness on one side of the body (Rathore et al., 2002); the term **hemiplegia** is applied when the disturbance is so severe that the one side of the body is paralyzed. In terms of cognitive-communication abilities, the hemiparesis is most problematic when the patient's dominant side is affected, as commonly occurs in patients with aphasia (i.e., right hemiparesis). This weakness of the dominant hand and/or arm, or dependence on the nondominant hand and/or arm, can negatively affect the accuracy and speed of these patients' writing, typing, drawing, and gesturing.

Limb apraxia is a motoric problem that is most frequently observed in patients with left hemisphere damage, particularly those with frontal or parietal lobe involvement, and that may or may not co-occur with other types of apraxia, such as oral apraxia or apraxia of speech (Heilman, Watson, & Rothi, 1997; Miller, 2002; Shatz, 1998). In fact, Donkervoort and colleagues (2000) found that approximately one-third of the left hemisphere stroke patients they evaluated presented with limb apraxia. Patients with limb apraxia have difficulty executing acquired and volitional movements of their fingers, wrists, elbows, and/or shoulders. As in apraxia of speech, these execution problems are not a product of muscular, sensory, or cognitive impairments. Typically, movements involving distal versus proximal body parts, and movements or actions involving a tool or instrument (i.e., transitive) versus no tool, are more difficult for patients with limb apraxia. Symptoms of limb apraxia include content errors in which the patient completes an incorrect movement or action (e.g., when asked to show how to blow a whistle, the patient gestures how to strike a match), and production errors in which the correct movement or action is attempted, but the spatial or temporal organization of the movement is in error (e.g., when gesturing how to brush his teeth, the patient performs the action with a flattened rather than gripped hand) (Rothi, Raymer, & Heilman, 1997).

Because limb apraxia can result in problems performing commands that involve purposeful moments, and sometimes even providing a reliable pointing or nodding response, clinicians should assess for limb apraxia prior to completing comprehension or other cognitive (e.g., memory, attention) testing to avoid misdiagnosing the problem. For a quick screen of possible limb apraxia, clinicians can administer the short apraxia subtests that many aphasia batteries include (e.g., *Aphasia Diagnostic Profiles*; Helm-Estabrooks, 1992). For a more in-depth and reliable evaluation (Butler, 2002), several protocols are described in the literature (e.g., Rothi et al., 1997), or there are also a few commercially available tests, such as the *Test of Oral and Limb Apraxia* (Helm-Estabrooks, 1991), the *Apraxia battery for Adults—2* (Dabul, 2000), and the *Naturalistic Action Test* (Schwartz, Buxbaum, Veramonti, Ferraro, & Segal, 2002).

There are a number of other motoric impairments that may compromise patients' ability to perform the types of movements and actions necessary to complete many linguistic and cognitive tests, and that consequently should be identified early in the assessment process (Krauss & Jankovic, 2002; Mayer, Keenan, & Esquenzi, 1999). These other motoric impairments are more frequently observed in patients with TBI or in patients who have progressive neurological disease. For example, many patients with TBI or Parkinson's disease have **bradykinesia,** a motoric problem related to excessive muscle tone that causes decreases in the speed and range of these patients' movements and, in particular, negatively affects their ability to manipulate small objects such as a pen or pencil. Patients who have cerebellar involvement may present with ataxia, in which the accuracy, force, and timing of movements is disturbed. For example, when asked to point to a certain object on a comprehension test, the patient with ataxia might overshoot the target object and end up giving what appears to be an incorrect pointing response. Excessive and involuntary movements disorders such as chorea, hemiballismus, and tics may occur following TBI and are a defining characteristic of some progressive diseases (e.g., Huntington's disease). The abrupt and uncontrollable movements associated with these disorders may affect patients' ability to complete certain linguistic and cognitive test procedures, as well as their communicative skills (e.g., writing, facial expressions, speech).

Screening for Perceptual Problems

Following brain damage, and in particular bilateral brain damage, patients may present with a variety of perceptual difficulties that must be identified so that these difficulties can be accounted or accommodated for during subsequent assessment procedures. These perceptual problems are not due to sensory loss (e.g., a hearing loss) but rather a breakdown in interpreting and applying meaning to sensory information.

Auditory Perceptual Problems

When patients have difficulty recognizing auditory information despite accurate recognition of the same stimuli in other modalities, they are diagnosed with **auditory agnosia** (Bauer & Zawacki, 1997). A number of different types of auditory agnosia have been identified, including: (1) pure word deafness, or impaired recognition of spoken language but relatively preserved recognition of other auditory stimuli; (2) auditory sound agnosia, or impaired recognition of nonverbal or environmental sounds (e.g., telephone ringing, frog croaking); and (3) amusia, or impaired recognition of musical rhythms or passages (Gates & Bradshaw, 1977; Vignolo, 2003; Wee & Menard, 1999). These auditory agnosias are typically rare, but when they do occur, they are more likely to be observed in patients with right or bilateral temporal lesions. Additionally, problems perceiving pitch and loudness have been identified in patients with neurogenic language disorders, most frequently those with RHD (Tompkins, 1995); although these types of auditory perceptual disorders are traditionally associated with RHD or bilateral brain damage, recent research suggests that patients with aphasia also may experience difficulty processing nonverbal sounds (Saygin, Dick, Wilson, Dronkers, & Bates, 2003; Tanaka, Nakano, & Obayashi, 2002; Vignolo, 2003).

Currently, there is a limited number of tests available to identify auditory perceptual disorders (Table 4-7). Clinicians, therefore, must work closely with other team members, particularly the audiologist, when assessing for the presence of these types of perceptual problems. Regardless of which test or tests are used, it is important to rule out hearing loss, language comprehension and expression problems, and a lack of familiarity with test items prior to giving a diagnosis of auditory agnosia (this also applies to diagnosing agnosias in other sensory modalities).

Visual Perceptual Problems

There are many visual perceptual problems with which adults with neurogenic language disorders might present. Typically these problems are more prevalent among patients with RHD or with bilateral brain damage (e.g., Alzheimer's disease) than those with unilateral left hemisphere damage (i.e., aphasia). First, many forms of **visual agnosia,** a disturbance in recognizing visual stimuli even though visual sensitivity is adequate to see the stimuli, have been identified, including: (1) visual object agnosia, or impaired recognition of actual or pictured objects; (2) prosopagnosia, or impaired recognition of familiar faces; (3) autopagnosia, or impaired recognition of body parts; (4) environmental agnosia, or impaired recognition of familiar environments (e.g., one's own home); and (5) propopagnosia, or impaired recognition of pictures or a mirror image of oneself (De Renzi, 1997a; Farah & Feinberg, 1997; Shatz, 1998). Second, patients with neurogenic language disorders may have complex visual discrimination and perception difficulties (De Renzi, 1997b; Tompkins, 1995). For example, patients who can match pictures of objects viewed at the same angle may have difficulty matching or recognizing those objects when viewed from an unusual angle (e.g., identifying a cup viewed from the top vs. the side), when provided an incomplete or obstructed view (e.g., hatch marks cover part of the picture), or when presented with lots of competing, background visual information (e.g., a figure-ground task). Problems with depth perception, visual scanning, and color perception (including achromotopsia, in which all colors are perceived to be dull or as shades of grey) are also possible.

Obviously, the presence of one or more of these visual perception deficits could confound a patient's performance of many linguistic and cognitive test procedures, such as naming, describing, recalling, drawing, or copying objects or pictures or geometric figures. Fortunately, there are a number of tests available to screen for the presence of visual perceptual difficulties (see Table 4-7). Many of these tests must be adapted when administering them to adults with neurogenic

Table 4-7. Tests of Auditory and Visual Perceptual Abilities

TEST	SOURCE	BRIEF DESCRIPTION
Hidden Figures Test	Talland (1965)	Assesses visuoperceptual closure (i.e., identification of target geometric figures) in the presence of a distracting, visual background.
Hooper Visual Organization Test	Hooper (1983)	Assesses visual integration or the ability to identify pictures of objects that have been cut up and rearranged. Multiple-choice format also available (Schultheis et al., 2000).
Judgment of Line Orientation	Benton et al. (1983)	Measures visuospatial judgment or the ability to identify a target line orientation from an array of lines.
Kent Visual Perceptual Test	Melamed (2000)	Assesses visual discrimination and visuomotor skills by requiring identification and copying, respectively, of various target visual stimuli.
Letter or Star Cancellation	Wilson et al. (1987)	Measures visual search and scanning abilities by requiring the discrimination of target letters or stars, respectively, from an array of distracting visual stimuli.
Phoneme Discrimination	Benton et al. (1983)	Assesses the auditory perceptual ability of discriminating pairs of nonsense syllables as being the same or different.
Seashore Tonal Memory Test	Seashore et al. (1960)	Assesses the ability to discriminate tonal changes in previously heard tonal patterns.
Tennessee Test of Rhythm and Intonation Patterns	Koike & Asp (1981)	Assesses auditory perception by requiring imitation of and Intonation nonsense syllable stimuli that differ in terms of number of syllables and prosody pattern.
Test of Auditory Perception	Williams (1990)	Measures the ability to discriminate and localize tone, word, and environmental sound stimuli.
Test of Facial Recognition	Benton et al. (1983)	Assesses the ability to match unfamiliar faces under different visual conditions (e.g., simple matching vs. matching target face with faces shown at different viewing angles).
Visual Object and Space Perception Test	Warrington & James (1991)	Assesses the ability to identify images of objects, animals, or letters that have been degraded or are blackened silhouettes, and the ability to complete visual spatial tasks such as counting arrays of joined cubes.

language disorders who may have problems understanding test instructions, or who may be unable to provide accurate verbal responses due to their linguistic deficits. Importantly, researchers are beginning to acknowledge the need for these test adaptations, and modified versions of these tests can frequently be found in the research literature (e.g., Schultheis, Caplan, Ricker, & Woessner, 2000).

Screening for Psychiatric Disorders

Psychiatric disturbances regularly co-occur with neurogenic language disorders. For example, estimates of the prevalence of psychotic symptoms in patients with dementia often exceed 70% (Paulsen et al., 2000), and depression is reported to occur in more than 60% of patients with TBI (Ponsford, Olver, & Curran, 1995). Regardless of etiology, patients with neurogenic language disorders may present with one or more of the following emotional or psychiatric problems: delusions, hallucinations, agitation, anxiety (including agoraphobia), apathy, mania, disinhibition, irritability, aggression, **lability** (i.e., difficulty controlling one's emotions that can manifest as excessive or inappropriate crying or laughing), sexual inappropriateness/dysfunction, low self-esteem, personality disorders (e.g., paranoid, schizoid), catastrophic reaction, and **depression** (Bakheit et al., 2004; Bishop & Pet, 1995; Burvill et al., 1995; Cummings, 1997; Cummings et al., 1994; Keponen et al., 2003). Of these various psychiatric disturbances, depression is frequently reported to be the most prevalent among adults with neurogenic communication disorders (Keponen et al., 2003; Mayberg & Solomon, 1995; Maynard, 2003; Stern, 1999). That is, whereas it is expected that patients who have suffered brain damage or have been diagnosed with a progressive neurological disease will experience some depression related to dealing with the negative effects of their brain damage or disease, many demonstrate significant and persistent depression, which in turn compromises their ability to profit from rehabilitation and participate in daily activities and social interactions.

Psychiatric problems of patients with neurogenic communication disorders can originate from a number of factors, including premorbid psychiatric disorders, medication side-effects, physiological changes associated with brain damage, nutritional problems, and psychological reactions to dealing with an acquired communication and other possible cognitive, physical, and behavioral impairments. Identifying and remediating psychiatric problems is imperative given that these problems have been shown to increase mortality rates, impact negatively patients' cognitive and communicative abilities, treatment outcomes, caregiver stress levels, quality of life, and, in patients with progressive diseases, increase the rate of disease progression (Clark & Smith, 1999; King, 1996; Ramasubbu & Patten, 2003; Stern et al., 1994).

Despite the prevalence of and negative consequences associated with psychiatric problems, there are few appropriate tools for diagnosing these problems in patients with neurogenic communication disorders (Hart et al., 2003; Shankar &

Orrell, 2000; Spencer, Tompkins, & Schulz, 1997; Stern, 1999). Reliable assessment of psychiatric problems in patients with neurogenic communication disorders is diffi-cult for several reasons. First, because most currently available assessment instru-ments were developed for psychiatric rather than neurological patient populations, many of them have linguistic, attention, memory, or executive function demands that exceed the capabilities of patients with neurogenic communication disorders (Table 4-8). For example, patients with aphasia may lack the linguistic skills necessary to comprehend or respond to interview-based or even checklist types of assessment tools, whereas patients with RHD, TBI, or dementia may have inadequate insight to complete accurately self-rating scales. A second confound to accurate assessment is that many of the signs used to diagnose psychiatric disorders may be obscured by the neurogenic communication problem or other concomitant neurological symptoms. For instance, diminished prosody and flat facial expression are common among not only patients with RHD, TBI, or Parkinson's disease, but also those with depression. Likewise, many dementing illnesses cause sleep disturbances (e.g., Alzheimer's dis-ease), another symptom used to diagnose depression. Consequently, depression and other psychiatric problems are often under-diagnosed in patients with neurogenic communication disorders because symptoms of the psychiatric problem are mis-attributed to the neurogenic disorder rather than a possible co-existing psychiatric problem (Shankar & Orrell, 2000; Stern, 1999; Witol, Kreutzer, & Sander, 1999). Lastly, identifying psychiatric disorders in patients with neurogenic communication problems has proven difficult because of their variable presentation among this patient population. Whereas there have been primarily consistent findings with respect to the positive relationship between frontal lobe involvement and psychotic symptoms such as aggression and irritability (e.g., Paulsen et al., 2000), variables such as lesion location and time post onset of brain damage or disease have proven to be relatively unreliable predictors of whether patients will or will not present with psy-chiatric problems such as depression and anxiety (Shankar & Orrell, 2000; Hosking, Marsh, & Friedman, 2000; Thomsen, 1984).

Despite these obstacles to accurate identification of psychiatric problems, there are a few steps clinicians can follow to help assure that the emotional stabil-ity of their patients is evaluated. First, as indicated in Table 4-7, there are some recently published tests developed specifically for patients with acquired brain damage that clinicians might use. These tests are more appropriate because they have taken into consideration the above discussed testing confounds. For example, many of these tests incorporate both self- and observer-ratings to examine for the possible influence of patient self-awareness deficits. There are now even some assessment protocols, such as the Stroke and Aphasia Depression Scale (SADS; Smollan & Penn, 1997), Stroke Aphasic Depression Questionnaire (Sutcliffe & Lincoln, 1998), *Visual Analog Mood Scales* (VAMS; Stern, 1998), and Visual Analogue Self-Esteem Scale (VASES; Brumfitt & Sheeran, 1999), which have minimal lin-guistic and cognitive demands. The SADS, VAMS, and VASES utilize visual analog scales that are anchored by both picture and printed word stimuli; therefore, even

Table 4-8. Measures of Psychiatric Well-Being

MEASURE	SYMPTOM ASSESSED	FORMAT	LINGUISTIC DEMANDS
Measures Originally Developed for Psychiatric Patients			
Beck Depression Inventory II (Beck et al., 1996)	depression	self-rated	sentence-level
Brief Symptom Inventory (Derogatis, 1975)	multidimensional	self-rated	sentence-level
Centre for Epidemiological Studies Depression Scale (Radloff & Terri, 1986)	depression	self-rated	sentence-level
Geriatric Depression Scale (Yesavage et al., 1983)	depression	self-rated	sentence-level
Hamilton Anxiety Rating Scale (Hamilton, 1959)	anxiety	observer-rated	n/a
Hamilton Rating Scale for Depression (Hamilton, 1960)	depression	observer-rated	n/a
Katz Adjustment Scale (Katz & Lyerly, 1963)	multidimensional	observer-rated	n/a
Minnesota Mutliphasic Personality Inventory-2 (Butcher et al., 1989)	multidimensional	self-rated	sentence-level
Profile of Mood States (McNair et al., 1981)	multidimensional	self-rated	word-level
Measures Originally Developed for Neurological Patients			
Cornell Scale for Depression in Dementia (Alexopolous et al., 1988)	depression	self- and observer-rated	sentence-level
Dementia Mood Assessment Scale (Sunderland et al., 1988)	depression	observer-rated	n/a
Frontal Behavioral Inventory (Kertesz et al., 1997)	multidimensional	observer-rated	n/a

(continues)

Table 4-8. *Continued*

MEASURE	SYMPTOM ASSESSED	FORMAT	LINGUISTIC DEMANDS
Frontal Lobe Personality Scale (Grace & Malloy, 1992)	multidimensional	observer-rated	n/a
Neurobehavioral Functioning Inventory (Kreutzer et al., 1999)	multidimensional	self- and/or observer-rated	sentence-level
Neuropsychiatric Inventory (Cummings et al., 1994)	multidimensional	observer-rated	n/a
Neuropsychology Behavior and Affect Profile (Nelson et al., 1989)	multidimensional	self- and observer-rated	sentence-level
Post-Stroke Depression Rating Scale (Gainotti et al., 1997)	depression	observer-rated	n/a
Rating Anxiety in Dementia (Shankar et al., 1999)	anxiety	observer-rated	n/a
Stroke and Aphasia Depression Scale (Smollan & Penn, 1997)	depression	self-rated	word-level
Stroke Aphasic Depression Questionnaire (Sutcliffe & Lincoln, 1998)	depression	observer-rated	n/a
Visual Analogue Self-Esteem Scale (Brumfitt & Sheeran, 1999)	self-esteem	self-rated	word-level
Visual Mood Analogue Scales (Stern, 1998)	multidimensional	self-rated	word-level

patients with severe linguistic impairments have been shown to be able to indicate accurately and reliably their self-perceptions of their current emotional status. Second, even if clinicians do not administer formal tests to identify psychiatric problems in their patients, they should, at the very least, assure that each of their patients' psychiatric well-being is evaluated in some fashion and on a regular basis, and be aware of symptoms and behaviors that are indicative of psychiatric problems so that appropriate referrals for psychological or psychiatric assessment and/or treatment can be made when necessary.

FORMAL TEST PROCEDURES

Formal or structured tests allow clinicians to compare their patients' communicative and cognitive performances to normative standards. Currently, a plethora of formal tests are available to assess the linguistic and cognitive status and functional outcome of adults with neurogenic language disorders (see Chapters 5 through 7). These tests differ on a variety of levels including length (e.g., a bedside aphasia screening vs. a detailed aphasia battery), scope (e.g., a test of verbal working memory vs. a memory test battery that assesses verbal and nonverbal short-, working, and long-term memory), and format (e.g., caregiver ratings vs. stimulus-response test) (Little & Doherty, 1996). Each test format has certain advantages and disadvantages associated with its use. Consequently, there is no ideal test or battery for a given patient population or neurogenic disorder, and clinicians must be well informed regarding which test or tests would be most appropriate given the general and specific goals they have generated for a specific patient. Likewise, it is important for clinicians to keep abreast of new test developments, such as the release of new tests or new versions of existing tests by manufacturing companies, and the publishing of new normative data in the research literature for existing tests. Often clinicians may grow comfortable with administering a certain test or battery of tests, but these measures often can quickly become outdated in terms of the test's theoretical framework, normative data, and even stimulus items.

For the vast majority of neurogenic patients, with the exception of those whose deficits are related to progressive brain damage, administration of formal test procedures, or, at the very least, outcome predictions based on formal test data should be postponed until they emerge from the acute stages of illness. For example, it is inappropriate to submit patients with TBI to an in-depth, formal cognitive-communicative examination while in the post-traumatic amnesia phase of recovery because of the widespread effects of this typically temporary confusional state. Likewise, many patients who have had strokes, particularly those with medical complications or those receiving numerous medications, are extremely confused and fatigued immediately following their brain attack. Consequently, formal test data from acute assessment sessions are typically confounded by the patients' current medical problems, and thus are inaccurate reflections of the nature and severity of the linguistic and cognitive consequences of their brain damage (Johnson, Valachovic, & George, 1998; Marshall, 1997).

Psychometric Properties and Considerations

Prior to administering any formal measure, clinicians should review the psychometric properties of the test to understand how best not only to utilize the test (e.g., can repeated administrations of the test be used to document treatment effects) but also to interpret test data. Basic psychometric properties with which clinicians should be familiar include test reliability, validity, and standardization.

Reliability

Reliability refers to how similar test results are across repeated administrations of the test under comparable testing conditions (Carmines & Zeller, 1979; Cronbach, 1990). The more consistent the data are from the repeated measurements, the more reliable the test is. To optimize reliability, tests should provide a thorough description of administration and scoring procedures to help clinicians reduce the occurrence of intra- (i.e., repeated test administrations by the same examiner) and inter-examiner (i.e., repeated test administrations by different examiners) measurement error from negatively affecting test reliability. Generally, clinicians should look for tests that report intra- and inter-examiner reliability coefficients that equal or exceed .80, as most researchers consider this to be an acceptable level of reliability. Clinicians should also be sure to check the reliability of not only the overall test, but also individual subtests. This is particularly important when clinicians opt to administer only certain portions of comprehensive test batteries (e.g., *Wechsler Memory Scales—III*). The test-retest reliability of a given measure should also be reviewed, particularly when the clinician wants to re-administer a test to monitor recovery. High test-retest reliability means that performance changes due to possible practice or artifactual improvements are minimal. Lastly, as previously noted, the reliability of linguistic and cognitive tests is compromised when these tests are administered during the early, acute phases of recovery from sudden brain damage (e.g., stroke, TBI) because of the extensive physiologic changes that typically occur during this time period.

Validity

When examining the psychometric adequacy of a test, clinicians need to review several types of **validity,** in particular, content-, construct-, and criterion-related validity. **Content validity** refers to how well a test measures all of the behaviors that it purports to measure (Carmines & Zeller, 1979). For example, an aphasia test should assess all language behaviors that are viewed to be theoretically and functionally necessary for successful communication. **Construct validity** concerns how well a test relates to other measures of the same construct (e.g., working memory, syntax). For example, a naming test would be said to have good construct validity if patients' scores on that test correlated well with their scores on another naming test. **Criterion-related** or **predictive validity** refers to how well a test predicts whether a patient has a deficit. For example, an aphasia test that distinguishes patients with aphasia from patients and adults without aphasia and with no brain damage, or a test of visual neglect that distinguishes patients with neglect from those without neglect would have good criterion-related validity. Recently, there has been increasing interest in a certain type of predictive validity—**ecological validity.** This type of validity refers to how well patients' test performances predict their behavior in daily, real-world settings (Sbordone, 1996).

Across most linguistic and cognitive tests, validity is usually the most problematic psychometric property (Murray & Chapey, 2001; Murray & Ramage, 2000). For example, the content validity of many tests of executive functioning has been questioned because these tests fail to include clear operational descriptions of what executive function or functions are being tested or what specific model of executive functioning upon which the test was developed. Similarly, many linguistic and cognitive tests have unacceptable ecological validity because scores on these tests do not help clinicians reliably predict which clients are at risk for daily activity limitations, social participation restrictions, or both (Ross & Wertz, 1999; Sbordone, 1996).

Standardization

To reduce measurement error and assure valid comparison of patients' performances to published normative data, test administration procedures should be standardized (Cronbach, 1990). **Standardization** is achieved by giving the test to a large sample of individuals who represent the cross-section of the population with whom the test will be used in clinical practice. Over time, a test should be revised to improve or update its sampling procedures and, consequently, expand its normative data to a greater variety of reference groups (e.g., greater minority representation in the normative sample). Sometimes these standardization updates are published as commercially available, revised tests (e.g., *Wechsler Memory Scales–III* vs. *Wechsler Memory Scales* or *Wechsler Memory Scales–Revised*). Other times the updated normative data can only be found in the research literature. For example, numerous journal articles have been published to extend the normative sample for the *Boston Naming Test* to a wider population in terms of age, education, type of residence (i.e., community vs. institution), racial background, and socioeconomic status (Henderson,

Frank, Pigatt, Abramson, & Houston, 1998; Neils et al., 1995). Further extension of the norms for many published linguistic and cognitive tests (e.g., *Western Aphasia Battery*; *Scales of Cognitive Ability for Traumatic Brain Injury*; *Arizona Battery for Communication Disorders of Dementia*) remains an area of need given that the demographic characteristics of the neurogenic patient population in North America continues to evolve slowly over time (Neils-Strunjas, 1998).

Ethnocultural Considerations

Another important factor to consider when selecting a formal test is whether or not the test conforms to the ethnocultural background of the patient being assessed. Variables such as length of residency in the United States, English proficiency, education level, health beliefs and practices, and the value that a given culture places upon different linguistic and cognitive skills, test stimuli, and tasks have been found to influence patients' test performances, and thus must be considered when deciding upon assessment priorities and procedures (Daker-White, Beattie, Gilliard, & Means, 2002; Kennepohl et al., 2004; Payne, 1997; Ross & Wertz, 2001). That is, clinicians must determine if the stimuli and procedures involved in a given test are salient and appropriate for the cultural groups regularly represented on their caseload. To do so, clinicians should review standardization information for the given test, familiarize themselves with the traditions and values of the ethnocultural population with whom they will be working, and/or conduct their own standardization and perhaps modification of the given test so that it does correspond with the ethnocultural backgrounds of their patient population.

Side Bar

Ethnocultural Variables

The issue of ethnocultural background may extend beyond typical conceptions, which are frequently limited to race or ethnicity. Additional factors such as age, education, and vocational background, however, also contribute to individuals' ethnoculture. For example, one of the first patients I evaluated as a clinical fellow was the former chief of staff of the hospital where I was employed. A well-educated, proud, and powerful man, he had strong feelings regarding what types of tasks were "worthy" of his time. Specifically, he refused to participate in any assessment tasks that included simple stimuli or responses. Instead, he would respond with a statement such as, "Well, everyone can do that."

In his case, most standardized tests failed to include items *salient* to his background and/or personality. Furthermore, few standardized tests include normative data from samples representative of individuals of his educational and professional history.

Test Batteries

A test is considered a test battery if it consists of several tasks or subtests, each designed to examine independently a different linguistic and/or cognitive ability. With respect to neurogenic language disorders, there are test batteries available for each patient population (i.e., aphasia, RHD, TBI, and dementia). Aphasia test batteries (e.g., *Western Aphasia Battery*) typically include subtests to evaluate basic skills in each language modality (i.e., listening, speaking, reading, writing). Test batteries for RHD (e.g., *Mini Inventory for Right Brain Damage–II*; MIRBI-II), TBI (e.g., *Scales of Cognitive Ability for Traumatic Brain Injury*), and dementia (e.g., *Arizona Battery for Communication Disorders of Dementia*) include subtests to evaluate language as well as other cognitive abilities such as memory, attention, and executive functioning because of the diverse processes that may be compromised in these neurogenic language disorders.

The main advantage to using test batteries is their efficiency and scope: They provide information concerning the integrity of a number of linguistic and/or cognitive functions in a relatively short period of time. Consequently, test batteries are often a good choice for an initial assessment to document general deficits and to identify areas that may require more in-depth testing. A disadvantage of test batteries is that they often lack a sufficient number of items to provide a precise and reliable characterization of a patient's abilities in each of the modalities or functions evaluated. Additionally, test batteries are often unsuitable for measuring change or recovery because areas in which the patient improved or deteriorated may be underrepresented in the overall test score. Take, for example, the MIRBI that contains only one item to assess reading comprehension. Because only one reading item is included, it becomes difficult for a clinician to determine whether the failure on this item of a patient with RHD should be attributed to a reading comprehension deficit, or perhaps to visual neglect or one of the other cognitive deficits with which that patient presents. Likewise, during an initial evaluation, a patient might fail this item because of a severe reading deficit; following treatment, he might continue to fail this item because, even though his reading abilities improved, they did not improve to the level necessary to pass this item. Accordingly, use of test batteries is associated with a trade-off in that the benefits of their efficiency and scope are countered by their limitations of assessment depth and detail.

Tests of Specific Linguistic and Cognitive Functions

In the ideal clinical setting, which unfortunately has all but disappeared, the clinician should examine in detail all factors that may affect the communicative performance of a patient with a neurogenic language disorder. Therefore, clinicians often need to augment and in some cases substitute test batteries with tests of more specific linguistic or cognitive functions. For example, specific tests are essential when a patient bottoms (i.e., fails all items) or ceilings out (i.e., passes all items) on a test battery: These test performance patterns provide the clinician with little information concerning the patient's areas of relative strength or weakness, and consequently must be supplemented with additional testing to allow for treatment planning. Compared to test batteries, tests of specific functions tend to provide a more precise quantification as well as qualification of the target linguistic or cognitive process, often by including more test items and, importantly, a more diverse range of item difficulty. As will be reviewed in Chapters 5 through 7, a plethora of tests for measuring specific linguistic and cognitive functions have been developed and are available both commercially and in the research literature. Whereas most of these tests discriminate problems at only the ICF body function level, there has been a recent thrust to develop tools for identifying activity and participation limitations as well.

When trying to choose which of these various tests might be most suitable for a given patient, clinicians should bear in mind some of the previously discussed patient characteristic, psychometric, and ethnocultural considerations. For example, a clinician trying to assess the memory abilities of a patient with aphasia will need to select a memory test that has relatively few linguistic demands so that the patient's score reflects that patient's memory rather than memory and language abilities. Likewise, a clinician assessing an elderly patient must pay special attention to the test's normative data, as few tests provide norms for individuals over the age of 80 years. As previously mentioned, in addition to checking test manuals for normative data, clinicians can also search the research literature, where expanded normative data for many tests have been published. For instance, updated and more comprehensive norms for verbal fluency tests such as the *Controlled Oral Word Association Test* (Benton, Hamsher, Rey, & Sivan, 1994) and the *Thurstone Word Fluency Test* (Thurstone & Thurstone, 1962) can be found in several recent research publications (e.g., Ivnik, Malec, Smith, Tangalos, & Petersen, 1996; Gladsjo, Miller, & Heaton, 1999).

Qualitative Assessment Considerations

Most formal, standardized tests provide primarily quantitative information in that they compare a given patient's performance to normative data. Therefore, these tests are most useful for documenting the presence or absence of a neurogenic language disorder. Clinicians must also keep in mind that in terms of treating neurogenic language disorders, it is equally important to collect **qualitative information** about the patient's communication and cognitive skills. Qualitative information pertains to *how* a patient performs a given task and thus concerns the identification of influential task parameters and of patient strategies.

Qualitative information can be gleaned by completing informal observations (as described earlier in this chapter), taking notes about patients' behaviors during standardized testing (e.g., during a spoken naming test, the clinician notes that even though the patient with aphasia cannot verbally name many test items, he is able to write with his finger on the table the first letter of many of these items), interviewing patients after they complete an assessment task (e.g., after completing an auditory comprehension test, the clinician asks the patient whether he had difficulty on the test because he did not understand the words or the grammar, because he forgot the information as the test went on, or both), or implementing test modifications to determine how these modifications influence patients' performances. Common stimulus and administration modifications that might be considered when testing patients with neurogenic language disorders include: (1) shifting the location of visual test stimuli to the unaffected hemispace or to a vertical versus horizontal display for patients with unilateral neglect or visual field deficits; (2) providing both written and verbal instructions for patients with unaided hearing losses, visual problems (e.g., cataracts), or premorbid reading problems; (3) allowing for written or pointing responses for patients with motor speech deficits; (4) enlarging visual stimuli for patients with visual problems; and (5) using auditory trainers or other amplified headphones to help patients compensate for uncorrected hearing loss. Although some of these modifications may negate the use of test norms, the qualitative information gained by implementing these alterations is often more valuable in terms of making prognostic and treatment recommendations than basing prognosis and treatment recommendations on misinterpreted performance and inaccurate information.

CAREGIVER ASSESSMENT

Given the increasing frequency and intensity with which caregivers are expected to participate in the rehabilitation process, it is important that clinicians collect some information about the caregivers of their patients with neurogenic disorders to see if they are willing and capable of participating. This information is very important, given that the caregiver's willingness and ability to provide help have been found to be a more important predictor of functional outcome than brain damage factors such as lesion size or severity of cognitive deficits (Kramer & Coleman, 1999). Likewise, there is a large literature indicating that caring for patients with neurogenic language disorders can have negative effects on the physical and emotional well-being of not only the patient, but also the patient's spouse, family, and other loved ones (Hooker et al., 2002; Le Dorze & Brassard, 1995; Machamer, Temkin, & Dikmen, 2002). Common negative consequences associated with caregiving include depression, guilt, anxiety, anger, and increased drug use, as well as the physical problems that can accompany these emotional problems (e.g., sleep and eating disturbances). Consequently, Le Dorze and Brassard (1995) recommended that caregivers should "not merely be considered as partners in rehabilitation. They may in fact require specific attention for dealing with their problems. Failure to attend to their problems may also lead to further handicaps for both the aphasic person and his or her family and friends" (p. 252).

When a clinician is concerned about the emotional and/or physical health of a caregiver, a screening tool might be used to identify or substantiate quickly if there is reason for concern. An alternate or additional approach would be to refer the caregiver to a family physician, psychiatrist, psychologist, or social worker for an assessment. In terms of screening tools, clinicians could choose among the measures listed in Table 4-8 or described in Chapter 7 if the caregiver's emotional well-being or quality of life, respectively, are of concern. In terms of making referrals, it is useful if the clinician can identify health care professionals in the caregiver's community that are knowledgeable about the neurogenic language disorder with which the caregiver's loved one presents. That is, if the caregiver of a patient with aphasia is having problems with depression, it is often most helpful if the psychologist or counselor to whom the caregiver is referred has an understanding of not only what aphasia is, but also common social and emotional consequences of aphasia.

SHARING ASSESSMENT RESULTS

A good assessment is achieved by not only selecting and completing the most appropriate and efficient assessment procedures, but also by organizing and condensing assessment results into a coherent and concise report. A well-written assessment report serves as the basis of intervention planning by specifying whether a patient requires treatment services and, if so, what treatment priorities and procedures may be most appropriate. Information in the following general areas should be included in a diagnostic report:

1. Background Information—a brief description of the patient's premorbid abilities and daily activities, current living and social situation, vocation, etiology and onset of the neurogenic language disorder, previously identified concomitant symptoms, and previous speech-language pathology services.

2. Assessment Results—a summary of current linguistic and cognitive strengths and weaknesses. This section should include the identification of factors that facilitate and hinder the patient's linguistic and cognitive abilities. Although typically it is not necessary to describe the observation and assessment procedures that were used, under some circumstances (e.g., a litigation case) this information may need to be included in the report.

3. Summary and Recommendations—a synopsis of the assessment findings, including statements regarding the diagnosis or, more specifically, the presence, type, and severity of the neurogenic language disorder. Recommendations regarding whether or not treatment is needed, and if so, provision of suggestions regarding the treatment goals and therapy approach or procedures.

Importantly, these reports must be written so that team members outside the field of speech-language pathology as well as caregivers and patients can understand the contents, and thus the use of professional jargon, slang, and vague terminology must be avoided. Likewise, the length of diagnostic reports should be curtailed as much as possible. As Golper (1996) wrote, "brief notes get read and long narratives do not" (p. 69).

When sharing assessment results with the patient, family, and significant others, clinicians should provide a verbal account at a family conference as well as a written summary. If medical or other professional terminology (e.g., vocabulary related to the etiology or site of brain damage) is to be introduced to the patient and caregivers, the clinician might consider using visual illustrations to define and explain these terms. For example, when reviewing with a patient and his spouse what parts of his brain have been damaged by his traumatic head injury, the clinician might outline those areas on a diagram or model of the brain. Because patients and their caregivers can easily be overloaded with too much information at one time (e.g., receiving reports from physical therapy, neuropsychology, physiatry, and occupational therapy all at the same time) and are often overwhelmed and anxious because of the many issues they are currently facing (e.g., uncertain prognosis, financial concerns, the effects of the medical diagnosis on loved ones), clinicians should also consider reviewing assessment results on more than one occasion to ensure that patients and caregivers understand the results and their implications and that they have had ample time to raise questions about these results (Luterman, 2001).

SUMMARY

As Little and Doherty (1996) concluded "There can be no 'ideal' measure or battery of measures which will provide the information required as economically and acceptably as possible in a psychometrically rigorous way" (p. 495). Therefore, for each patient, the clinician must begin by specifying the purpose of the assessment in terms of what information is needed and why. Only after the purpose of the assessment has been stipulated and complicating conditions (e.g., sensory or motoric problems) have been identified should a clinician begin to choose which formal linguistic and cognitive assessment procedures to use for a given patient. Likewise, clinicians must avoid relying solely on test scores, but also take into consideration the patient's motivation, attitude toward formal testing, coping style, environmental support, and other additional physical, behavioral, and social variables (e.g., fatigue, depression, side effects of medications) when making diagnostic and prognostic decisions. Finally, and perhaps most importantly, clinicians must acknowledge that assessment is an ongoing component of treatment and must occur at every phase of rehabilitation.

Chapter 5

Assessment of Function: Quantifying and Qualifying Linguistic Disorders

LEARNING OBJECTIVES

After reading this chapter you should be able to:

- Specify why observations must precede formal language testing procedures.

- Identify clinical situations in which screening of language abilities is appropriate.

- Compare and contrast test batteries designed for patients with aphasia with those designed for patients with dementia, or cognitive-communicative disorders associated with right hemisphere brain damage or traumatic brain injury.

- List the pros and cons of aphasia classification systems.

- Identify patient populations for whom testing of specific language functions is typically essential.

- Describe tests that evaluate specific linguistic abilities, including comprehension and production of phonology and orthography, lexical-semantics, morphosyntax, and pragmatics and discourse.

- Identify tests that evaluate gesture and drawing abilities.

- Explain the cognitive neuropsychological and neurolinguistic approach to linguistic assessment.

- Explain factors that may confound the administration or interpretation of language tests.

- Describe biographic, medical, and cognitive variables that should be considered when making prognoses about linguistic outcomes.

KEY TERMS

ageism
canonical
circumlocution
cohesion
derivational affix
discourse genre

inflectional affix
informativeness
neologism
paraphasia
relational or closed
   class words

segmental versus
   suprasegmen-
   tal phonology
speech acts
substantive or open
   class words

INTRODUCTION

As reviewed in Chapter 1, language consists of a number of linguistic functions, each of which may be compromised by acquired brain damage or disease. Because the nature (e.g., focal vs. diffuse; static vs. progressive) and location (e.g., cortical vs. subcortical; right vs. left hemisphere; frontal vs. posterior) of brain damage varies among the different neurogenic patient populations, clinicians must be able to assess and treat a variety of circumscribed (i.e., impairment of one specific linguistic process) and broad (i.e., impairment of several linguistic processes) linguistic deficits. For example, a patient who suffers a small, focal stroke to the left parietal lobe might present with only one linguistic symptom: a reading deficit due to impaired access to the orthographic input lexicon (see the model illustrated in Figure 1-1). In contrast, a patient who suffers a severe traumatic brain injury (TBI) and diffuse cortical and subcortical damage to both hemispheres might present with not only this same reading deficit but additional semantic problems that affect his comprehension and production abilities in other language modalities.

The purpose of this chapter, therefore, is to describe assessment procedures specific to evaluating the linguistic components of neurogenic language disorders with an emphasis on procedures and tools that allow quantifying and qualifying linguistic symptoms at the body function level of the International Classification of Functioning, Disability, and Health (ICF) framework (World Health Organization; WHO, 2001). First procedures pertaining to the initial steps of a language assessment, that is, collecting case history and completing unstructured observations, are described. Next, more formal or structured methods for quantifying and qualifying language skills at the ICF level of body function are reviewed, including the administration of test batteries designed to evaluate general language ability and tests that assess more circumscribed linguistic functions. Lastly, factors that should be considered when making prognoses regarding linguistic outcomes are reviewed.

GENERAL ASSESSMENT PROCEDURES

Although the exact format of a language assessment will vary depending on the clinical setting (e.g., acute care hospital vs. skilled nursing facility vs. outpatient rehabilitation) as well as the patient's current needs and abilities, language evaluations designed to quantify and qualify problems at the ICF level of body function generally begin with the completion of a case history and informal observations followed by more formal or structured assessment procedures. The structured component of a language assessment may consist of one or more of the following: (1) a test that only screens general language abilities, (2) a test battery that evaluates a number of language processes and modalities, and/or (3) a test that examines in detail only one or two specific linguistic functions. Regardless of what procedures are selected, clinicians must remain flexible, as each step of the assessment process may reveal new patient strengths and weaknesses that will either negate the use of certain tests and procedures or highlight the need for additional tests and procedures. Likewise, even once the initial evaluation is completed, plans for further assessment are typically necessary to document treatment progress.

CASE HISTORY AND OBSERVATIONS

The collection of case history information is the first essential step of the assessment process, as it aids clinicians in their subsequent selection of informal procedures as well as structured tests. In addition to reviewing medical charts or files, clinicians will need to obtain additional information from patients and, ideally, their caregivers and other health care team members (see Chapter 4 for suggestions regarding what case history information should be accumulated). This information can be acquired by asking patients and caregivers to complete questionnaires or, if time permits, by interviewing them in person. The latter method is preferable, as observations pertaining to patients' communicative strengths and weaknesses as well as their caregivers' communication styles and strategies also can be attained. Figure 5-1 provides an example of a case history or patient intake form that clinicians might adapt for their clinical setting. Clinicians also may consult published tools such as the *Caregiver Administered Communication Inventory* (Tanner & Culberston, 1999a), the *Neurobehavioral Functioning Inventory* (Kreutzer, Seel, & Marwitz, 1999), or the La Trobe Communication Questionnaire (Douglas, O'Flaherty, & Snow, 2000), which require patients and/or caregivers to rate the occurrence or frequency of common cognitive and communicative disorders. Additionally, guidelines for structuring interviews of patients with aphasia or cognitive impairments and their caregivers can be found in *Conversation Analysis Profile for People with Aphasia* (Whitworth, Perkins, & Lesser, 1999a) or *Conversation Analysis Profile for People with Cognitive Impairment* (Perkins, Whitworth, & Lesser, 1997), respectively.

Regardless of how case history information is acquired, clinicians should ensure that some observation of their patients is completed prior to selecting and administering any formal tests. These observations should focus on documenting patients' positive and negative communicative behaviors, as well as the conditions (e.g., environmental conditions, communicative partners, time of day, conversational topic, language modality) under which language successes and failures occur. Clinicians should not limit their observations to just patients' language behaviors, but should also take note of how caregivers interact with the patients. For example, clinicians may watch for whether caregivers utilize strategies that facilitate (e.g., use short, simple commands or reduce ambient noise to enhance the patient's auditory comprehension) or impede (e.g., correct the patient's output or ask for multiple repetitions that lead to patient frustration) the patients' language abilities. Observations are particularly important in certain clinical settings and for assessing certain patient populations. For example, in acute care facilities, patients with neurogenic conditions are often unable to complete structured or formal language tests because of their physical limitations and/or emotional reactions to the onset of their neurological insult and subsequent symptoms (Holland & Fridriksson, 2001; Marshall, 1997). Observations also may be the primary means for assessing patients who present with a broad range of severe impairments (e.g., severe hemiparesis, aphasia, apraxia, and cognitive deficits), as most formal language tests will

Demographic/Backgrouund Information

1. Name _____ 2. Birthplace _____

3. Address _____ 4. Birth date _____

5. Phone Number _____ 6. Date of Report _____

7. Patient's native language(s) _____ If not English, at what age did the patient learn
   English? _____ What other languages does the patient speak, read, and/or write?

   _____

8. Patient's ethnocultural background _____

9. Patient's highest level of education _____

10. Patient's current, or, if retired, previous, primary occupation _____

11. List patient's interests or favorite activities _____

    _____

    _____

12. Marital status: single _____ widowed _____ separated _____

                             married _____ divorced _____ remarried _____

13. List patient's primary caregiver and/or immediate family members:

Name	Age	Relationship	Phone Number	E-Mail
_____	_____	_____	_____	_____
_____	_____	_____	_____	_____
_____	_____	_____	_____	_____
_____	_____	_____	_____	_____
_____	_____	_____	_____	_____

Medical History

1. Date of injury or onset of symptoms _____

2. Patient's handedness (before stroke or disease onset): Right _____ Left _____
   Ambidextrous _____

3. Does the patient wear glasses? _____ See well enough to read _____ Have any other visual problems, such as right/left visual field cut, cataracts, or macular degeneration? _____

4. Does the patient have a hearing loss? _____ Wear a hearing aid? _____ If yes, in the right ear
   _____, left ear _____, or both _____?

Figure 5-1. Example of a case history or patient intake form.

5. Describe the patient's general health _____

_____

_____

6. List the patient's current medications and dosages:

_____

_____

_____

7. Has the patient had or currently have any of the following?

Onset Date and Current Status

Stroke	Yes	No	_____
Aphasia	Yes	No	_____
Other Communication Disorder	Yes	No	_____
Right or Left-Sided Weakness	Yes	No	_____
Neglect	Yes	No	_____
Dementia	Yes	No	_____
Memory Impairment	Yes	No	_____
Other Neurological Disease	Yes	No	_____
Head Injury	Yes	No	_____
Seizure Disorder	Yes	No	_____
Clinical Depression	Yes	No	_____
Other Psychiatric Problems	Yes	No	_____
Alcohol Abuse/Problems	Yes	No	_____
Other Substance Abuse	Yes	No	_____
Other Major Illness	Yes	No	_____

Communication and Cognitive Status and Needs

1. Patient's current or suspected communication and/or cognitive problems _____

_____

2. What communication and/or cognitive problems, if any, are of concern to the patient and caregiver?

_____

_____

_____

Figure 5-1. *Continued.*

3. Cause of current or suspected communication and/or cognitive problems _____

_____

4. Date of onset of communication and/or cognitive problems _____

5. Describe the patient's ability to communicate:

   Preferred output language modality _____

   Most successful output language modality _____

   Most successful input language modality _____

   Pragmatic strengths/weaknesses _____

   _____

6. Current commnication strategies used by:

   Patient _____

   Caregivers _____

7. Describe the patient's cognitive status:

   Attention _____

   Memory _____

   Executive Functioning _____

8. Has the patient received previous:

	Dates	Agency	Address
a. speech-language therapy	_____	_____	_____
b. audiology	_____	_____	_____
c. cognitive assessment	_____	_____	_____
d. cognitive therapy	_____	_____	_____

Figure 5-1. *Continued.*

be beyond their ability level, resulting in basal level test performances (i.e., at or near 0% accuracy) (Beaumont, Marjoribanks, Flury, & Lintern, 1999). Likewise, patients whose language problems are primarily reflective of high level cognitive deficits typically perform well on structured tasks and in controlled environments (Bernicot & Dardier, 2001; Murray & Ramage, 2000); therefore, failure to observe their language behaviors in less predictable settings may result in an overestimation of their language skills. Accordingly, for at least some patients, observation may provide the most valid, reliable, and thus informative means of qualifying a neurogenic language disorder.

SCREENING OR BEDSIDE PROCEDURES

Typically, screening tests are used in acute health care settings, or when there is little time available for assessment and only general information concerning a patient's linguistic abilities is needed (e.g., is the patient aphasic or not aphasic?). The purposes of screening or bedside tests are to establish efficiently the presence or absence of language disorders, and to identify language skills in need of further assessment or that will be the focus of initial treatment (Al-Khawaja, Wade, & Collin, 1996). Because of these tests' short length and tendency to sample only a narrow range of language functions, clinicians must keep in mind that screening tests do not provide a complete depiction of patients' language profiles. Instead, they are useful when: (1) in the early and acute stages of recovery from stroke, TBI, or other abrupt-onset neurological disorder, patients are too ill or fatigued to undergo a lengthy evaluation; (2) the patients' length of stay in the clinical facility is brief; or (3) cost containment dictates immediate clinical information without extensive testing.

Clinicians have two options for screening language abilities: They may create their own screening or bedside tools, or utilize commercially available tests. Those interested in developing their own screening protocol should consult Holland and Fridriksson (2001). These researchers provided suggestions for developing brief as well as functional diagnostic activities such as: (1) having patients read their get well cards to evaluate reading aloud and/or comprehension skills; (2) making mistakes such as calling the patient by the wrong name to determine if the error is caught and, if so, how is it addressed (i.e., does patient respond in a pragmatically appropriate manner); and (3) encouraging patients to complete their daily hospital menu to assess reading and basic writing abilities. A strength of informal protocols is that they can be developed to reflect the specific needs of the primary patient profile. For example, items on a protocol designed to screen patients being admitted to an Alzheimer's disease unit would most likely differ from those on a protocol for screening patients being admitted to a stroke rehabilitation unit. A weakness of informal protocols is that often the validity and reliability of the data gleaned from these measures cannot be determined because clinicians have not established observation or measurement consistency within and across clinicians or over time (Peach, 2001).

Because of their convenience and typically stronger psychometric properties (Davis, 2000), many clinicians utilize published screening tests versus informal protocols. As shown in Table 5-1, most language screening instruments that are

Table 5-1. Screening or Bedside Tests of Linguistic Disorders

INSTRUMENT	SOURCE
Acute Aphasia Screening Protocol	Crary et al. (1989)
Aphasia Language Performance Scales	Keenan & Brassell (1975)
Aphasia Screening Test	Reitan (1991)
Bedside Evaluation Screening Test–II	West et al. (1998)
Cognistat	Kiernan et al. (1995)
Frenchay Aphasia Screening Test	Enderby et al. (1997)
In-Patient Functional Communication Interview	McCooey et al. (2000)
Mississippi Aphasia Screening Test	Nakase-Thompson et al. (2003)
Sheffield Screening Test for Acquired Language Disorders	Syder et al. (1993)
Shortened Porch Index of Communicative Ability	Holtzapple et al. (1989)
Sklar Aphasia Scale	Sklar (1983)
The Aphasia Screening Test–II	Whurr (1997)
Quick Assessment for Aphasia	Tanner & Culbertson (1999)

commercially available or described in the research literature have been specifically developed for patients with aphasia. For example, the *Bedside Evaluation Screening Test–2* (BEST-2; West et al., 1998) was designed to evaluate in 20 minutes or less the listening, speaking, and reading skills of both high- and low-level aphasic patients. BEST-2 was standardized on approximately 200 patients, has acceptable reliability and validity, and provides two sets of norms: those for patients less than 75 years of age and those for patients over the age of 75. Because BEST-2 does not assess writing, clinicians may instead select the *Aphasia Language Performance Scales* (ALPS; Keenan & Brassell, 1975), as this screening test has four scales (i.e., Listening, Talking, Reading, Writing), each of which has 10 items of increasing difficulty. Another benefit of the ALPS is that a Spanish version is available.

Another option for screening language is using shortened versions of more comprehensive language test batteries. For instance, shorter versions of several aphasia test batteries, including the *Minnesota Test for Differential Diagnosis of*

Aphasia (Powell, Bailey, & Clark, 1980) and the *Porch Index of Communicative Ability* (Holtzapple, Pohlman, LaPointe, & Graham, 1989), can be found in the research literature. Likewise, a short version of the *Boston Diagnostic Aphasia Examination* (BDAE-3; Goodglass et al., 2000) can be purchased by itself or along with this comprehensive test battery. The short form is a truncated version of the BDAE-3 that assesses spoken and written language production and comprehension skills in 30 to 45 minutes.

Whereas there are many test options available for screening for the presence of aphasia or basic language impairments, there remains a need to develop tools that are appropriate for identifying the high-level language difficulties (e.g., impaired comprehension of implied information; inefficient or disorganized discourse production) that are characteristic of patients with TBI, with right hemisphere brain damage (RHD), or who are in the early stages of certain dementing illnesses (e.g., Parkinson's disease). Even screening instruments such as *Cognistat* (Kiernan, Mueller, & Langston, 1995), which were standardized on patients representing a broad spectrum of neurogenic disorders, focus on assessing lower-level language abilities. An exception is the La Trobe Communication Questionnaire (Douglas et al., 2000), which measures the perceptions of patients with TBI and their caregivers regarding the patients' communicative abilities. It consists of two forms, one for the patient and one for the caregiver to complete. Each form has the same 30 items that are rated on a four-point scale to indicate whether the discourse-level, cognitive-communicative problems occur never or rarely, sometimes, often, or usually or always. Sample items include "Go over and over the same ground in conversation," "Switch to a different topic of conversation too quickly," "Carry on talking about things for too long in your conversations," "Keep track of the main details of conversations," and "Answer without taking time to think about what the other person has said." Although this questionnaire has been found reliable for evaluating the perceived communicative abilities of young adults, its suitability for older individuals has not yet been established. Accordingly, when clinicians suspect and want to document the presence of high-level language difficulties in older patients, they will need to rely on observations or informal protocols that allow them to quantify and qualify their patients' interactions in a variety of contexts and with a number of conversational partners.

Side Bar

Screening: A Good Place to Start but a Bad Place to End

Clinicians must always keep in mind that a pass on a screening test does not invariably signify that the patient has intact linguistic abilities. For example, Mr. Russell suffered a left hemisphere stroke that affected small portions of his parietal and occipital lobes. At two days post-stroke, he accurately completed the ALPS. Although his clinician noted that some of his test responses were slow, she attributed this to fatigue, as Mr. Russell had complained

(continued)

of feeling extremely tired since his stroke. Because no one, including Mr. Russell, his family, or other health care team members, voiced any concerns regarding Mr. Russell's communication abilities, the clinician concluded that further speech-language therapy services were not needed. Unfortunately, upon discharge to home, Mr. Russell began to experience significant communication problems, including word retrieval difficulties, problems reading the newspaper, and difficulties completing daily e-mail and online chatroom activities. Had his clinician extended Mr. Russell's initial language assessment to include observation of him discussing controversial issues or talking in noisy environments, his word-finding difficulties would have been evident. Likewise, had the clinician included reading and writing tasks reflective of his daily reading and writing needs in his screening, his written word retrieval difficulties and visual scanning problems would also have been exposed.

○ TEST BATTERIES

In rehabilitation and long-term health care settings or when more assessment time is available and patients have adequate stamina, clinicians may begin a language assessment by administering a test battery specific to their patient's documented or presumed neurogenic language diagnosis. For instance, a clinician would administer an aphasia battery to a patient who has already been diagnosed with aphasia or whom she suspects has aphasia based on initial assessment data. Whereas aphasia test batteries have been around for over 40 years, the development of test batteries for patient populations with RHD, TBI, and dementia has only occurred over the last 15 years; consequently, fewer test battery options are available for these patient populations (Table 5-2). When utilizing test batteries, clinicians must keep in mind that even though these tools provide more comprehensive data than screening tests, their primary functions are to identify the presence and severity of a language disorder and to highlight language functions that may be compromised. In most cases, they are not designed to indicate the specific linguistic or cognitive locus of the identified language disorder. Consequently, test battery results should ideally be supplemented by findings from tests of specific linguistic and/or cognitive functions prior to specifying treatment goals and procedures.

APHASIA TEST BATTERIES

Aphasia test batteries consist primarily of tasks designed to assess basic language functions (e.g., semantics, syntax) in each communication modality (i.e., speaking, listening, reading, writing, gesturing). As shown in Table 5-2, a number of batteries are currently available, each having its own distinct strengths and weaknesses. Those batteries that are particularly popular in clinical and research settings in the

Table 5-2. Test Batteries for Specific Neurogenic Language Disorders

TARGET NEUROGENIC LANGUAGE DISORDER	INSTRUMENT	SOURCE
Aphasia	Aphasia Diagnostic Profiles	Helm-Estabrooks (1992)
	Assessment of Communicative Effectiveness in Severe Aphasia	Cunningham et al. (1995)
	Assessment of Language-Related Functional Activities	Baines et al. (1999)
	Bilingual Aphasia Examination	Paradis & Libben (1987)
	Boston Assessment of Severe Aphasia	Helm-Estabrooks et al. (1989)
	Boston Diagnostic Aphasia Examination, 3rd Ed.	Goodglass et al. (2001)
	Burns Brief Inventory of Communication and Cognition: Left Hemisphere Inventory	Burns (1997)
	Comprehensive Aphasia Test	Swinburn et al. (2004)
	Examining for Aphasia–III	Eisenson (1994)
	Minnesota Test for Differential Diagnosis	Schuell (1965b)
	Multilingual Aphasia Examination, 3rd Ed.	Benton et al. (2001)
	Neuropsychological Assessment Battery– Language Module	Stern & White (2003)
	Neurosensory Center Comprehensive Examination for Aphasia	Spreen & Benton (1977)
	Porch Index of Communicative Ability	Porch (1981)
	Western Aphasia Battery	Kertesz (1982)
Right Hemisphere Disorders	Assessment of Language-Related Functional Activities	Baines et al. (1999)
	Burns Brief Inventory of Communication and Cognition: Right Hemisphere Inventory	Burns (1997)
	Mini Inventory of Right Brain Injury–II	Pimental & Kingsbury (2000)
	Right Hemisphere Language Battery–II	Bryan (1995)
	RIC Evaluation of Communication Problems in Right Hemisphere Dysfunction–Revised	Halper et al. (1996)
Traumatic Brain Injury Disorders	Brief Test of Head Injury	Helm-Estabrooks & Hotz (1991)
	Burns Brief Inventory of Communication and Cognition: Complex Neuropathology Inventory	Burns (1997)

(continues)

Table 5-2. *Continued*

TARGET NEUROGENIC LANGUAGE DISORDER	INSTRUMENT	SOURCE
Traumatic Brain Injury Disorders (*continued*)	OWLS: Oral and Written Language Scales	Carrow-Woolfolk (1995–96)
	Repeatable Battery for the Assessment of Neuropsychological Status	Randolph (1998)
	Scales of Cognitive Ability for Traumatic Brain Injury	Adamovich & Henderson (1992)
	Test of Adolescent and Adult Language–3	Hammill et al. (1994)
Dementia	Arizona Battery for Communication Disorders of Dementia	Bayles & Tomoeda (1993)
	Burns Brief Inventory of Communication and Cognition: Complex Neuropathology Inventory	Burns (1997)
	Functional Linguistic Communication Inventory	Bayles & Tomoeda (1994)
	Repeatable Battery for the Assessment of Neuropsychological Status	Randolph (1998)
	Severe Impairment Battery	Saxton et al. (1993)

United States and Canada for assessing acute and chronic aphasia (Katz et al., 2000) include the *Minnesota Test for Differential Diagnosis of Aphasia* (MTDDA; Schuell, 1965b), the *Boston Diagnostic Aphasia Examination* (BDAE; Goodglass & Kaplan, 1983; Goodglass et al., 2001), the *Western Aphasia Battery* (WAB; Kertesz, 1982), and the *Aphasia Diagnostic Profiles* (ADP; Helm-Estabrooks, 1992).

The MTDDA (Schuell, 1965b) is one of the oldest and most thorough aphasia batteries, consisting of 46 subtests for assessing spoken and written language production and comprehension abilities. Unfortunately, many aspects of this test are now outdated, including its stimuli and aphasia classification system. Furthermore, the texts that contain MTDDA normative data and guidelines for interpreting test results (e.g., *Differential Diagnosis of Aphasia with the Minnesota Test*; Schuell, 1965a) are no longer commercially available. Given that several other more recently developed aphasia batteries are now available, use of the MTDDA is no longer advocated.

The remaining popular aphasia batteries evaluate all language modalities and were designed to categorize patients' language profiles into connectionist aphasia syndromes (e.g., Broca's, Wernicke's, transcortical motor). For example, the WAB (Kertesz, 1982) consists of 10 oral language subtests, which assess spoken language production and comprehension, and an additional seven other subtests, which evaluate written language production and comprehension, praxis, and construction skills. Aphasia types are assigned on the basis of specific test scores, and three summary scores can be calculated to quantify WAB performances: (1) the Aphasia Quotient, based on scores from the oral language subtests, (2) the Language Quotient, based on scores from the oral, reading, and writing subtests (for specific instruction for calculating this score, see Shewan & Kertesz, 1984), and (3) the Cortical Quotient, based on scores from all subtests. A software program, The Western Aphasia Battery Scoring Assistant (Kertesz, 1993), is currently available to facilitate data reporting and calculation of the Aphasia and Cortical Quotient summary scores. Whereas Kertesz (1982; Shewan & Kertesz, 1980) reported that the WAB possesses strong psychometric properties in terms of both reliability and validity, Ross and Wertz (2001) identified significant correlations between age and Aphasia and Cortical Quotients. These findings indicate that additional assessment data must be acquired to assist in interpreting the WAB outcomes of elderly patients, and to avoid underestimating their language abilities.

With the ADP (Helm-Estabrooks, 1992), clinicians may identify the nature and severity of aphasia, monitor language recovery, and document the general social-emotional status of their patients. The ADP consists of 10 subtests that assess speaking, listening, reading, writing, and gestural modalities, and has a faster administration time of approximately 30 minutes (at least for mildly impaired patients), compared to the other aphasia batteries. It is quicker in part because its reading and writing sections are short, and thus follow-up testing in these language modalities will be necessary for at least some patients. The ADP also contains a list of behaviors that clinicians can use to screen for social-emotional problems such as lability, anxiety, and impulsiveness. ADP raw scores are converted to subtest and summary standard scores, which in turn can be used to determine aphasia type. Furthermore, confidence ranges (i.e., standard error of measurement intervals) can be plotted for each subtest and summary standard score so that clinicians can identify significant changes in their patients' language abilities over time. The ADP is a suitable test choice for many patients, as it was standardized on a large sample of neurological patients (primarily those with left hemisphere stroke) who represented a broad range of ages and education levels.

The BDAE-3 (Goodglass et al., 2001) represents an updated and expanded version of Goodglass and Kaplan's (1983) earlier and extremely popular BDAE. The Standard Test of the BDAE-3 has many of the same subtests found in earlier BDAE editions for evaluating conversational and narrative speech (e.g., description of the Cookie Theft Picture), auditory and reading comprehension (e.g., Commands), oral and written expression (e.g., Responsive Naming), and repetition; the Standard Test also utilizes similar rating scales and scoring procedures to determine aphasia severity and type. Like its predecessors, the BDAE-3 manual describes supplementary tests to examine nonverbal skills, such as drawing to command and finger agnosia. Most new subtests are part of the BDAE-3's Extended Test and include retelling Aesop's Fables, Word Comprehension by Categories,

Semantic Probe (i.e., comprehension of semantic features of target nouns), Syntactic Processing (i.e., comprehension of semantically reversible and complex syntactic forms), Naming in Categories, Lexical Decision, Phonics (e.g., identifying homophones), Derivational and Grammatical Morphology, spelling Nonsense Words, and Limb/Hand and Bucco-Facial/Respiratory Praxis. These Extended subtests allow clinicians to form more precise linguistic explanations of their patient's communication difficulties. There also is a BDAE-3 Short Form that may be utilized when time or patient factors such as fatigue necessitate only screening patients' language abilities. Another addition is the Language Competency Index that can be calculated if the Standard Test and the *Boston Naming Test* (Kaplan, Goodglass, & Weintraub, 2001) have been given. This index is calculated from percentile scores from expressive syntax, auditory comprehension, and naming measures, and was designed to provide a quantitative indicator of the severity of patients' language impairment, although guidelines regarding the interpretation of this index are not provided. Despite many improvements (e.g., choice of administering Standard, Extended, or Short Test Forms, addition of new subtests), the psychometric properties of the BDAE-3 remain weak. For example, its standardization sample is relatively small, ranging from 85 to only 33 aphasic subjects across subtests, and demographic characteristics of the standardization sample are not provided. Likewise, the test manual provides no information pertaining to intra- or inter-rater or test-retest reliability, or construct validity.

In addition to the above frequently used aphasia batteries, there also are comprehensive tests for special populations of patients with aphasia. For example, when assessing patients who do not speak English or speak it as a second language, clinicians may choose from aphasia tests created in another language (e.g., Aachen Aphasia Battery; Huber et al., 1983, 1984), translated versions of aphasia tests originally developed in English (e.g., Hua et al., 1997; Mazaux & Orgozo, 1981), or aphasia tests that offer several language versions that are functionally and culturally equivalent in content (versus simply direct translations), such as the *Bilingual Aphasia Test* (Paradis & Libben, 1987, 1993) or the *Multilingual Aphasia Examination* (Benton et al., 2001; Rey, Sivan, & Benton, 1991). Of these options, the first and last are preferred, as direct translations of English tests do not take into consideration language and/or cultural differences. For example, items on a naming subtest may vary from high to low word frequency in English, but when translated to another language, only represent low frequency words.

Aphasia test batteries specific to patients with severe language impairments, including the *Boston Assessment of Severe Aphasia* (BASA; Helm-Estabrooks, Ramsberger, Morgan, & Nicholas, 1989) and the Assessment of Communicative Effectiveness in Severe Aphasia (Cunningham, Farrow, Davies, & Lincoln, 1995), also are available. These tests tend to probe simpler language functions and have more liberal response requirements so that patients with severe aphasia do not simply receive basal-level scores, which in turn do not provide insight into language areas of relative strength but only indicate areas of weakness. For instance, whereas on other aphasia batteries only verbal responses are scored as correct or incorrect, on the BASA *both* gestural and verbal responses are scored in terms of whether they are *partially* or *fully* communicative, and clinicians also record refusals, perseverations, and affective responses. Therefore, more qualitative and quantitative information regarding the language abilities of patients with severe aphasia can be obtained using these special tests versus traditional aphasia batteries.

Aphasia Classification: Pros and Cons

As just described, most aphasia test batteries (e.g., WAB, ADP, BDAE-3), in addition to identifying the presence and severity of language impairments, help clinicians categorize their patients' language profiles into aphasia types (see also Chapter 2). The most common classification system to which most aphasia test batteries adhere is anatomically based and includes Broca's, Wernicke's, conduction, anomic, transcortical motor, transcortical sensory, transcortical mixed, and global aphasia types. Even when the test battery does not assist with aphasia classification (e.g., *Burns*), clinicians often will still qualify their patients' language symptoms using the dichotomous classifications of fluent versus nonfluent aphasia (some physicians also still use the dichotomous categories of receptive vs. expressive aphasia).

As touched upon in Chapter 2, however, there are several negatives associated with these aphasia classification systems (Byng, Kay, Edmundson, & Scott, 1990; Caplan, 1993; Gordon, 1998; Varney, 1998; Wertz, 1984). First, as many practicing clinicians can attest, many patients' language symptoms do not neatly fit into just one aphasia type, with some clinicians and researchers estimating that they have difficulty assigning an aphasia classification to up to 70% of their patients. Second, the language symptoms of patients within a given aphasia type are not truly homogenous (e.g., some patients with Wernicke's aphasia have greater reading than auditory comprehension deficits, whereas other Wernicke's patients show the inverse profile). Third, dichotomous classification systems (e.g., receptive vs. expressive; sensory vs. motor) are often misleading, as both language comprehension and production are impaired, at least to some degree, in most patients with aphasia. Fourth, aphasia classification may be influenced by which aphasia test battery is used (e.g., the aphasia type assigned to a given patient may differ depending on whether the ADP, WAB, or BDAE-3 was used). Fifth, aphasia classifications do not specify the nature of the patients' underlying linguistic problems (e.g., a semantic vs. lexical access problem), and consequently do not provide a sufficient basis for selecting treatment goals and procedures. Despite these limitations, use of classification systems will likely persist in both clinical practice and research because, for at least some patients, use of an aphasia type succinctly describes their language syndrome to other clinicians or researchers. That is, when other clinicians or researchers read this label in the medical chart, clinical report, or published study, they will have a good general idea of what specific language symptoms to expect in the patient.

RIGHT HEMISPHERE TEST BATTERIES

A few standardized test batteries are available for assessing cognitive-communicative disorders associated with RHD (see Table 5-2). RHD test batteries contrast with aphasia batteries in two significant ways. First, RHD batteries assess not only language abilities but also cognitive functions, such as attention, that are commonly compromised by RHD. Second, whereas aphasia batteries evaluate basic language processes, RHD batteries examine higher-level language processes (e.g., interpretation of figurative language) and pragmatic skills that are more frequently affected by RHD. Accordingly, clinicians should avoid administering aphasia test batteries to their RHD patients, as most RHD patients will either ceiling out on the language tasks (perform at or near 100% accuracy) or display difficulties that are cognitively versus linguistically based. For example, a patient with RHD who errs on matching spoken words to pictures, a common task on aphasia test batteries, might be making mistakes because of visual neglect rather than poor auditory comprehension.

The *Mini Inventory of Right Brain Injury* (MIRBI; Pimental & Kingsbury, 1989) and the more recently updated MIRBI-II (Pimental & Kingsbury, 2000) were designed to identify quickly patients with RHD between the ages of 20 and 90 who are having difficulties in one or more of the following areas: visuoperception, neglect, affect, orientation, memory, behavior, and language. MIRBI-II test items are arranged into the following 10 sections: visual scanning, integrity of gnosis, integrity of body image, visuoverbal processing (i.e., reading and writing), visuosymbolic processing, integrity of visuomotor praxis (i.e., drawing), higher-level language skills (e.g., interpretation of humor), expressing emotion, general affect, and general behavior. Because only a few items are dedicated to assessing each section, this test is actually more similar to a screening test than a comprehensive test battery and typically can be completed in less than 30 minutes. Integrity of body image, general affect, and general behavioral processing sections are based on clinicians' ratings versus patients' performance of specific test procedures; for example, to quantify general affect, a plus/minus rating is used to indicate whether or not patients display flat effect (i.e., decreased intonation, little variation in facial expression). Total raw scores on the MIRBI-II can be converted to standardized scores, percentiles, and an overall severity rating that ranges from normal to profound impairment. The psychometric properties of the MIRBI-II exceed those of the original version in terms of reliability, validity, and size and description of the RHD normative sample (e.g., 128 vs. 30 RHD subjects for the MIRBI-II vs. MIRBI). In summary, MIRBI findings may be used to determine the presence and general severity of RHD-related cognitive-communicative problems, but must be supplemented by additional observational and test findings before treatment goals and procedures should be specified.

The *Burns Brief Inventory of Communication and Cognition* (Burns, 1997) consists of three sections: a Left Hemisphere Inventory for patients with aphasia, a

Complex Neuropathology Inventory for patients with TBI or dementia, and a Right Hemisphere Inventory for patients with RHD. The Right Hemisphere Inventory is designed to identify attention, visuospatial perception and construction, and communicative impairments, and consists of 12 tasks such as visual scanning, clock drawing and recognizing familiar faces to assess attention and visuospatial skills, and interpreting implied information and idioms to assess abstract language abilities. Scores for each task are plotted on a grid to indicate whether for that particular skill, the patient has a severe deficit (i.e., impaired to a degree that rapid improvement in treatment is unlikely), moderate deficit (i.e., impaired but likely to respond to treatment), mild deficit (i.e., unlikely to be an immediate treatment priority), or no deficit (i.e., perfect score on the task). The test manual also provides standard error of measurement for each task so that meaningful changes in patients' performances across repeated testings can be determined. Like the other *Burns* inventories, the Right Hemisphere Inventory takes approximately 30 minutes to administer and is suitable for patients between the ages of 18 and 80. The *Burns* was validated on a sample of 333 individuals representing a spectrum of neurogenic disorders (i.e., left or right stroke, TBI, dementia) and reports acceptable levels of reliability and validity. Because most tasks consist of only five items, follow-up testing is frequently essential to qualify problem areas.

Although there are at least four test batteries currently available that were developed specifically for assessing the cognitive-communicative abilities of patients with RHD (see Table 5-2), all have content and/or standardization weaknesses that limit their usefulness. For example, as Tompkins and Lehman (1997) cautioned: "Theoretical foundations for these measures are often underdeveloped and out-of-date," "Standardization samples are typically small and poorly characterized," and "Reliability and validity data also are diluted by questionable evidence and methods for deriving them" (pp. 282–283). Whereas some tests have been revised to address, at least in part, some of Tompkins and Lehman's critique (e.g., MIRBI-II), clinicians should avoid relying solely on the results of these test batteries when attempting to quantify and qualify cognitive-communicative disorders related to RHD.

TRAUMATIC BRAIN INJURY TEST BATTERIES

To date, a limited number of test batteries have been developed to assess the presence and severity of cognitive-communicative deficits associated with TBI (see Table 5-2). In fact, prior to the 1990s, clinicians relied upon tests developed for other patient populations (particularly aphasia tests) or utilized their own informal assessment protocols (Schwartz, 1989). Aphasia tests, however, are only appropriate for the minority of TBI patients who present with frank language deficits (Sarno, Buonaguro, A., & Levin, 1986), as they were not designed to assess the types of high-level language and discourse problems that are a more common consequence of TBI (Chapman et al., 1992; Duff et al., 2002; McDonald & Pearce, 1998). Generally, TBI test batteries evaluate not only high-level language abilities, but also a range of basic cognitive functions, as these too are commonly compromised by head injury and may contribute to these patients' communicative difficulties (e.g., Turkstra & Holland, 1998).

In 1992, a more suitable TBI test option became available, the *Scales of Cognitive Assessment for Traumatic Brain Injury* (SCATBI; Adamovich & Henderson, 1992). The SCATBI is appropriate for patients representing a spectrum of TBI severities, and consists of five sections: Organization (e.g., Sequencing Words subtest), Recall (e.g., Recall of Oral Paragraphs subtest), Orientation (e.g., Pre- and Post-morbid Questions subtests), Reasoning (e.g., Inductive Reasoning: Analogies subtest), and Perception/Discrimination (e.g., Shape Discrimination subtest). Test administration time will fluctuate depending on the severity of the patient's symptoms, varying from 30 minutes for mildly impaired patients to over 2 hours for those with more severe impairments. Clinicians have the option of administering individual subtests or the entire battery, depending on the patient's needs and time constraints. Raw scores for each test section as well as a total test score can be converted to percentiles and standard scores, and can be used to determine an overall severity rating (i.e., severe, moderate, mild, borderline normal, and normal). Standard errors of measurement are also available so that clinicians can determine whether changes in patients' performances over time are meaningful or significant. The test was standardized on a large sample of patients with TBI whose demographic and medical characteristics matched those representative of the population of patients with TBI; for instance, most had suffered a closed head injury, were male, and were younger than 50 years old (median age = 30). Whereas certain psychometric properties appear acceptable and are given adequate discussion in the test manual (e.g., concurrent validity), others receive only cursory attention (e.g., inter-rater reliability).

The *Brief Test of Head Injury* (BTHI; Helm-Estabrooks & Hotz, 1991) also was developed specifically for patients with TBI, but particularly those with more severe or acute injuries. The BTHI takes approximately 30 minutes to administer and assesses orientation/attention, auditory (e.g., following commands) and reading comprehension, spoken language production (e.g., naming, picture description), memory (e.g., word recall), and visuospatial abilities (e.g., matching of abstract designs). Stimuli and response demands were designed to be suitable for patients with concomitant motor symptoms or visual neglect. In terms of scoring, either verbal or gestural responses can receive full credit on several test items, again indicating the suitability of this test for more severely impaired patients. BTHI performances can be converted into cluster standard scores (i.e., scores for each cognitive-communicative domain) or a total standard score. The total test score can also be interpreted as a Severity Score (i.e., Severe, Moderate, Mild, Borderline Normal). Confidence intervals also can be plotted, making the BTHI suitable for repeated testings. It was standardized on a large sample of patients with TBI (*n* =

265) and small sample of healthy controls ($n = 29$), most of whom were less than 50 years old and male. Acceptable levels of several forms of reliability and validity are reported in the test manuals, although specific statistical data for some psychometric properties such as inter-rater reliability are not provided.

Another option, particularly for younger patients who have TBI, is the *Test of Adolescent and Adult Language–3* (TOAL-3; Hammill, Brown, Larsen, & Wiederholt, 1994). This test evaluates semantic and syntactic aspects of listening (i.e., spoken word-to-picture and spoken sentence-to-picture matching), speaking (i.e., generating spoken sentences using a target word, repetition of grammatically complex sentences), reading (i.e., identifying semantically related written words, identifying written sentences that convey similar meanings), and writing skills (i.e., generating written sentences using a target word, combining two or more sentences into one written sentence). To speed test administration, basals and ceilings are used. A basal occurs when the patient achieves five consecutive, correct responses; all items below this basal are then assumed to be correct and are not administered. A ceiling occurs when the patient makes five consecutive errors; all items above this point are assumed to be incorrect and are not administered. Composite standard scores for each language modality (i.e., listening, speaking, reading, writing), for spoken versus written language skills, for semantic versus syntactic skills, for receptive versus expressive language skills, and for general language ability can be calculated. To help determine areas of strength and weakness, difference scores are provided so that clinicians can identify meaningful differences among the various composite scores, For instance, only when the difference between expressive and receptive composite scores exceeds a difference score of 8 should that difference be considered significant. The TOAL-3 was standardized on an extensive sample of individuals up to the age of 24 years, 11 months. Although the test manual reports strong psychometric properties, recent research suggests that the construct validity of certain subtests is suspect. For example, Turkstra and Holland (1998) identified a significant influence of working memory on performances of the listening/grammar subtest, indicating that memory skills are also evaluated by this subtest.

Despite the current availability of test batteries specifically designed for populations of patients with TBI, survey data indicate that many clinicians continue to utilize tests standardized on other patient populations. For example, Frank and Barrineau (1996), Duff et al. (2002), and more recently the Academy of Neurological Communication Disorders and Sciences (2004) found that the BDAE was one of the most frequently utilized test batteries when clinicians were assessing cognitive-communicative disorders associated with TBI. This is unfortunate given that (1) the BDAE was only standardized on patients with aphasia (i.e., primarily left hemisphere stroke patients), (2) this test does not evaluate the types of cognitive-communicative problems that patients with TBI frequently endure (i.e., pragmatic communication deficits), and (3) more appropriate test batteries are now available. As Duff et al. (2002) warned, clinicians using aphasia tests "will not have clinically valid information on the individual [with TBI] and the extent of his/her deficits.

Ultimately, this may prevent detection and administration of proper information and treatment referrals" (p. 782).

DEMENTIA TEST BATTERIES

Similar to RHD and TBI test batteries, dementia test batteries are limited in number and evaluate language as well as cognitive skills (see Table 5-2). They contrast with RHD and TBI batteries, however, in that the content of their language subtests focuses more on basic rather than high-level language skills. Clinicians should note that because Alzheimer's disease is the most frequent cause of dementia, most dementia test batteries were designed to identify and quantify the types of language and cognitive impairments associated with this dementing disease. This means that these tests may not be suitable for patients with other forms of dementia, as the types and progression of language and cognitive symptoms are not uniform across all dementing illnesses (see Chapters 2 and 3). For example, an aphasia battery may be more appropriate for patients in the early stages of frontotemporal dementia, as many of their initial symptoms are language-based, including problems with syntax (Grossman, 2002), a deficit that would not be quantified by current dementia test batteries. This point highlights the need for clinicians always to assure that the demographic and clinical characteristics of their patients match those of the subject sample on which the tests they use were developed and standardized.

The *Arizona Battery for Communication Disorders of Dementia* (ABCD; Bayles & Tomoeda, 1993) represents the first commercially available test battery for assessing communication disorders associated with dementing diseases. The ABCD has 14 subtests that assess language comprehension (e.g., Following Commands, Comparative Questions, Reading Comprehension subtests), language production (e.g., Repetition, Confrontation Naming, Object Description subtests), memory (e.g., Mental Status, Story Retelling Immediate and Delayed, Word Learning subtests), and visuoconstruction abilities (e.g., Generative Drawing, Figure Copying subtests), and that take between 45 to 90 minutes to complete, depending on the severity of the patient's dementia. ABCD performances can be interpreted in terms of individual subtests, construct scores (i.e., Mental Status, Episodic Memory, Linguistic Expression, Linguistic Comprehension, Visuospatial Construction), or overall total test score. The ABCD was standardized on patients with Alzheimer's disease, patients with Parkinson's disease (the majority of whom did not have dementia), and young and age-matched healthy adults. According to the test authors, young adults were included in the control group as this test also may be suitable for some patients with TBI. Although certain forms of reliability and validity appear adequate, others, such as inter-rater reliability, are not discussed at all in the test manual.

Another option for assessing the overall cognitive-communicative abilities of dementia patients is the *Repeatable Battery for the Assessment of Neuropsychological*

Status (RBANS; Randolph, 1998). It has 12 subtests designed to evaluate visuospatial (e.g., Figure Copy subtest), memory (e.g., Story Memory and Recall subtests), attention (e.g., Digit Span), and language (e.g., Picture Naming) abilities in approximately 30 minutes in patients between the ages of 20 and 89 years. Compared to the ABCD, the RBANS provides a less comprehensive examination of language abilities, but it does have strong psychometric properties and offers parallel test forms, which makes it more appropriate for repeated testing, and thus for monitoring dementia progression.

Test batteries such as the *Functional Linguistic Communication Inventory* (FLCI; Bayles and Tomoeda, 1994) and *Severe Impairment Battery* (Saxton, Swihart, & Boller, 1993) also are available, but for a specific dementia patient population—those with moderate to severe dementia. These tests were developed because patients in the later stages of dementia are often too impaired to complete the ABCD or other standard tests of language and cognition. For example, to assess more basic communication skills, the FLCI consists of ten subtests, including Greeting and Naming, Comprehension of Signs (e.g., stop sign, exit sign), Object-to-Picture Matching, Word Reading and Comprehension, Following Commands, and Pantomime. Subtest scores and the total test score can be compared to the standardization sample's scores to determine a severity level. The FLCI is shorter than the ABCD, taking between 20 to 30 minutes to complete. Although acceptable test-retest reliability and criterion validity are reported, other forms of reliability and validity are not addressed in the test manual, and the standardization was limited to a relatively small sample of 40 patients, all of whom had Alzheimer's disease. In the test manual, Bayles and Tomoeda (1994) mentioned that studies regarding the use of the FLCI with other dementia patient populations were planned, and that clinicians would be able to obtain these updated norms at no cost from the authors when they become available.

TESTS OF SPECIFIC LINGUISTIC FUNCTIONS

As listed in Table 5-3, there are many test options available for evaluating the integrity of specific language functions in patients with neurogenic language disorders. For most patients, these tests are needed to delineate the nature of language difficulties identified during earlier steps of the assessment process (e.g., observations, screening test, language test battery). Use of these tests will be particularly important when evaluating patients with mild language impairments, as they often perform at ceiling levels on test batteries (Ross & Wertz, 2003; 2004). Because test batteries for RHD are generally psychometrically weak (Tompkins & Lehman, 1997), tests of specific linguistic (and cognitive) functions also should be included when evaluating patients with cognitive-communicative disorders related to RHD. Likewise, assessment beyond the use of test batteries is essential when pragmatic and discourse-level deficits are suspected because these language abilities are frequently not evaluated or receive only cursory attention on language test batteries

Table 5-3. Tests of Specific Language Functions

LANGUAGE FUNCTION	INSTRUMENT	SOURCE
Phonology/Orthography		
Suprasegmental Phonology	Seashore Tonal Memory Test	Seashore et al. (1960)
	Florida Affect Battery	Blonder et al. (1991)
	Tennessee Test of Rhythm and Intonation Patterns	Koike & Asp (1981)
Phonemic Perception	Psycholinguistic Assessments of Language Processing in Aphasia	Kay et al. (1997)
Orthography/ Reading	Johns Hopkins University Dyslexia Battery	Goodman & Caramazza (1986b)[1]
	Peabody Individual Achievement Test–Rev.	Markwardt (1997)
	Psycholinguistic Assessments of Language Processing in Aphasia	Kay et al. (1997)
	Reading Comprehension Battery for Aphasia–2	LaPointe & Horner (1998)
	Test of Word Reading Efficiency	Torgesen et al. (1999)
Orthography/ Writing	Johns Hopkins University Dysgraphia Battery	Goodman & Caramazza (1986a)[1]
	Psycholinguistic Assessments of Language Processing in Aphasia	Kay et al. (1997)
Lexical-Semantics		
Comprehension	Comprehensive Receptive and Expressive Vocabulary Test–2	Wallace & Hammill (2002)
	Gray Diagnostic Reading Tests–2	Bryant et al. (2004)
	Gray Oral Reading Tests–4	Wiederholt & Bryant (2002)
	Gray Silent Reading Test	Wiederholt & Blalock (2001)
	Johns Hopkins University Dyslexia Battery	Goodman & Caramazza (1986b)[1]
	Peabody Individual Achievement Test–Rev.	Markwardt (1997)
	Peabody Picture Vocabulary Test–3	Dunn & Dunn (1997)
	Putney Auditory Comprehension Screening Test	Beaumont et al. (2002)
	Psycholinguistic Assessments of Language Processing in Aphasia	Kay et al. (1997)
	Pyramids and Palm Trees	Howard & Patterson (1992)
	Reading Comprehension Battery for Aphasia–2	LaPointe & Horner (1998)
	Revised Token Test	McNeil & Prescott (1978)
	Test of Reading Comprehension–3	Brown et al. (1995)
	Test of Word Knowledge	Wiig & Secord (1992)

(continues)

Table 5-3. *Continued*

LANGUAGE FUNCTION	INSTRUMENT	SOURCE
Comprehension (continued)	Test of Word Reading Efficiency	Torgesen et al. (1999)
	Verb and Sentence Test	Bastiaanse et al. (2002)
	Wide Range Achievement Test–3	Wilkinson (1993)
Production	Action Naming Test	Obler & Albert (1979)
	Auditory Naming Test	Hamberger & Seidel (2003)
	Armstrong Naming Test	Armstrong (1996)
	Boston Naming Test, 2nd Ed.	Kaplan et al. (2001)
	Comprehensive Receptive and Expressive Vocabulary Test–2	Wallace & Hammill (2002)
	Controlled Oral Word Association Test	Benton et al. (2001)
	Johns Hopkins University Dysgraphia Battery	Goodman & Caramazza (1986a)[1]
	Object Naming Test	Newcombe et al. (1971)
	OWLS Written Expression Scale	Carrow-Woolfolk (1996)
	Psycholinguistic Assessments of Language Processing in Aphasia	Kay et al. (1997)
	Slosson Oral Reading Test–Revised 3	Slosson et al. (1990)
	Test of Adolescent and Adult Word-Finding	German (1990)
	Test of Word Knowledge	Wiig & Secord (1992)
	Test of Written Language–3	Hammill & Larson (1996)
	The Naming Test	Williams (1996)
	The Word Test 2–Adolescent	Bowers et al. (2005)
	Thurstone Word Fluency Test	Thurstone & Thurstone (1962)
	Verb and Sentence Test	Bastiaanse et al. (2002)
	Wide Range Achievement Test–3	Wilkinson (1993)
Syntax **Comprehension**	Auditory Comprehension Test for Sentences	Shewan (1979)
	Psycholinguistic Assessments of Language Processing in Aphasia	Kay et al. (1997)
	Putney Auditory Comprehension Screening Test	Beaumont et al. (2002)
	Revised Token Test	McNeil & Prescott (1978)
	Test of Reading Comprehension–3	Brown et al. (1995)
	Test for Reception of Grammar	Bishop (1983)
	Verb and Sentence Test	Bastiaanse et al. (2002)

(continues)

Table 5-3. *Continued*

LANGUAGE FUNCTION	INSTRUMENT	SOURCE
Production	OWLS Written Expression Scale	Carrow-Woolfolk (1996)
	Northwestern Syntax Screening Test	Lee (1971)
	Shewan Spontaneous Language Analysis	Shewan (1988a, 1988b)
	The Reporter's Test	DeRenzi & Ferrari (1978)
	Test of Written Language–3	Hammill & Larson (1996)
	Verb and Sentence Test	Bastiaanse et al. (2002)
Pragmatics/Discourse[2]		
Comprehension	D-KEFS Word Context subtest	Delis et al. (2001)
	Facial Expression Stimuli and Test	Young et al. (2002)
	Functional Auditory Comprehension Task	LaPointe & Horner (1978)
	Discourse Comprehension Test	Brookshire & Nicholas (1997)
	Gray Diagnostic Reading Tests–2	Bryant et al. (2004)
	Gray Oral Reading Tests–4	Wiederholt & Bryant (2002)
	Gray Silent Reading Test	Wiederholt & Blalock (2001)
	Nelson Reading Skills Test	Hanna et al. (1977)
	Reading Comprehension Battery for Aphasia–2	LaPointe & Horner (1998)
	Test of Language Competence–Expanded	Wiig & Secord (1989)
	Test of Reading Comprehension–3	Brown et al. (1995)
	The Awareness of Social Inference Test	McDonald et al. (2002)
Production	Conversation Analysis Profile for People with Aphasia	Whitworth et al. (1997)
	Conversation Analysis Profile for People with Cognitive Impairment	Perkins et al. (1997)
	OWLS Written Expression Scale	Carrow-Woolfolk (1996)
	Peabody Individual Achievement Test–Rev.	Markwardt (1997)
	Test of Language Competence–Expanded	Wiig & Secord (1989)
	Test of Written Language–3	Hammill & Larson (1996)
Gesture Comprehension and/or Production	Apraxia Battery for Adults–2	Dabul (2000)
	Assessment of Nonverbal Communication	Duffy & Duffy (1984)
	Pantomime Recognition Test	Benton et al. (1993)
	Test of Oral and Limb Apraxia	Helm-Estabrooks (1991)

[1]A complete listing of these tests' stimuli and tasks can be found in Beeson and Hillis (2001).
[2]These discourse-level tests assess multiple linguistic and cognitive functions, including syntactic and semantic processing as well as attention, memory, and high-level cognitive skills such as inferencing.

(e.g., MIRBI, SCATBI, *Burns* Complex Neuropathology Inventory) (Turkstra, 1999). Finally, as a caveat, clinicians must keep in mind that many tests designed to evaluate specific language functions actually assess additional perceptual, linguistic, and cognitive functions. For example, a test designed to evaluate comprehension of complex syntactic structures that involves matching spoken sentences to pictures will require, in addition to syntactic processing, verbal memory (i.e., temporarily retain the sentence while scanning the picture stimuli), lexical-semantic (i.e., understanding the vocabulary in the target sentence), and visuoperceptual (i.e., discriminating visual differences between the picture stimuli) skills. Therefore, before utilizing one of these tests with a given patient, clinicians must determine what demands the test makes on other linguistic and cognitive abilities, as well as have an understanding of whether these additional linguistic and cognitive abilities are problematic for their patient.

PHONOLOGICAL AND ORTHOGRAPHIC PROCESSES

Further assessment of phonological and orthographic processes is typically only necessary when evaluating patients with aphasia. Whereas other neurogenic patient populations may display difficulties with these levels of language processing, these difficulties are usually cognitively or motorically based, or will not be a treatment priority. For example, although patients with RHD can have difficulties identifying or producing letters, these difficulties are unlikely to reflect problems in selecting or using graphemes, but rather visuospatial or attentional deficits (e.g., neglect dyslexia or dysgraphia; spatial dysgraphia) (Ardila & Rosselli, 1993; Friedman, Ween, & Albert, 1993; Hillis & Caramazza, 1995). Likewise, in patients with TBI, phonological and orthographic deficits are possible, but treatments for these deficits are typically inappropriate as remediation of other language (i.e., pragmatic problems), cognitive (e.g., memory, attention), and behavioral (e.g., disinhibition) impairments will have a greater impact on their daily functioning.

Phonology

Both **segmental** (i.e., processing the sound elements of words or syllables) and **suprasegmental** (i.e., processing intonation, stress, and pauses) aspects of phonology may be compromised in patients with aphasia, particularly those with concomitant dysarthria and/or apraxia of speech (Blumstein, 1998). Whereas some aphasia test batteries include subtests to evaluate segmental phonology in terms of production of syllables or the influence of the phonological composition of words on repetition skills (e.g., BDAE-3; ADP), there are no commercial tests available for examining just this component of language in adults. Clinicians may, however, use the following procedures to quantify and qualify segmental phonology production difficulties (Murray & Chapey, 2001): (1) identify phonemic errors in discourse samples and on word retrieval tests, and attend to the phonological context of those errors; (2) utilize stimulability testing to determine what contexts and cueing variables may assist patients' production of error phonemes; and (3) identify problems with patients' peripheral speech mechanism that may be contributing to their phonology difficulties.

Difficulties with phonemic perception are also possible in neurogenic language disorders (Franklin, 1989). To identify problems processing language at this level, tasks that involve discriminating nonword and/or word minimal pairs may be used. Such tasks can be found on the *Psycholinguistic Assessments of Language Processing in Aphasia* (PALPA; Kay, Lesser, & Coltheart, 1997). As the name indicates, this test is based on a psycholinguistic model of aphasia (similar to that depicted in Figure 1-1), and consists of 60 sets of stimuli designed to identify what level or levels of the model are impaired and affecting production or comprehension of spoken and written language. It was not designed to be given in its entirety, but rather based on other assessment data, clinicians should select only certain subtests to delineate further their patients' language impairment. A major limitation of the PALPA is that there has been nominal exploration of the reliability or validity of its subtests. When validity has been explored, insufficiencies have been identified (e.g., Cole-Virtue & Nickels, 2004). Furthermore, normative data are limited to the means and standard deviations of a small group (i.e., $n = 32$) of non-brain-damaged adults of unspecified age, education, or ethnocultural background, and are provided only for certain subtests. A recent investigation was conducted to establish normative accuracy and response time data for some PALPA subtests that lacked this information (Nickels & Cole-Virtue, 2004); however, this study too included a relatively small sample and included predominantly young participants. Collectively, these psychometric weaknesses make interpretation of PALPA subtest performances difficult.

Early research suggested that patients with RHD have problems processing suprasegmental components of phonology (e.g., Ross, 1984; Weintraub, Mesulam, & Kramer, 1981). More recent findings, however, indicate that, as in aphasia, problems producing suprasegmentals subsequent to RHD may, at least in part, reflect a concomitant dysarthria (Ryalls, Joanette, & Feldman, 1987). Likewise, researchers have questioned whether problems perceiving suprasegmentals following RHD are truly linguistic in nature (Robin, Tranel, & Damasio, 1990; Tompkins & Flowers, 1985). That is, evidence has accumulated to suggest that lower level auditory perceptual problems as well as cognitive limitations may underlie difficulties on prosodic comprehension tasks for patients with RHD. Additionally, if impaired production of prosody or suprasegmentals is suspected, clinicians must attempt to assure that they have an adequate description of patients' premorbid suprasegmental abilities; for instance, patients might have always spoken with flat intonation and excessive pausing, and thus, failure to determine this information would lead to unnecessary assessment procedures.

In terms of assessment, some RHD test batteries have items dedicated to evaluating comprehension and production of certain aspects of suprasegmental phonology (e.g., production of various emotional intonations on the MIRBI-2), although the reliability of these tasks is suspect. There also are some specific tests for examining this aspect of language (see Table 5-3). For example, the Florida Affect Battery (Blonder, Bowers, & Heilman, 1991) evaluates skills such as discriminating facial emotions, emotional and nonemotional (e.g., statement vs. question intonation) prosody, and matching facial emotions with spoken emotional prosody. To assure that other impairments are not confounding performance of these tests, however, motor speech and cognitive assessment results must be considered before final decisions regarding the presence of suprasegmental phonology difficulties are made.

Orthographic Processing

Orthographic or graphemic processing problems can result in deficits of reading, writing, or both, and do occur in a number of neurogenic language disorders (e.g., aphasia, dementia). Patients with difficulties at this level of language processing have problems converting graphemes to phonemes (i.e., letter-to-sound) or phonemes to graphemes (i.e., sound-to-letter) for reading or writing, respectively.

Several tests are available to help determine whether patients' reading or writing difficulties reflect problems with graphemic decoding, phonemic-to-graphemic conversion, and/or lexical-semantic access (e.g., whole word reading) (see Table 5-3). Typically, these tests include tasks that involve writing, reading aloud, or identifying nonwords (e.g., "plif," "forgel"), as nonword stimuli can only be decoded using grapheme-to-phoneme conversion or written using phoneme-to-grapheme conversion. For example, the *Test of Word Reading Efficiency* (Torgesen, Wagner, & Rashotte, 1999) has two subtests: Sight Word Efficiency, which assesses the number of real words an individual can identify within 45 seconds, and Phonetic Decoding Efficiency, which assesses the ability to read aloud nonwords in a brief time period (45 s). Equivalent forms are available to help control for practice effects when repeated administrations are necessary. Although the test only has norms for individuals up to the age of 25, it may still be useful for older patients, as clinicians may interpret their performances in terms of grade equivalent scores. Some core and supplemental subtests of the *Reading Comprehension Battery for Aphasia–2* (RCBA-2; LaPointe & Horner, 1998) also evaluate whether patients display graphemic and/or lexical-semantic reading difficulties, although no reliability or validity studies have been completed on the supplemental subtests (see Lexical-Semantic Processes section of this chapter for a further description of the RCBA-2). For writing, several subtests of the PALPA (e.g., Nonword Spelling; Letter Length Spelling) allow assessment at the grapheme level (Kay et al., 1997); as previously mentioned, because of undocumented psychometric properties and limited normative data, interpreting PALPA findings can be difficult, particularly if clinicians fail to obtain information regarding their patients' premorbid spelling abilities.

LEXICAL-SEMANTIC PROCESSES

As reviewed in Chapter 1 and depicted in Figure 1-1, lexical-semantic processing involves the phonological input and output lexicons (i.e., the stores of previously heard or produced spoken word forms), the orthographic input and output lexicons (i.e., the stores of previously read or written word forms), and the semantic system. Problems with lexical-semantic processing are universal in aphasia and frequent in other neurogenic language disorders as well (Murray, 2000; Sarno et al., 1986). Accordingly, numerous test choices are available to evaluate the integrity of lexical-semantic comprehension or production abilities (see Table 5-3). These tests vary in terms of which language modalities (i.e., speaking, listening, reading, and/or writing) and contexts (i.e., isolated words vs. sentence level vs. discourse level) are evaluated. Although test batteries for each neurogenic patient population will typically include lexical-semantic subtests, specific tests will often delineate the effects of influential variables on patients' lexical-semantic comprehension and production skills (see Table 5-4); the direction (e.g., positive vs. negative influence) and magnitude of these effects are important when selecting treatment stimuli and procedures. Examples of commercially published tests as well as research protocols for assessing lexical-semantic skills are described below.

Lexical-Semantic Comprehension

Common procedures for evaluating patients' understanding of lexical-semantic information at the word level include identifying real or pictured objects, actions, attributes, categories, or relationships that match or are associated with a spoken or written word or another pictured object, action, or attribute. For example, to determine whether patients have a general semantic or modality-specific impairment, clinicians may utilize *Pyramids and Palm Trees* (Howard & Patterson, 1992). By manipulating whether stimulus and response modalities involve pictures or written or spoken words, six versions of this test are possible. The basic task involves presenting patients with three stimuli, one of which they need to match with one of the others in terms of the strongest or closest semantic association. For example, for the stimuli "pyramid," "pine tree," and "palm tree," "palm tree" should be selected to match best with "pyramid." A number of semantic relationships, such as function and location, are assessed. Because of its forced-choice response format, the test has proven appropriate for a spectrum of patient severity levels. Guidelines for identifying performance patterns indicative of semantic- versus lexical-level impairments are provided in the test manual. No normative data for

Table 5-4. Variables that may Influence the Lexical-Semantic Processing Abilities of Patients with Neurogenic Language Disorders

VARIABLE	*RELATIONSHIP TO LEXICAL SEMANTIC ABILITIES	SOURCE EXAMPLES
length of linguistic stimulus	negative	Nickels & Howard (1995); Weidner & Lasky (1976)
semantic similarity of response choices	negative	Duffy & Watkins (1984)
word frequency	positive	Deloche et al. (1996); Kremin et al. (2001)
imageability	positive	Kay et al. (1990)
concreteness	positive	Nickels (1995)
age of acquisition	negative	Kremin et al. (2001)
salience (i.e., main idea vs. detail)	positive	Nicholas & Brookshire (1995)
part of speech (e.g., nouns vs. verbs)	variable	Caramazza & Hillis (1991); Zingeser & Berndt (1990)
semantic category	variable	Kremin et al. (2001); Laiacona et al. (2001)
stimulus modality (e.g., visual vs. auditory)	variable	Benton et al. (1972); Hamberger & Seidel (2003)
sentence constraint	positive	Murray (2000); Puskaric & Pierce (1997)
cognitive demands of the task (e.g., attention, memory)	negative	Funnell & Hodges (1995); Murray (2000)
stimulus presentation rate	negative	Blumstein et al. (1985)
visual complexity of picture stimuli	negative	Kremin et al. (2001)

*Clinicians must keep in mind that these relationships were established via group studies, in which significant effects were not observed for all subjects. Therefore, it remains possible that a given patient's lexical-semantic skills may not be influenced by these variables or even may be inversely affected (Laiacona et al., 2001).

patient populations are available, but the test manual does indicate that scores of 90% correct or better should be considered indicative of adequate semantic processing, at least on this test; cut-off scores for chance-level performance also are provided.

Because many test batteries (e.g., ADP, MIRBI, ABCD, SCATBI) include only a cursory evaluation of reading abilities, additional testing to quantify and qualify reading comprehension is often necessary. If problems at the word level are suspected, clinicians might select the *Reading Comprehension Battery for Aphasia–2* (RCBA-2; LaPointe & Horner, 1998), as it has 17 subtests that require silent or oral reading, eight of which evaluate reading at the word level (e.g., Synonyms) and the remainder of which evaluate reading at the letter (e.g., Letter Naming), sentence (e.g., Sentence Comprehension), or paragraph level (e.g., Paragraph–Factual Comprehension). Raw scores for each subtest and the total test score can be converted to percentiles. The nominal information in the test manual pertaining to the RCBA-2's psychometric properties consists of brief descriptions of previous studies utilizing the original version of this test; therefore, interpreting RCBA-2 findings will be difficult for clinicians who are unable to access copies of these earlier studies. Other tests that evaluate reading at the word level include the *Wide Range Achievement Test–3* (Wilkinson, 1993) and *Test of Word Reading Efficiency* (Torgesen et al., 1999).

Some tests evaluate lexical-semantic understanding at the sentence or discourse levels versus receptive vocabulary or word level abilities. Because of the length and complexity of stimuli on many of these tests, however, clinicians must keep in mind that test completion may stress, in addition to lexical-semantic comprehension, other linguistic (e.g., morphosyntax) and cognitive (e.g., memory) functions. For instance, the *Revised Token Test* (RTT; McNeil & Prescott, 1978) requires patients to complete auditory commands that vary in terms of length and syntactic complexity with a set of tokens of various shapes, sizes, and colors. A strength of this test is its 15-point multidimensional scoring system that provides qualitative as well as quantitative information pertaining to the accuracy, completeness, promptness, and motoric efficiency of patients' responses, as well as patients' need for stimulus repetitions or cues. The RTT has normative data for healthy adults and patients who have had a left or right hemisphere stroke, and also reports acceptable levels of reliability and validity. Another option is the Putney Auditory Comprehension Screening Test (Beaumont et al., 1999; 2002), which was specifically developed for patients with severe motor and/or visual problems who are unable to complete the response requirements of more traditional comprehension tests (e.g., manipulating and pointing to objects as on the RTT; completing commands with body parts like on the BDAE-3). This test is designed to determine an optimal language complexity level for maximizing patients' auditory comprehension by utilizing 60 yes-no questions (e.g., "Do judges earn less than milkmen?"; "Is orange a color and a fruit?"), which patients are allowed to answer via whatever modality they can (e.g., verbally, buzzer, pointing, eye movements). Additionally, stimuli have been developed to minimize orientation and memory demands. Accordingly, this test would be appropriate for a number of neurogenic patient populations, particularly those with severe motoric or visual impairments (e.g., Huntington's disease, brain stem stroke, TBI).

Lexical-Semantic Production

Numerous tests are available for evaluating spoken and written production of lexical-semantic information, including the ability to retrieve and produce labels or names of objects, actions, events, attributes and relationships, or categories (see Table 5-3). Most of these tests use highly structured tasks to evaluate word retrieval skills, including confrontation naming (i.e., providing the name of a real or pictured stimulus), providing definitions, superordinate or category naming, verbal fluency (i.e., name as many exemplars of a semantic category or that start with a certain letter as possible in a short time period), phrase completion or closure, production of rote or over-learned material (e.g., naming the months of the year, reciting the Pledge of Allegiance), repetition or copying, and recognition naming (i.e., choosing the correct label from a small set of stimuli).

Without question, the *Boston Naming Test* (BNT; Kaplan et al., 1983) is the most frequently used test for evaluating word finding in both clinical and research settings (e.g., Katz et al., 2000). It consists of 60 black-and-white drawings that depict nouns, which decrease in familiarity as the test progresses. If patients are unable to name a picture, the test examiner provides a semantic or function cue and then, if the target is still not named, a phonemic cue. In 2001, a revised edition of the BNT was published (Kaplan, Goodglass, & Weintraub, 2001). This new version differs from the original BNT in that it includes a Short Form that can be used to screen naming abilities, and it allows for providing multiple choice cues after semantic and phonemic cues have been given when patients are having difficulty naming an item. Close examination of the content and statistical qualities of both versions of the BNT raises several concerns and questions about their popularity. First, both BNT editions examine only noun retrieval, even though production of other parts of speech (e.g., verbs, adverbs, adjectives) is frequently problematic in neurogenic language disorders (Murray & Karcher, 2000; Kim & Thompson, 2004). Second, neither BNT manual provides information regarding any aspect of reliability, which is particularly problematic given that there is insufficient description of how to administer and score either test. Finally, the normative data that are listed in the first version's manual are outdated and only extend up to the age of 59 years. This last weakness can be remediated by consulting more recently published norms in the research literature that take into consideration a number of influential demographic (e.g., education, residence) and cultural variables (e.g., Barker-Collo, 2001; Tombaugh & Hubley, 1997; Welch, Doineau, Johnson, & King, 1996). Updated norms for adults between the ages of 18 and 79 are provided in the new edition of the BNT, but description of this normative sample is limited to education level only.

Compared to the BNT, several other commercially available word-finding tests have stronger psychometric characteristics. For example, the *Comprehensive Receptive and Expressive Vocabulary Test – II* (CREVT-II; Wallace & Hammill, 2002) has two subtests, one that evaluates vocabulary comprehension via a picture pointing task and one that assesses vocabulary production via a definition task. A variety of word types, including nouns, verbs, and adjectives, serve as stimuli for the receptive subtest, and can be elicited on the expressive subtest because of its task format (i.e., providing definitions of nouns and verbs vs. just labeling pictures of objects). This test is suitable for a wide variety of patients, as its test items have been found unbiased for gender and ethnicity, its norms extend from age four through 90 years, and it has strong reliability and validity. Furthermore, it has two equivalent forms so that repeated testing can be conducted to monitor patient progress over time.

Because many language test batteries do not include a comprehensive assessment of writing abilities (e.g., *Burns,* ADP, SCATBI), additional evaluation of written lexical-semantic skills is frequently needed. The Spelling subtests of the *Wide Range Achievement Test–3* (Wilkinson, 1993) require patients to write the names of pictures, as well as individual letters and words from dictation. Strengths of this test include that it offers equivalent forms and thus is appropriate for documenting changes in writing over time, and that it has computer software to facilitate scoring; however, a limitation is that its normative data extend only up to age 75.

For patients in whom more abstract aspects of semantic processing are compromised, tests such as *The Word Test 2: Adolescent* (TWT; Bowers, Huisingh, LoGiudice, & Orman, 2005) or *Test of Word Knowledge* (TWK; Wiig & Secord, 1992) might be used. Both tests allow evaluating a broad spectrum of word-finding skills, including the ability to generate synonyms, antonyms, definitions, or multiple meanings. Both tests underwent extensive standardization and have strong psychometric properties. Although both were developed only for children up to age 18, these tests' authors acknowledge that these assessment tools may additionally provide valuable information regarding the word retrieval abilities of adults.

Whereas the above tests utilize structured tasks to evaluate lexical-semantic abilities at primarily the single word level, other assessment tools involve less controlled activities to examine lexical-semantic aspects of patients' connected language. Assuring that language assessments include the examination of spontaneous, connected language output is necessary because for many patients there is only a weak relationship between their word- and discourse-level lexical-semantic abilities (King, Hough, Walker, Rastatter, & Holbert, 2004; Mayer & Murray, 2003; Tingley, Kyte, Johnson, & Beitchman, 2003). Although picture description tasks are most frequently used to elicit spoken and written language samples, clinicians might also use conversation, story-retelling, role playing, video-narration, procedural description (e.g., "How do you make scrambled eggs?"), or explaining picture sequences (Bracy & Drummond, 1993; Cherney, 1998; Hartley & Jensen, 1991; Ulatowska, Doyel, Freedman-Stern, Macaluso-Hayes, & North 1983). Use of these other elicitation methods instead of or in addition to picture descriptions is recommended because picture description tasks can elicit labeling behavior, which in turn restricts the number and variety of lexical-semantic, syntactic, and discourse behaviors in the language sample (Li, Ritterman, Della Volpe, & Williams, 1996; Shadden, Burnette, Eikenberry, & DiBrezzo 1991; Shadden, 1998). Additionally, language samples should be minimally 300 to 400 words in length to ensure adequate test-retest stability of whatever measures are being used to quantify and qualify language output (Brookshire & Nicholas, 1994).

There are a number of approaches to analyzing lexical-semantic content in spoken or written language samples. One of the most frequently used approaches quantifies how informative samples are using measures such as "content units" (Yorkston & Beukelman, 1980), "discourse clarity measures" (Sherratt & Penn, 1990), "main concepts" (Nicholas & Brookshire, 1995b), and "correct information units" (CIUs; Nicholas & Brookshire, 1993). For example, Nicholas and Brookshire (1993) described a series of rules for calculating and comparing the number of words and CIUs, which are words that are "accurate, relevant and informative relative to the eliciting stimulus" (p. 340). To determine the **informativeness** and efficiency of patients' language samples, Nicholas and Brookshire advised clinicians to determine the number of words per minute as well as the percentage of CIUs (i.e., number of CIUs/number of words). Subsequent research has supported the use and reliability of CIU analysis for quantifying communicative informativeness and efficiency on a variety of discourse tasks (Doyle et al., 1995; Murray, Holland, & Beeson, 1998), and indicates that CIUs and other content measures predict well how unfamiliar listeners will rate the informativeness of (Doyle et al., 1996) and socially relevant changes in (Ross & Wertz, 1999) the verbal output of patients with aphasia. A study by Oelschlaeger and Thorne (1999), however, indicated that the reliability of the CIU approach may be inadequate for analyzing samples of "naturally occurring conversation" (p. 636); these researchers suggested that there are insufficient guidelines for using CIU analysis with conversational samples (vs. narrative or picture description samples), and recommended obtaining additional training with this measurement technique before applying it to naturally occurring conversation.

In addition to documenting lexical-semantic retrieval accuracy, the nature and pattern of content errors made by patients in their verbal or written output should be evaluated. For example, word retrieval errors can be classified as: (1) **phonemic or literal paraphasias,** which contain substitutions, additions, omissions, and/or rearrangements of target word phonemes, (2) **semantic paraphasias,** which are substitutions of words that are semantically related to the target words, (3) **random paraphasias,** which are substitutions of words that lack apparent semantic relations to the target words, (4) **circumlocutions,** which involve the use of descriptions or definitions for the target words, (5) **neologisms,** which involve the use of nonsense versus target words, (6) **indefinite substitutions,** which involve the use of nonspecific words or descriptions for target words, and (7) **no responses.** Additionally, clinicians may monitor for other word-finding difficulty symptoms in the spoken and written discourse of their patients, including the use of fillers (e.g., "um," "well," "you know"), part-word, word, or phrase repetitions, silent pauses, false starts or abandoned utterances, and metalinguistic comments about the task or language ability (e.g., "I know it but I can't say it.") (Brookshire & Nicholas, 1995; Tingley et al., 2003) (see Table 5-5 for further examples). Tingley et al. (2003) cautioned, however, that these disruptions may reflect not only lexical-semantic retrieval difficulties, but also problems with syntactic or pragmatic aspects of discourse production or even the patients' emotional status or knowledge of the discourse topic.

Table 5-5. Examples of Types of Paraphasias and Discourse-Level Symptoms of Word-Finding Difficulty

ERROR OR SYMPTOM TYPE	EXAMPLES
phonemic/literal paraphasia	"Canadan" for "Canadian"; "picinica" for "picnic"
semantic paraphasia	"puppy" for "cat"; "train" for "bus"
random paraphasia	"September" for "hungry"; "jumping" for "washing"
circumlocution	"It's red and grows on trees" for "cherry"
indefinite substitution	"there" for "my house"; "thing" for "clock"
neologism	"tember" for "happy"; "banertine" for "soccer"
no response	
nonword, word, or phrase fillers	"I lost my um. . . uh. . . wallet." "I lost my. . . you know. . . wallet."
part-word, word, or phrase repetitions	"She went to the. . . the. . . the. . . islands."
silent pauses	"My. . . . . friend gave it to me."
false starts	"He had. . . the girl had the wrong number."
abandoned utterances	"Dylan was practicing for. . . ."
metalinguistic comments	"I just can't think of it."

Cognitive Neuropsychological and Neurolinguistic Approaches

Cognitive neuropsychological and neurolinguistic approaches to evaluating lexical-semantic processing abilities aim to identify which component or components of language models (see Chapter 1 and Figure 1-1) have been compromised (Caplan, 1993; Kay et al., 1996; Beeson & Hillis, 2001). For example, lexical-semantic comprehension problems could emerge from impaired access to or organization of the phonological or graphemic input lexicon and/or the semantic system. To identify the locus or loci of impairment, clinicians can use the PALPA (Kay et al., 1997), one of the first commercially available tests based solely on psycholinguistic theory; even though this is a published test, however, information pertaining to its psychometric properties is currently unavailable, and only nominal normative data are provided. Another option is to consult assessment protocols described in the research literature (e.g., Hillis, Rapp, Romani, & Caramazza, 1990; Raymer & Rothi, 2001; Rothi, Raymer, Maher, Greenwald, & Morris, 1991). Most frequently, these protocols involve a set of tasks that differ in terms of input modality (e.g., spoken word vs. written word vs. picture) and mode of response (e.g., repetition vs. written naming vs. pointing to a picture), and one set of stimuli that have been carefully selected to control or examine a number of linguistic factors (e.g., word frequency, length, semantic category, spelling regularity). Patients' performances of these various comprehension (e.g., matching semantically related pictures; spoken word-to-picture matching) and production tasks (e.g., writing to dictation, naming to spoken definitions) are then contrasted to identify the level(s) of impairment. The consistency of patients' errors across modalities, tasks, and sessions also is evaluated, as access deficits are associated with inconsistent errors, whereas loss of linguistic representations is associated with consistent errors.

MORPHOLOGICAL AND SYNTACTIC PROCESSES

Further assessment of morphological and syntactic skills is most frequently necessary when evaluating the language abilities of patients with aphasia or TBI who have suffered focal dominant hemisphere lesions, as morphosyntactic impairments are common in these patient populations. A more detailed morphosyntactic evaluation also may be informative when trying to determine dementia type, as certain dementing illnesses can be distinguished, at least in part, by their differential effects on morphosyntax. For example, an agrammatic language profile is common in Pick's disease and frontotemporal dementia, but rare in Alzheimer's disease (e.g., Grossman, 2002).

Morphosyntactic Comprehension

Comprehension of morphosyntactic processes may be evaluated at both word and discourse levels. At the word level, understanding of **substantive or open class** (e.g., verbs, nouns, adjectives, adverbs) and **relational or closed class words** (e.g., prepositions, pronouns, determiners, conjunctions) should be evaluated. Because comprehension of nouns is invariably evaluated on test batteries for aphasia, RHD, TBI, and dementia, further assessment is typically only necessary to evaluate other substantive and relational words. Likewise, few test batteries examine patients' comprehension of grammatical morphemes, including **derivational** (i.e., morphemes that transform words into different types of form words; e.g., "sleep" into "sleepy") or **inflectional** (i.e., morphemes that provide syntactic information; e.g., "s" on "sleeps" indicates subject-verb agreement) affixes.

There is only a limited choice of commercial tests for examining understanding of form words (beyond nouns) or derivational and inflectional morphemes (Table 5-3). The *Verb and Sentence Test* (VAST; Bastiaanse, Edwards, & Rispens, 2002) has one subtest dedicated to evaluating auditory comprehension of 40 verbs that vary in transitivity (i.e., whether or not the verb may take an object), word frequency, and name relatedness with a noun. Another option, the PALPA (Kay et al., 1997), has a few listening and reading subtests for assessing understanding of verbs, adjectives, and locative prepositions (e.g., Written Comprehension of Locative Relations) and recognizing a variety of grammatical morphemes (e.g., Auditory Lexical Decision: Morphological Endings). Although the BDAE-3 (Goodglass et al., 2001) also has a few Extended Subtests that evaluate recognition of written form words (e.g., prepositions, auxiliary verbs) and words with derivational or inflectional affixes, only a limited number of items are included, and thus further testing is often necessary. Another possibility is research protocols described in the literature. For example, Caplan and Bub (1990) created a test that includes lexical decision, word-picture matching, and similarity judgment tasks to evaluate recognition and comprehension of morphologically complex words.

Assessing morphosyntactic comprehension at the sentence level primarily involves identifying problems understanding a range of simple (e.g., active) and complex sentence forms (e.g., passives, object-relative clauses). For example, the VAST (Bastiaanse et al., 2002) has two subtests, Grammaticality Judgment and Sentence Comprehension, which examine recognition and understanding of spoken **canonical** (e.g., active sentences) and **noncanonical** (e.g., passives) sentence types. This test also assesses morphosyntactic production abilities at the word (i.e., Verb Production) and sentence levels. The sentence level subtests include Sentence Construction, Sentence Anagrams with and without Pictures, and *Wh*-Anagrams subtests, which require patients to produce grammatically complete declarative and interrogative sentences. The anagram tasks involve more complex sentence forms than are typically elicited by picture description tasks. For these anagram subtests, patients are given a set of word and phrase cards, and asked to create a sentence (e.g., "the bike," "is fixed by," "the man" cards to form a target passive sentence); in the Sentence Anagrams with Pictures and *Wh*-Anagrams subtests, the sentence that they form should match the target picture that they are given. Whereas administration of the entire VAST may take as long as two to three hours, clinicians may opt to give only two to four subtests, which should require only approximately 30 minutes. Because this test was developed and standardized in Europe, there may be certain items that need to be adapted to reflect American English vocabulary.

Other structured tests available for examining syntax comprehension include the *Revised Token Test* (McNeil & Prescott, 1978), PALPA (Kay et al., 1997), and *Auditory Comprehension Test for Sentences* (Shewan, 1979). Some of these tests, however, have been criticized because they do not assess a broad enough range of sentence types, do not allow distinguishing between syntax comprehension and working memory problems, or both (Caplan, 1993; Thompson, 2001). Clinicians may therefore choose to utilize protocols described in the literature (e.g., Caplan & Bub, 1990; Caplan, Waters, & Hildebrandt, 1997; Thompson, 2001). These tests typically involve sentence-picture matching (e.g., Thompson, 2001) or object manipulation or acting out (e.g., Caplan et al., 1997) tasks, and evaluate a variety of syntactic forms that vary in sentence canonicity (e.g., active sentences with Subject-Verb-Object order vs. passives with noncanonical, Object-Verb-Subject order) and number of verbs and propositions (e.g., active vs. conjoined sentences). Additionally, to assure that patients are not using lexical-semantic processing or world knowledge to interpret the sentences, semantically reversible stimuli are preferable (e.g., "The woman was served by the man." vs. "The customer was served by the waiter.")

Morphosyntactic Production

Morphosyntactic production abilities can be evaluated using structured or constrained tasks, by analyzing samples of patients' spoken and written language, or both. As with word-level comprehension tests, most formal tests of word-level, morphosyntactic production abilities evaluate retrieval of nouns more than other word forms. Exceptions include the VAST (Bastiaanse et al., 2002), which assesses verb production, and the CREVT-II (Wallace & Hammill, 2002), *Test of Adolescent and Adult Word-Finding* (German, 1990), and PALPA (Kay, Byng, Edmundson, & Scott, 2001), which require production of a range of form words including verbs, adjectives, and prepositions. The PALPA (Kay et al., 2001) additionally includes repetition, reading aloud, and spelling subtests that evaluate production of a variety of grammatical morphemes. A few research protocols also are available that use sentence completion (Caplan & Bub, 1990; Goodglass & Berko, 1960), spelling (Goodman & Caramazza, 1986a), or oral reading (Goodman & Caramazza, 1986b) to evaluate production of a range of form words or inflectional and derivational affixes.

There are only a few structured tests for assessing sentence-level morphosyntactic abilities. For example, the VAST (Bastiaanse et al., 2002), as previously described (see Morphosyntactic Comprehension section of this chapter), includes three subtests for evaluating production of declarative and interrogative sentence forms. For identifying morphosyntactic problems in patients' written output, clinicians may select the *OWLS Written Expression Scale* (Carrow-Woolfolk, 1996), which was designed for individuals between the ages of five and 22 and evaluates word (e.g., spelling, punctuation), syntactic (e.g., phrase and sentence structure, modifiers), and discourse-level writing abilities (e.g., cohesion, organization). Oral, written, and pictorial prompts are used to elicit the writing samples, and the entire test takes about 15 to 25 minutes to administer. This test was standardized on a large sample (i.e., $n = 1700$) and has strong psychometric properties. Although normative data are limited to young adults, this OWLS scale may still prove informative for older patients, as their performances can be converted to age- and grade-based standard scores.

Another approach to evaluating morphosyntactic production is to analyze the accuracy, types, and frequency of form words, grammatical morphemes, and syntactic structures used by patients in their spoken and/or written discourse. Numerous scoring systems are available for this purpose in the research literature (Edwards, 1995; Menn, Ramsberger, & Helm-Estabrooks, 1994; Saffran, Berndt, & Schwartz, 1989; Thompson et al., 1995). Because some of these systems were created to quantify and qualify agrammatic output (e.g., Saffran et al., 1989; Thompson et al., 1995) and others for fluent or paragrammatic output (e.g., Edwards, 1995), the types of structural forms analyzed across these systems can vary. Most systems, however, include sufficient description of language sample collection and analyses procedures, and thus have been associated with acceptable levels of intra- and inter-rater reliability (Prins & Bastiaanse, 2004).

In addition to determining what morphosyntactic forms patients are producing, clinicians should also examine what types of errors are being made. That is, clinicians should document whether their patients are omitting certain form words, grammatical morphemes, or sentence forms (e.g., leaves out auxiliary verbs), substituting incorrect form words, grammatical morphemes, or sentence forms (e.g., uses "she" for all subject pronouns), or both. Likewise, the consistency of morphosyntactic errors should be determined. If patients are inconsistently making errors, clinicians should additionally explore whether or not linguistic (e.g., vocabulary familiarity), patient (e.g., fatigue), or task variables (e.g., story retelling vs. unconstrained conversation) are influencing their patients' language output.

PRAGMATICS AND DISCOURSE SKILLS

Assessing pragmatics and discourse abilities is essential when evaluating the language abilities of patients with RHD or TBI, given that these aspects of language are frequently compromised in these patient populations (Chapman et al., 1994; Hartley & Jensen, 1991; Tompkins et al., 1994), but typically inadequately addressed by RHD (e.g., MIRBI) and TBI (e.g., SCATBI) test batteries. Likewise, it is important to document the integrity of these language skills in patients with dementia, as early pragmatic impairment is indicative of certain forms of dementia (e.g.,

Pick's disease, frontotemporal dementia; Grossman, 2002). Although in aphasia pragmatic skills are often assumed to be an area of relative strength, pragmatic difficulties and discourse deficits may occur (Coelho, Liles, Duffy, Clarkson, & Elia, 1994; Holland, 1996). Accordingly, a comprehensive language assessment of any neurogenic patient should include pragmatic and discourse-level tasks. Furthermore, it is important to keep in mind the complex nature of these language areas; that is, deficits in other linguistic (e.g., lexical-semantic processing), emotional (e.g., depression), and cognitive (e.g., attention, memory) functions may underlie or contribute to pragmatic and discourse impairments (Hartley & Jensen, 1991; Murray et al., 1998; Tompkins et al., 1994; Welland, Lubinski, & Higginbotham, 2002). Therefore, assessment of these other areas is necessary before making conclusions about the presence and nature of pragmatic and discourse difficulties.

Pragmatic and Discourse Comprehension

As shown in Table 5-3, several commercially available tests evaluate patients' understanding of pragmatic and discourse rules and conventions. Most of these tests examine one or more of the following: (1) whether patients can glean main ideas from spoken or written discourse, (2) whether patients can process main ideas as well as detailed information in spoken or written discourse, and (3) whether patients can make inferences, resolve ambiguities or discrepancies, or revise interpretations based on the spoken or written text to which they were exposed, contextual cues (e.g., communication partner's facial expression), and/or their general world knowledge. For example, the *Discourse Comprehension Test* (DCT; Brookshire & Nicholas, 1993) was developed to evaluate comprehension of spoken or written discourse in patients with aphasia, RHD, or TBI. Patients listen to or read story passages, and then after each story answer a set of yes/no questions that evaluate their understanding and retention of directly stated or implied main ideas and details. The stories and questions are audiotaped to allow for reliable test administration; furthermore, the speaker's rate and prosody on the audiotapes were controlled to maximize auditory processing in patients with aphasia. Unfortunately, the DCT's standardization sample is quite limited, consisting of only 40 adults with no brain damage, and 60 adults with brain damage (i.e., 20 with aphasia, 20 with TBI, and 20 with RHD); reliability and standard error data were established on an even smaller sample size (i.e., 14 adults with aphasia and seven with RHD). A recent investigation by Welland et al. (2002) provided data regarding the DCT performances of patients in the early or middle stages of Alzheimer's disease, but again sample size was small and limited to only eight individuals per patient group.

Another formal test option is the *Test of Language Competence–Expanded Edition* (TLC-E; Wiig & Secord, 1989). Although the TLC-E was developed for adolescents, it has proven suitable in several research studies aimed at quantifying and qualifying high-level language comprehension and production problems in adults with a variety of disorders, including Alzheimer's disease, depression, Parkinson's disease, and Huntington's disease (e.g., Chenery, Copland, & Murdoch, 2002; Murray, 2002). The TLC-E consists of three comprehension subtests, Ambiguous Sentences, Making Inferences, and Figurative Language, which evaluate understanding of lexical and structural ambiguities, alternative inferences, and metaphors, respectively. It also has one expressive subtest, Recreating Sentences, which requires the generation of sentences that are appropriate to the pictured context and that contain a prescribed set of words. The TLC-E was standardized on a large sample of students (i.e., $n = 1796$) between the ages of nine and 19, and has acceptable levels of validity and reliability. Depending on their patients' ages and premorbid abilities, clinicians may choose to interpret their patients' TLC-E performances in terms of standard scores for the oldest normative group on the test, age-equivalent scores, or data reported for healthy, older adults in the research literature (e.g., Murray, 2002).

Some cognitive test batteries have subtests that are suitable for evaluating pragmatic or discourse comprehension skills. For example, the *Delis-Kaplan Executive Function System* (DEFS; Delis, Kramer, Kaplan, & Ober, 2001), a battery of executive function tests, includes a Word Context subtest that assesses comprehension of language in context. On this subtest, patients are told that they need to figure out the meaning of some words from a "different language" (the words are actually nonsense words), and then are given sentence clues to help them generate an answer. For example, for the item "gesh," clues include "You *gesh* a space," "Loud music can *gesh* a room," and "You *gesh* a bucket with water." Bardo, Delis, and Kaplan, (2002) found that this subtest better discriminated patients with frontal lobe lesions from their healthy peers than the DKEFS Proverb Interpretation subtest, and concluded that the Word Context subtest requires a greater degree and more realistic integration of information than proverb interpretation tasks.

If problems reading connected text are suspected, clinicians should opt to use reading tests developed for academic purposes, as those developed for neurogenic patient populations are often too easy, tend to evaluate only understanding of basic language forms and explicitly stated information, or have content weaknesses. For example, patients whose reading difficulties are restricted to the discourse level typically perform at ceiling levels on the RCBA-2, perhaps in part because the most difficult paragraph falls below the seventh-grade level. Likewise, paragraph-level reading subtests on aphasia test batteries have been found to have relatively low passage dependency, meaning that patients can correctly respond to questions about these paragraphs *without* reading the paragraphs (Nicholas et al., 1986).

Accordingly, tests such as the *Nelson Reading Skills Test* (Hanna et al., 1977) or *Gray Diagnostic Reading Tests–2* (GDRT-2; Bryant, Wiederholt, & Bryant, 2004), which have more acceptable levels of passage dependency and offer a broader range of complexity/grade levels, are more appropriate test choices for patients whose reading abilities break down beyond the sentence level. For example, the GDRT-2, which subsumes several previously published reading tests, namely the *Gray Oral Reading Test–4* (Wiederholt & Bryant, 2002) and the *Gray Silent Reading Test* (Wiederholt & Blalock, 2001), evaluates not only understanding of graphemic-phonemic relations and word-level reading skills, but also comprehension of passages that increase in complexity, oral reading rate, and oral reading accuracy. Passage comprehension is assessed via questions pertaining to main ideas, details, and possible inferences. Strengths of the GDRT-2 include its comprehensive quantification and qualification of reading skills, strong psychometric properties including an absence of gender or ethnocultural bias, and parallel forms so that changes in reading ability over time can be monitored. Although the GDRT-2 was only standardized on individuals up to the age of 18, clinicians assessing adults may still be able to establish the presence and severity of a reading disorder through the calculation of grade- or age- equivalent scores.

McDonald and colleagues' (2002) *The Awareness of Social Interference Test* (TASIT) represents one of the few tests available to identify problems processing pragmatic or social contextual information. This test consists of three subtests, Emotion Evaluation, Social Inference-Minimal, and Social Inference-Enriched, that use videotaped vignettes and standardized response probes to examine patients' perceptions of basic (e.g., fear, anger, happiness) and more subtle (e.g., sincerity, sarcasm, deception) visual and vocal emotional demeanors. TASIT includes alternate forms of each subtest to allow reliable, repeated testing. So far, this test has been normed on primarily young adults (i.e., mean age of standardization sample was 22.9 years), making it more suitable for the typically younger population of patients with TBI than the typically older populations of patients with stroke and dementia.

In addition to or instead of the above formal tests, clinicians could develop their own probe tasks based on activities described in the literature to evaluate patients' understanding of other pragmatic and discourse functions (e.g., Tompkins, 1995; Hartley, 1995). For example, the general format of these probes could involve patients listening to or reading different types of discourse samples (e.g., procedural, conversational, news editorial), and then requiring them to complete one or more of the following: (1) answering a series of yes/no questions that probe understanding of main ideas versus details and/or explicitly versus implicitly stated information; (2) summarizing the main idea by providing a title for the sample; (3) ranking statements from the sample in terms of importance to the main idea; (4) identifying factual versus opinion statements; and/or (5) providing a plausible conclusion to an incomplete sample. A variety of variables may be manipulated to increase or decrease the difficulty level of these probe tasks, including length of discourse sample, topic, context, and vocabulary familiarity, number or density of propositions, extent of semantic redundancy, and ratio of essential to nonessential propositions (for a comprehensive description of influential variables and development of probe tasks, see Tompkins, 1995).

Pragmatic and Discourse Production

Although extensive research has been dedicated to characterizing pragmatic and discourse production in a variety of neurogenic language disorders (e.g., Arkin & Mahendra, 2001; Glosser & Deser, 1990; McDonald, 1993; Myers & Brookshire, 1994), nominal resources have been devoted to developing standardized procedures for assessing these language skills. Accordingly, only a limited number of commercial tests and discourse analysis procedures are listed in Table 5-3. For instance, there are a few academically-based tests, such as the *Test of Written Language–3* (TOWL-3; Hammill & Larsen, 1996), that can evaluate both the word- and discourse-level writing skills of patients who are expected to ceiling out on more basic writing tasks, like those found on aphasia test batteries. The TOWL-3 was developed for children up to the age of 18, but may be used with adults as raw scores can be converted to grade and age equivalents in addition to percentiles and standard scores. A Story Construction subtest provides information regarding discourse-level writing (e.g., plot, character development, general composition), whereas other subtests such as Vocabulary, Spelling, and Logical Sentences assess writing at the word and sentence levels. Equivalent forms also are available for repeated testing.

Given this limited choice of commercially available tools, clinicians will also or instead need to exploit procedures described in the research literature to evaluate the pragmatic and discourse production abilities of their patients. A plethora of tasks and analysis procedures have been developed reflecting the broad range of abilities that are encompassed by these areas of language processing (e.g., Arkin & Mahendra, 2001; Florance, 1981; Glosser & Deser, 1990; Hartley & Jensen, 1991; Lubinski, 1994; Penn, 1988; Prutting & Kirchner, 1987; Simmons-Mackie & Damico, 1996; Togher, 2001). Because a description of assessment activities for each area of pragmatic and discourse production is beyond the scope of this textbook, only those areas deemed to apply to a variety of neurogenic language disorders, that have ecological importance, and that have been used frequently in previous empirical studies will be addressed (for more comprehensive reviews see Cherney, Shadden, & Coelho, 1998, Joanette & Brownell, 1990, or McDonald, Togher, & Code, 1999). Specifically, procedures for collecting discourse samples and assessing cohesion, speech acts, and discourse and topic management strategies will be reviewed briefly.

Collecting Discourse Samples

As mentioned previously in the Lexical-Semantic Production section of this chapter, formal test batteries and, thus, clinicians tend to utilize primarily picture description tasks to elicit spoken and written discourse samples. As several researchers have warned, however, relying solely on descriptive discourse samples will result in a skewed assessment of patients' abilities, given that only a limited range of pragmatic and discourse behaviors are being elicited (Shadden, 1998; Togher, 2001).

Instead, language samples collected from a variety of **genres,** or types of discourse, should be analyzed to determine patients' pragmatic and discourse strengths and weaknesses. These genres include the more traditional narrative (i.e., storytelling), procedural (i.e., explaining how to complete a procedure such as changing a tire), and expository (e.g., "Where were you when President Kennedy was assassinated?" or "Why are you in the hospital?") discourse types, as well as more recently advocated and perhaps ecologically valid service encounters (e.g., making telephone calls to get information on a product or service), expert interviews (e.g., being interviewed by student clinicians about the consequences of RHD), and gossiping discourse tasks (Arkin & Mahendra, 2001; McDonald, 1992; Togher, 2001). Likewise, incorporating different communication partners (e.g., familiar vs. unfamiliar; authority figure vs. peer) into these discourse tasks will also allow examining patients' flexibility in adapting their pragmatic and discourse output to different contexts (Hartley, 1995; Togher, 2001).

Side Bar

Language Sampling: The Benefits of Going Beyond Picture Description

Collecting and analyzing only one discourse sample can easily result in an inaccurate characterization of a patient's discourse production abilities. For example, Mr. Leggat is a patient with moderate nonfluent aphasia who has been attending our clinic's aphasia support group for several years. In conversation, he is a rather passive participant in that he primarily only responds to questions and rarely initiates new topics or provides elaborated responses. His picture description samples are similar in that he provides very limited output that primarily consists of labeling objects and people in the picture rather than providing a story about what is going on in the picture. In contrast, if Mr. Leggat is asked to describe his vocational history or hobbies, the mean length of his utterances, the informativeness of his verbal output, and his use of discourse repair strategies increase significantly. Accordingly, if a clinician had only included a picture description or conversation sample as part of Mr. Leggat's initial assessment, his spoken discourse skills would have been appreciably underestimated.

Cohesion Analysis

Cohesion refers to the linguistic means by which words and sentences are meaningfully linked to each other within a text or spoken discourse sample. A variety of cohesive devices have been identified, including (Coelho, 1999; Glosser & Deser, 1990): (1) reference markers such as personal (e.g., "he," "our," "us") and demonstrative (e.g., "these," "here," "that") pronouns that refer to preceding or shortly following unambiguous antecedents; (2) lexical markers such as reiteration (e.g., repeating exact words, or using synonyms or superordinates to tie to previously stated or written vocabulary); (3) conjunctive devices such as causal (e.g., "because," "otherwise"), temporal (e.g., "then," "while"), and additive (e.g., "and," "likewise," "additionally") conjunctions; and, (4) ellipsis, in which previously stated or written words are omitted because they can be presupposed from the preceding text (e.g., in response to "Where did Dylan leave his lunch box?", answering "At the front door." is acceptable even though "He left the lunch box" was omitted from the response). When analyzing discourse samples for cohesion, clinicians should identify not only the types of cohesive devices that patients are using, but also the extent and adequacy of their use. That is, use of cohesive markers can be quantified by calculating the number of cohesion ties per utterance, and qualified by determining whether these ties were appropriately used and complete (e.g., unambiguous and easily determined antecedent), inappropriately used and incomplete (e.g., antecedent is missing), or inaccurate (e.g., ambiguous antecedent) (for more specific information about cohesion analysis, see Cherney et al., 1998).

Speech Acts

Speech acts refer to theoretical units of communication that encompass "what the message-sender means, what the message (or other linguistic elements) means, what the message-sender intends, what the message-receiver intends, what the message-receiver understands, and what the rules governing the linguistic utterance are" (Murray & Chapey, 2001, p. 94). Several classification systems have been developed to describe the range of intentions available (Dore, 1974; Halliday, 1994; Searle, 1969). Some intents encountered most frequently on a daily basis include requests for information or goods and services, greetings, responses, protests, and assertions. Although called speech acts, these communication units can be expressed through any modality (e.g., facial expressions, intonation, body movements). Accordingly, because our words alone do not always express intent, some speech acts are "indirect," as they require processing of not only linguistic information but also contextual cues.

A few discourse analysis systems described in the literature, including Prutting and Kirchner's (1987) Pragmatic Protocol, Penn's (1988) Profile of Communicative Appropriateness, and Terrell and Ripich's (1989) Discourse Abilities Profile, involve tallying and/or rating patients' use of speech acts. For instance, to use the Pragmatic Protocol, clinicians collect a 15-minute, unstructured conversational sample between the patient and a familiar communication partner, and then rate the appropriateness of 30 pragmatic parameters that encompass a number of speech acts as well as discourse and topic management skills (e.g., topic initiation and maintenance). The adequacy of nonverbal (e.g., body language or kinesics) and paralinguistic (e.g., prosody) behaviors also are rated. To summarize Protocol findings, the proportion of appropriate to inappropriate pragmatic behaviors is calculated. High inter-rater reliability has been reported, but only when raters received between eight and 10 hours of training with the Protocol. Prins and Bastiaanse (2004) raised additional concerns with the Pragmatic Protocol, including the lack of information regarding its validity and test-retest reliability and that each pragmatic parameter is rated on only a two-point scale (i.e., "appropriate" vs. "inappropriate").

Discourse and Topic Management Strategies

Effective use of each discourse or genre type (e.g., narrative, procedural, expository, casual conversation) requires an understanding of and adherence to a set of discourse rules or format regularities. For example, successful storytelling or narrative discourse requires organizing and producing one or more story episodes, each of which should at minimum specify the setting (i.e., characters, location, time), an initiating event (that leads a character to develop a plan), an action, and an outcome (related to the character's plan) (Stein & Glenn, 1979). Likewise, successful conversations and other **discourse genres** (e.g., service encounters) require effective use of behaviors such as: (1) topic initiation, including topic selection, introduction, and switching; (2) topic maintenance, which is achieved through turn-taking (i.e., appropriate use and comprehension of verbal and nonverbal cues to indicate the beginning and end of a conversational turn) and elaborations; and (3) repair and/ or revision strategies, including use of repetitions, simplifications, and other forms of revision, and requests for repetitions or revisions (Mentis & Prutting, 1991; Prutting & Kirchner, 1987; Terrell & Ripich, 1989).

A number of rating scales and analysis protocols are described in the literature to assist clinicians in quantifying and qualifying their patients' use of these various discourse and topic management behaviors (e.g., Arkin & Mahendra, 2001; Murray, 1998; Prutting & Kirchner, 1987; Sherratt & Penn, 1990; Terrell & Ripich, 1989). For example, Hartley (1995) developed an Analysis of Topic rating form that can be used to determine the frequency with which patients and their communication partners use positive (e.g., "New-appropriate topic initiation," "Clarification of own information") as well as negative (e.g., "Noncoherent topic change," "Evasion of question") discourse and topic skills during conversation. Before adopting one of these analysis tools, clinicians should determine how much training is necessary to achieve acceptable levels of intra- and inter-rater reliability, or alternatively whether or not the tool authors even reported any measures of reliability. Likewise, because many analysis protocols were developed for select patient populations (e.g., Sherratt & Penn's [1990] system was devised to analyze discourse samples of a patient with RHD), it is unlikely that one protocol will be able to characterize sufficiently the discourse and topic management strengths and weaknesses associated with the spectrum of neurogenic language disorders.

GESTURE AND DRAWING

Assessing whether gesture and drawing are viable communication modalities is necessary when patients have severe language deficits that significantly restrict their spoken and written language abilities (Daniloff, Noll, Fristoe, & Lloyd, 1982; Lyon & Helm-Estabrooks, 1987; Varney, 1982; Ward-Lonergan & Nicholas, 1995). In terms of gestures, research indicates that iconic gestures (i.e., gestures having a relatively direct correspondence with the concepts that they represent, such as pantomiming the function of objects) and AmerInd signs (i.e., a modified version of American Indian Hand-Talk; see also Chapter 11) are easier to perceive and produce than American Sign Language by naive viewers or users, respectively; consequently, these types of gestures are more appropriate assessment and treatment stimuli (Campbell & Jackson, 1995; Christopoulou & Bonvillian, 1985; Daniloff, Fritelli, Buckingham, Hoffman, & Daniloff, 1986). The *Assessment of Nonverbal Communication* (Duffy & Duffy, 1984) evaluates gestural recognition and production abilities; however, this test is no longer available from the publisher, so only clinicians who already have access to this test will be able to make use of it. Furthermore, although some aphasia test batteries include gesture subtests, these typically (1) do not evaluate comprehension skills and (2) have only a limited number of test items to evaluate production abilities (e.g., ADP). Accordingly, many clinicians will need to rely upon non-standardized tasks described in the research literature (e.g., Bell, 1994; Benton et al., 1983; Daniloff et al., 1982; Rothi et al., 1997), or develop their own probe tasks. A typical gesture comprehension task will involve presenting gestures either live or in the more reliable videotaped format, and then requiring patients to point to the correct picture in a multiple-choice format that matches the gesture stimulus. It also may be informative to assess the influence of gestural information on patients' auditory comprehension abilities (Records, 1994). In this case, the clinician could complete the following additional versions of the above probe task: present just an auditory stimulus (i.e., evaluate spoken word-to-picture matching), and present both the auditory and gestural versions of the stimulus. For assessing gesture production, published apraxia tests such as Dabul's (2000) *Apraxia Battery for Adults–2* can provide some information. Likewise, clinicians could present real or pictured objects and ask patients to produce or imitate gestures for these objects.

To determine if drawing may be a suitable means of communication, Helm-Estabrooks and colleagues (Helm-Estabrooks & Albert, 2004; Helm-Estabrooks & Lyon,1987) recommended first establishing that patients have the following: (1) relatively intact visuosemantic processing skills, at least for the concepts to be drawn, (2) sufficient access to symbols within their visuosemantic system, (3) adequate visual attention, (4) sufficient motor and praxic skills for holding a writing implement and drawing, (5) skill at revising and augmenting drawing to facilitate communication interactions, and (6) a willingness to use drawing as a means of communication. Accordingly, a drawing assessment should evaluate not only patients' ability to depict a variety of concepts and events, but also their ability to copy, draw from memory, and perform hand and limb motoric and praxic skills. Although several RHD and dementia batteries include drawing subtests, these tasks were designed to evaluate primarily visuoperceptual and visuoconstruction abilities, and thus should be augmented by an evaluation of more advanced drawing abilities. One tool that will allow such an evaluation is the Daily Mishaps Test (Helm-Estabrooks & Albert, 1991). This test examines how well patients draw enacted scenarios that contain one- to three-part scenes. Because standardized scoring criteria are not provided, clinicians must either create their own or use procedures described in the research literature (e.g., Murray, 1998).

TEST CONFOUNDS

Clinicians must be cognizant of a number of factors that may confound the interpretation of language test results. Two particularly influential factors are age and education. That is, because strong negative effects of age and education on language abilities have been found (MacKenzie, 2000; Tombaugh & Hubley, 1997; Ulatowska et al., 1995), clinicians must always try to assure that the normative samples of the language tests they use match the age and education backgrounds of their patients closely. The normative data of many language tests, however, are based on population samples that fail to represent a broad enough age or education range to be suitable for all patients. In terms of age, normative samples often do not extend to represent the oldest age group, whereas in terms of education, those with low education levels are often under-represented (Hawkins & Bender, 2002; MacKenzie, 2000). This is particularly important when assessing high-level language abilities (e.g., proverb explanation, understanding of implied information), as age and education effects are most apparent on tests of these language skills. Most frequently, failure to identify tests with suitable normative data results in the misdiagnosis of impaired language abilities.

Another important factor to consider when assessing language skills, in particular pragmatic and discourse abilities, is ethnocultural background (Kennepohl et al., 2004). For example, a growing literature has documented that the variety and frequency of discourse and topic management strategies used by adults varies as a function of their ethnocultural background (e.g., Molrine & Pierce, 2002; Ulatowska et al., 2000). Failure to consider these ethnocultural differences could result in (1) inappropriate interpretation of certain discourse behaviors as linguistic symptoms or (2) failure to document compromised usage of certain discourse behaviors.

If the normative sample of a given test or discourse analysis procedure does not match the demographic background of a given patient, clinicians should consult the research literature to determine if additional normative information pertaining to that test or procedure is available. Often, extended normative data for commercially available tests become available subsequent to these tests' initial publication as investigators explore these tests' suitability for additional patient populations (e.g., Gladsjo et al., 1999).

PROGNOSTIC FACTORS FOR LINGUISTIC OUTCOMES

Once language assessment procedures have been completed and assessment findings interpreted, speech-language pathologists must be prepared to make prognoses about their patients' language recovery. Not only will patients, their caregivers, and other health team members be interested in expected language outcomes, so too will medical insurance companies, which utilize this information to approve treatment services (see Chapter 12). Rather than providing generic "will get better" or "won't get better" prognoses, clinicians should try to be as specific as possible (e.g., the patient will be able to tolerate intensive treatment at this time; the patient will require at least two months of biweekly outpatient treatment to show meaningful gains on the ADP; the patient will be able to return to an independent living conditions). To do so, a number of the prognostic indicators must be taken into consideration. The various predictor variables identified in the research literature include those related to biographical, medical, and linguistic and cognitive factors, each of which are described below and summarized in Table 5-6.

BIOGRAPHICAL FACTORS

Biographical factors that clinicians should consider include the patient's age, gender, education, premorbid intelligence, personality, support systems, usual or daily activities, and level and type of life participation. Although a significant negative relationship between age and treatment outcomes has been observed for patients with TBI (Cifu et al., 1996), mixed findings have been reported for aphasic and dementia patient populations (Boller et al., 1991; de Riesthal & Wertz, 2004; Ferro, Mariano, & Madureira, 1999; Ogrezeanu, Voinescu, Mihailescu, & Jipescu, 1994). These equivocal results no doubt reflect that many variables such as personal attitude, general medical health, and level and type of daily activities and social participation may confound the influence of age on recovery (Murray & Chapey, 2001; Tompkins, Jackson, & Schulz, 1990). Therefore, final prognoses should never be based solely upon a patient's age. This is particularly important to keep in mind, given that **ageism,** the systematic stereotyping and discrimination of people on the basis of their age, is still pervasive in health care.

Side Bar

Even Old People Like to Get Better!

In our university clinics, we continue to receive requests for assessment, treatment, or both from patients who have received no or minimal services from a variety of health care facilities (e.g., acute-care, long-term care, home health). Unfortunately, patient age often appears to underlie why these patients never received a speech-language pathology referral or were

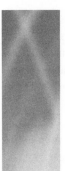

(continued)

provided an inadequate course of speech-language therapy. For example, we recently worked with Mrs. Stroffolino, who in her mid-80s suffered a closed head injury from a fall. She was admitted and treated in an acute care hospital for her orthopedic injuries. Although she reported to her doctor difficulties thinking of words and remembering recent events, she was never given a speech-language pathology or neuropsychological evaluation during her hospital stay. Her doctor instead told Mrs. Stroffolino and her family that these problems were typical for someone of Mrs. Stroffolino's age and that no rehabilitation services were therefore necessary. Fortunately, Mrs. Stroffolino and her family were not satisfied with this doctor's feedback and sought additional information from our clinic.

Table 5-6. **Prognostic Indicators for Language Recovery**

FACTORS SUGGESTING BETTER PROGNOSIS	FACTORS SUGGESTING POORER PROGNOSIS	NONPREDICTIVE FACTORS
Younger age (TBI only)	Etiology:	Age (etiologies other than TBI)
High premorbid intellectual ability	Stroke (vs. TBI)	Gender
Adequate patient motivation	Ischemic stroke	Education level
Appropriate family and caregiver attitudes	Progressive disease	
Communication symptoms:	Lesion Location:	
Awareness of deficits	Dominant hemisphere	
Less severe language impairment	Multiple lesions	
Anomic or conduction aphasia	Bilateral lesions	
Stimulability and self-cueing ability	Cortical (vs. subcortical)	
	Frontal lobe (in TBI)	
	Concomitant medical, physical, or psychiatric problems:	
	Apraxia of speech	
	Depression	
	Medications:	
	Those that cause confusion or fatigue	
	Those with communication side effects	
	Communication symptoms:	
	Auditory comprehension deficits	
	Global or severe Wernicke's aphasia	
	Cognitive deficits:	
	Anosognosia	
	Memory impairments	
	Neglect	

The influence of gender on language outcomes also remains unresolved. In some studies, gender and outcome are linked with better recovery in males (Holland, Greenhouse, Fromm, & Swindell, 1989), whereas in other studies females are favored (Basso, Capitani, & Moraschini 1982; Pizzamiglio, Mammucari, & Razzano, 1985). In still other studies, no significant differences in the language recovery or, in the case of progressive diseases, rate of language deterioration of female versus male patients have been observed (Bayles et al., 1999; Ogrezeanu et al., 1994). Given these mixed findings, gender does not appear to be an influential prognostic variable.

Although education level can affect patients' performances of language tests (Hawkins & Bender, 2002; MacKenzie, 2000), it is not clear whether it affects the degree or rate of their language recovery (Connor et al., 2001; de Riesthal & Wertz, 2004; Ferro et al., 1999). Instead, clinicians should consider patients' overall premorbid intellectual ability, which appears to have more predictive power than education level (Lecours, Mehler, Parente, & Beltrami, 1988; Tompkins et al., 1990). To obtain estimates of premorbid intelligence, clinicians can use easy-to-calculate equations published in the research literature that are based on statistical weightings of patients' age, education, gender, occupation, race, and other demographic information (Barona, Reynolds, & Chastain, 1984; Wilson, Rosenbaum, & Brown, 1979).

Research indicates that personality variables and levels of social support are strongly associated with overall health, morbidity, mortality, and treatment prognosis in many health conditions, including stroke and head injury (Andersson & Fridlund, 2002; Tompkins et al., 1990). For instance, patients' motivation, desire, and determination to improve will clearly influence the course and outcomes of their treatment (Wressle, Eeg-Olofsson, Marcusson, & Henriksson, 2002). As van Harskamp and Visch-Brink (1991) noted, "the patient's motivation is of utmost importance: patients need to exert themselves to make progress" (p. 533). Likewise, family or caregiver attitudes regarding patients' improvement potential and treatment program, as well as their emotional well-being, will affect intervention outcomes (Evans, Bishop, & Haselkorn, 1991; Freed, 2004; Tompkins et al., 1990). Accordingly, to foster patients' and caregivers' willingness to participate actively in treatment, clinicians must assure that patients and their caregivers are well educated about the patients' symptoms, have the opportunity to contribute to treatment planning, and are provided support to minimize negative emotional reactions (Patterson & Wells, 1995; Wressle et al., 2002).

MEDICAL FACTORS

Influential medical factors that should be considered when making prognoses include the etiology and duration of the neurogenic language disorder, the site and extent of brain damage, and the presence and severity of concomitant physical and mental health problems.

Different language outcomes are associated with the different neurological etiologies. For example, there is better recovery from aphasia subsequent to TBI than aphasia subsequent to stroke or other vascular disorders (Basso et al., 1980; Gil et al., 1996; Sarno et al., 1986). Better communication outcomes also may be expected if a patient survives a hemorrhagic rather than an ischemic (i.e., thrombotic or embolic) stroke, because hemorrhages tend to produce less permanent brain damage, particularly within cortical areas (Basso, 1992; Ferro et al., 1999; Holland et al., 1989; Nicholas, Helm-Estabrooks, Ward-Lonergan, & Morgan, 1993). With respect to dementia, certain dementing illnesses are associated with greater compromise of language abilities than others. For instance, initial symptoms of Alzheimer's disease, Pick's disease, and frontotemporal dementia are often language-based, whereas in Huntington's, Parkinson's, and dementia with Lewy bodies, cognitive symptoms often precede and are more severe than language symptoms (Grossman, 2002; Sutton-Brown & Suchowersky, 2003).

With respect to stroke, TBI, and other non-progressive neurological disorders, the greatest language recovery rate is most frequently observed during the first few months post onset, a time line that overlaps with spontaneous physiological recovery processes such as the resorption of edema (Basso, 1992; Pedersen, Jorgensen, Nakayama, Raaschou, & Olsen, 1995). Patients and caregivers, however, must be reminded that patients with static neurological disorders can continue to demonstrate significant progress for years beyond the period of spontaneous recovery (Blomert, 1998). Similarly, with treatment, patients with progressive neurological disorders can slow the rate and extent of their disease progression for many years following symptom onset (Arkin & Mahendra, 2001).

Site and extent of brain damage also may influence language outcomes. Generally, poor language prognosis, in terms of amount and rate of recovery (or in the case of progressive diseases, rate of deterioration), is associated with large dominant-hemisphere lesions or multiple lesions (Ferro, 1992; Goldenberg & Spatt, 1994; Karbe, Kessler, Herholz, Fink, & Heiss, 1995); that is, the larger the lesion, the poorer the language outcome. More specifically, severe or more enduring aphasia may be expected if brain damage: (1) encompasses the central core of the dominant-hemisphere language area subserved by the middle cerebral artery (Holland et al., 1989); (2) affects dominant-hemisphere temporobasal areas (Goldenberg & Spatt, 1994; Naeser & Palumbo, 1994); (3) extends deep into underlying white matter pathways or other subcortical structures of the dominant-hemisphere (Ferro et al., 1999); or (4) involves bilateral lesions (Naeser et al., 1998). In RHD, communicative disorders are more likely if patients suffer cortical versus subcortical brain damage (Joanette et al., 1990), whereas in TBI, they are more frequent and significant following a severe frontal lobe or closed head injury (Chapman et al., 1992; 1994).

An extensive literature documents that patients suffering from concomitant medical, physical, or psychiatric complications are more likely to have longer hospital stays, and less likely to achieve the extent or rate of recovery as that obtained by patients without these conditions (Holland et al., 1989; Jorgensen et al., 1995). For example, patients with TBI who develop a hardening of connective tissue called heterotopic ossification have been found to have longer inpatient rehabilitation stays, poorer functional outcomes by discharge, and less frequent discharges to home, compared to patients with TBI who had similar severities of head injury but no heterotopic ossification (Johns, Cifu, Keyser-Marcus, Jolles, & Fratkin, 1999). Likewise, aphasia recovery is compromised by the presence of motor speech disorders such as apraxia of speech (Ogrezeanu et al., 1994). Patients with neurogenic disorders who have depression, anxiety, or other psychological problems also are at risk for poorer rehabilitation outcomes than their cohorts without these mental health problems (Ben-Yishay & Daniels-Zide, 2000; Diamond, Holroyd, Macciochi, & Felsenthal, 1995; Herrmann, Britz, Bartels, & Wallesch, 1995; Paolucci et al., 1998). It is important to note, however, that this risk of poorer outcome can be reduced if depression is diagnosed and treated as soon as possible (van de Weg, Kuik, & Lankhorst, 1999).

Medications also may negatively affect patients' communicative functioning. For example, the side effects of some antidepressants and anticonvulsant drugs include dysarthria and stuttering (O'Sullivan & Fagan, 1998). Furthermore, a number of medications frequently prescribed to neurogenic patients, including anticonvulsants, sedatives, and antihypertensives, may cause confusion, fatigue, and decreased arousal or alertness, which in turn can affect patients' ability to complete language activities, and more generally reduce their rate of recovery (Small, 2002; Vogel, Carter, & Carter, 2000; Zafonte, Elovic, Mysiw, O'Dell, & Watanabe, 1999). Accordingly, clinicians should review what medications their patients are taking to ascertain whether these drugs have the potential to inhibit or enhance their patients' current communication abilities.

LINGUISTIC AND COGNITIVE FACTORS

A number of linguistic and cognitive factors should be considered when attempting to provide prognostic information. In terms of language, variables such as language stimulability and severity and type of aphasia have been found influential. For instance, several studies have found initial severity of aphasia to be a strong predictor of language recovery (de Riesthal & Wertz, 2004; Ogrezeanu et al., 1994; Pedersen et al., 1995): More severe initial language impairments are associated with less positive language outcomes. Furthermore, patients with severe auditory recognition and comprehension problems tend to demonstrate less recovery than those with less severe impairments in this language modality (Schuell et al., 1964; Smith, 1971).

Strong links also have been reported between aphasia type and the extent of recovery or the residual pattern of language impairment. Generally, patients with anomic or conduction aphasia have the best language prognosis, and those with global or severe Wernicke's have the worst prognosis (Ferro et al., 1999; Ogrezeanu et al., 1994; Paolucci et al., 1998); given the previous discussion of the relationship between aphasia severity and language prognosis, this pattern of outcomes might be predicted, as anomic and conduction aphasias produce less severe language symptoms than global and severe Wernicke's aphasias. Patients who continue to present with global aphasia beyond three months post-onset are at greatest risk for poor language outcomes (Kertesz, 1979). In addition to making predictions regarding the extent of language improvement, clinicians may also make predictions regarding changes in aphasia type. With recovery, Broca's, Wernicke's, conduction, or transcortical (sensory, motor, or mixed) aphasia types should evolve toward anomic aphasia (Ferro et al., 1999; Ogrezeanu et al., 1994), and global aphasia hopefully resolves toward Broca's aphasia (Mohr, 1976).

The extent to which patients may profit from cues, that is, the extent to which the patients are stimulable, should also be considered when making language outcome predictions. Some research has indicated that patients with aphasia who are initially responsive to prompts and cues have better spoken language recovery than patients for whom cueing is unproductive (Keenan & Brassell, 1974). Likewise, several researchers have hypothesized that patients who can learn to cue themselves will display better language outcomes and generalization of trained language skills than patients who must rely on others for cues (Murray & Chapey, 2001; Singer & Bashir, 1999).

Generally the presence of cognitive deficits is associated with greater levels of disability and higher rates of institutionalization (Patel et al., 2003). More specifically, there is growing evidence to support the contention that language recovery and rehabilitation outcomes, including generalization of trained skills or compensatory strategies, may be negatively affected by the presence of concomitant cognitive impairments (Helm-Estabrooks, 1998; Murray et al., 2004; Ramsberger, 1994; Sinotte et al., 2003). For example, the executive functions of self-awareness and self-monitoring appear closely linked to language outcomes and therapy progress, as patients with poor awareness of their language or other symptoms, or of situations that enhance and degrade their language skills, have a poorer prognosis than patients without these cognitive deficits (Joanette et al., 1990; Keenan & Brassell, 1974; van Harskamp & Visch-Brink, 1991). Patients with aphasia who have bilateral lesions or damage to temporobasal regions, and therefore concomitant impairments of memory and/or executive functioning, also are less successful in speech-language therapy than patients whose brain damage did not affect these areas (Goldenberg & Spatt, 1994; Naeser et al., 1998). Likewise, stroke patients with neglect have longer hospitalizations and less favorable rehabilitation outcomes than those without this cognitive symptom (Paolucci et al., 1998; Pedersen, Jorgensen, Nakayama, Raaschou, & Olsen, 1997). Finally, significant associations between the discourse problems of patients with RHD or TBI and deficits of working memory or executive functioning (McDonald & Pearce, 1998; Tompkins et al., 1994) also indicate that the integrity of cognitive abilities should be considered when making prognoses regarding language outcomes.

SUMMARY

Over the past two decades, advances in our understanding of linguistic impairments associated with aphasia, RHD, TBI, and dementia have led to the development of numerous approaches and procedures for evaluating neurogenic language disorders at the ICF level of body function. A key to managing this broad spectrum of test options is acknowledging that the evaluation of linguistic abilities is a multistep process that cannot be completed via the administration of a single language test. Instead, the assessment process must begin with the collection of case history information and completion of observations. On the basis of those data, clinicians next select and administer tests of general and specific linguistic functioning. The last step of the assessment process involves interpreting linguistic test findings in light of cognitive test results (see Chapter 6), findings from participation and activity evaluations (see Chapter 7), and the consideration of certain influential biographic and medical variables. Only when all of these assessment procedures have been completed should final recommendations regarding linguistic outcomes and treatment goals and procedures be made.

Chapter 6

Assessment of Function: Quantifying and Qualifying Cognitive Disorders

LEARNING OBJECTIVES

After reading this chapter you should be able to:

- Provide a rationale for assessing the cognitive abilities of patients with neurogenic language disorders.

- Identify formal and informal procedures that may be used to help collect case history information pertaining to a cognitive assessment.

- Describe the purpose and format of cognitive screening tests.

- Differentiate between test batteries for evaluating general cognitive abilities and those for assessing attention, memory, or executive functioning

- Describe tests that evaluate specific attention, memory, or executive function abilities at the ICF level of body structure and function.

- Identify test batteries and tests of specific cognitive

KEY TERMS

cognitive flexibility
divided attention
inhibition

orientation
selective or focused
    attention

sustained attention
working memory

functions that are suitable for patients with concomitant language disorders.

- Explain factors that may confound the administration or interpretation of cognitive tests.

- Describe biographic, medical, and cognitive variables that should be considered when making prognoses about cognitive outcomes.

INTRODUCTION

It is well established that patients with neurogenic language disorders frequently, if not always, have concomitant cognitive impairments including deficits of attention, memory, and/or executive functioning (Bayles, 2003; MacDonald, 2000; Murray, 2002; Murray, Ramage, & Hopper, 2001; Stierwalt & Murray, 2002; see also Chapter 2). Additionally, caregivers and neurogenic patients who are cognizant of the severity and breadth of their symptoms typically voice most concern over cognitive problems associated with the onset of brain damage or disease (Marsh, Kersel, Havill, & Sleigh, 2002; Visser-Kiezer, Meyboom-de Jong, Deelman, Berg,

& Gerritsen, 2002). As discussed in Chapter 2, cognitive impairments also may be the sole cause of communication problems (as is commonly the case in patients who have suffered a traumatic brain injury or right hemisphere brain damage), or may exacerbate linguistic problems (as may occur in patients with aphasia or certain forms of dementia) (Bayles, 2003; Murray, 2000; Murray & Stout, 1999; Turkstra & Holland, 1998).

In addition to their negative influences upon communication, cognitive deficits may have dire effects upon the rehabilitation process. For example, patients with concomitant cognitive deficits are less likely to benefit from behavioral treatments and, accordingly, have a slower recovery or poorer functional outcomes compared to their peers without these coexisting problems (Chen et al., 1998; Goldenberg, Dettmers, Grothe, & Spatt, 1994; Kalra, Perez, Gupta, & Wittink, 1997; Pedersen et al., 1996). More specifically, patients with anosognosia tend to do poorly in rehabilitation because they fail, at least acutely, to recognize their need for therapy, their expectations for treatment outcomes far exceed their true potential, or both (Jehkonen et al., 2000; Melamed, Grosswasser, & Stern, 1992). Likewise, one group of researchers found that attention test performance was a strong predictor of brain-injured patients' use of memory aids (Evans et al., 2003).

Just as rehabilitation can be negatively affected by cognitive problems, so too can social and vocational outcomes (Nybo & Koskiniemi, 1999). For instance, several studies have found a negative relationship between neglect and the social and vocational outcomes of stroke patients (Appelros, Karlsson, Seiger, & Nydevik, 2002; Jehkonen et al., 2000), and one investigation reported that attentional abilities were most influential on the ability of patients with aphasia to return to work, even more so than their language abilities (Ramsing, Blomstrand, & Sullivan, 1991). Finally, there is evidence supporting a positive association between neglect or executive function deficits and caregiver burden (Appelros et al., 2002; Marsh et al., 2002; Rymer et al., 2002; Watanabe & Taki, 2000). Consequently, including a cognitive assessment aimed at the ICF level of body function may result in improved estimations of the extent and type of treatment needed by patients with neurogenic language disorders, as well as the type of support and training needed by their caregivers.

Whereas it is clear that most patients with neurogenic language disorders will benefit from a comprehensive cognitive evaluation, it is less clear which health care professional should complete that evaluation. That is, the scopes of practice for several disciplines currently encompass assessing at least some cognitive functions. For example, in hospital and rehabilitation settings, occupational therapists, neuropsychologists, and speech-language pathologists may all be capable of assessing cognitive skills. Likewise, in school settings, resource teachers or learning specialists, speech-language pathologists, and school psychologists may have been trained to complete cognitive testing. Accordingly, an essential first step to a cognitive evaluation is to determine whether cognitive skills will be assessed by one or several health care team members: Failing to predetermine team member responsibilities could result in redundant or, conversely, inadequate testing.

As mentioned in Chapter 4, it also is important to review state and national professional association guidelines to determine what assessment tools each health care team member is allowed to administer. For example, in some states and provinces, only psychologists are licensed to use and interpret the results of certain cognitive tests, particularly those that evaluate memory and executive functioning. Even in the presence of these professional restrictions, a speech-language pathologist's input is recommended, especially when patients have language impairments that may confound standardized assessment administration and scoring procedures. Speech-language pathologists have the most professional training related to assessing and treating language disorders, and thus often have the greatest insight regarding how best to adapt testing procedures, interpret test findings, or both when assessing the cognitive abilities of patients with neurogenic language disorders.

Side Bar

Dementia due to Inaccurate Test Results versus Impaired Cognition

The failure to acknowledge the influence of communication impairments upon the outcomes of cognitive tests can result in inaccurate interpretation of test results. For example, during an initial speech-language diagnostic session with a patient presenting with a degenerative cerebellar disorder, the patient's wife, Mrs. Ashcroft, was interviewed to determine the previous services that Mr. Ashcroft had received. She was asked whether or not Mr. Ashcroft had received any prior cognitive testing, and about the outcome of that testing. Mrs. Ashcroft replied that Mr. Ashcroft's neurologist had completed a short cognitive test on several occasions, but she did not know the name of the test. She did know, however, that the neurologist had concluded that Mr. Ashcroft was presenting with dementia, based on the results of that cognitive testing. Following further questioning, we were able to determine that Mr. Ashcroft had received the *Mini-Mental State Examination* (MMSE; Folstein, Folstein, & McHugh, 2001; see Cognitive Status and Dementia Screening Tools section of this chapter for further description of this test). This was alarming to us, given that Mr. Ashcroft had been presenting with severe ataxia, severe ataxic dysarthria, and mild anomia for some time and, consequently, that his performance on the MMSE would no doubt have been confounded by these motor and communication problems. That is, basing a diagnosis of dementia only on MMSE results was inappropriate, as it is difficult to determine whether or not Mr. Ashcroft's verbal and written MMSE responses were inaccurate because of possible cognitive problems or because of his severe motor and communication difficulties.

Regardless of whether speech-language pathologists fulfill a direct or indirect role in evaluating cognitive skills, they must be knowledgeable of cognitive tests and assessment procedures to assure an appropriate understanding of their patients' cognitive strengths and limitations. Accordingly, the purpose of this chapter is to overview the components of a cognitive evaluation and to provide an introduction to the multitude of commercially available tests and research protocols that are currently available to quantify and qualify the cognitive abilities of patients with neurogenic disorders at the ICF level of body function.

○ ASSESSMENT PROCEDURES

Cognitive evaluations should follow the same format as that utilized to complete language evaluations: Begin with the compilation of the case history and observational data, and then, based on that information, select and administer formal or structured tests of cognition. Recall that assessment must be considered a continual process, as initial tests may reveal new areas of cognitive strength or weakness, or patients' cognitive profiles or functional needs may change as a result of spontaneous recovery or treatment.

CASE HISTORY AND OBSERVATIONS

Prior to giving structured or formal tests of cognition, an imperative first step to assessment is the assemblage of case history and observational information to help make decisions regarding test selection as well as subsequent interpretation of test results. Interviewing both patients and their caregivers to collect the case history can be particularly valuable when completing a cognitive evaluation. For instance, a comparison of patient and caregiver responses can provide information regarding the patient's long-term memory limitations (e.g., is the patient able to recall accurately information encoded prior to the onset of the brain damage or disease?). Likewise, executive problems such as anosognosia can be identified by noting whether or not patients specify the same types and severities of problems as their caregivers. Indeed, research indicates that compared to their significant others, patients who have suffered a traumatic brain injury (TBI), regardless of head injury severity, under-report cognitive, emotional, and behavioral symptoms (Sbordone, Seyranian, & Ruff, 1998). Information pertaining to other cognitive abilities also can be accrued during the patient interview. For example, the clinician might suspect attention problems if the patient appears distractible and requires continuous prompts to stay on task. For a listing of more information to accrue during the case history, refer to Chapter 4.

Several confounds necessitate that cognitive assessments include direct observations of patients in a variety of contexts. First, the external structure of formal test procedures may minimize or even completely obscure certain cognitive problems (Dugbartey et al., 1999; Murray & Ramage, 2000). For example, formal assessments are typically conducted in a quiet environment (e.g., a testing room with just the examiner and patient present), and thus are accommodating for patients with attention problems; likewise, patients often are provided supports such as the repetition of task instructions and cues to stay on task or to switch to the next task, which can help some patients compensate for memory impairments or disinhibition and other executive function deficits. Accordingly, failing to observe patients in informal and unstructured environments may lead to an over-estimation of their cognitive abilities. Inversely, formal testing situations may negatively affect the performance of patients who are unfamiliar with such procedures, such as those with little formal education or the elderly (Nussbaum, 1998); in these cases, omitting the observational aspect of the assessment may lead to overestimation of the presence and/or severity of cognitive problems.

Clinicians may consult protocols in the research literature or commercially available tools to help interview patients and caregivers, and to assist in collecting, organizing, and summarizing observational data pertaining to patients' cognitive abilities. For instance, when executive function deficits are suspected, a clinician might use the Problems Checklists of Parenté and Herrmann (2003), Executive Interview (Royall, Mahurin, & Gray, 1992), or Dysexecutive Questionnaire of the *Behavioral Assessment of Dysexecutive Syndrome* (BADS; Wilson, Alderman, Burgess, Emslie, & Evans, 1996) to interview the patient, caregiver, and/or other health care team members. Rating scales for other cognitive domains are also available, including the Attention Questionnaire (Sohlberg et al., 2001) and the *Brown Attention-Deficit Disorder Scales* (Brown, 1996). As an example of these tools, the Dysexecutive Questionnaire consists of 20 items (e.g., "She/he loses his/her temper at the slightest thing," "She/he has difficulty thinking ahead or planning for the future."), each of which is rated on a scale from zero, which equals "never," to four, which equals "very often," to determine the frequency with which common symptoms of executive dys-functioning occur (e.g., personality changes such as aggressiveness, behavior problems such as impulsivity, cognitive impairments such as planning difficulties). There are two versions, one to be used with patients and one for caregivers, so that clinicians can compare patients' self-ratings to those of their caregivers. Importantly, high correlations between the Dysexecutive Questionnaire ratings of caregivers and the performances of their brain-damaged relatives on formal tests of executive functioning have been reported (Burgess, Alderman, Evans, Emslie, & Wilson, 1998).

The *Profile of Executive Control System* (PRO-EX; Braswell et al., 1992) represents an assessment tool available to help clinicians structure the observational component of a cognitive assessment. More specifically, PRO-EX provides suggestions for: (1) unstructured situations in which to observe patients (e.g., hospital cafeteria, hospital room), (2) set-up tasks to elicit executive function behaviors (e.g., the patient is asked to make telephone calls to obtain information such as how to get a building permit), and, (3) patient and caregiver interview questions. To help qualify the observational data, clinicians identify their patients' highest level of functioning on a number of executive behaviors via the PRO-EX Rating Protocol. For example, ratings for initiation skills can vary from the lowest, "Able to initiate only with physical prompting," to the highest, "Independently initiate a variety of complex tasks even if they do not feel motivated" (p. 2). Braswell et al. reported acceptable inter-rater reliability when the PRO-EX was used to observe and rate the executive function abilities of 32 clients who had suffered either a TBI or stroke. Tools such as PRO-EX offer clinicians a means by which to help verify the reliability of data gleaned from fully unstructured observations of their patients' cognitive abilities.

COGNITIVE STATUS AND DEMENTIA SCREENING TOOLS

Following completion of the case history, interviews, and observations, formal or structured test procedures can be implemented. Formal testing often begins with administration of a bedside or screening test, particularly when patients are in an acute care setting. The purposes of these tools are to determine the presence or absence of cognitive impairments or dementia, and to identify cognitive functions in need of further evaluation. As shown in Table 6-1, many bedside or screening tests are currently available, each of which invariably includes a limited number of items to assess a variety of cognitive functions including **orientation** (e.g., oriented to time, person, and place), visuoperception and visuoconstruction, verbal and nonverbal memory, language, attention, and some executive functions. Because these tests are short in length and only sample a limited number of cognitive functions, their results have limited usefulness in terms of planning treatment or evaluating treatment effects.

The *Mini-Mental State Examination* (MMSE; Folstein et al., 1975; 2001) is perhaps the most widely used and researched cognitive screening tool. It consists of brief set of questions and tasks designed to assess orientation to time and place (e.g., what is the year?), mental calculation (e.g., subtract seven from 100 and then keep subtracting by seven), verbal short-term memory (i.e., recall three words after a short delay), language (e.g., write a sentence.), and visuoconstruction skills (i.e., copy a design). A cutoff score of 23 out of a maximum of 30 is recommended to indicate impaired cognitive status. To help classify the severity of cognitive impairment, Folstein et al. (2001) have provided score ranges in which normal = 27–30, mild impairment = 21–26, moderate impairment = 11–20, and severe impairment = zero–10.

Although numerous studies attest to the reliability and validity of the MMSE (for a review see Tombaugh & McIntyre, 1992), its use with certain patient populations should be avoided or, at the very least, its scores must be interpreted cautiously. For example, because of its heavy language and motor speech demands, the MMSE is inappropriate for many patients with neurogenic language disorders, as poor performance might reflect aphasia, dysarthria, and/or apraxia rather than cognitive problems (Golper, Rau, Erskins, Langhans, & Houlihan, 1987). Likewise, research suggests that the MMSE is insensitive to cognitive symptoms associated with right hemisphere brain damage (Dick et al., 1984; Nelson, Fogel, & Faust,

Table 6-1. Bedside and Screening Tests of Cognitive Disorders

INSTRUMENT	SOURCE
Addenbrooke's Cognitive Examination	Hodges (2004)
Alzheimer's Disease Caregiver's Questionnaire	Solomon (2002)
Alzheimer's Quick Test	Wiig et al. (2002)
Blessed Dementia Scale	Blessed et al. (1968)
Clock Drawing	Freedman et al. (1994)
Cognistat	Kiernan et al. (1995)
Cognitive Behavior Rating Scales	Williams (1987)
Cognitive-Linguistic Quick Test	Helm-Estabrooks (2001)
Community Screening Interview for Dementia	Hall et al. (1996)
Cross-Cultural Cognitive Examination	Glosser et al. (1993)
Dementia Rating Scale–2	Mattis (2001)
Frontal Behavioral Inventory	Kertesz et al. (1997)
Galveston Orientation and Amnesia Test	Levin et al. (1979)
Julia Farr Services Post-Traumatic Amnesia Scale	Forrester & Geffen (1995)
Middlesex Elderly Assessment of Mental State	Golding (1989)
Mini-Mental State Examination	Folstein et al. (1975; 2001)
Minnesota Cognitive Acuity Screen	Knopman et al. (2000)
Modified Mini-Mental State Exam (3MS)	Teng & Chui (1987)
Qualitative Evaluation of Dementia	Royall et al. (1993)
Rancho Los Amigos Levels of Cognitive Functioning	Hagen (1981)
Repeatable Battery for the Assessment of Neuropsychological Status	Randolph (1998)
Short Portable Mental Status Questionnaire	Pfeiffer (1975)
Telephone Interview for Cognitive Status	Brandt et al. (1988)
Wechsler Abbreviated Scale of Intelligence	Wechsler (1999)

1986), and may miss patients experiencing the earliest stages of dementing diseases (Feher et al., 1992). MMSE scores are influenced by variables such as low education, ethnocultural background, and poor health (Escobar et al., 1986), and thus this test also may be inappropriate for patients presenting with several of these variables (Barrie, 2002; Nussbaum, 1998). Therefore, clinicians should consult the research literature to determine if normative data are available for the specific patient population with which they work (e.g., Crum, Anthony, Bassett, & Folstein, 1993).

The additional tools listed in Table 6-1 are similar to the MMSE, but in some cases are more suitable for identifying cognitive problems in a broader spectrum of patients. For example, the Minnesota Cognitive Acuity Screen (Knopman, Knudsen, Yoes, & Weiss, 2000) and the Telephone Interview for Cognitive Status (Brandt, Spencer, & Folstein, 1988) are similar in length and content to the MMSE, but were developed for administration over the phone to individuals with motoric, emotional, or financial limitations that may impede their ability to attend an in-person assessment; similarly, caregivers can complete the Alzheimer's Disease Caregiver's Questionnaire (Solomon, 2002) online. Tools such as the Cross-Cultural Cognitive Examination (Glosser et al., 1993) and Community Screening Interview for Dementia (Hall, Ogunniyi, Hendrie, & Brittain, 1996) were developed for administration to patients representing diverse ethnocultural and educational backgrounds. Other screening tests vary from the MMSE by evaluating a wider range of cognitive ability levels (e.g., *Dementia Rating Scale–2* [Mattis, 2001]), including more refined scoring systems (e.g., Modified Mini-Mental State Exam [Teng & Chui, 1987]) and/or providing parallel forms so that repeated testing can be completed without the confound of learning or repetition effects (e.g., *Repeated Battery for the Assessment of Neuropsychological Status* [Randolph, 1998]). Although these tests tend to take longer to administer and score than the MMSE, they have been found, at least in some studies, to yield more accurate screening results (McDowell, Kristjansson, Hill, & Hebert, 1997).

A few cognitive screening tools have been developed for specific patient populations. For example, the *Alzheimer's Quick Test* (Wiig, Nielsen, Minthon, & Warkentin, 2002) consists of five sets of timed naming tasks (i.e., Color-Form, Color-Number, Color-Letter, Color-Animal, and Color-Object Naming). Based on previous research, these tasks have been shown effective at identifying the presence of mild to moderate parietal lobe dysfunction, which, as mentioned in Chapters 2 and 3, is associated with Alzheimer's disease, even early in the disease process. Each naming task is completed three times: once to name each single-dimension of the visual stimuli, and once to name both dimensions of the visual stimuli. For instance, on the Color-Form task, patients first name as quickly and accurately as possible the color of each shape stimulus depicted on the test page. Next, they name as quickly and accurately as possible the name of each shape stimulus; finally, they are required to name as quickly and accurately as possible both the color and shape of each stimulus. Both naming accuracy and response time are evaluated to determine if patients are performing within a normal range, slower- or less-accurate-than-normal range, or non-normal or pathological range. These performance ranges were based upon a standardization sample that represented a fairly broad range of ages (i.e., 15 to 72 years) and ethnocultural backgrounds. Although the test manual states that the same criterion ranges of naming accuracy and response time can be used for individuals "between 15 and 75+," use of the test with individuals over the age of 72 appears inappropriate, as adults over that age did not participate in the standardization process.

Finally, one of the quickest and easiest to administer cognitive screening tools is Clock Drawing (see Figure 6-1). Although it was initially developed to assess visuo-constructional abilities, subsequent research has found that it also evaluates attention, memory, and executive function abilities (Royall, Cordes, & Polk, 1998; Freedman et al., 1994). Several versions of the clock drawing task and scoring are available (for a review see Barrie, 2002). For example, the task can be administered as a free-drawn condition in which patients are asked to "Draw a clock, put in all the numbers, and set the hands to. . .," or a pre-drawn condition in which they are given a piece of paper with a pre-drawn circle representing a clock and asked to write in the numbers and set the hands to a specified time (usually "ten past eleven"). While patients complete the task, clinicians can observe the patients' planning strategies (e.g., placing anchor numbers—12, three, six, and nine—before placing other numbers), areas of difficulty as evidenced by over-writing or latencies, and whether repetition of instructions is necessary (suggesting possible memory problems). Clock drawing performance correlates well with other cognitive screening tools, including the MMSE, and has been shown to be more suitable than the MMSE for patients who are not native English speakers or have low education levels (Barrie, 2002; Royall et al., 2003).

In summary, a variety of screening tests are available to establish the presence or absence of cognitive impairment. For patients whose screening test outcomes indicate cognitive problems, the next step of the evaluation may be completing a more in-depth and/or comprehensive cognitive test battery or tests of specific cognitive functions. Alternately, in cases in which the clinician has ample assessment time available and the patient has already been determined to have cognitive difficulties, the screening step of the evaluation may be skipped, with the clinician instead opting to begin with one of the cognitive test batteries described below.

TEST BATTERIES

Administration of a test battery is frequently the next step of a cognitive evaluation if the cognitive screening or other initial assessment procedures suggest impaired cognitive functioning. Two basic types of cognitive test batteries are available: those designed to evaluate a range of cognitive functions and thus provide an overview of patients' general cognitive abilities or intelligence, and those designed to evaluate a range of cognitive behaviors within only one domain of cognition

a)

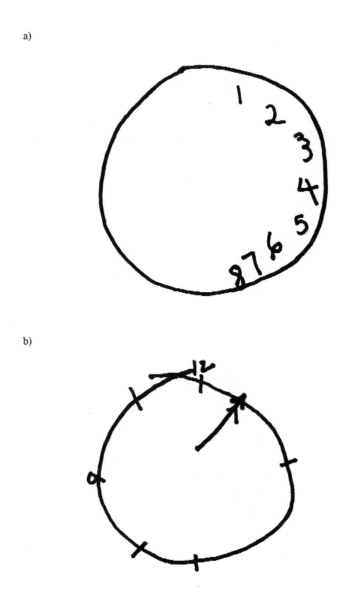

b)

Figure 6-1. Examples of clock drawings by (a) a patient with left neglect and perseveration (i.e., extra loops on "3") and (b) a patient with Alzheimer's disease and visuoconstruction problems. In both examples, patients were asked to set the clock to 1:45.

(e.g., a memory battery that assesses short- and long-term memory skills). Examples of each of these types of test batteries are described below.

General Cognitive Functioning Test Batteries

A number of general cognitive test batteries are currently available (Table 6-2). Speech-language pathologists should check with other health care team members and state requirements before utilizing these tools, as administration of these batteries often falls under the purview of psychology or neuropsychology. Typically,

Table 6-2. Cognitive Test Batteries

TARGET COGNITIVE FUNCTION	INSTRUMENT	SOURCE
General Cognitive Functioning	Halstead-Reitan Neuropsychology Test Battery	Reitan & Wolfson (1985)
	Kaplan Baycrest Neurocognitive Assessment	Kaplan et al. (2000)
	Neuropsychological Assessment Battery	Stern & White (2003)
	Severe Impairment Battery	Saxton et al. (1993)
	Severe Cognitive Impairment Profile	Peavy (1998)
	Ross Information Processing Assessment–2	Ross-Swain (1996)
	Ross Information Processing Assessment–Geriatric	Ross-Swain & Fogle (1996)
	Wessex Head Injury Matrix	Shiel et al. (2000)
	Wechsler Adult Intelligence Scales–III	Wechsler (1997a)
Attention	APT Test	Sohlberg & Mateer (2001)
	Test of Everyday Attention	Robertson et al. (1994)
Memory	Rivermead Behavioral Memory Test–II	Wilson et al. (2003)
	Rivermead Behavioral Memory Test–Extended Version	Wilson et al. (1998)
	Wechsler Memory Scales–III	Wechsler (1997b)
	Wide Range Assessment of Memory and Learning–II	Adams & Sheslow (2003)
Executive Functioning	Behavioral Assessment of the Dysexecutive Syndrome	Wilson et al. (1996)
	Behavior Rating Inventory of Executive Function	Gioia et al. (2001)
	Delis-Kaplan Executive Function System	Delis et al. (2001)
	Executive Control Battery	Goldberg et al. (2000)
	Executive Interview (EXIT)	Royall et al. (1992)

speech-language pathologists utilize these test batteries only when neuropsychology services are unavailable (which is the case in many rural communities and nursing homes), and even then, they typically only give certain subtests rather than the entire battery. Regardless of whether speech-language pathologists play a direct or indirect role in administering these batteries, they should be familiar with them so that they can accurately interpret neuropsychology reports and, if need be, appropriately select and utilize specific subtests.

The most widely applied batteries of overall cognitive functioning are the *Wechsler Adult Intelligence Scales–Revised* (WAIS-R; Wechsler, 1981) and its most recent update, the *Wechsler Adult Intelligence Scales–III* (WAIS-III; Wechsler, 1997). Although these batteries or portions of them are a common component of psychology and neuropsychology evaluations, our clinical experiences indicate that they are infrequently included in speech-language pathology assessments. The WAIS-III consists of 14 subtests, 11 of which made up the WAIS-R. These subtests evaluate a range of verbal and nonverbal, or "performance," skills, including language (e.g., Comprehension, Vocabulary), auditory verbal memory (e.g., Digit Span, Letter-Number Sequencing), visuoconstruction (e.g., Block Design, Object Assembly), and executive function abilities (e.g., Similarities, Matrix Reasoning). Compared to the WAIS-R, the WAIS-III provides more extensive norms covering ages 16 through 89, updated items and visual stimuli (e.g., visual stimuli were enlarged to facilitate administration to patients with impaired visual acuity), and extended floors on several subtests to provide a more informative assessment of patients with severe cognitive impairments. The entire test takes approximately 60 to 90 minutes to complete and allows calculation of three types of intelligence quotients (i.e., Verbal, Performance, and Full Intelligence), four index scores (i.e., Verbal Comprehension, Perceptual Organization, Working Memory, and Processing Speed), and scaled scores for individual subtests. Of greatest interest for identifying more specific areas of strength and weakness are individual subtest scores, patterns of performance across subtests, and index scores, rather than the intelligence quotient outcomes.

One of the most recently developed cognitive test batteries is the *Neuropsychological Assessment Battery* (NAB; Stern & White, 2003). It consists of 33 subtests grouped into six modules: Screening (e.g., Screening Mazes, Screening Word Generation), Attention (e.g., Digits Forward, Driving Scenes), Language (e.g., Oral Production, Writing), Memory (e.g., List Learning, Story Learning), Spatial (e.g., Visual Discrimination, Figure Drawing), and Executive Functions (e.g., Judgment, Categories). Importantly, each module, with the exception of the Screening module, contains one subtest that is more functional in nature. For example, the Daily Living Memory subtest requires patients to learn and then recall and recognize information such as medication instructions, an address, and a phone number. Whereas it takes approximately four hours to administer the entire battery, the NAB was developed so that clinicians may choose to administer individual modules or subtests. The NAB provides two alternative forms to reduce practice effects, has excellent psychometric properties, was extensively standardized (i.e., *n* =

1,448), and offers two sets of norms: (1) Demographically Corrected Norms that allow comparison of a patient's score to that of age-, sex-, and educationally matched peers, and (2) U.S. Census-matched Norms that allow comparison of a patient's score to that of an age-matched group representative of the current U.S. population in terms of education levels, ethnocultural background, and geographic region.

Based on our clinical experiences and previous research conducted by Frank and Barineau (1996), the *Ross Information Processing Assessment* (RIPA; Ross, 1986) appears to be the most frequently utilized cognitive test battery by speech-language pathologists, particularly when assessing the cognitive status of patients with TBI. In addition to the original RIPA, a revised version, RIPA-2 (Ross-Swain, 1996), and a version for geriatric in-patient populations, RIPA-Geriatric (RIPA-G; Ross-Swain & Fogle, 1996), are currently available. All versions of the RIPA evaluate orientation, short- and long-term verbal memory, auditory comprehension, and reasoning skills. Clinicians should avoid use of the original RIPA because of its psychometric weaknesses. Whereas the RIPA-2 has better reliability and validity qualities than its earlier version, it too has psychometric limitations including construct validity problems. The RIPA-2 test manual also states that it is appropriate for patients up to age 90, but the oldest participants in the standardization sample were only 72 years of age; therefore, calculating standard scores and percentiles for patients over the age of 72 may be inappropriate. Instead, use of the RIPA-G appears more appropriate when evaluating elderly patients.

Some general cognitive test batteries have been designed for specific patient populations. For example, the *Wessex Head Injury Matrix* (Shiel, Wilson, McLellan, Horn, & Watson, 2000) represents one of the few assessment options available to document initial status as well as slow and subtle progress in patients with severe head injuries. This test requires a health care team member to rate patients on 62 items to monitor the integrity of cognitive as well as communicative and social skills. These items can be rated by just observing, or by testing the patient on certain tasks that involve everyday objects. Other cognitive test batteries have been developed primarily for patients with dementia. For instance, the *Severe Impairment Battery* (SIB; Saxton, Swihart, & Boller, 1993) was designed for patients with severe cognitive and behavioral impairments associated with dementia. Like other cognitive test batteries, the SIB evaluates attention, orientation, memory, and other cognitive skills; it differs, however, from other batteries in that SIB items are easier, and clinicians are allowed to give gestural cues. Furthermore, patients may receive credit for partial or gestural responses to help avoid a test performance profile referred to as a **basement or floor effect,** in which patients predominantly receive scores of zero.

Test Batteries for Specific Cognitive Domains

When it is clear based on observation, interview, and screening data that the patient is displaying difficulty in only one or two cognitive domains, clinicians may opt to utilize test batteries that comprehensively assess only one cognitive domain. For example, if early assessment findings suggest that a patient has primarily memory problems, a memory test battery that evaluates a number of memory functions (e.g., verbal working memory, nonverbal short term memory, episodic memory) might be selected rather than a general cognitive test battery that evaluates all cognitive domains. These batteries for specific cognitive domains typically consist of subtests that represent shorter versions of a collection of specific cognitive function tests. For instance, the *Delis-Kaplan Executive Function System* (D-KEFS; Delis, Kaplan, & Kramer, 2001) consists of nine tests, most of which were or are available as separate tests (e.g., Trail Making, Verbal and Design Fluency, Color-Word Interference [similar to the Stroop test], and Proverb tests). The strength of cognitive domain batteries is that they evaluate a number of skills within one cognitive area (e.g., separate subtests for sustained, focused, and divided attention skills), and thus provide the clinician with detailed information regarding strengths and weaknesses within that cognitive domain, which in turn will help identify specific treatment goals and procedures.

Attention Test Batteries

Presently, clinicians have a limited choice of attention test batteries (Table 6-2). Of those available, the *Test of Everyday Attention* (TEA; Robertson, Ward, Ridgeway, & Nimmo-Smith, 1994) has been the most frequently used and evaluated in the research literature (e.g., Bate, Mathias, & Crawford, 2001), and is gaining acceptance in both speech-language pathology and neuropsychology clinical practice (e.g., Kinsella, 1998; Murray, 2002a). The TEA consists of eight subtests designed to evaluate a number of attention functions in adults 16 to 80 years of age (Robertson et al., 1994). Example subtests are as follows: (1) to assess attention switching, the Visual Elevator subtest requires patients to switch between counting forwards and backwards to figure out at which floor an elevator arrives; (2) to assess sustained attention, the Lottery subtest requires patients to listen for a target lottery number among a long list of numbers; (3) to assess focused attention, the Elevator Counting with Distraction subtest requires patients to count one type of tone stimulus and ignore another to figure out at which floor an elevator arrives; and (4) to assess divided attention abilities, the Telephone Search While Counting subtest requires patients to complete a counting and a visual scanning task at the same time. In contrast to most other attention tests, the TEA utilizes everyday life materials and tasks, and accordingly has been found to have good ecological validity. For example, the Map Search subtest, which evaluates visual selective attention, requires patients to scan a large map of a city to locate all the symbols indicative of a restaurant. Other advantages of the TEA over other attention tests are that it provides parallel forms to facilitate measuring changes in attention abilities over time, and that it has been standardized on adults with hearing impairments (Robertson et al., 1994) as well as patients representing a range of neurological disorders, including stroke, head injury, and progressive dementing diseases (Robertson, Ward, Ridgeway, & Nimmo-Smith, 1996).

Memory Test Batteries

Of the various memory batteries currently available, the *Wechsler Memory Scale–Revised* (WMS-R; Wechsler, 1987) and its successor, the *Wechsler Memory Scale–III* (WMS-III; Wechsler, 1997b), are certainly the most frequently used. Both versions evaluate auditory and visual learning, and auditory and visual short- and long-term memory functions. An example auditory memory subtest is Logical Memory of the WMS-R and WMS-III, which requires patients to retell a story immediately and then after a 25- to 35-minute delay. One of the visual memory subtests is the WMS-III Faces, on which patients indicate which in a series of photographs of faces are those they have already been shown and those which are new; delayed recognition of these faces also is required 25 to 35 minutes later. Although several memory indexes can be calculated (e.g., Auditory Immediate, Auditory Delayed, Visual Immediate, Working Memory), clinicians often only examine individual subtest scores because of the continuing debate over the reliability and validity of the indexes (for further discussion of this debate, see Stout & Murray, 2001). Improvements in the newer version include expanded norms for adults up to age 89 and, for several subtests, the addition of extended floors and recognition formats to allow more informative evaluation of patients with severe cognitive impairments (Wechsler, 1997b). Computerized scoring and a training video are also available for the WMS-III.

In an attempt to develop a memory test with greater ecological validity, Wilson and colleagues (1985) created the *Rivermead Behavioral Memory Test* (RBMT) and, more recently, the *Rivermead Behavioral Memory Test–Extended* (RBMT-E; Wilson et al., 1998) and RBMT-II (Wilson, Cockburn, & Baddeley, 2003). These tests utilize tasks analogous to everyday memory activities such as remembering a short route, the name of a person, or that an appointment needs to be made, and can be administered fairly quickly in about 25 minutes. Consequently, performances of these tests have been found to predict accurately functional independence and employment outcomes in many cultures and countries (Fraser, Glass, & Leathem, 1999; Man & Li, 2001). The RBMT-II provides more extensive norms than the original RBMT, with data on individuals varying from age 16 to 96 years (Wilson et al., 2003); furthermore, this test provides four alternate forms so that it can be administered repeatedly to monitor treatment effects and avoid practice effects. Although the RBMT-E has less extensive norms, it too has parallel forms and was designed for use with relatively mildly impaired patients who would likely perform at or near **ceiling,** or 100% accuracy, on the easier RBMT (Wilson et al., 1998).

Executive Functioning Test Batteries

Executive function test batteries are particularly useful because, as Delis and colleagues (2001) noted, "The single-score method is especially problematic with executive-function tasks because such tests typically tap a host of fundamental and higher-level cognitive skills. Patients perform poorly on executive-function tests for vastly different reasons, and the single score provided by most of the existing instruments often fails to provide useful data for capturing the neurocognitive mechanisms of the impairment" (p. 4–5). That is, relying on just one test of executive functioning might result in over- or underestimating the integrity of a given patient's executive function abilities. For example, overestimation may result because only one or a limited number of executive skills were evaluated, and those executive skills were not those that are problematic for the patient. Underestimation may occur when a patient displays difficulty on an executive function test, not because of a deficit in that executive skill, but rather because of impairments in other, more basic cognitive abilities such as attention; likewise, many other executive function abilities may be relatively intact in that patient, but if these were not evaluated, the clinician remains unaware of these areas of strength. Accordingly, clinicians should consider administering an executive function test battery (or a number of executive function tests) so that a range of executive skills is assessed. They also should assure that tests of more basic cognitive abilities have already been administered so that performances of executive function tests can be interpreted in the light of these other cognitive test results.

A number of executive function test batteries have been published recently (Table 6-2). The *Delis-Kaplan Executive Function System* (D-KEFS; Delis et al., 2001) has nine subtests that can be used alone or in combination with other D-KEFS subtests, and that are designed to evaluate a number of verbal and nonverbal executive function abilities such as cognitive flexibility, inhibition, and problem solving. Specific subtests include the Trail Making, Verbal and Design Fluency, Color-Word Interference, Sorting, Twenty Questions, Word Context, Tower, and Proverb tests. Several of these subtests represent versions of tests that were previously available separately, either commercially or in the research literature. For example, D-KEFS' Sorting Test was previously known as the California Card Sorting Test (Delis et al., 1992). Advantages of using D-KEFS versus individual executive function tests include: (1) to improve the reliability of repeated testing, D-KEFS provides alternate forms for three subtests, Sorting, Twenty Questions, and Verbal Fluency; (2) D-KEFS normative data encompasses ages 8 through 89 years; and (3) in terms of severity, D-KEFS is sensitive to the full spectrum of executive function deficits (Delis, Kaplan, & Kramer, 2001). In terms of scoring, many D-KEFS subtests provide several measures to reflect the variety of basic and complex cognitive abilities assessed by these subtests. Clinicians also may calculate indices for key executive function abilities, including initiation, verbal concept-formation, nonverbal concept-formation, cognitive flexibility, and behavioral response flexibility based on performance of a number of subtests.

The seven subtests of the *Behavioral Assessment of Dysexecutive Syndrome* (BADS; Wilson et al., 1996) were designed to evaluate executive functioning via tasks that are more similar to daily activities than those of the D-KEFS. For example, the Key Search Test assesses planning and self-monitoring by asking patients to draw the route they would take to find a lost set of keys in a large field (illustrated by a square on a piece of paper); the Zoo Map Test examines planning and **cognitive flexibility** by requiring patients to draw the route they would take to visit a number of prescribed locations on a map of a zoo while also following a set of stipulations such as traveling on certain paths only once. The BADS is suitable for a broad range of patients and provides normative data for healthy adults 16 to 87 years of age and individuals with brain damage 19 to 76 years of age. Additionally, certain BADS subtests have been shown to be useful in other languages and cultures (e.g., Chan & Manly, 2002).

TESTS OF SPECIFIC COGNITIVE FUNCTIONS

There are numerous choices available when clinicians are looking for tests to assess specific attention, memory, or executive function abilities. Table 6-3 contains only a sample of tests that can be found commercially or in the research literature, and that are appropriate for one or more neurogenic patient populations. Clinicians should base their test selections on previous observation, interview, or test battery findings, and on patients' concomitant symptoms. For example, when attempting to assess a patient with reduced visual acuity, the clinician should rely upon tests that utilize auditory stimuli. Likewise, clinicians assessing cognitive abilities in patients with severe aphasia may choose tests with relatively low language demands, both in terms of test stimuli and response requirements. Clinicians also must keep in mind that many well-established measures purported to evaluate a specific cognitive function actually are multifactorial in nature. This means that several cognitive skills are needed to complete, and thus are assessed by, these tests (Lezak, 1995; Murray & Ramage, 2000). For example, several attention tests such as the *Paced Auditory Serial Addition Test* (Gronwall, 1977) and *Criterion-Oriented Test of Attention* (Williams, 1994a) exploit not only attention, but also complex language and math skills for completion; therefore, before using these tests' findings to make final conclusions regarding the integrity of attention, clinicians also must have accrued additional assessment data concerning the integrity of these other skills.

Test of Specific Attention Functions

Given that attention encompasses a number of cognitive skills including sustained attention, focused or selective attention, attention switching, and divided attention, tests that assess one or a few specific attention functions in the modality of audition, vision, or both are available (Table 6-3). Examples of tests that evaluate

Table 6-3. Measures of Specific Cognitive Functions

COGNITIVE FUNCTION	INSTRUMENT	SOURCE
Attention	Brief Test of Attention	Schretlen (1997)
	*Color Trails Test	D'Elia et al. (1996)
	Comprehensive Trail-Making Test	Reynolds (2002)
	Criterion-Oriented Test of Attention	Williams (1994a)
	*d2 Test of Attention	Brickenkamp & Zillmer (1998)
	Expanded Trail Making Test	Stanczak et al. (1998)
	Paced Auditory Serial Addition Test	Gronwall (1977)
	SCAN-A: A Test for Auditory Processing Disorders in Adolescents and Adults	Keith (1993)
	Trail Making Test	Reitan & Wolfson (1985)
	Vigil Continuous Performance Test	The Psychological Corporation (1996)
Neglect	*Balloons Test	Edgeworth et al. (1998)
	*Behavioral Inattention Test	Wilson et al. (1987)
	Burning House Test	Marshall & Halligan (1988)
	*Comb and Razor Test	Beschin & Robertson, (1997)
	Indented Paragraph Test	Caplan (1987)
	*Test of Visual Field Attention	Williams (1994b)
	*Verbal and Nonverbal Cancellation Test	Weintraub & Mesulam (1985)
	Visual Search and Attention Test	Trenerry et al. (1990)
Nonverbal Memory	*Benton Visual Retention Test	Sivan (1992)
	*Brief Visuospatial Memory Test–Revised	Benedict (1997)
	*Continuous Visual Memory Test	Trahan & Larrabee (1988)
	*Location Learning Test	Bucks et al. (2000)
	*Rey Complex Figure Test and Recognition Trial	Meyers & Meyers (1995)
	*Visual Patterns Test	Della Sala et al. (1997)
Verbal Memory	Auditory-Verbal Working Memory Test	Tompkins et al. (1994)
	California Verbal Learning Test–II	Delis et al. (2000)
	Contextual Memory Test	Toglia (1993)
	Hopkins Verbal Learning Test–Revised	Brandt & Benedict (2001)
	Paced Auditory Serial Addition Test	Gronwall (1977)
	Selective Reminding Test	Buschke (1973)
	Sentence Repetition Test	Spreen & Strauss (1998)
	Wechsler Test of Adult Reading	Wechsler (2001)

(continues)

Table 6-3. *Continued*

COGNITIVE FUNCTION	INSTRUMENT	SOURCE
Verbal and Nonverbal Memory	* Cambridge Test of Prospective Memory	Wilson et al. (2005)
	*Doors and People	Baddeley et al. (1994)
	*Recognition Memory Test	Warrington (1999)
Executive Functions	*Beta III	Kellogg & Morton (1999)
	Booklet Category Test	DeFilippis & McCampbell (1997)
	*Butt Non-Verbal Reasoning Test	Butt & Bucks (2004)
	Cognitive Failures Questionnaire	Broadbent et al. (1982)
	*Color Trails Test	D'Elia et al. (1996)
	*Comprehensive Test of Nonverbal Intelligence	Hammill et al. (1997)
	Executive Function Route-Finding Task	Boyd & Sauter (1994)
	FAS/Controlled Oral Word Association Test	Benton et al. (2001)
	Hayling and Brixton Tests	Burgess & Shallice (1997)
	Object Sorting Test	Goldstein & Sheerer (1953)
	Photocopy Tasks	Crepeau et al. (1997)
	*Porteus Maze Test	Porteus (1965)
	Rapid Assessment of Problem Solving	Marshall et al. (2003)
	*Raven's Progressive Matrices	Raven (1998)
	*Ruff Figural Fluency Test	Ruff (1996)
	Stroop Color and Word Test	Golden (2002)
	Stroop Neuropsychological Screening Test	Trenerry et al. (1989)
	Test of Problem Solving–Adolescent	Bowers et al. (1991)
	*Test of Nonverbal Intelligence–3	Brown et al. (1997)
	*The Category Test	Williams (1994c)
	Tinkertoy Test	Lezak (1995)
	*Tower of Hanoi	Simon (1975)
	*Tower of LondonDX: Research Version	Cullbertson & Zillmer (1999)
	Wheelbarrow Test	Butler et al. (1989)
	*Williams Inhibition Test	Williams (1994d)
	*Wisconsin Card Sorting Test	Grant & Berg (1993)

Note. * indicates that subtests or entire test may be suitable for patients with language production and/or comprehension impairments.

these different attention functions are described below. Because it is difficult to isolate specific cognitive skills, however, clinicians are reminded that some attention tests assess additional cognitive abilities. This is why certain tests are listed as both attention and executive function tests in Table 6-3.

Sustained attention tests typically involve completing mundane tasks (e.g., monitoring for a visual or auditory target in the absence or presence of foils) for extended time periods. Many recently developed sustained attention tests are computer-based. For example, the *Vigil Continuous Performance Test* (The Psychological Cooperation, 1996) provides computerized administration and scoring of several sustained attention tasks, each of which takes about eight minutes to complete. These tests can be varied in terms of complexity (e.g., rate of stimulus presentation) and stimulus type (e.g., verbal vs. nonverbal targets), and are suitable for a broad age range of six to 90 years. Whatever test is used to evaluate sustained attention, the clinician should monitor not only the amount of time patients are on task, but also whether they can maintain performance quality over time.

Focused or selective attention tests are similar to complex sustained attention tasks in that they require identifying target stimuli while rejecting irrelevant stimuli. One of the long-standing tests used to evaluate focused attention as well as attention switching is the Trail-Making Test (Reitan & Wolfson, 1995). This test has normative data for elderly patients (Spreen & Strauss, 1998), and has been found sensitive to even subtle deficits associated with mild TBI (Brooks, Fos, Greve, & Hammond, 1999). Currently several versions of this test are available, including the *Color Trails Test* (D'Elia, Satz, Uchiyama, & White, 1996), the *Comprehensive Trail-Making Test* (Reynolds, 2002), and the Expanded Trail Making Test (Stanczak, Lynch, McNeil, & Brown, 1998). Basically, Trails tests involve connecting a series of stimuli (e.g., numbers written as numerals or, in words, letters) in a set order as quickly as possible. In one condition, patients typically are asked to connect one stimulus series, whereas in the other, more complex condition, they must switch between connecting a stimulus from one series with that from the other. For example, in the simpler condition, patients might be required to connect numbers in increasing order, whereas in the more complex condition, they would have to connect numbers and letters in increasing order by alternating between the numbers and letters (e.g., 1 – A – 2 – B – 3 – C etc.). The *Color* (D'Elia et al., 1996) and Expanded versions (Stanczak et al., 1998) were developed for patient populations who have communication disorders that may confound their performance of the original test, which requires connecting letters and numbers. For example, in the Expanded version (Stanczak et al., 1998), patients connect a series of clock faces drawn with clock hands and tick marks rather than numbers in ascending time order (e.g., 12:00, 12:15; 12:30) or a series of black dots in order of increasing size. Because of its low language demands, this version of the Trails would be appropriate for patients with number or letter recognition problems.

Few test options are available for assessing **divided attention.** Dual-task procedures are typically used because divided attention refers to the ability to complete more than one task at the same time (Murray, 2002). Although several dual-task protocols are described in the research literature (e.g., Holtzer, Burright, & Donovick, 2004; Murray, 2000), currently there appears to be only one commercially available dual-task test, the Telephone Search While Counting subtest of the TEA (Robertson et al., 1994). On this subtest, patients must, at the same time, count strings of audio-taped tones, and search a replica of a page from a telephone book for pre-specified target businesses; their dual-task performances are then quantified in terms of accuracy and total response time. There remains a clear need to develop more tests of divided attention, particularly those with minimal language demands, as only patients with mild aphasia may be able to perform this TEA subtest without their language deficits significantly impeding their performance.

Neglect Tests

As neglect is considered a disorder of attention (Cherney, 2002; see also Chapter 2), tests for identifying the presence and severity of neglect are discussed here. Even though patients with neglect can often have relatively intact speech, language, and memory skills, they still have a much poorer prognosis for an independent outcome compared to patients without neglect (Jehkonen et al., 2000). Consequently, it is important not only to document the presence of neglect, but also to determine which environmental conditions exacerbate or ameliorate neglect symptoms. Clinicians also are reminded that although neglect is most frequently associated with right hemisphere brain damage (Cherney, 2002), it also can occur following left hemisphere damage, and thus may be a possible symptom in a variety of neurogenic disorders, including aphasia (Appelros et al., 2002), dementia (Foldi, LoBosco, & Schaefer, 2002), and cognitive-communicative impairments associated with traumatic brain injury (Cocchini, Beschin, & Della Sala, 2002).

A number of tests and research protocols are available to identify the presence of neglect. These assessment tools invariably involve one or more of the following tasks (Cherney, 2002; Golisz, 1998; Rapport, Farchione, Dutra, Webster, & Charter, 1996): (1) line bisection, in which patients try to divide a line in half (patients with neglect will mark the line toward their ipsilesional side); (2) cancellation tasks, in which patients cross out or identify a target letter, number, object, or shape among an array of stimuli (patients with neglect will fail to cross out more stimuli on their contralesional vs. ipsilesional side); (3) drawing or copying of symmetrical objects or shapes, or preferably asymmetrical stimuli, as these have been found to be more sensitive to subtle forms of neglect (patients with neglect will leave out more details on the contralesional vs. ipsilesional side of their drawing); and (4) reading aloud or copying of words, sentences, and/or paragraphs (patients with neglect may omit or make substitution errors when reading or writing letters, syllables, or words on their contralesional side). Clinicians can manipulate a number of variables to increase or decrease the complexity of neglect tasks (Table 6-4). Complexity should be increased when mild neglect problems are suspected.

Table 6-4. Variables to Manipulate the Complexity of Neglect Tests

TYPE OF TASK	VARIABLES TO INCREASE TASK COMPLEXITY	VARIABLES TO DECREASE TASK COMPLEXITY
Cancellation Tasks	similar targets and foils	dissimilar targets and foils
	scattered distribution of stimuli	arranged display (e.g., rows, columns)
	complex stimuli (e.g., letters)	simple stimuli (e.g., basic shapes)
	dense stimulus presentation	dispersed stimulus presentation
	many foils	few foils
Line Bisection	long line	short line
	extrapersonal space (e.g., on wall with light pointer)	peripersonal space (e.g., table top)
	vertical or radial line orientation	horizontal line orientation
	no anchor	anchor placed at left end of line
Drawing/Copying	asymmetrical stimulus	symmetrical stimulus
	spatially separated (e.g., two objects)	spatially integrated or meaningful scene (e.g., two men shaking hands)
Writing	pseudowords	real words

Commercially available tests of neglect vary in length and, consequently, comprehensiveness (Table 6-3). For example, for a quick visual neglect screening tool, clinicians might consider the *Balloons Test* (Edgeworth et al., 1998). This cancellation task only takes about six minutes to administer. Its first subtest requires canceling out line drawings of balloons from amongst line drawings of circles; the second subtest is a more complex, inverse version of the first subtest, and involves canceling out the circles (which perceptually do not "pop out" as much) from among the balloons. On the other end of the length spectrum is the *Behavioral Inattention Test* (BIT; Wilson, Cockburn, & Halligan, 1987), which consists of (1) six conventional paper-and-pencil subtests such as line bisection, drawing, and figure copying that take about 10 minutes to complete, and (2) several more functional or "behavioral" subtests such as telephone dialing, menu and article reading, telling and setting the time, and map navigation, which take about 45 minutes to complete. Patients' scores on the conventional and behavioral portions are calculated, and cut-off scores are provided to determine the presence of unilateral visual neglect. Recent research indicates that the conventional and behavioral portions of the BIT are significantly correlated (Cassidy, Lewis, & Gray, 1998; Cherney & Halper, 2001), suggesting that administering only the conventional portion may be adequate if clinicians are faced with significant assessment time constraints.

Whereas the above tests document response accuracy, a few tests also allow collecting reaction times, which in turn may provide a more sensitive measure of neglect. For example, Williams' (1994b) *Test of Visual Field Attention* is a software program through which patients indicate via a mouse-press response whenever they see a simple visual stimulus on the computer screen. The visual stimuli are presented at random locations, so that by the end of the test, the patients' accuracy and response times for stimuli presented to each visual quadrant or central versus peripheral fields can be determined. Similarly, Potter et al. (2000) developed computerized methods for administering several standard visual neglect tasks, such as line bisection and cancellation. Their software also permits recording of accuracy and reaction time differences between responses to the left versus right hemispace. Potter et al. noted that some patients who did not display accuracy differences when responding to stimuli presented on the left versus right side did display response time differences, underscoring the sensitivity of their protocol to subtle neglect symptoms.

Although several test options are available for assessing the presence and severity of neglect, few of these go beyond evaluating visuospatial neglect and thus may overlook other neglect symptoms, such as sensory extinction, auditory neglect, or hemiakinesia (Azouvi et al., 2002; Bowen, McKenna, & Tallis, 1999; see also Chapter 2). Another criticism of most neglect tests is their questionable ecological validity. That is, patients who perform within the normal range on many of these paper-and-pencil tests may still display or report significant neglect problems in their daily environments. Accordingly, it is recommended that clinicians not rely on just one paper-and-pencil neglect measure, but rather administer at least two to three tasks, assuring that (1) one of those tasks allows documenting response times as well as accuracy, and/or (2) these test performances, along with observations for neglect symptoms in daily activities and environments (e.g., dressing, eating, hygiene activities), are used to make final decisions regarding the presence and severity of neglect.

Tests of Specific Memory Functions

There are a myriad of memory tests available, some that focus more on evaluating verbal memory skills, and others that aim to evaluate nonverbal or visual memory skills. Selection from these should be based on specific assessment goals, time availability, and, depending on the patient's communication and physical abilities, test adaptability. For example, patients with neurogenic language or motor speech disorders often are given nonverbal or visual memory tests that use drawings and objects versus linguistic stimuli in an attempt to circumvent these patients' communicative problems and, consequently, to allow an unconfounded view of their memory abilities. Healthy adults, however, often exploit their verbal skills (e.g., subvocalization of object names) to aid their performance on these "nonverbal," visual tests; consequently, clinicians must be vigilant in determining whether the poor visual memory test performances of patients with communication disorders reflect impaired language, a true memory deficit, or perhaps a combination of both.

Verbal Memory Tests

One of the more frequently administered tests of verbal memory is the *California Verbal Learning Test–II* (CVLT; Delis, Kramer, Kaplan, & Ober, 2000). This test, as well as those similar to it, such as *Hopkins Verbal Learning Test-Revised* (Brandt & Benedict, 2001), is popular because it provides information regarding a number of auditory verbal memory functions, including recall and recognition accuracy, encoding strategies (e.g., ability to use semantic clustering), learning rates, and error types (e.g., perseverative responses, false-positive errors). Basically, the CVLT requires patients to learn, recall, and, lastly, recognize a 16-item "shopping list" of words that represent four semantic categories (e.g., clothes, fruits) (Delis et al., 2000). Over five consecutive trials, patients listen to the list read by the examiner, and then immediately try to recall as many items as possible. After these trials, a new "shopping list" of 16 items is read aloud for patients to recall; this second list allows the clinician to evaluate proactive interference, in which patients use words from the first list while trying to recall the second list, and retroactive interference, in which patients use words from the second list while trying to recall the first list during subsequent delayed trials. Next, patients are instructed to recall as many items as possible from the first list, followed by a cued recall task in which they are given category cues for items that they fail to recall; these free and cued recall tasks are then repeated 25 minutes later to evaluate unstructured and structured retrieval, respectively, from long-term memory. The final step of the CVLT is a recognition task in which clients listen to a word list and indicate which items are from the first shopping list. This test also provides a short form that may be useful when there are time constraints or the patient fatigues easily. Finally, the CVLT may be used with commercially available software to aid in scoring and comparing test performances to normative data.

Other verbal memory tests are less comprehensive and examine only a subset of the memory abilities evaluated by the CVLT. For example, there are a variety of span tasks available that only assess immediate verbal memory span. These span tasks are sometimes categorized as tests of basic attention ability, as span performance can be affected negatively by concentration problems (Butters, Delis, & Lucas, 1995; Lezak, 1995). Verbal span tasks can be found on several test batteries as well as in the research literature, and typically require the patient to repeat back a series of digits (e.g., Digit Span of the WMS-III or WAIS-III), syllables (see Lezak, 1995 for examples), phrases (e.g., Repetition subtest of the *Arizona Battery of Communication Disorders of Dementia* [ABCD]; Bayles & Tomoeda, 1993), or sentences (e.g., Sentence Repetition Test; Spreen & Strauss, 1998) in the same order as the clinician presented them. A more functional span task is the Telephone Test, which requires patients to recall seven- and 10-digit strings that are presented visually in a format akin to telephone numbers (Crook, Ferris, McCarthy, & Rae, 1980). Generally, forward span measures by themselves are not informative, as many neurogenic patient populations adequately perform these tasks, particularly if they have suffered only mild to moderate degrees of brain damage or are in the early to middle stages of a dementing disease (Lezak, 1995; Murray, 2002b).

Verbal **working memory** tests are similar to span tasks in that they require the temporary storage and then recall of verbal information. They differ from span tasks, however, in that they also impose some form of interference on patients while they are trying to hold that information temporarily. For example, backward span tasks such as the Digits Backwards subtest of WAIS-III or WMS-III are proposed to assess working memory because not only must patients temporarily retain a list of items, but then they also must switch the order of those items before responding. Another example is Tompkins and colleagues' (1994) auditory-verbal working memory test, in which patients listen to sets of audiotaped sentences that increase over time in terms of the number of sentences within a set (see Figure 6-2). For each sentence set, patients must try to recall the last word of each sentence *and* also indi-

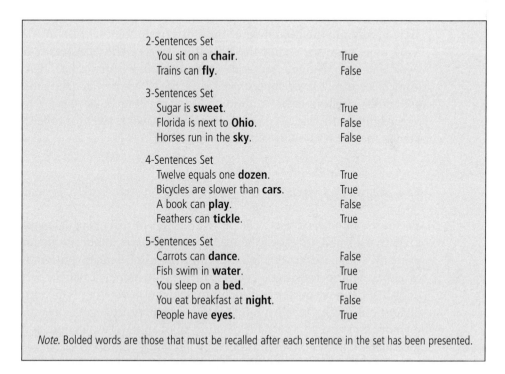

2-Sentences Set	
You sit on a **chair**.	True
Trains can **fly**.	False
3-Sentences Set	
Sugar is **sweet**.	True
Florida is next to **Ohio**.	False
Horses run in the **sky**.	False
4-Sentences Set	
Twelve equals one **dozen**.	True
Bicycles are slower than **cars**.	True
A book can **play**.	False
Feathers can **tickle**.	True
5-Sentences Set	
Carrots can **dance**.	False
Fish swim in **water**.	True
You sleep on a **bed**.	True
You eat breakfast at **night**.	False
People have **eyes**.	True

Note. Bolded words are those that must be recalled after each sentence in the set has been presented.

Figure 6-2. Sample stimulus items from Tompkins and colleagues' (1994) auditory-verbal working memory test.

cate whether each sentence is true or false (i.e., the interference component of the task). Clinicians then tally the number of word recall and true/false errors, and can compare their patients' performances to those reported for healthy adults or individuals with left or right hemisphere brain damage by Tompkins and colleagues (Lehman & Tompkins, 1998; Tompkins et al., 1994). Other working memory tests can be found in the research literature (e.g., Baddeley, Emslie, Kolodny, & Duncan, 1998) or as subtests on cognitive or memory test batteries (e.g., WAIS-III Letter-Number Sequencing). Establishing the integrity of working memory in patients with neurogenic language disorders is important because a growing research literature has documented a positive relationship between working memory and language abilities in a number of neurogenic patient populations (Bayles, 2003; Caspari, Parkinson, LaPointe, & Katz, 1998; Tompkins et al., 1994; Turkstra & Holland, 1998).

Story retelling tasks also are used to evaluate immediate and delayed verbal memory. In many cases, these tasks are preferable to span tests because they represent a more realistic, daily memory activity (Lezak, 1995). In these tasks, patients are asked to retell, word-for-word if possible, a story immediately after they have heard it. After a 20- to 30-minute delay, patients are again asked to recall the story word-for-word, if possible. Patients' responses are then typically analyzed in terms of the number of correctly recalled story "ideas" versus words. Patterns of recall also may be evaluated, such as presence of a primacy effect, in which patients recall more ideas from the beginning of the story, or a recency effect, in which patients recall more from the end of the story. Interference effects also may be examined if patients are required to recall more than one story. The Logical Memory Immediate and Delayed subtests of the WMS-III are perhaps the most frequently used story retelling tasks. Additional story retelling tasks may be found in the research literature (e.g., Mapou, Kramer, & Blusewicz, 1989) or other test batteries such as the Story Retelling subtests of the ABCD.

Nonverbal Memory Tests

There are a number of tests available to assess nonverbal or spatial memory abilities (Table 6-3). Familiarity with these tests is particularly important if clinicians work primarily with patients with aphasia whose linguistic deficits contraindicate the use of verbal memory tests; that is, when patients with linguistic deficits perform poorly on verbal memory tests, it is difficult to distinguish whether poor verbal memory, linguistic deficits, or both underlie this poor performance. Nonverbal or spatial memory tests also are a valuable component of an RHD evaluation, as this memory modality is commonly compromised by RHD (e.g., Lewis-Jack et al., 1997).

Many nonverbal memory tests parallel those already described with respect to assessing verbal memory abilities, except that they require the recall of object locations, symbols, or matrix patterns specifically designed to minimize verbal coding, and thus minimize use of verbal memory skills. For example, there are a few visual span tasks with forward and backward recall versions, such as the Visual Memory Span subtest of the WMS-R, that are akin to the previously described verbal span tasks, except that rather than recall verbal stimuli, patients point to a series of colored shapes or blocks in a specified order. Likewise, *Rey's Visual Design Learning Test* (RVDLT; Spreen & Straus, 1998) approximates the CVLT by requiring patients to learn a series of 15 visual designs over several trials, and by providing information regarding visual learning and recall.

Several nonverbal or visual memory tests, including the RVDLT, require drawn responses. Another example is the Complex Figure Test, on which patients first copy, then recall immediately after a 30-second to three-minute delay, and finally recall after a 20- to 30-minute delay a complex, abstract design; the copy task provides information about visuo-perceptual and construction skills, whereas the latter two tasks yield information pertaining to immediate and delayed visual memory abilities, respectively. Several versions of this test are available commercially, such as the *Rey-Osterrieth Complex Figure Test* (Meyers & Meyers, 1995) and in the research literature (e.g., Corwin & Blysma, 1993) such as the scoring system of Stern et al. (1999). These versions vary in terms of task and scoring procedures, and normative data. Clinicians must assure that the task instructions and procedures they use match those on which their selected scoring system and normative data were based.

If patients' motoric deficits negate the use of a drawing task, another test option is the *Continuous Visual Memory Test* (CVMT; Trahan & Larrabee, 1988). This test examines immediate and delayed visual memory by requiring patients to view a series of complex, abstract designs and indicate for each design whether it is a "new" design that they have not yet been shown during the test, or an "old" design that they have already seen during the test. Once patients have viewed all of the 112 designs, there is a 30-minute delay, and then patients are asked to identify which designs they had previously viewed several times (i.e., which are the "old" designs). There also is a visual discrimination subtest to assure that visuoperceptual difficulties were not affecting patients' performances negatively. The CVMT comes with a new manual supplement that provides updated norms for individuals seven though 80 years of age.

The newer *Location Learning Test* (Bucks, Willison, & Burn, 2000) utilizes a more functional nonverbal memory task to assess visuospatial learning and recall. In this test, patients are shown an array of pictures depicting everyday objects that are commonly misplaced, such as glasses, keys, and a purse, and are asked to learn the location of each object. The pictures are then removed, and patients are asked to replace the pictures in their appropriate location; there also is a recognition task to determine if visual perceptual problems are confounding test results. Scoring documents the degree of displacement error, not just the number of correctly placed pictures. This test was specifically designed for older adults, particularly those with suspected dementia, and has normative data for the ages of 50 through 96 years.

Test of Specific Executive Functions

Because the cognitive domain of executive functioning is considered a multidimensional construct, it is most appropriate to administer several tests that assess a number of executive functions (Burgess et al., 1998; Murray & Ramage, 2000). Before administering these tests, however, clinicians must consider the following caveats (Delis et al., 2000; Murray & Ramage, 2000; Wilson, Watson, Baddeley, Emslie, & Evans, 2000). First, clinicians must recognize that completing any executive function test will invariably evoke a combination of basic (e.g., attention, perception, language) and high-level cognitive abilities (e.g., planning, inhibition); consequently, poor performance on an executive function test could be indicative of problems at any cognitive processing level. It is therefore highly inappropriate to administer executive function tests without having previously administered tests of other linguistic and cognitive functions. Second, clinicians must keep in mind that most executive function tests have poor test-retest reliability. This is not necessarily a fault of test developers, but rather reflects the nature of executive functioning. That is, many executive function tests examine how well patients can cope with novel or unusual situations or problems. Therefore, after they have completed these tests once, performing these tests again will not necessarily be as informative, as the tests' situations or problems will no longer be novel. To avoid this problem, clinicians should select, when possible, executive function tests that include alternate or equivalent forms. Finally, clinicians are reminded that there is little agreement regarding either the vernacular or composition of the domain of executive functioning. Therefore, to help clinicians become familiar with the variety of executive function tests currently available (Table 6-3), we have adopted the following categorization of executive function tests, acknowledging that these categories are not completely distinct, that some tests could be applied to more than one category, and that other authors may describe different categories or domains of executive functioning: (1) planning tests that evaluate formulation of strategies and sequencing of strategy steps to meet intended goals; (2) organization tests that assess structuring or categorizing external stimuli and one's own responses; (3) **inhibition** tests that evaluate control over automatic, habitual, or irrelevant processing or responding; (4) cognitive flexibility tests that examine the ability to change or revise one's own responses in the event of failure; (5) problem-solving tests that assess problem identification as well as generation and selection of possible solutions; and (6) self-monitoring tests that examine the evaluation and regulation of one's own performance, including the identification of one's own strengths and weaknesses.

Planning Tests

Planning tasks include maze completion, tower tests, and clock drawing (described in the Cognitive Status and Dementia Screening Tools section of this chapter). To complete these tasks efficiently, patients must plan the sequence of their responses before executing those responses. For example, maze completion tests, which are similar to maze tasks found in children's activity books, require patients to solve a series of mazes that increase in complexity (e.g., more incorrect path options, longer path between the beginning and the end of the maze). Because of their minimal language demands, these tasks are suitable for patients with neurogenic language disorders. Both accuracy and completion time can be recorded to quantify and qualify patients' performances. The two most frequently used maze tests are the *Porteus Maze Test* (Porteus, 1965) and the Mazes subtest of the *Wechsler Intelligence Scale for Children–III* (WISC-III; Wechsler, 1991). The newer *Cognitive-Linguistic Quick Test* (CLQT; Helm-Estabrooks, 2001) also has a maze subtest. Although the WISC-III mazes only have norms up to the age of 15 years, 10 months, Lezak (1995) noted that because its most difficult maze is approximately as complex as the most difficult *Porteus* maze, and because it offers an easy administration and scoring format, the WISC-III Mazes are a suitable choice for adult patients. Research suggests that maze tasks may be most appropriate for moderately to severely impaired patients, as patients with mild degrees of brain damage often perform as well as their healthy peers on these tasks (e.g., Brooks et al., 1999).

A number of tower tests are available both commercially (e.g., *Tower of London DX: Research Version*; TOL:RV; Culbertson & Zillmer, 1999) and in the research literature (e.g., Tower of Hanoi, Simon, 1975). These tests require patients to develop an efficient plan in order to use the fewest moves to complete a spatial arrangement task. For example, on the TOL:RV, which provides norms for both children and adults, patients must rearrange colored wooden beads from their initial position on two of three upright rods, or "towers," to a target configuration on another rod using as few moves as possible. Trial difficulty is manipulated by increasing the number and complexity of steps necessary to reconfigure the beads, and test performance can be evaluated in terms of the number of moves necessary to achieve a solution, and the number of task trials that were solved. Tower tests described in the research literature offer a number of procedural and scoring options to manipulate task complexity and provide more test measures, respectively (Kafer & Hunter, 1997; Shallice, 1982). For example, the tower test can be made more difficult by increasing the number of towers and beads, or can be made easier by requiring patients to estimate the minimum numbers of moves they would need to solve the task prior to completing the task (i.e., cueing patients to plan their solution ahead of time to help minimize trial-and-error moves). Likewise, additional data can be collected, such as the amount of time patients take to plan their solution and the amount of time they take to implement their solution.

A more functional planning test is the Executive Function Route-Finding Task (Boyd & Sautter, 1994). This test requires patients to find their way from a starting point to a target location, such as an unfamiliar office within the building in which testing is taking place. No specific instructions regarding how patients should find their final location are provided, other than they are asked to find the destination as quickly and efficiently as possible and are told they cannot ask the clinician any questions. The clinician accompanies the patient throughout the test so that the patient can be rated on a four-point scale in the following areas: (1) task understanding (e.g., does not ask clinician questions, begins task spontaneously), (2) incorporation of information seeking (e.g., asks building staff for directions, looks for signs), (3) retaining directions (e.g., takes notes to remember directions), (4) error detection (e.g., checks signs to assure that directions are being followed correctly), (5) error correction (e.g., realizes when an error has been made and attempts to self-correct independently), and, (6) on-task behavior (e.g., avoids chatting with familiar staff or patients to complete task as quickly as possible). If necessary, the clinician may provide nonspecific cues such as "What should you be doing?" or specific cues such as "Maybe you should ask someone for help." Whatever cues are provided, clinicians should make note of what level of assistance was necessary for the patient to complete the test. Whereas this test provides qualitative information about patients' planning skills, quantitative interpretation (i.e., severity of impairment) is not possible, as normative data are unavailable.

Organization Tests

One of the most popular organization tests is the *Wisconsin Card Sorting Test* (WCST; Grant & Berg, 1993), no doubt in part because it has relatively low language demands, and thus is suitable for a variety of neurogenic patient populations. Although often referred to as an organization or categorization task, the WCST actually evaluates a number of executive functions, including whether a patient can develop a strategy to sort or categorize a deck of cards (i.e., organization or categorization), maintain that strategy (i.e., inhibition of impulsive responses), and switch to a new strategy when feedback indicates to do so (i.e., cognitive flexibility). Cards in the WCST deck vary in terms of the symbols on them (e.g., circles vs. stars), the color of the symbols (e.g., red vs. green circles), and/or the number of symbols (e.g., one vs. four circles), and thus can be sorted by form, color, or number. Based on the clinician's limited feedback of "correct" or "incorrect," patients must figure out how to sort the cards, one-by-one, under the three stimulus or key cards that represent each of the possible categories. Following 10 consecutive correct sorts, the target category is switched so that patients must deduce the new correct sorting strategy, again based on only the clinician's feedback. Because the WCST can be exceedingly frustrating and time consuming for neurogenic patients (Nussbaum, 1998), several modified versions have been developed that use fewer cards, ease the requirements for task discontinuation, or remove cards that share more than one stimulus characteristic with the key cards to reduce confusion and make discerning the correct sorting strategy easier (Haaland, Vranes, Goodwin, & Garry, 1987; Nelson, 1976). Normative data for these modified versions are available in the research literature (Axelrod, Jiron, &

Henry, 1993; Haaland et al., 1987). Merrick and colleagues (2003) recommended that modified versions are more appropriate for evaluating organization efficiency (e.g., how quickly patients can identify the sorting strategy, do they have a deficit) whereas the original WCST is better for determining if patients can, when given enough time and opportunity, learn to identify sorting strategies, and thus have the rehabilitation potential to improve with practice.

Other examples of organization or categorization tests include the *Booklet Category Test–II* (DeFilippis & McCampbell, 1997), the computerized *The Category Test* (Williams, 1994c), and the Object Sorting Test (Goldstein & Sheerer, 1953). The latter test differs from the WCST and many other organization tests because it utilizes a set of 30 common objects, and thus compared to the abstract, visual stimuli found on other tests, these stimuli should be familiar to most patients. To complete the task, patients are asked to sort these objects and then explain their strategy. Next, they are asked to group the objects again, but in a different way. This process can be repeated several times, given that the objects can be classified according to a number of features including object function, color, composition, and location, or where the object would normally be found. An advantage to this test is that clinicians can adapt the basic sorting task to elicit other responses. For instance, the clinician could (1) group a subset of objects together and ask the patient to figure out the clinician's sorting strategy, (2) select one object and ask the patient to find other objects similar to it, or (3) dictate by which category the patient should sort the objects. Regardless of what response format is utilized, clinicians should require patients to give verbal explanations of their actions to provide more insight into the patients' organization strategies.

Inhibition Tests

Inhibition tests evaluate patients' ability to disregard irrelevant information, to avoid automatic response tendencies, or to prevent use of previously acceptable responses (Murray & Ramage, 2000). Most frequently, Stroop tasks (e.g., Golden, 2002; Trenerry, Crosson, DeBoe, & Leber, 1989; Wiig et al., 2002) are used to assess these forms of inhibition. These tests typically consist of at least two timed tasks, one in which patients read aloud color names, and the other in which they name the color of ink in which the word is written (for a grayscale version, see Figure 6-3). The second task should take patients longer to complete because they must inhibit the more frequent response of reading aloud words; they should experience the greatest interference when the written word and color conflict. To quantify how well patients deal with this interference, their response accuracies on the two tasks are compared: The greater the difference between the two trials, the more interference and thus greater problems with inhibition the patient experienced. Of the various commercially available Stroop tasks, Golden (2002) provided the most extensive normative data for patients ranging in age from 15 to 90 years.

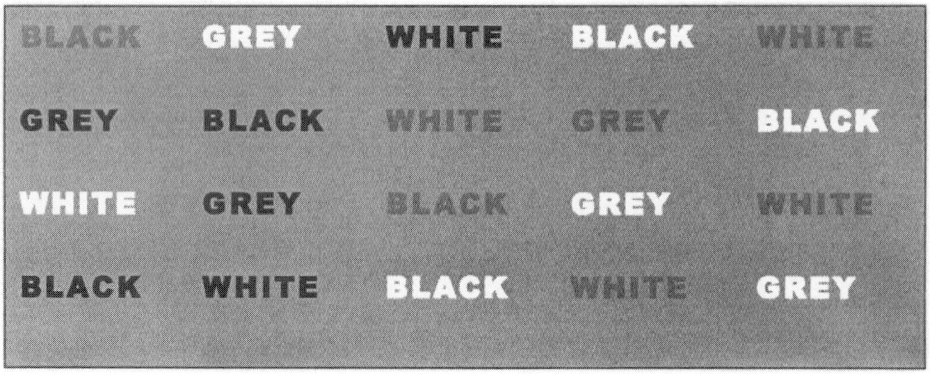

BLACK	GREY	WHITE	BLACK	WHITE
GREY	BLACK	WHITE	GREY	BLACK
WHITE	GREY	BLACK	GREY	WHITE
BLACK	WHITE	BLACK	WHITE	GREY

Note. The traditional Stroop task involves colored ink and color words (e.g., red, green, yellow), which were not possible to reproduce in this book.

Figure 6-3. **Example of a grayscale Stroop-like test.**

Because of its high speech and language demands, the Stroop task is highly inappropriate for many patients with dysarthria, aphasia, or both. For these patients, clinicians must look for inhibition test protocols in the research literature. For example, Guitton and colleagues (1985) developed an antisaccade, inhibition task that has nominal speech or language demands. Their task requires patients to focus on a center fixation point on a computer. Visual cues are then randomly flashed to the right or left of the fixation point, and patients are asked to direct their eyes in the direction opposite to the cue. Inhibition is tested, as the automatic response of looking in the same direction as the cue (i.e., saccade) must be avoided (i.e., antisaccade). Performance is quantified by determining the patient's percentage of incorrect saccades.

Cognitive Flexibility Tests

Cognitive flexibility is closely related to the cognitive functions of attention switching and inhibition, as it refers to how well patients can shift from one task to another when internal or external feedback indicates the need to change. Consequently, many tests traditionally described as cognitive flexibility tasks, such as Trail-Making tests, have already been described in other sections of this chapter. Additional cognitive flexibility tasks, such as copying alternating figures or letters (e.g., alternate between writing cursive "n" then "m") and repetitive sequential hand movements (e.g., quickly switching among a fist, edge, and palm hand positions), are included as subtests in cognitive test batteries such as the *Dementia Rating Scales* (Mattis, 2001), or can be found in research studies (e.g., Grigsby, Kaye, & Robbins, 1992; Rende, 2000).

Problem Solving Tests

There are many test options available to evaluate problem-solving skills, including the *Test of Problem Solving–Adolescent* (Bowers, Barrett, Huisingh, Orman, & LoGiudice, 1991), Tinkertoy Test (Lezak, 1995) and Rapid Assessment of Problem Solving (Marshall, Karow, Morelli, Iden, & Dixon, 2003). Several of these tests have nominal language demands, and thus are appropriate for a broad range of neurogenic patient populations. For example, tests such as *Raven's Progressive Matrices* (Raven, 1998), *Test of Nonverbal Intelligence–3* (TONI-III; Brown, Sherbenou, & Johnsen, 1997), and *Comprehensive Test of Nonverbal Intelligence* (Hammill, Pearson, & Widerholt, 1997) involve showing patients a design or series of designs with a piece of the design or design series missing. Patients then must determine which symbol or design from an array of possibilities best completes the design or design series. All of these tests provide extensive norms for children and adults. Both the *Raven's* and TONI-III also have equivalent forms, which make them useful when multiple test administrations are needed for monitoring treatment effects.

Problem-solving tasks that more closely resemble daily activities can be found in the research literature. For example, the photocopy task (Crepeau, Scherzer, Belleville, & Desmarais, 1997) requires patients to learn how to use a photocopier and then complete some more complex tasks, such as copying a picture without reproducing the surrounding text or copying a document that is longer than the common 8.5 × 11.5-inch letter format. In the wheelbarrow test (Butler, Anderson, Furst, & Namerow, 1989), patients are asked to assemble a full-scale wheelbarrow following an instruction sheet. Data that can be gleaned from these types of tasks include: (1) how accurately and independently patients completed the task(s), (2) how long it took them to complete the task(s), (3) what strategies they used to complete the tasks (e.g., did they ask the clinician or others for assistance?), (4) whether they self-corrected, and/or (5) whether clinician cues were required, and if so how many and what kind (e.g., general or specific cues).

Self-Monitoring Tests

Fluency tasks are frequently considered measures of self-monitoring because they require patients to provide responses on a continuous basis while keeping track of responses they have already produced, as well as those they are not allowed to produce. Fluency tasks that require verbal or nonverbal responses are available. For example, many aphasia and dementia test batteries, such as the *Western Aphasia Battery* (Kertesz, 1982) and ABCD, respectively, have a verbal fluency subtest on which patients list as many exemplars as possible in one or two minutes, without repeating themselves, from a prescribed semantic category (e.g., animals, means of transportation). Verbal fluency tasks also may require the generation of words that begin with a certain letter. For instance the FAS or *Controlled Oral Word Association*

Test (Benton et al., 2001), which has been widely used and standardized, requires patients to name as many words as possible beginning with the letter F, then A, and then S, given one minute for each letter. Not only must patients avoid repeating themselves on this test, but they also must avoid listing proper names or numbers. Whereas verbal fluency performance is often quantified in terms of how many correct exemplars were generated, clinicians also may examine whether or not patients utilized any organization strategies, such as semantic clustering (e.g., first naming domestic animals, then naming zoo animals), to aid their performance.

If the patients' speech or language deficits preclude the use of a verbal fluency task, clinicians can instead administer a test such as the *Ruff Figural Fluency Test* (RFFT; Ruff, 1996), which has nominal verbal demands. To complete the RFFT, patients must create as many unique designs as possible in a minute on a sheet of paper with a grid of 35 squares, each of which contains five dots. Patients are instructed to make a design in each square by using straight lines to connect at least two dots. Five trials are completed with different dot configurations, some of which include pre-drawn lines so that the effects of interference can be evaluated. Scoring consists of calculating the number of novel patterns and perseverative errors. Clinicians also can examine whether patients utilized any strategies such as pattern rotation. Although the RFFT is standardized, the normative sample is somewhat limited, as age norms only extend up to 70 years.

Related to self-monitoring is the awareness of one's own strengths and weaknesses. As mentioned in Chapter 2, many patients with neurogenic language disorders have anosognosia, or an impaired awareness of the nature, severity, and/or consequences of their physical, linguistic, and/or cognitive symptoms. Accordingly, clinicians may need to quantify and qualify awareness disorders. Although there are no standardized measures available for assessing awareness, clinicians can obtain information pertaining to the integrity of their patients' self-awareness via interviews and observations. For example, as mentioned in the Case History and Observations section of this chapter, interviewing or giving questionnaires to both patients and their caregivers will allow the clinician to compare responses for any disparities in perceptions of the patients' weaknesses and strengths. In addition to the previously described BADS Dysexecutive Questionnaire (Wilson et al., 1996), there are several questionnaire and interview protocols in the research literature to help clinicians structure this aspect of an executive function assessment (e.g., Giacino & Cicerone, 1998). For example, the Self-Awareness of Deficits Interview (Fleming, Strong, & Ashton, 1996), which has recently received empirical support (Bogod, Mateer, & McDonald, 2003), provides questions regarding three areas of awareness: self-awareness of deficits, self-awareness of the functional implications of one's deficits, and the ability to set realistic goals. The clinician then rates responses using a four-point scale on which zero represents appropriate awareness and four indicates impaired awareness.

A caveat to relying on just the comparison of patient and caregiver reports to quantify and qualify self-awareness is that caregivers, like patients, can provide unreliable responses. For instance, factors such as caregivers' stress levels, personality, and personal involvement, or the patients' time post onset may influence the accuracy of caregivers' responses (Bogod et al., 2003). Accordingly, clinicians should augment interview/questionnaire responses with data collected from other awareness assessment strategies, such as requiring patients to make predictions regarding their performance of standardized tests and then comparing their predicted and actual test scores (Fischer, Trexler, & Gauggel, 2004; Sohlberg, 2000); lack of awareness is indicated when patients frequently overestimate their performance. Another option is to watch for certain behaviors indicative of anosognosia throughout the cognitive assessment (Sohlberg, 2000). These behaviors include minimal or no self-correcting behaviors, failure to use compensatory strategies, and poor motivation or lack of cooperation during structured assessment tasks because the patient does not see the need for an assessment.

TEST CONFOUNDS

Although numerous cognitive test choices are available, not all of these will be appropriate for all patients with neurogenic language disorders. Consequently, clinicians must carefully read test manuals to determine if the tests they are considering using were standardized on a normative sample that is representative of their patients. In particular, clinicians should always check for the age, education, ethnocultural, and language backgrounds of tests' normative samples, as these variables have been found to influence outcomes on formal cognitive tests (Vanderploeg, Axelrod, Sherer, Scott, & Adams, 1997; Kennepohl et al., 2004). Unfortunately, because of narrow normative samples, many tests, particularly those published 15 or more years ago, have limited use for patients who are elderly, have low education, speak English as a second language, or represent an ethnocultural minority. To avoid this confound, some new tests provide standardized versions for individuals who speak English as a second language (e.g., *Cognitive Linguistic Quick Test*), were developed for a specific language (e.g., *Evaluación Neuropsicológica Breve en Español*, Ostrosky-Solis, Ardila, & Rosselli, 1997), and/or have normative data that are stratified by age and education (e.g., NAB). Likewise, although the normative data in many tests' manuals may be restrictive, extended norms often are available in research studies conducted subsequent to these tests' initial publication (e.g., Duff et al., 2003; Heaton, Miller, Taylor, & Grant, 2004; Llinas Regla et al., 1995).

Clinicians also must ensure that the instructions and response demands of cognitive tests are compatible with the physical, sensory, and language abilities of their patients. For example, cognitive tests that require understanding of long, complex task instructions would be inappropriate for many patients with language comprehension difficulties due to aphasia or dementia; likewise, cognitive tests that require drawing complex designs may be unsuitable for patients with hemiparesis who must use their nondominant hand to draw or write. Use of tests that exceed the physical, sensory, and/or language skills of patients will produce invalid results, as the clinician will be unsure whether poor performance on these tests was reflective of a true cognitive deficit, or was rather the product of these other symptoms.

QUALITATIVE ASSESSMENT CONSIDERATIONS

If time limitations or other confounds obstruct administering formal cognitive tests, clinicians should keep in mind that information regarding the integrity of their patients' cognitive abilities can be gleaned informally while completing language assessment procedures. More specifically, cognitive abilities may be informally evaluated by observing the presence of certain behaviors indicative of cognitive problems, and by administering language tests in formats that vary the cognitive demands of the language tasks or assessment environment.

Clinicians may monitor for possible cognitive problems while completing their initial observations and interviews, or while administering formal language tests. For example, attention impairments might be suspected if patients appear easily distracted (i.e., sustained and/or selective attention problems), the quality of their performance quickly deteriorates (i.e., sustained attention problems), they have difficulty switching between language tasks (i.e., attention shifting problems), or their performance breaks down when they attempt to process more than one modality or information source or to complete more than one task at a time (i.e., divided attention problems). Signs of memory problems include the need for frequent reminders about task instructions, or when patients' comprehension abilities appear to be more influenced by the length of the material rather than by linguistic factors such as grammatical complexity or vocabulary familiarity. Likewise, clinicians should consider the possibility of impaired executive functioning when patients appear impulsive, inappropriate, perseverative, concrete, or unaware of their deficits, the extent of their deficits, or the implications of their deficits.

Another option is to adapt language tests so that the cognitive demands of the language tasks are varied. For example, a reading comprehension test could be administered both in quiet and noisy, distracting environments to determine whether focused attention demands negatively affect patients' reading rate or comprehension accuracy. To evaluate the effects of increased memory demands on the repetition abilities of patients with aphasia, patients could be instructed to repeat immediately after the clinician on some items, to repeat only after a five-second delay on other items, and to count to five and then repeat on still other items (i.e., filled delay condition). Whatever manipulations are introduced to evaluate the effects of high and low cognitive demands on language task performance, clinicians must remember to keep the linguistic complexity of the stimuli similar across the various task conditions; for instance, for the repetition test example, the repetition items for the immediate, delayed, and filled delay response conditions must be similar in length and phonological, syntactic, and semantic complexity. Failure to do so will result in ambiguous findings, as clinicians will not be able to determine whether their patients' poor performances were a product of linguistic or cognitive factors.

PROGNOSTIC FACTORS FOR COGNITIVE OUTCOMES

A final step of assessment is to formulate prognoses regarding patients' rehabilitation potential, recovery rate, or eventual outcome. Several of the biographical, medical, and cognitive prognostic factors noted in Chapter 5 to influence language outcomes also may relate to cognitive outcomes (see Tables 5-6 and 6-5). Clinicians are reminded that predictions regarding patients' recovery patterns or outcomes must be based on the consideration of many prognostic variables, as by themselves these variables provide only weak and thus possibly inaccurate approximations of patients' future cognitive status.

In terms of biographical variables, age appears to be a strong cognitive outcome predictor, as many studies have found that older patients with neurogenic disorders tend to have more severe cognitive problems and poorer functional outcomes than their younger counterparts (Cifu et al., 1996; Fischer & LaFleche, 1998;

Table 6-5. Prognostic Indicators for Rehabilitative Outcome Related to Cognitive Impairments

FACTORS SUGGESTING BETTER PROGNOSIS	FACTORS SUGGESTING POORER PROGNOSIS
Younger age	Lesion Variables:
Good premorbid physical health	Lesion severity (as evidenced by coma length, duration of post-traumatic amnesia)
Regular exercise	Large lesions
	Frontal lobe involvement
	Early right hemisphere involvement in Parkinson's Disease
	Concomitant medical, physical, or psychiatric problems:
	Diabetes
	Depression
	Anxiety
	Presence of certain linguistic/cognitive deficits:
	Anosognosia
	Neglect
	Early language symptoms in Alzheimer's Disease

Hier, Mondlock, & Caplan, 1983; Teri, Borson, Kiyak, & Yamagishi,1989); some researchers contend, however, that normal age-related changes in cognition may contribute, at least in part, to poor neuropsychological outcomes among elderly patients (Johnstone, Childers, & Hoerner, 1998). Controversy persists regarding the relationship between education and cognitive outcomes: Some studies report that well-educated adults show fewer or less progressive cognitive impairments than their less-educated peers (Lyketsos, Chen, & Anthony, 1999), whereas other studies find no significant association between education and cognitive outcomes (Gilleard, 1997). Christensen et al. (2001) noted that in many investigations in which a strong relationship between education and cognitive changes was identified, researchers failed to control for practice or retest effects; this is particularly problematic because adults' test-taking skills are linked to their education level, and thus highly educated adults tend to show larger practice effects when completing multiple administrations of the same tests.

Medical variables also should be considered, as patients who have one or more medical, physical, or psychiatric complications are at risk for poorer outcomes compared to patients without these concomitant conditions. For instance, diabetes should be considered a complicating factor, as patients with diabetes have slower recovery rates (Lukovits, Mazzone, & Gorelick, 1999); slower recovery in these patients may be related to severe hypoglycemic episodes, in which loss of consciousness may compromise cerebral functioning, or to daily fluctuations in glucose levels, which can negatively affect attention and other cognitive abilities (Fujioka et al., 1997; Hertanu & Moldover, 1996). In contrast, patients who had good premorbid physical health, and who exercise regularly subsequent to the onset of their brain damage or disease, are more likely to have positive cognitive and emotional outcomes than their out-of-shape peers (Bassey, 2000; Hill, Wahlin, Winblad, & Backman, 1995). Emotional or psychiatric health also is an influential prognostic indicator, as patients with psychiatric disorders such as depression or anxiety, or who adopt negative coping strategies such as denial or avoidance, tend to have less success in rehabilitation than patients without psychiatric problems or those who utilize positive coping strategies such as problem-oriented coping or seeking education about their symptoms or disease (Ben-Yishay & Daniels-Zide, 2000; Ehmann, Beninger, Gawel, & Riopelle, 1990).

Lesion variables also appear influential. In TBI, the greater the severity of the brain injury, as indexed by length of coma and duration of post-traumatic amnesia, as well as extent of brain damage, the more likely the patient will experience slow cognitive recovery or enduring cognitive impairments (Dikmen & Machamer, 1995; Zafonte et al., 1996). More generally, regardless of etiology, large brain lesions and frontal lobe damage are most detrimental to overall cognitive abilities and outcomes (Ferro et al., 1999; Robertson & Murre, 1999). Links between lesion location and presence or recovery of specific cognitive deficits also have been reported. For example, neglect recovery is more likely if frontoparietal or, more generally, cortical areas are spared (Hier et al., 1983). In Parkinson's disease, patients who demonstrate initial left-sided motor symptoms and thus early right hemisphere involvement tend to present with more diverse and severe cognitive problems than patients who initially experience right-sided motor symptoms and thus early left hemisphere involvement (Lee, Harris, Atkinson, & Fowler, 2001). As with language recovery, greatest and most rapid cognitive improvements are observed within the first few months post onset of nonprogressive brain damage (Ferro et al., 1999; Stone, Patel, Greenwood, & Halligan, 1992).

In general, the presence of any cognitive deficit may compromise patient recovery and subsequent functional outcome (Kayser-Jones, Schell, Porter, Barbaccia, & Shaw, 1999; Kalra et al., 1997; Tatemichi et al., 1994), and more severe initial cognitive deficits are associated with poorer outcomes (Dikmen & Machamer, 1995; Ferro et al., 1999). Certain cognitive deficits, however, appear to be more detrimental to long-term outcomes. For example, findings from several studies indicate that patients with neglect and/or executive dysfunctioning, particularly impaired self-awareness, will have poorer overall cognitive recovery and rehabilitation outcomes than patients without these cognitive symptoms (Chen et al., 1998; Fischer & LaFleche, 1998; Patel, Coshall, Rudd, & Wolfe, 2003; Pedersen et al., 1997; Sherer et al., 1998). Similarly, in progressive diseases, early demonstration of executive deficits is associated with rapid cognitive deterioration (Butters, Lopez, & Becker, 1996). There also appears to be a link between language skills and cognitive or rehabilitation outcomes. In Alzheimer's disease, patients who demonstrate language deficits such as confrontation naming problems or impaired semantic categorization abilities as an early or initial symptom show faster cognitive deterioration than patients without these language problems (Chan, Salmon, Butters, & Johnson, 1995), and in TBI, patients with aphasia often have more severe cognitive impairments than their non-aphasic peers (Gil et al., 1996).

SUMMARY

A growing body of research indicates that patients with neurogenic language disorders often present with concomitant deficits of attention, memory, and executive functioning, and that these deficits may negatively affect not only their language abilities, but also their rehabilitation and functional outcomes. Accordingly, this chapter reviewed the basic format of a cognitive evaluation by describing a number of informal and formal procedures and tests that may be used to assess general as well as specific cognitive abilities. Currently the role of speech-language pathology in assessing and treating neurogenic cognitive disorders continues to evolve and varies depending on the clinical setting. Regardless, however, clinicians must be prepared to evaluate the cognitive abilities of their patients or, even if they are not directly involved in the cognitive assessment, be able to interpret the results of cognitive evaluations in order to plan and provide effective treatment of their patients' cognitive and linguistic disorders.

Chapter 7

Assessment of Activity and Participation and Quality of Life

INTRODUCTION

In Chapters 5 and 6, strategies for assessing the underlying impairments contributing to cognitive and communicative activity limitations were described. These assessment techniques allow the clinician to describe the nature of language and cognitive-communicative disorders as well as design treatment programs. In addition to understanding the underlying impairments and activity limitations experienced by our patients, we also need to appreciate the impact of these conditions on their ability to participate in desired activities, as well as on their overall quality of life. Assessment of participation and quality of life serves two main purposes. First, understanding the impact of communication and cognitive deficits on "real-life" activities informs treatment planning. That is, patients who experience significant participation restrictions related to their neurogenic language disorder may be more likely to be motivated to pursue treatment than patients whose quality of life has been impacted minimally by their impairments.

Second, participation and quality of life measures are critical when determining treatment effectiveness. Whereas improvements on impairment level measures suggest that treatment has been beneficial, only when we demonstrate that treatment has had a positive effect on the patient's functional performance, societal participation, and/or quality of life can we be sure treatment has been truly effective. More complete discussions of issues related to treatment efficacy are included in Chapter 8 and Chapter 12. In this chapter, we will highlight strategies for assessing functional performance, societal participation, and quality of life, for the purposes of planning treatment and evaluating treatment efficacy.

DEFINING TERMS

The tools described in this chapter are variably termed **functional measures, measures of participation,** or **measures of quality of life.** In some literature, these terms are used interchangeably, but in this chapter, each term will be used to denote a specific aspect of "real life" performance.

Functional measures of performance are used in all areas of rehabilitation and typically target "real life" activities such as self-care and ambulation. With respect to communication, functional assessment refers to describing a "person's ability to communicate despite the presence of impairments such as aphasia, dysarthria, or hearing loss" (Frattali, 1994, p. 306). For example, a functional measure may assess a patient's success in communicating with a family member. Within this framework, functional measures assess the ICF level of activity limitations (as defined in Chapter 1) and address communication in ways unlike those targeted by the impairment level measures described in Chapters 5 and 6. Whereas those measures help describe underlying impairments of language and other cognitive domains, as well as communication behaviors during structured tasks, functional measures attempt to describe communication behaviors during daily life activities. In this respect, functional measures are similar to participation-level measures.

Measures of participation are those that assess the degree to which individuals participate in the activities characteristic of their daily lives. For example, the measure may assess whether a patient attends sporting events, performs job duties, or participates in social activities. The focus of participation measures *is* participation. Other measures address how the individuals *feel* about their participation (Hirsch & Holland, 2000). Such **quality of life measures** target factors beyond participation and include issues of feelings, attitudes, and beliefs related to the ability to enjoy life. Quality of life measures often include items such as "I am generally happy" or "My life is satisfying."

All three of these assessment targets (i.e., functional communication, participation, and quality of life) contribute to our understanding of how a neurogenic language disorder impacts the lifestyle of any given patient. Furthermore, by addressing these factors, we are better able to make recommendations regarding the need for treatment and potential treatment procedures, and to evaluate the effectiveness of the treatment that is provided. Figure 7-1 lists the measures reviewed in this chapter as well as additional measures available through the research literature.

Affect Balance Scale (ABS; Bradburn, 1969) [3]

Amsterdam-Nijmegen Everyday Language Test (ANELT; Blomert et al., 1987, 1994) [1]

ASHA Functional Assessment of Communication (ASHA FACS; Frattali et al., 1995) [1]

ASHA Quality of Communication Life (CQL; Paul-Brown, Frattali, Holland, Thompson, Caperton and Slater, 2004).) [2, 3]

Assessing Disability and Handicap (Swigert, 1997) [2]

Behaviour, Emotion, Attitude, Communication Questionnaire (Hoen et al., 1997) [3]

Burden of Stroke Scale (BOSS; Doyle et al., 2004) [1, 2, 3]

Communication Profile (Gurland et al., 1982) [1]

Communication Profile: Functional Skills Survey (Payne, 1994) [1]

Communicative Activities of Daily Living – 2 (CADL-2; Holland et al., 1999) [1]

Communicative Effectiveness Index (CETI; Lomas et al., 1989) [1]

Communicative/Competence Evaluation Instrument (Houghten et al., 1992) [1]

Community Integration Questionairre (CIQ; Willer et al., 1993) [2]

Craig Handicap Assessment and Reporting Technique (CHART; Whiteneck et al., 1992) [2]

Dartmouth COOP Functional Assessment Charts (Nelson et al., 1987) [3]

Functional Communication Profile (FCP; Sarno, 1969) [1]

Functional Independence Measure (FIM; State University of New York, 1993) [1]

Functional Life Scale (FLS; Sarno et al., 1973) [2]

Pragmatic Protocol (Prutting and Kirchner, 1987) [1]

Psychosocial Well-Being Index (PWI; Lyon et al., 1997) [3]

Ryff Scales of Psychological Well-Being (Ryff et al., 1989) [3]

Satisfaction with Life Scale (SWLS; Diener et al., 1985) [3]

Sickness Impact Profile (SIP; Bergner et al., 1981) [2, 3]

Stroke and Aphasia Quality of Life Scale- 39 (SAQLS-39; Hilari, Byng, Lamping, and Smith, 2003) [1, 2, 3]

Stroke-Specific Quality of Life Scale (SS-QOL; Williams, Weinberger, Harris, Clark, and Biller, 1999) [1, 2, 3]

---

[1] Measures Communication Function
[2] Measures Participation
[3] Measures Quality of Life

Figure 7-1. **Published Measures of Communication Function, Participation, and Quality of Life.**

FUNCTIONAL MEASURES

Of the measures to be discussed in this chapter, functional measures have the longest history in health care settings, and are likely the most widely used by speech-language pathologists. Functional measures are typically used for two main purposes (Brookshire, 1997). The first purpose, for which these measures are more commonly used, is to document program effectiveness. The second purpose, which is of greater importance to this discussion, is to assess changes in the performance of individual patients.

FUNCTIONAL MEASURES DESIGNED FOR PROGRAM EVALUATION

Most rehabilitation programs conduct ongoing evaluation of program effectiveness. Often termed "continuous quality improvement," the process of systematically evaluating program effectiveness is required by accreditation agencies (e.g., Joint Council for the Accreditation of Healthcare Organizations). Historically, programs could document quality by verifying that established policies and procedures were monitored and administered consistently (i.e., **process measures**). Process measures were convenient for administrators because performance data (e.g., average delay between the time a referral was received and when the evaluation was completed) were readily obtained, and thus improvements in quality could be documented easily. Unfortunately, process measures are insensitive to some important aspects of program quality, such as improved patient function or reduced treatment costs. In recognition of these limitations, accrediting agencies began requesting that programs document quality **outcomes.**

Side Bar

Process Measures in Acute Care: An Example

Evaluating quality through the use of process measures can be very helpful in some situations. In an acute care setting, we wanted to verify that hospital staff members were following speech-language pathology's recommendations for maximizing communication with individual patients. To study this, we asked each staff member involved with the patient to initial a form indicating he or she understood not only the unique needs of this patient but also what procedures to use to communicate best with this patient. When we analyzed the documentation collected from many patients over time, we found that a good proportion of the staff initialed the forms. Our process measure indicated that the procedures we had in place were appropriate for our goal of facilitating effective communication between our patients with neurogenic language disorders and their hospital care providers.

What we were unable determine from our data, however, was whether the patients *actually communicated* more effectively when hospital staff members were made aware of the patients' unique communication needs. Information about this level requires outcome measures.

Outcomes, as the term suggests, refer to the end results of program efforts, specifically, changes in patients' communicative and cognitive functioning. Whereas impairment level measures such as those discussed in Chapters 5 and 6 might serve to document outcomes, such measures do not serve well for program evaluation for one main reason: Not all patients exhibit the same impairments. To demonstrate that a *program* is effective, the measure used must be appropriate for all patients who participate in the program. To this end, the most frequently used functional measures for program evaluation (i.e., outcome measures) are very general so as to be applicable to all patients regardless of their medical diagnosis or type of neurogenic language disorder. Additionally, these functional measures tend to be brief and simple, allowing them to be administered to patients as they enter a program and again at discharge, ideally by any member of the health care team. What follows is a description of some of the outcome measures most frequently utilized in today's health care systems.

Functional Independence Measure

Perhaps the most well-known and widely used functional outcome measure is the *Functional Independence Measure* (FIM; State University of New York at Buffalo Research Foundation, 1993). Developed specifically to document rehabilitation outcomes, it consists of a seven-point scale for evaluating six performance domains: self-care, sphincter control, mobility, locomotion, communication, and social cognition (Figure 7-2). Each domain includes two or more specific performance areas (e.g., locomotion includes walking and stairs) that are rated according to level of independence. The communication domain consists of two performance areas: comprehension and expression. Social interaction, problem-solving, and memory are the three behaviors included in the social cognition domain. It is clear that these performance areas are broad enough to be applicable to all patients with neurogenic language disorders. Unfortunately, because the behaviors are so broadly defined, and because the independence rating scale is neither particularly sensitive nor reliable (Adamovitch, 1990; Warren, 1992), the FIM has not been widely acclaimed by speech-language pathologists. Despite the documented limitations of the FIM, however, it continues to be a popular outcome measure for program evaluation.

ASHA FACS

In recognition of the FIM's limitations in identifying changes in functional performance in the areas of communication, the American Speech-Language-Hearing Association (ASHA) developed a functional measure specifically for communication. The *ASHA Functional Assessment of Communication Skills for Adults* (ASHA

L e v e l s	7 Complete independence (timely, safely) 6 Modified independence (device)	NO HELPER
	Modified dependence 5 Supervision 4 Minimal Assist (Subject = 75%) 3 Moderate Assist (Subject = 50%) Complete dependence 2 Maximal Assist (Subject = 25%) 1 Total Assist (Subject = 0%+)	HELPER

	ADMIT	FOLLOW-UP
Self-Care		
A. Eating		
B. Grooming		
C. Bathing		
D. Dressing-Upper Body		
E. Dressing-Lower Body		
F. Toileting		
Sphincter Control		
G. Bladder Management		
H. Bowel Management		
Mobility		
Transfer:		
I. Bed, Chair, Wheelchair		
J. Toilet		
K. Tub, Shower		
Locomotion		
L. Walk/wheelchair		
M. Stairs		
Communication		
N. Comprehension: Auditory Visual		
O. Expression: Verbal Nonverbal		
Social Cognition		
P. Social Interaction		
Q. Problem Solving		
R. Memory	Total FIM:_____	Total FIM:_____

NOTE: Leave no blanks; enter 1 if patient not testable due to risk.

Adapted from Research Foundation. (1990). Guide for use of the Uniform Data Set for Medical Rehabilitation. Buffalo, NY: Research Foundation, State University of New York.

Figure 7-2. Functional Independence Measure (FIM).

FACS; Frattali, Thompson, Holland, Wohl, & Ferketic, 1995) is similar to the FIM in several ways. First, it includes a seven-point rating scale assessing level of independence. Additionally, the ASHA FACS targets several specific behaviors grouped into related domains: social communication (e.g., uses names of familiar people), communication of basic needs (e.g., recognizes familiar faces/voices), daily planning (e.g., dials telephone numbers), and reading/writing/number concepts (e.g., follows written directions). However, unlike the FIM, the ASHA FACS assesses independence in 33 cognitive-communicative behaviors, making it potentially more sensitive to changes in communicative skill. Additionally, the ASHA FACS allows examiners to assess performance qualitatively in each domain, in terms of adequacy, appropriateness, promptness, and communicative sharing. Finally, the ASHA FACS has been standardized for patients with left hemisphere damage as well as those with traumatic brain injury.

Because the ASHA FACS and the FIM provide similar independence scores, some speech-language pathology programs may choose to use the ASHA FACS instead of the FIM to evaluate program effectiveness. Moreover, the ASHA FACS scores reported by the speech-language pathology program can be compared to those submitted by other rehabilitation programs. The high number of items assessed and the complex qualitative scoring system, however, dictate that only trained individuals administer the tool.

FUNCTIONAL MEASURES DESIGNED FOR PATIENT EVALUATION

Measures designed for program evaluation may not be particularly useful when applied to individual patients. That is, measures such as the FIM do not readily inform treatment planning, nor are they necessarily sensitive to treatment-related changes. Therefore, when the purpose is to assess the functional communication skills of individual patients, other tools may be more appropriate. Whereas a number of scales have been described in the research literature (see Figure 7-1 and Murray & Chapey, 2001), the discussion here will be limited to the most well-known and widely applied functional measures.

ASHA FACS

Because the ASHA FACS describes in detail patient behaviors across a variety of domains, it may be used to evaluate patient performance as well as program effectiveness. When used for patient evaluation, the qualitative rating scale assessing adequacy, appropriateness, promptness, and communicative sharing is employed to a greater extent than for program evaluation. The independence rating scale may be used for both patient and program evaluation, but the qualitative scale may provide information more valuable for treatment planning and evaluating treatment effectiveness.

Functional Communication Profile

The *Functional Communication Profile* (FCP; Sarno, 1969) is one of the earliest measures of functional communication. Similar to the functional measures described above, the FCP includes a rating scale targeting several performance domains. The clinician rates the patient's ability to perform specific tasks in the areas of movement (e.g., ability to imitate oral movements), speaking (e.g., saying noun-verb combinations), understanding (e.g., understanding television), reading (e.g., reading newspaper headlines), and other cognitive and communicative areas (e.g., writing name, calculation, money skills). The FCP's rating system is scored not according to level of independence, but rather as the proportion of the patient's ability to perform the tasks prior to neurological injury or disease onset. This scoring method may be challenging because clinicians may not be fully aware of patients' premorbid abilities. The rating scale of the next instrument addresses this limitation.

Communicative Effectiveness Index

Lomas and her colleagues (1989) developed a functional measure of communication that differs from those described above in that the rating scales of their *Communicative Effectiveness Index* (CETI) are scored by the spouse or caregiver of the individual with the neurogenic language disorder. Like the FCP, the CETI is based on comparing the patient's current communicative performance with his or her premorbid abilities. Because caregivers likely have greater knowledge than the clinician about premorbid abilities, as well as more opportunities to observe patients in their current functional communication situations, CETI ratings might be expected to be particularly valid for assessing functional communication skills. Patients with adequate comprehension skills at the sentence level may be able to complete the CETI rating scales themselves. In these cases, the clinician may wish to have the caregivers as well as the patient complete the CETI to identify any differences in perceptions regarding treatment effectiveness.

Communicative Activities of Daily Living–2

In addition to rating scales such as the CETI and FCP, functional communication skills may be assessed by directly eliciting target behaviors. The *Communicative Activities of Daily Living–2* (CADL-2; Holland, Frattali, & Fromm, 1999), a standardized test for patients with aphasia or right hemisphere damage due to stroke or traumatic brain injury (TBI), was designed to elicit communicative behaviors in structured yet functional interactions. It includes items targeting divergent, contextual, and nonverbal communication, social interaction, and other functional skills such as sequential relationships and humor. Whereas several items utilize scenarios to elicit communicative behaviors (e.g., "You need shoelaces, but you can't find them. If a clerk asked, 'May I help you?' what would you say?"), others elicit responses in a more spontaneous way (e.g., asking the patient to complete a form but not offering a writing utensil, to determine if the patient notices the anomaly and attempts to correct it). An earlier version of the CADL (Holland, 1980) included role-playing tasks that simulated functional communication interactions, which is yet another way to assess functional skills.

Assessment of Language-Related Functional Activities

Another tool that directly elicits functional communication behaviors is the *Assessment of Language-Related Functional Activities* (ALFA; Baines, Martin, & Heeringa, 1999). Addressing a diverse array of activities involving the use of language (e.g., telling time, counting money, using a calendar, understanding medicine labels), ALFA items were designed to incorporate scenarios representative of functional activities. For example, one item requires the patient to write a check for a specific bill, being sure to include the current date. The ALFA yields an independent functioning rating that estimates the probability the patient will exhibit independent functioning. Clinicians may consider the independent functioning rating when developing treatment goals and prognoses.

A strength of the ALFA is that the standardization sample was relatively large (i.e., *n* = 495 patients and 150 normal controls) and diverse, including patients with stroke, TBI, and dementia. Thus, the ALFA may be appropriate for patients demonstrating neurogenic language disorders resulting from a variety of etiologies.

Informal Measures of Functional Communication

Clinicians may take advantage of the fact that "functional communication" often occurs spontaneously during interactions among the patient, family members, health care providers, and other patients. How such interactions are assessed may vary from the primarily subjective (e.g., successful, inefficient) to systematic and objective (e.g., conversational analysis; Crockford & Lesser, 1994). Tools assessing discourse effectiveness (see Chapter 5) might be employed to assist in the description and analysis of functional communication samples. There is some evidence that informal assessment strategies are helpful in revealing changes in functional communication, and that they also hold the potential benefit of revealing the functional communication strengths and weaknesses of patients' communication partners (Crockford & Lesser, 1994).

Selecting Functional Measures for Patients with Neurogenic Language Disorders

Before leaving the discussion of functional measures, it is important to note that we have highlighted the use of these tools to address neurogenic language disorders. Some tools, however, may be more or less suited for documenting functional skills in patients with different communication disorders. For example, the highly generic items on the FIM may be appropriate for patients with aphasia, apraxia of speech, or dysarthria, but less sensitive to changes in patients with disorders such as right hemisphere damage (Odell & Flynn, 1998). Both the ASHA FACS and FCM are heavily weighted with items most appropriate for individuals with aphasia including only a few items relevant to motor speech or cognitive disorders (e.g., "saying own name" and "using writing instead of speech."). The CETI predominately includes items that address communication limitations commonly experienced by patients with either aphasia or motor speech disorders (e.g., "giving 'yes' and 'no' answers appropriately."), although a few key items (e.g., "describing or discussing something at length.") are appropriate for individuals with cognitive disorders as well. Accordingly, when selecting a functional outcome measure, clinicians should carefully consider the impairments of the patient as well as the features of the outcome measure to determine the most appropriate match.

PARTICIPATION MEASURES

A common characteristic of functional communication measures is that they attempt to assess communication skills as they are observed in activities outside of the therapeutic setting. A related, but separate, strategy is to assess the degree to which individuals with neurogenic language disorders participate in typical daily activities. Participation measures have not been used as frequently as functional measures during initial assessment or to evaluate treatment effectiveness, but they do offer unique information about how patients' communication or cognitive limitations are impacting their ability to participate in the activities enjoyed premorbidly.

Existing participation measures were not designed specifically for patients with neurogenic language disorders. Instead, most target activities for which participation might be restricted due to any number of conditions. For example, the Craig Handicap Assessment and Reporting Technique (CHART; Whiteneck, Charlifue, Gerhart, Overholser, & Richardson, 1992) includes, among others, items related to economic self-sufficiency. Clearly, this factor might be impacted by limited communication or cognitive skills, as well as other impairments such as reduced mobility. In contrast to CHART, the Community Integration Questionnaire (CIQ; Willer, Rosenthal, Kreutzer, Gordon, & Rempel, 1993) is an example of a participation measure targeting a specific diagnostic group: in this case, patients with TBI. Although both the CHART and CIQ provide information about an individual's degree of participation in standard daily activities, they have been criticized for being more sensitive to participation restrictions related to physical rather than communication limitations (Hirsch & Holland, 2000).

Perhaps the best evidence that a participation measure is appropriate for individuals with neurogenic language disorders is when that measure has been successfully used to demonstrate improvement as a result of speech-language treatment. One such measure is the *Functional Life Scale* (FLS) developed by Sarno, Sarno, and Levita (1973). This tool targets several activity domains, including cognition (e.g., orientation to time, able to shift from one task to another with relative ease), activities of daily living (e.g., feeds self, dresses self), activities in the home (e.g., performs light housekeeping chores, uses television), outside activities (e.g., goes shopping for food, uses public transportation alone), and social interaction (e.g., participates in games with other people, attends social functions outside of home). Items within each activity domain are rated along the four dimensions of self-initiation, frequency, speed, and overall efficiency. Using the FLS, Sarno (1997) reported that individuals with aphasia participating in a rehabilitation program showed improvement in several domains (e.g., cognition and outside activities), as well as with respect to quality of activity performance (e.g., speed and efficiency). Whereas the complex nature of the rating scale enhances the FLS's sensitivity to changes as a result of treatment, it also increases the amount of time and skill required to administer the instrument and score it reliably. That is, clinicians will require training and should determine the consistency of their ratings prior to using this tool independently.

INFORMAL MEASURES OF PARTICIPATION

Many clinicians will find it advantageous to include informal measures of participation as part of the complete evaluation process. A distinct advantage of informal measures is that the clinician can tailor the content and form to meet the unique presentation of each patient. For example, if a clinician is aware of a patient's premorbid interests and activities, assessment activities can be devised that carefully document that patient's participation in these specific areas.

Informal assessment of participation might include asking the patient, family members, or both about participation in typical activities. Many questions utilized in the formal measures described above might serve as a model for the types of questions clinicians could include in an informal interview. For example, Swigert (1997) described a four-question interview to address participation. In this approach, patients are asked to identify situations in which communication is most difficult and to describe how communication difficulties have impacted interactions with friends, family, and at work. A unique item asks the patient, "Do you avoid situations because of your speech?" (p. 59). These questions could easily be incorporated into the clinical interview.

Additionally, useful information regarding participation can be gained through direct observation of the patient during typical activities. Ideally, these observations would take place in naturalistic settings such as social events, vocational activities, or other activities the patient had been involved in premorbidly. A clear advantage of direct observation is that the clinician may gain valuable insights into the interactions between the patient and the communication situation. That is, many times it will become clear that the key factor limiting a patient's participation in a particular activity is not the communication disorder, but rather the environment. For instance, factors such as background noise or pacing of the activity, which may have a strong influence on the success with which patients with neurogenic language disorders participate in activities, are often difficult to ascertain from an interview alone.

QUALITY OF LIFE MEASURES

Whereas participation measures contribute unique information to our understanding of the impact of neurogenic language disorders on our patients' lives, they do not address a key component of treatment effectiveness, that of quality of life. That is, the inability to balance the checkbook or select items at a grocery store (i.e., participation measures) may have little or no impact on the quality of life of a patient who has never been responsible for these tasks or perhaps never enjoyed being responsible for these tasks. Similarly, some patients may participate in highly unique activities that are not addressed by standardized participation measures (e.g., participation in a foreign language club). Quality of life measures allow clinicians to assess more directly the impact of communication and cognitive limitations on patients' overall well-being.

Just as overlap exists among measures of function and participation, the same is true for measures of participation and quality of life. The unique aspect of quality of life measures is the attempt to characterize patients' emotional response to disruptions in function and participation. Quality of life and well-being may be assessed both formally and informally (Figure 7-1). We will first review some formal measures targeting quality of life.

Side Bar

Quality of Life: The Patient's Priority

Assessing both participation and quality of life may reveal patient experiences that are surprising, yet quite relevant, to the clinical process. Ray is a 64-year-old man with severe aphasia characterized by limited auditory comprehension and fluent, empty speech. He presented for outpatient evaluation approximately one year after his left hemisphere stroke. Through interviews with Ray's neighbor, who graciously accompanied Ray to the evaluation, we learned that following his stroke, Ray had been committed to a psychiatric hospital by his (now) ex-wife, who had then proceeded to obtain authority over Ray's finances.

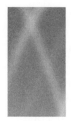

(continued)

We further learned that even though Ray continued to participate in nearly all the activities he enjoyed, his quality of life was limited by the loss of his driver's license resulting from his inappropriate committal and his inability to adequately defend his legal rights. Ray's goals for therapy were very specific: to pass the written test to regain his driver's license, and to develop strategies for effectively communicating with his ex-wife and legal representatives.

GENERAL QUALITY OF LIFE MEASURES

Many measures have been devised to assess quality of life. In this section we first discuss a select sample of such general measures that have been used to assess quality of life in individuals with neurogenic language disorders. Second, a sample of quality of life measures developed specifically for individuals experiencing communication disorders will be presented.

Sickness Impact Profile

The *Sickness Impact Profile* (SIP; Bergner, Bobbitt, Carter, & Gibson, 1981) includes items describing activities in 12 categories of daily living: sleep and rest, emotional behavior, body care and movement, home management, mobility, social interaction, ambulation, alertness behavior, communication, work, recreation and pastimes, and eating. Patients identify each of the 136 items that are impacted by their health. Based on the overall number as well as the type of items identified, the SIP provides scores representing overall dysfunction, dysfunction in each activity category, and dysfunction in psychosocial and physical domains.

The SIP may be self-scored by the patient or administered as an interview. In either case, the patient must have adequate comprehension skills to understand the items and how to rate them. The items are heavily weighted with respect to daily activities, making the SIP very similar to participation measures. However, the items related to emotional behavior may provide some insight into patient well-being. Hirsch and Holland (2000) recommended supplementing the SIP with additional questions addressing life satisfaction.

Dartmouth COOP Functional Assessment Charts

The SIP described above may be somewhat taxing to administer because of its length. Additionally, it may be inappropriate for individuals with disrupted communication or cognitive abilities because of the sheer number, as well as the linguistic complexity, of the items. An alternative measure that addresses these limitations is the Dartmouth COOP Functional Assessment Charts (Nelson, Fogel, & Faust, 1987). In this measure, patients respond to a single question on each of nine charts that target physical fitness, feelings, daily activities, social activities, pain, changes in health, overall health, social support, and quality of life. For each chart, the patient is asked to respond by rating the question along a five-point scale that is depicted both verbally and visually.

Because of the limited number of items, the Dartmouth Charts may be administered in less than five minutes. Additionally, the visually depicted rating scale may facilitate the responses of individuals with even severe communication limitations. Another benefit is that items addressing feelings and quality of life provide insight into well-being and life satisfaction, in addition to the information provided with respect to participation.

Affect Balance Scale

Whereas rating scales often directly ask patients about the impact of impairments on their quality of life, another strategy for assessing qualify of life is to ask patients to respond to items that indirectly reflect well-being. One measure utilizing this strategy is the Affect Balance Scale (ABS; Bradburn, 1969).

Similar in length to the Dartmouth Charts, the ABS requires patients to respond to ten questions regarding their experience of a variety of feelings during the past few weeks. For example, one item asks, "During the past few weeks did you ever feel depressed or very unhappy?" The patient responds with a simple "yes" or "no" answer. Five items, including the item above, denote negative feelings. The remaining five denote positive feelings (e.g., "During the past few weeks did you ever feel particularly excited or interested in something?"). Bradburn (1969) suggested that a score reflecting the difference between the negative and positive affect items is an indication of overall well-being.

Because ABS questions do not specify that health issues are necessarily the cause of positive or negative feelings, the scale can be used for a variety of purposes outside of rehabilitation (Bradburn, 1969). When the ABS has been employed in studies examining the effectiveness of communication treatment, it has failed to reveal differences in ratings as a result of aphasia treatment (Lyon et al., 1997) or between young adults with or without a history of specific language impairment (Records, Tomblin, & Freese, 1992). Although it is impossible to determine whether the lack of significant change reflected a true lack of difference due to therapy or between the clinical groups of interest, additional evidence is needed to support the use of the ABS or other emotional assessment tools (e.g., depression or anxiety scales such as those listed in Chapter 3) as effective means of demonstrating change related to communication or cognitive treatment.

Satisfaction with Life Scale

The *Satisfaction with Life Scale* (SWLS; Diener, Emmons, & Larsen, & Griffen, 1985) involves even fewer items than the Dartmouth Charts or the ABS. The SWLS requires patients to respond to five items using a seven-point rating scale. The items are quite general and, like the ABS, do not relate specifically to medical issues. For example, one item is "In most ways my life is close to my ideal." Originally designed to assess quality of life in populations without medical concerns (e.g., college students, prison inmates), it can be used effectively to assess well-being in medical populations as well (Arrindell, Meeuwesen, & Huyse, 1991). Hirsch and Holland (2000) proposed that the ABS and SWLS might complement each other in the assessment of overall quality of life, given that the ABS focuses on affect whereas the SWLS focuses on satisfaction. Together, the two measures may provide insight into the well-being of patients with communication or cognitive limitations.

Using General Quality of Life Measures for Patients with Neurogenic Language Disorders

Limited information is available regarding which quality of life measures may be most appropriate for individuals with neurogenic language disorders. Hirsch and Holland (1999) attempted to identify the strengths and weaknesses of several tools for addressing the quality of life of individuals with aphasia. These authors examined five measures: Dartmouth COOP Charts, the Affect Balance Scale (ABS), Behavior, Emotion, Attitude, and Communication questionnaire (BEAC), the *Sickness Impact Profile* (SIP), and the OneQ, an informal measure of quality of life that involves only one question. Examiners and patients both rated the scales according to a variety of characteristics including item wording, response format, and amount of assistance needed for patients to complete the measure. Additionally, examiners rated overall appropriateness of each measure, and patients provided ratings regarding item wording, validity, and like/dislike.

Of the measures studied, the SIP had the longest (average 36 minutes) and the OneQ had the shortest administration time (average one minute). The three remaining measures had average administration times of less than 13 minutes. The examiners rated the OneQ and ABS the most favorably with respect to item wording. The SIP and BEAC were rated the least favorably, with items that were long, complex, and/or ambiguous.

With respect to response format, the BEAC was rated least favorably by the examiners. The ratings of the other measures did not differ significantly from each other. Hirsch and Holland (1999) proposed that several features of the favorably rated measures facilitated administration, including vertical arrangement of scales, limited response options, and pictorial representations of responses.

Patients completing the OneQ and ABS required less assistance than when completing the remaining measures. These two measures were also rated most favorably with respect to overall appropriateness, with the OneQ rated above the ABS. The factors affecting ratings of overall appropriateness included ease of administration, reliability of subject responses, appropriateness of content, and face validity.

When all examiner ratings were summed, the OneQ measure was rated most favorably and the SIP least favorably.

The patients judged the various measures to be no different from one another with respect to item wording, validity, or like/dislike. Even when all patient ratings were summed, no differences among measures were identified. These findings suggest that whereas patients may not prefer any measure to another, examiners reported a strong preference for the OneQ. Speech-language pathologists might consider these findings when selecting a tool for assessing the quality of life of patients with neurogenic language disorders.

COMMUNICATION RELATED QUALITY OF LIFE

The following measures were designed specifically to address the needs of individuals experiencing communication disorders. The clear advantage of these tools over general quality of life measures is that each has published psychometric data supporting their use with patients with communication disorders. Unfortunately, because these scales were developed only recently, their application to some patient groups (e.g., TBI, dementia) has not yet been studied.

Stroke-Specific Quality of Life Scale

Stroke-Specific Quality of Life Scale (SS-QOL; Williams, Weinberger, Harris, Clark, & Biller, 1999) and its shorter version, *Stroke and Aphasia Quality of Life Scale–39* (SAQLS-39; Hilari, Byng, Lamping, & Smith, 2003), are two scales designed to address the unique needs of individuals experiencing aphasia following stroke. Although described as quality of life measures, these tools involve patient ratings of function (e.g., trouble with preparing food, trouble with speaking), participation (e.g., going out less, doing hobbies less), and quality of life (e.g., feeling discouraged). The SS-QOL and SAQLS-39 include items related to physical (e.g., trouble with walking), psychosocial (e.g., feeling irritable), communication (e.g., trouble with finding words), and energy (e.g., feeling tired often) domains. Although these domains target issues commonly disrupted following stroke, the items are also relevant for patients with neurogenic language disorders resulting from other etiologies (e.g., TBI, dementia). Thus, it is likely that future research will explore the validity of using these instruments to assess quality of life in individuals with etiologies other than stroke.

Burden of Stroke Scale

A quality of life measure very similar to the SS-QOL and SAQLS-39 is the *Burden of Stroke Scale* (BOSS; Doyle et al., 2004). Like the SS-QOL and SAQLS-39, the BOSS incorporates items addressing function, participation, and quality of life.

The BOSS is unique, however, in the way its items are combined to address each level of description. For example, in the communication domain, the examiner asks, "Because of your stroke, how difficult is it for you to talk with a group of people?" The patient then responds according to a five-point scale (i.e., not at all, a little, moderately, very, cannot do). If the patient indicates difficulty with that particular area of function, follow-up probes addressing participation and quality of life are administered (e.g., "You indicated that you have some difficulties communicating. How often do difficulties communicating cause you to feel anxious, unhappy, or frustrated?" and "How much do difficulties communicating prevent you from doing the things in life that are important to you?").

The BOSS includes items in the domains of mobility (e.g., balance), self-care (e.g., dressing), communication (e.g., writing a letter), cognition (e.g., concentrating), swallowing (e.g., swallowing liquids), social relations (e.g., maintaining family roles), energy and sleep (e.g., staying awake through the day), and negative (e.g., loneliness) and positive mood (e.g., confidence). Similar to the SS-QOL and SAQLS-39, these domains are relevant to patients experiencing cognitive or communication disorders resulting from etiologies other than stroke, but additional research is needed to evaluate their application to these other patient groups.

ASHA Quality of Communication Life Scale

Given the value of determining the impact of communication disorders on relationships and participation in daily life activities, the American Speech-Language-Hearing Association published the *Quality of Communication Life Scale* (QCLS; Paul-Brown et al., 2004). The QCLS consists of 18 statements for which patients are asked to state their agreement. Unlike other quality of life scales, patients are instructed that the statements are specifically concerned with communication. For example, the clinician instructs, "Think about how you feel now. For each statement, first ask yourself: 'Even though I have difficulty communicating. . .', then read the statement." (p. 35). Several items address participation issues (e.g., 'I stay in touch with family and friends," "People include me in conversations"), whereas others address well-being and quality of life (e.g., "I am confident that I can communicate," "I like myself"). Patients indicate their agreement with each statement by placing a mark on a five-point printed vertical scale (i.e., the top of the scale indicates the statement describes the patient well). The clinician then calculates the average rating, excluding the final item, "In general, my quality of life is good," to provide an overall estimate of patients' quality of communication life.

The QCLS can be administered in less than twenty minutes, with patients completing the scale either independently or with clinician assistance. Although the standardization sample was relatively small (i.e., $n = 57$), patients with aphasia, cognitive-communicative disorders, or dysarthria were included, suggesting that the QCLS may be appropriate for a variety of patients.

INFORMAL MEASURES OF QUALITY OF LIFE

Informal measures of quality of life will most likely take the form of an interview focusing on the patient's emotional response to impairments, activity limitations, and participation restrictions. The informal measure shown in Figure 7-3 asks patients to rate the impact of their disorder on various aspects of their life. Alternatively, clinicians might assess quality of life using a single, carefully worded question such as, "Overall, how would you rate your current lifestyle?" (Hinckley, 1998). Regardless of the precise format, informal measures of quality of life should aid the clinician in determining the unique impact of communication and cognitive limitations for each individual patient.

RELATIONSHIPS AMONG MEASURES OF IMPAIRMENT, FUNCTION, PARTICIPATION, AND QUALITY OF LIFE

The preceding discussion was organized to highlight the unique features of assessment tools addressing functional communication, participation, and quality of life. It is notable, however, that many assessment tools, even those purporting to target only one of these ICF levels of description, in fact address two or more of the constructs as they have been defined here. This phenomenon likely reflects partially the subjectivity with which individual authors categorize various behaviors, but also leads to the question of whether these various tools actually measure different underlying constructs (Irwin, Wertz, & Avent, 2002). Surprisingly few studies have explored the relationships among measures of impairment, activity, and participation/quality of life. Additionally, such studies addressing neurogenic language impairments in adults have focused on aphasia more so than cognitive communicative disorders associated with right hemisphere brain damage, TBI, or dementing diseases.

How well are you able to perform your job duties?

Do you do the things you used to do for enjoyment with friends and family?

Are you able to understand what people say, and can others understand you?

Do you feel tired or ill?

Do you feel strong emotions—sadness, anger, frustration—because of your impairments?

Adapted from Verdolini (1994). Voice disorders. In J. B. Tomblin, H. L. Morris, & D. C. Spriestersbach (Eds.), *Diagnosis in speech-language pathology* (pp. 247–297). San Diego: Singular Thomson Learning.

Figure 7-3. **Example of questions to include in an informal assessment of quality of life.**

The nature of the relationships among various levels of measurement has varied across studies, as has the interpretation of the findings. Ross and Wertz (2002) investigated relationships among two language impairment tests (*Western Aphasia Battery*, *Porch Index of Communicative Ability*—see Chapter 5), two tests of functional communication (CADL-2, ASHA FACS), and two measures of quality of life, neither of which were reviewed in this chapter but were similar in nature to those summarized in preceding sections. The battery of tests was administered to a group of adults with chronic aphasia and a control group of age-matched healthy aging adults. For the aphasic group, no significant relationships were observed between language impairment and quality of life, or between functional communication and quality of life. The authors interpreted these findings to suggest that because quality of life was not related to language impairment or functional communication, language therapy targeting quality of life could not be justified. Alternately, the findings might suggest that each level of description is unique, so it is therefore worthwhile to address each construct during assessment and potentially during treatment.

Two additional studies (Aftonomos, Steele, Appelbaum, & Harris, 2001; Irwin et al., 2002) examining relationships among similar instruments reported significant correlations between scores on impairment-level (e.g., *Western Aphasia Battery*) and activity-level tools (e.g., CETI). Aftonomos et al. (2001) further reported, however, that the changes in scores over time were not the same across measurements, supporting the clinical value of including measures of impairment and function when reporting patient response to treatment.

Nonetheless, as Irwin et al. (2002) recommended, additional research utilizing appropriate statistical methods is needed to describe more clearly the relationships among the measures targeting the various ICF constructs. Our understanding of these issues will be further strengthened as measures of impairment and function in patients with cognitive communicative disorders (e.g., Fromm & Holland, 1989) are included in such studies. Finally, given that performance on measures of language impairment, functional communication, and quality of life has been shown to be influenced by the patient's age, gender, and/or educational level (Ross & Wertz, 2001), it is likely that additional research will identify further factors that influence the relationship among the constructs of impairment, activity, participation, and quality of life.

AUTHENTIC ASSESSMENT AND ETHNOGRAPHY

The final section of this chapter addresses a method of assessing communication function, life participation, and quality of life without the use of formal measures such as those outlined previously. Simmons-Mackie and Damico (1996) developed the Communicative Profiling System (CPS), a form of **authentic assessment** based on ethnographic and conversational analysis research methods. CPS incorporates five basic assessment principles: (1) assessment addresses communication in real-life situations, (2) assessment considers the contexts in which communication takes place, (3) systematic data collection procedures are employed, (4) data are subjected to systematic qualitative analyses, and (5) conclusions are developed specifically for planning intervention.

Each of the four phases of CPS involves data collection and analysis. In Phase One, the clinician develops a broad perspective of the patient's communication behaviors by interviewing individuals who communicate with the patient. From these interviews, the clinician identifies behaviors, contexts, and interactants that will serve as the framework for viewing the communicative abilities of the patient. The second phase involves direct observation of communicative interactions. Simmons-Mackie and Damico suggested that the clinician engage in participant-observation rather than attempting to contrive situations that mimic real-life contexts. Also included in Phase Two is collection of anecdotal reports of specific communicative interactions (e.g., the patient's spouse may describe the patient's attempt to order at a restaurant). The clinician considers the information gained in Phases One and Two to identify communicative patterns that warrant closer assessment.

Phase Three involves collecting and analyzing videotaped samples of communication in authentic contexts selected based on the communicative behaviors, contexts, and interactants deemed most relevant during earlier CPS phases. Further examination of the information obtained in Phases One through Three allows the clinician to explore more fully the interactions between communication behavior and context (Phase Four) as a means of identifying the purposes specific communicative behaviors might serve, as well as noting the communication strategies the patient may select in different contexts. When the authentic assessment process is complete, the clinician will likely have obtained information regarding the ICF constructs of activity and participation, as well as environmental factors. The assessment will inform treatment planning, as well as serve as a baseline against which the effectiveness of treatment can be judged.

The authentic assessment process described by CPS may be particularly useful when standardized tools are deemed inappropriate, inadequate, or both for addressing a specific patient's concerns. For example, a young adult experiencing a stroke, a patient who is deaf or multilingual, or a patient who has family members who also exhibit communication impairments will each likely demonstrate unique needs that may not be addressed by tools designed for more typical patient groups. CPS provides a system for identifying and gaining an understanding of unique contexts and interactants that impact the patient's communication function, life participation, and quality of life. Nonetheless, given the time required to utilize CPS, clinicians should balance the value of gaining potentially unique clinical insights against the costs in terms of the clinician's, patient's, and family members' time.

SUMMARY

This chapter concludes the discussion of assessment of neurogenic language disorders. The assessment strategies described will help clinicians identify the impairments contributing to the communication limitations experienced by patients, as well as the impact of these limitations on their function, life participation, and overall quality of life. Only when information about all of these factors is obtained can a complete diagnosis be determined, a reliable prognosis established, and an effective treatment program planned. Furthermore, the assessment process does not end here. As previously stated in Chapter 4, continued assessment throughout the treatment process is critical both to ensuring that treatment is effective and to monitoring the patient for signs of disease progression or new disease onset. The methods described in Chapters 4 through 7 are appropriate for initial evaluation, as well as for ongoing assessment and evaluation of treatment efficacy. The remaining chapters will focus on developing and evaluating treatment strategies that address the impairments, activity limitations, and participation restrictions identified in the assessment process.

Chapter 8

Evidence–Based Practice

By William H. Irwin

Appalachian State University

LEARNING OBJECTIVES

After reading this chapter you should be able to:

- Discuss the purpose and philosophy of evidence-based practice (EBP).

- Define outcomes and discuss the relationship between outcomes and EBP.

- Identify sources of evidence for asking EBP questions.

- Define and discuss the relationships among treatment efficacy, effectiveness, and efficiency.

- Describe the phases of outcomes research.

- Summarize levels of evidence scales and apply them to the critical appraisal of evidence.

- Discuss strategies for evaluating the benefit of treatment for individual patients.

KEY TERMS

clinical trial
critical appraisal
dose
effectiveness

efficacy
efficiency
evidence-based
practice

outcome
outcomes measurement

INTRODUCTION

Before beginning the discussion of intervention for neurogenic language disorders (Chapters 9 through 11), it is important to consider the processes by which clinicians determine which interventions to implement. Thus, this chapter describes evidence-based practice and its application to the management of neurogenic language disorders.

Evidence-based practice (EBP), "the conscientious, explicit, and judicious use of current best evidence in making decisions about the care of individual patients" (Sackett, Rosenberg, Gray, Haynes, & Richardson, 1996, p. 71), is a framework for integrating clinical expertise, patient values, and the best available evidence into the clinical decision-making process that informs patient care. That is, EBP requires that clinicians apply critical appraisal to determine the relevance, validity, and accuracy of available evidence to determine what constitutes *the current best evidence and, consequently, to make decisions about which treatments will be most appropriate for which patients.* The conscientious and judicious use of clinical evidence requires persistent review of current clinical research and maintenance of clinical skills by clinicians seeking to improve patient-centered outcomes (Reilly, 2004b). Evidence-based clinical practice in speech-language pathology (SLP) is not an entirely new way of doing business, but rather an updated one that demands more accountability for clinical decision making.

OVERVIEW OF EBP

Evidence-based practice has become a widely used term, presumably reflecting the interest in and need for the application of its methodology, not only in SLP but in other allied health disciplines, as well as medicine, education, mental health, social services, early intervention, and other fields (Dunst, Trivette, & Cutspec, 2002). EBP has gained momentum as an integral component of clinical service in health care, and its practice and teaching have spread across the globe, both in clinical practice and medical and allied health education (Mykhalovskiy & Weir, 2004; Reilly, 2004b). EBP represents the formalization of a perspective that has traditionally been considered the benchmark of exemplary clinical practice—applying the science-base to the art of clinical care. Indeed, Cash (2004) suggested that EBP is the ideal to which all clinicians should aspire.

A basic tenet of EBP highlights acknowledging the limitations of relying on authority and dogma to make clinical decisions. Rather than solely rely on expert opinion EBP gives far more weight to rigorous scientific studies in the clinical decision-making process (Dollaghan, 2004). The essence of EBP is making explicit the process that guides clinical practice through careful evaluation of current evidence, filtered through the prisms of sound clinical judgment and patient values.

Professional reliance on a framework that integrates clinical expertise with scientific evidence provides a standard for evaluating interventions for neurogenic language disorders. Development of and reliance on an adequate evidence base has the potential to: (1) reduce variations in clinical practices that may negatively affect patient outcomes; (2) increase the cost effectiveness of patient care services, and (3) provide compelling rationale for allocating limited health care resources that may increase the perceived value of and consistent reimbursement for SLP services by third-party payers.

Clinicians benefit from EBP because "reliance on evidence-based practices allows clinicians to be accountable, ethical, and responsible, not only to their clients, but to their profession and themselves . . . when reporting to clients, their families, and third party payers" (Apel & Self, 2003, p. 8). Clinical researchers benefit as systematic literature reviews shed light on specific areas in which practices are based solely on expert opinion and/or convention, with EBP providing a standard approach for identifying and documenting evidence deficiencies as well as an impetus for generating more and better evidence. Finally, graduate education, in its move toward competency-based education, benefits by having a framework for teaching the skills needed to develop competency in the knowledge base. When clinical practices are supported by quality evidence and sound theory, there is added justification for acquiring the knowledge and skills necessary to adopt those practices. It is neither sufficient nor possible to know or teach everything in a given area of communication sciences and disorders; new information is added to the database continually. It is possible and desirable, however, to teach and learn the tools necessary to answer the clinical questions that arise in current as well as future everyday practice. EBP provides a sound methodological toolbox for doing so.

HISTORY AND DEVELOPMENT OF EBP

EBP was originally termed evidence-based medicine, or EBM (Sackett, Richardson, Rosenberg, & Haynes, 1997). The term EBM was coined in the early 1990s by clinical epidemiologists at McMaster University in Hamilton, Ontario, Canada. This group formalized an approach to the clinical practice of medicine based on careful review and application of the current best evidence in the clinical research literature. In its short but influential history, EBM has expanded dramatically into nursing, allied health professions, health care policy, and outside of health care into education and beyond. As Mykhalovskiy and Weir (2004) pointed out, the evidence-based movement has been met with remarkable enthusiasm.

Although SLP as a discipline has promoted the use and development of the science base to improve clinical care, until recently there was no formal model for applying the existing evidence base and integrating that evidence with clinical practice. Plante (2004) observed that "an increasing emphasis on evidence, rather than intuition, for guiding clinical practice signals disciplinary maturation" (p. 389). Regardless of the level of disciplinary development signaled by a move toward EBP, there are major gaps in the evidence base for common clinical SLP practices. If EBP is to provide the pathway for filling these knowledge gaps, the first step is to provide the education necessary to develop the skills needed to apply this new model of clinical decision making.

DESCRIPTION OF EBP

The most compelling argument for employing EBP is that it increases the likelihood of better outcomes for patients. Moreover, in a recent technical report, the Research and Scientific Affairs Committee of the American Speech-Language Hearing Association (ASHA, 2004) acknowledged EBP as a key component of its research mission, with an anticipated importance in providing direction for clinical research needs. The report specified that EBP may not only help guide the clinical research agenda but also enhance the quality of the evidence base in communication disorders research.

Philosophy of EBP

The EBP model is about solving clinical problems using a set of systematic guidelines. The fundamental goal is to guide clinical decisions about patient care by integrating patients' clinical information with the best evidence available from clinical research and experience. EBP de-emphasizes intuition, unsystematic clinical experience, and pathophysiologic rationale as adequate grounds for clinical decision making (Frattali & Worral, 2001). Likewise, ASHA (2004) has encouraged adoption of the EBP framework to increase awareness of the limitations of expert opinion as the sole basis for clinical decision making.

Guyatt and colleagues (2000) proposed two primary principles to guide clinicians practicing EBP. The first principle, *evidence is never enough*, implies that there are other important factors to consider when making clinical decisions. This simple but powerful statement suggests that clinical decisions about patient care must take into account both the best available external evidence and clinical expertise; this includes the skills necessary for "more thoughtful identification and compassionate use of individual patients' predicaments, rights, and preferences in making clinical decisions about their care" (Sackett, Richardson, Rosenberg, & Haynes, 1997, p. 2). In addition to patient considerations, clinical and societal values are brought to bear in the decision-making process. Thus, evidence alone does not dictate the decision to be made, but it instead informs the decision-making process.

The second principle concerns the nature of the evidence. The EBP model posits a hierarchy of the quality or strength of evidence that guides decision making. Classification of clinical research evidence is discussed in terms of levels or classes that are ordered from strong to weak on the basis of scientific and methodological rigor (Golper et al., 2001; Reilly, 2004b). Specific criteria for evaluating evidence differ somewhat according to the type of clinical decision to be made (e.g., screening, prevention, diagnosis, therapy, prognosis, or health care economics; ASHA, 2004). Consequently, there are numerous published evidence hierarchies or classifications for each type of clinical question; further discussion and examples will be presented below.

Two additional EBP principles, critical appraisal and systematic observation, shift the focus of the clinical process from judgment- to data-driven care (Frattali, 2001). The principle of critical appraisal applies to the process of determining the validity, impact, and applicability of the external evidence (Sackett, Strauss, Richardson, Rosenberg, & Haynes, 2000). Systematic observation requires that clinicians evaluate their own clinical processes using empirical methods and, in so doing, build an experiential database that provides objective data to guide clinical decision making.

THE PROCESS OF EVIDENCE-BASED PRACTICE

EBP is "a process of life-long self-directed learning in which caring for our own patients creates the need for clinically important information" (Sackett et al., 2000,

1. Convert the need for information into an answerable question
2. Identify the best evidence with which to answer that question
3. Critically appraise the evidence
4. Apply the results of this appraisal in clinical practice
5. Evaluate your performance

Figure 8-1. The five critical steps of EBP.

p. 2). The process consists of five critical steps: question formulation, searching for evidence, critical appraisal of the evidence, using the results of the critical appraisal in clinical practice, and performance evaluation (see Figure 8-1). The following description of each step is adapted from Sackett et al. (2000).

STEP 1. CONVERTING THE NEED FOR INFORMATION (ABOUT DIAGNOSIS, PROGNOSIS, TREATMENT, ETC.) INTO AN ANSWERABLE QUESTION.

This step requires focus on a specific aspect of practice. Reilly (2004a) suggested that "one of the most useful tools for developing clinical questions is the PECOT approach to question-framing (P = patient/population group; E = exposure or intervention if about therapy; C = control or comparison; O = outcome(s); and T = time-frame)" (p. 114). For example, we may ask the question "Has stimulation treatment been shown to improve the spoken language production of patients with chronic aphasia?" In this case, P = patients with aphasia, E = stimulation treatment, C = patients with aphasia who do not receive stimulation treatment, O = improved spoken productions, and T = in the chronic phase of recovery. Narrowing the question in this way to a specific focus on these aspects of a clinical question greatly facilitates performing Step 2.

STEP 2. IDENTIFYING, WITH MAXIMUM EFFICIENCY, THE BEST EVIDENCE WITH WHICH TO ANSWER THAT QUESTION.

Finding evidence efficiently requires knowledge and skills in using the available information databases. The vast increase in the SLP literature, as well as clinical research in related health care disciplines (e.g., neuropsychology, nursing, occupational therapy), requires that clinicians use effective search strategies to produce a good return on their time investment. The astute evidence-based practitioner knows where and how to look for the evidence if it is to be found. For example, searchable electronic databases such as those in Table 8-1 include research citations relevant to neurogenic language and other communication disorders. Journal

Table 8-1. Electronic Indexes in which Neurogenic Language Disorders Research Citations may be Found

INDEX	DESCRIPTION	ACCESS URL
CARL	Database of the Colorado Association of Research Libraries	www.carl.org
CINAHL	Database serving nursing and allied health disciplines	http://www.cinahl.com/
Cochrane	Database with emphasis on evidence-based reviews	http://www.cochrane.org/index
Dissertation Abstracts	Indexed doctoral dissertations across disciplines	http://library.dialog.com/bluesheets/html/bl0035.html
EM-BASE	Database serving biomedical and pharmacological disciplines	http://www.embase.com/
MEDLINE (PubMed) Also incorporates citations from BIOETHICSLINE	Comprehensive biomedical database provided by the National Library of Medicine	http://www.ncbi.nlm.nih.gov/entrez/query.fcgi
PsycInfo	Abstract database of psychological literature	http://www.psycinfo.com/
Science Citation Index	Index of science and technical journals	http://www.isinet.com/products/citation/sci/

Note. Many of these indexes may be accessed through university or health center libraries at no cost.

articles, book chapters, texts, instrument manuals, and bibliographies provide another, albeit less efficient, means of locating evidence. Generally, each source's utility will be dependent on the nature of the question posed.

Knowing where to look is only a start; next, clinicians must develop efficient search strategies to ensure that the search is broad enough to include all relevant sources but exclude those that do not directly address the question posed. Librarians can help educate clinicians about effective and efficient search strategies. Other sources of evidence may be found by asking specialists or experts knowledgeable in the area of interest who are likely to stay current with the literature. With the advent of online discussion forums, and e-mail contact information listed in journal articles, the experts are often accessible for questions and/or requests for relevant references and, in most cases, are enthusiastic about helping. Don't underestimate the value of this approach; in some cases, the expert's opinion may constitute the current best evidence!

STEP 3. CRITICALLY APPRAISE THE EVIDENCE FOR ITS VALIDITY, IMPORTANCE AND PRECISION, AND USEFULNESS.

Critical appraisal is the process of deciding whether a specific piece of evidence can help in answering the clinical question. EBP appraisal methods differ depending on the type of clinical practice question posed. For example, there are separate critical appraisal worksheets addressing diagnosis versus treatment versus prognosis. There also are critical appraisal guidelines for determining whether systematic reviews of the literature are valid, important, and useful for your clinical question.

EBP Applied to Diagnostic Questions

At present, EBP principles have been adopted most widely with respect to treatment, even though they apply to diagnostic issues as well. Although a detailed discussion of EBP concepts unique to assessment is beyond the scope of this chapter, the following illustration highlights how the process may be applied to diagnosing neurogenic language disorders.

Imagine we receive a referral for a patient who had a single left hemisphere stroke two weeks ago. Our own clinical experience may lead us to predict that a patient with this lesion site will exhibit aphasia, and we can further support this prediction with EBP. For example, a recent prospective study determined that in a group of 106 consecutively admitted stroke patients, 34% were diagnosed as having aphasia in the acute phase (Kauhanen et al., 2000). Thus, with only this knowledge and no additional data from the patient, 34% is a good estimate of the probability that this patient has aphasia. After conducting a brief initial interview, we may further suspect that the patient has mild aphasia. If we are considering using a formal test to determine whether the patient indeed has aphasia, we may want to know how well a specific formal test assists in diagnosing mild aphasia. A literature search reveals a study that applied EBP in determining the importance of selected formal tests for diagnosing mild aphasia (Ross & Wertz, 2004). Using the process and this empirical data, we determine that the ASHA FACS–Communication Dimensions score provides a 96% probability of correctly diagnosing mild aphasia, providing ample evidence to support using this tool.

Although additional issues must be considered when using EBP to answer diagnostic questions (e.g., whether the evidence employed independent, blind administration of a gold standard or included a large sample of patients), it is clear that the basic principles of identifying and critically evaluating available evidence will help inform assessment as well as treatment decisions.

Within the EBP framework, treatment questions center on the themes of validity, importance, and usefulness. Framing the empirical treatment literature in the broader context of outcomes research provides some guidance for making judgments about whether a specific treatment or treatment approach is valid, important, and useful. The following discussion provides an overview of outcomes research and establishes a context for considering the relevant questions to ask when judging treatment evidence.

Outcomes Research

In the preface to her book on measuring outcomes in speech-language pathology, Frattali (1998) quoted advice from this author's mentor, Terry Wertz, regarding a useful way of thinking about outcomes.

> The process requires answers to three fundamental questions:
>
> What do you mean? (thus, requiring operational definitions)
> How do you know? (requiring evidence to support the claim)
> What difference does it make? (placing the claim in a pragmatic context) (p. ix).

The EBP framework may help answer these fundamental questions. Outcomes research is the study of the outcomes of health care services and procedures used to prevent, diagnose, treat, and manage illness and disability (Agency for Healthcare Policy and Research, 1990). It is a multidimensional concept defined in terms of the agent. The agents can be clinicians, employers, educators, payers, or clients and their families. Frattali (1998) used the term **outcomes measurement** to include both outcomes and efficacy research. The conceptual framework for outcomes research and efficacy research will be elaborated below. Although outcomes research is not directly related to EBP, the concept is inherent in EBP practices (Cash, 2004).

Outcomes are often difficult to quantify and differ depending on the perspective taken. For example, outcomes may be clinical, functional, administrative, economic, societal, or client-centered (Frattali, 1998). Additionally, they may index changes that are desired or deleterious to a person's health-related quality of life. Wertz and Irwin (2001) defined **outcome** as the following:

> Outcome is a natural result; a consequence; or, generally, a comparison of an observation at a later point in time with an observation made earlier (Wertz, 1998). Thus, for aphasic people, comparison of performance observed after a period of spontaneous recovery and/or treatment with earlier performance, at onset or pretreatment, permits speculation about the influence of time and/or treatment on performance outcome. Unless specific conditions are met, outcome does not automatically index the efficacy, effectiveness, or efficiency of what did or did not occur between the earlier observation and the later one (p. 235).

For speech-language pathologists interested in treating and managing patients with neurogenic language disorders, clinical outcomes are paramount. Just as there are numerous outcome perspectives, within the domain of clinical outcomes there are many different and varied goals and objectives that drive decisions about outcomes measurement. For example, using the ICF framework (World Health Organization, 2001), clinical outcomes regarding treatment effects might rely upon measuring changes at the body structure or function, activity, and/or participation level. Another example is ASHA's National Outcomes Measurement System (NOMS), used to collect and analyze outcomes data in a variety of communication-disordered populations. The NOMS project provides data regarding changes in patient performance (using seven-point Functional Communication Measures; see Chapter 7) that occur between admission and discharge within specific disorders and across program settings (e.g., acute care, skilled nursing facility). NOMS data document changes between two points in time, but do not permit inferences about treatment efficacy or effectiveness. Therefore, relationships between outcomes and other variables are not obtainable with these data. Despite this limitation, the NOMS project provides a form of evidence that reflects what occurs in actual clinical practice and may suggest areas in which more research is needed (Mullen, 2003).

Robey (2004) suggested that although clinical outcomes play a central role in clinical practice and research, there is a difference in how outcomes data are gathered. Specifically, there are two distinct types of clinical outcomes research regarding treatment: (1) treatment efficacy research and (2) treatment effectiveness research. **Efficacy,** according to the Office of Technology Assessment (OTA; 1978), is: "[t]he probability of benefit to individuals in a defined population from a medical technology applied for a given medical problem under ideal conditions of use" (p. 16). Robey and Schultz (1998) stressed the constraints of this definition: Inference about efficacy is applicable to a population, not an individual, the treatment and the specific clinical population are clearly specified, and the conditions in which the treatment is administered are optimized. Thus, evidence of treatment efficacy indicates the *potential* maximum benefit of a particular treatment administered under ideal conditions and may not be equivalent to the actual benefits of treatment in clinical practice. For example, in many treatment studies, patients are provided treatment with intensity and frequency that surpass what is available in real-world contexts. Accordingly, it may be unreasonable to expect the same quantity and quality of improvement as was achieved in these treatment investigations in daily clinical settings.

In contrast, OTA (1978) specified that "evidence of treatment **effectiveness** establishes the value of a particular treatment protocol for effecting beneficial change under the conditions of routine clinical practice" (p. 6). According to the accepted standards of clinical outcomes testing used throughout the broader research community, research to establish a treatment's effectiveness should only be conducted after that treatment's efficacy has been established (Robey, 2004; Robey & Schultz, 1998; Wertz & Irwin, 2001).

Efficiency implies high productivity: a maximum effect for the effort expended. For example, a treatment determined to be efficacious and effective might be compared with another treatment to determine which results in the better or more *efficient* outcome. Another approach to evaluating efficiency might involve manipulating an efficacious and effective treatment to determine whether reductions in treatment intensity, duration, or both can still evoke similar positive outcomes. As Wertz and Irwin (2001) observed, it is necessary to establish a treatment's efficacy and effectiveness prior to evaluating its efficiency.

There is a widely accepted comprehensive model for organizing the programmatic research necessary for conducting clinical outcomes research. The model has five distinct phases that follow a logical progression from the small sample size studies of discovery in the first two phases to the efficacy, effectiveness, and cost-effectiveness studies of later phases. Robey and Schultz (1998) described an adapted five-phase model for aphasiologists that is applicable for clinical outcomes research not only in other neurogenic language disorders but also throughout speech-language pathology and audiology (Robey, 2004). Although each phase of the model is concerned with outcomes, efficacy and effectiveness research are tested in only specific phases (Wertz & Irwin, 2001). The following summary of each phase is adapted from Robey and Schultz (1998) and from other reviews and descriptions of the model (Robey, 2004; Wertz & Irwin, 2001).

Phase I. The fundamental purposes of Phase I are to select a treatment effect, identify if that effect is present, and, if so, estimate the magnitude of that effect. More generally, Phase I is considered a time of discovery. To determine if the treatment is active, researchers estimate the appropriate **dose** (i.e., treatment intensity and duration), and make a first approximation of the population definitions and treatment protocol. Additionally, hypotheses that will be tested at later stages are generated and developed. Because this is a "discovery" phase, researchers typically adopt liberal statistical significance levels to allow treatment effects to emerge if they are present. Phase I research includes case studies, single-subject studies, small group experiments, and retrospective studies, in which investigations are brief, employ small sample sizes, and do not require control groups.

Phase II. If the results of Phase I studies are promising, Phase II research is initiated to begin preparations for conducting a clinical trial. In this phase, optimization of the treatment protocol, the participants, the outcome measures, the dosage, and other important variables is determined. More specifically, Phase II studies are initiated to: (1) refine the primary hypothesis; (2) develop an explanation for why the treatment works; (3) refine the selection criteria (e.g., time post onset, type and/or severity of neurogenic language disorder) for the target population; (4) standardize the treatment protocol; (5) identify and select outcome measures that are proven to be valid and reliable; and (6) determine the optimal treatment dosage in terms of treatment intensity and duration. Like those in Phase I, Phase II studies are brief, employ small sample sizes, and do not require external control patients (e.g., patients who receive no or delayed treatment). As the research program matures, case studies and single-subject studies are followed by small-group studies.

Phase III. Phase III research consists of **clinical trials** designed to test the efficacy of treatments developed and optimized via Phase I and II investigations. Clinical trials are characterized by large sample sizes, typically involve multiple sites, and utilize conservative statistical significance criteria. Robey (2004) reported that the gold standard research design in the behavioral sciences is a parallel-groups design. This design involves a randomized controlled trial (RCT) in which selected participants are randomly assigned to either a treatment or no-treatment/control group. Random assignment provides control for treatment selection and other sources of systematic bias that may influence outcomes, and the treatment versus no-treatment comparison allows demonstrating that observed benefits can be attributed to treatment.

Phase IV. The purpose of Phase IV research is to examine the treatment's outcome in ordinary clinical practice (i.e., effectiveness) after having established the efficacy of the treatment. As in Phase III studies, large samples are required, but no-treatment control groups are not. Parallel group studies and multiple replications of single-subject studies are appropriate for effectiveness research. Phase IV research expands the applicability of the treatment protocol within the target population and with variations in the criteria. For example, researchers might evaluate treatment outcomes when the population definition (e.g., include patients, regardless of education background), service delivery model (e.g., include homework activities in addition to direct intervention), and/or extent of clinician training are varied.

Phase V. Effectiveness research continues in this phase and may expand to include explorations of efficiency. In Phase V research, the goals may include determining who benefits from the treatment (e.g., patients *and* caregivers), and evaluating the costs of providing the treatment at the individual and societal levels. Large group studies or multiple replications of single-subject studies are appropriate to address Phase V purposes. No-treatment/control groups are not required.

Applying this adapted five-phase model to adult neurogenic language disorders is controversial, especially considering RCT as the gold standard for establishing efficacy. This model, however, offers numerous advantages to recommend its adoption. First, the broader outcomes research and scientific community employs this model (Robey, 2004; Robey & Schulz, 1998; Wertz & Irwin, 2001). Second, its organization imposes a logical and standard sequence of progression and standardization of terms. Considering the human and fiscal expense of conducting programmatic research, it is imperative to impose a framework on the process that allows justifying the expense involved. Third, the status of the treatment protocol is apparent to consumers of the research provided the model is followed. Last, and directly applicable to the EBP framework, working within the five phase model, the relationships between different types and grades of evidence are made transparent.

Levels of Evidence

Another means of organizing and evaluating outcomes is through levels of evidence rating scales, also called quality of evidence rating scales. Numerous published scales offer structured hierarchies, from strongest to weakest, for rating the strength or quality of scientific evidence. To ensure that reviews of clinical research and related literature are scientifically and clinically robust, the Agency for Healthcare Research and Quality (AHRQ, 2002) has published an evidence-based technology assessment of systems to rate the strength of scientific evidence. The following outlines one of the earliest rating systems proposed by the Canadian Task Force on the Periodic Health Examination (1987):

I. Evidence obtained from at least one properly randomized controlled trial.

II-1. Evidence obtained from well-designed controlled trials without randomization.

II-2. Evidence obtained from well-designed cohort or case-control analytic studies, preferably from more than one center or research group.

II-3. Evidence obtained from multiple time series with or without the intervention. Dramatic results in uncontrolled experiments could also be regarded as this type of evidence.

III. Opinions of respected authorities, based on clinical experience, descriptive studies, or reports of expert committees.

Another classification system, provided by the Quality Standards Committee of the American Academy of Neurology (AAN, 1994), includes three levels of evidence. In an article rating the evidence for a speech-language pathology treatment, the evidence was classified according to the following scale:

Class I: Evidence from one or more well-designed, randomized controlled clinical trials.

Class II: Evidence from one or more randomized clinical studies such as case-control, cohort studies, etc.

Class III: Evidence from expert opinion, case series, case reports, and studies with historical controls.

Regardless of the rating system employed, the common feature is that the highest evidence rating includes at least one RCT, whereas the lowest level applies to evidence accrued from expert opinion (or similar authority) or studies without adequate external control. These scales allow a standard rating on the basis of study design. Inferring strength of evidence from study design alone, however, may be problematic in that other factors, which influence evidence quality, may not be adequately considered. For example, sample size, recruitment bias, losses to follow-up, atypical patient groups, and other threats to internal and external validity do not affect ratings on either of the above scales. Likewise, results from a single RCT with a small sample size do not necessarily provide more convincing evidence than consistent results with high precision from numerous high-quality trials with non-randomized designs (Guyatt, Sinclair, Cook, & Glasziou, 1999). Therefore, critical evidence appraisal must extend beyond study design to include additional issues concerning validity, importance, and usefulness.

Accordingly, ASHA (2004) identified five common themes that contribute to evidence quality: a) independent confirmation and converging evidence from multiple studies, b) experimental control, c) avoidance of subjectivity and bias, d) analysis of effect sizes and confidence intervals, and e) the relevance (to typical patients) and feasibility (applicability) of the results. That is, evaluating evidence from a treatment study does not end with assigning a level of evidence but rather must additionally include examining whether the study avoided both identified and unanticipated bias, and minimized confounds that could threaten the validity of its results (Dollaghan, 2004). When critically appraising a piece of evidence, issues of internal and external validity must be considered. Internal validity regards whether the treatment results are truly attributable to the experimental treatment, whereas external validity concerns whether the same results apply outside of the particular experimental circumstances in which the study was conducted.

Side Bar

ASHA and EBP

Clinicians may wonder how the policy statements issued by ASHA relate to EBP. In fact, many principles of EBP are typically incorporated into the development of Practice Guidelines, which recommend procedures for specific areas of practice based on research findings and expert opinion. Clinicians should nonetheless critically appraise the evidence cited in the Guidelines, particularly in light of new evidence that may become available after Guidelines are published.

Based on their review of the literature, Tompkins and Lustig (2001) proposed a checklist of questions that address some of the most important issues to consider when evaluating evidence (Figure 8-2). Their checklist addresses the issues of validity and importance, and shifts clinicians' focus from the Introduction and Discussion sections of studies to a focus on their Methods and Results sections, a crucial shift for appropriate critical appraisal and clinical integration (Frattali, 2001). Answering these questions about a particular study should facilitate an adequate appraisal of its validity and importance.

This is an obviously time-consuming process, and thus, this time commitment can present a barrier to its adoption. Fortunately, the EBP framework includes

1. Are convincing rationales and hypotheses provided?
2. Are the research questions answerable?
3. Do the participants represent the group(s) they are meant to represent?
4. Are participants sufficiently described for assessing the believability, replicability, and generability of the results?
5. Are procedures, conditions, and variables adequately described?
6. Are procedures, conditions, and variables reliable and valid?
7. Is the behavior sample adequate?
8. Are precautions taken to reduce potential, even unknowing bias, on the part of the participant and the examiner? (appropriate blinding)
9. Are the data interpreted appropriately?
10. Are maintenance and generalization programmed into and probed in the study?
11. Are individual participant characteristics related to the reported outcomes?
12. Is there some attempt to evaluate the clinical meaningfulness or importance of changes attributed to the experimental manipulation?

Figure 8-2. Checklist of questions for determining the validity and importance of evidence from treatment studies (Tompkins & Lustig, 2001).

considering pre-processed evidence in which evidence validity and importance have already been critically appraised. Researchers and clinicians in neurogenic communication and cognitive disorders are leading the way in their efforts to pre-process the evidence (see Figure 8-3). Critical appraisal must also be applied to pre-processed evidence, but much of the time-consuming work of searching and obtaining the evidence and evaluating its validity and importance has been performed according to specific criteria to ensure its quality.

The usefulness of a valid and important piece of evidence must be determined for each patient individually. To do so, clinicians should answer the following questions, adapted from Sackett et al. (1997).

1. Do the results apply to your patient?
   - Is your patient so different from those in the study that its results can't help you?
   - How great would the potential benefit of therapy be for your individual patient?

2. Are your patient's values and preferences satisfied by the treatment regimen and its likely outcomes?
   - Do your patient and you have a clear assessment of their values and preferences?
   - Are the patient's values and preferences met by this treatment and its likely outcomes?

The Academy of Neurologic Communication Disorders & Sciences: Evidence-Based Practice Guidelines for the Management of Communication Disorders in Neurologically Impaired Individuals

This resource is home to the EBP project, initiated to improve the quality of services to individuals with neurologic communication and cognitive disorders by assisting clinicians in decision making about the management of specific populations through guidelines based on research evidence. (http://www.ancds.org/practice.html)

Selected reports also published in journals include:

Kennedy, M. R., Avery, J., Coelho, C., Sohlberg, M., Turkstra, L., & Ylvisaker, M. (2002). Evidence-based practice guidelines for cognitive-communication disorders after traumatic brain injury: Initial committee report. *Journal of Medical Speech-Language Pathology, 10,* ix–xiii.

Sohlberg, M. M., Avery, J., Kennedy, M. R. T., Ylvisaker, M., Coelho, C., Turkstra, L., & Yorkston, K. (2003). Practice guidelines for direct attention training. *Journal of Medical Speech-Language Pathology, 11,* xix–xxxix.

Spencer, K. A., Yorkston, K. M., Beukelman, D. R., Duffy, J., Golper, L. A., Miller, R. M., Strand, E. A., & Sullivan, M. (2002, Oct. 2002). *Practice Guidelines for Dysarthria: Evidence for the Behavioral Management of the Respiratory/Phonatory System* (Technical Report 3). Minneapolis, MN: Academy of Neurologic Communication Disorders and Sciences.

Yorkston, K. M., Spencer, K. A., Duffy, J. R., Beukelman, D. R., Golper, L. A., Miller, R. M., Strand, E. A., & Sullivan, M. (2001b). Evidence-based practice guidelines for dysarthria: Management of velopharyngeal function. *Journal of Medical Speech-Language Pathology, 9,* 257–273.

Agency for Healthcare Research and Quality: Evidence-Based Practice Centers

The AHRQ's Evidence-Based Practice Centers develop evidence reports and technology assessments on topics relevant to clinical, social science/behavioral, economic, and other health care organization and delivery issues—specifically those that are common, expensive, and/or significant for the Medicare and Medicaid populations. (http://www.ahcpr.gov/clinic/epcix.htm)

ASHA: Selected Online Member Resources

Evidence-Based Practice: Practice Guidelines
(http://www.asha.org/members/slp/topics/ebp/evidence_guidelines.htm)

Evidence-Based Practice Articles
(http://www.asha.org/members/slp/topics/ebp/ebp_articles.htm)

Levels of Evidence
(http://www.asha.org/members/slp/topics/ebp/evidence_levels.htm)

The Cochrane Library

A source of reliable and up-to-date information on the effects of interventions in health care. Published on a quarterly basis, The Cochrane Library is designed to provide information and evidence to support decisions taken in health care and to inform those receiving care. The Cochrane Library consists of a regularly updated collection of evidence-based medicine databases. (http://www.cochrane.org/reviews/clibintro.htm)

(continues)

Figure 8-3. Annotated list of selected online EBP resources. Many of these sources include preprocessed evidence to help the clinician both identify and critically appraise treatment evidence.

Centre for Evidence-Based Medicine at the University of Toronto Health Network

An EBP center with the goal of helping to develop, disseminate, and evaluate resources that can be used to practice and teach EBP for undergraduate, postgraduate, and continuing education for health care professionals from a variety of clinical disciplines. Among the resources available are glossaries, tutorials, syllabi, and other resources for teaching EBP, a list of evidence resources, worksheets, calculators, appraisal checklists, and numerous links to other EBP resources. (http://www.cebm.utoronto.ca/)

The Centre for Health Evidence at the University of Alberta

An EBP center with the goal of providing support for rudimentary and advanced training in evidence-based practice. Among the resources available are extensive libraries of tips, help systems, resource summaries, quizzes, surveys, teaching scripts, reminders, and information games. This site is also the repository for the *User's Guides to the Medical Literature*, the seminal series of articles responsible for advancing EBP. (http://www.cche.net/che/home.asp)

The Oxford Centre for Evidence Based Medicine

An extensive resource center designed to promote evidence-based health care and provide support and resources to all practitioners. Among the resources available are glossaries, tutorials, tips for searching for evidence, a list of critically appraised topics, and numerous links to other EBP resources. (http://www.cebm.net/index.asp)

Scottish Intercollegiate Guidelines Network

Resources from an organization whose objective is to improve the quality of health care for patients in Scotland by reducing variation in practice and outcome, through the development and dissemination of national clinical guidelines containing recommendations for effective practice based on current evidence. Resources include published guidelines on a wide variety of clinical practices, EBP calculators, checklists, and other tools for evaluating papers. (http://www.sign.ac.uk/index.html)

Figure 8-3. *Continued.*

STEP 4. APPLY THE RESULTS OF THIS APPRAISAL IN CLINICAL PRACTICE

Implementing this step is self-evident, but deserves brief mention due to some issues involved. If the valid and important evidence is to be useful to your patient, the likelihood of its benefit is linked to administering the diagnostic measure or treatment in a manner consistent with the evidence. Adapting the techniques specified in the diagnostic or treatment protocol may be desirable or even necessary, but weakens the link to the evidence on which the clinical decision to use that protocol was based. Though this is the essence of individualization and clinical innovation, decisions to depart from published protocols require that these decisions be made explicitly and based on evidence—in this case clinical expertise provides the evidence—to be consistent with EBP principles. When a treatment is administered on the basis of evidence supplied by your own clinical expertise, the final step in the EBP model takes on additional significance.

STEP 5. EVALUATE YOUR PERFORMANCE

Self-evaluation of clinical performance is an important component of EBP. Using empirical methods to track clinical progress provides an additional source of evidence based on objective data rather than unsystematic intuition. Objective treatment data can be generated from individual patients using single-subject research design (for a comprehensive introduction, see McReynolds & Kearns, 1983), patient and caregiver satisfaction questionnaires, comparisons with outcomes data from the ASHA NOMS project, and consistent and reliable data collection during treatment administration. It also is important to collect objective data regarding program evaluation and quality and improvement initiatives (see Chapter 7). Clinicians must justify their practices by providing reliable and valid data as evidence in support of those practices.

CURRENT PRACTICES AND FUTURE DIRECTIONS

In its efforts to provide optimal care to people with communication and cognitive disorders, including those with neurogenic language disorders, ASHA (2004) has endorsed EBP principles and practices to improve the quality of evidence available to support clinical decision making. A perusal of the adult neurogenic language disorders treatment research published within the last several years demonstrates that EBP is being taken seriously and is having an impact within the research community. It remains to be demonstrated, however, how EBP will affect clinical practice and outcomes. One survey of speech-language pathologists indicated that most respondents placed a high value on the role of research, but generally had only a superficial understanding of the EBP process (Vallino-Napoli & Reilly, 2004). As EBP continues to be emphasized by associations such as ASHA, as well as funding agencies and training programs, it is likely that clinicians will become better informed and more effective practitioners of EBP.

SUMMARY

The concepts and processes of EBP described in this chapter provide clinicians with a systematic process for considering scientific evidence when making treatment decisions. The following chapters addressing specific treatment strategies will assist clinicians in their efforts to incorporate EBP by providing brief reviews of the available evidence supporting the treatments described. When appropriate, we also identify the nature of evidence still needed to assist clinicians with treatment decisions. Only when clinicians are well educated about not only the range of treatment options available, but also, as highlighted by EBP, the quality of research on which those treatments were developed and evaluated, will successful clinical management of adult neurogenic language disorders be achieved.

Chapter 9

Remediation of Function: Behavioral Approaches

LEARNING OBJECTIVES

After reading this chapter you should be able to:

- Compare and contrast stimulation and cognitive neuropsychological approaches to treating language impairments at the ICF level of body function.

- Describe specific behavioral treatment procedures for addressing phonological, orthographic, lexical-semantic, morphosyntactic, or pragmatic impairments.

- Describe specific behavioral treatment procedures for addressing attention, memory, or executive function impairments.

- Discuss strengths and weaknesses of utilizing commercially available workbooks and computer software programs when treating linguistic and/or cognitive disorders in patients with neurogenic language disorders.

- Discuss linguistic and cognitive treatment planning

KEY TERMS

barrier games
cognitive neuropsychological treatment
cueing hierarchy
errorless learning
mapping therapy
Melodic Intonation Therapy
mnemonic strategies
Multiple Oral Rereading
prospective memory
reauditorization
Response Elaboration Training
semantic feature analysis
spaced retrieval
stimulation treatments
Treatment of Underlying Forms
Voluntary Control of Involuntary Utterances

issues pertaining to the generalization and transfer of treatment effects.

INTRODUCTION

Clinicians face two challenges when planning and providing treatment for the linguistic and cognitive impairments of patients with neurogenic language disorders. First, clinicians must often prove to those making the referrals and those funding the therapy that linguistic and cognitive treatments do indeed work. Although a significant and growing research literature supports linguistic and cognitive treatment efficacy (e.g., Robey, 1994; Holland, Fromm,

254

DeRuyter, & Stein, 1996), speech-language pathology services continue to be declined or restricted by many insurers (Katz et al., 2000; Ruiz, 2000). Inadequate provision of cognitive and communicative therapy services is perhaps most pervasive with respect to the dementia patient population. As several investigators have noted, when clinicians do receive referrals for dementia patients it is typically for dysphagia assessment and treatment, as health care providers often (1) view cognitive and communicative intervention for these patients as inappropriate given the progressive nature of dementia, or (2) are unaware that intervention can produce significant improvements in these patients' abilities (Hopper, Bayles, Harris, & Holland, 2001; Mahendra & Arkin, 2003). Accordingly, it is imperative that clinicians keep abreast of the empirical findings that support the provision of linguistic and cognitive treatments for neurogenic language disorders, and have on hand a list of research citations that can be forwarded to referral sources or funding agencies when advocating for treatment services.

A second challenge clinicians face is selecting from the plethora of treatment approaches the technique or techniques that will be most appropriate for each individual patient. This selection will be facilitated in part by a comprehensive evaluation that provides data pertaining to patients' linguistic and cognitive strengths and weaknesses as well as their daily cognitive-communicative needs (see Chapters 4–7). Having a critical understanding of the variety of therapies currently available also is essential to selecting and providing the most suitable and efficient treatment for a given patient, particularly when the clinician's initial treatment choice proves ineffective.

To help resolve these challenges, the purpose of this chapter is to review a variety of treatment procedures that have been developed to remediate impairments of communication, cognition, or both at the ICF level of body function in patients with neurogenic language disorders. The first half of the chapter describes behavioral treatments designed to address linguistic impairments associated with aphasia and, to a lesser degree, other neurogenic language disorders. The second half of the chapter summarizes behavioral therapies aimed at facilitating recovery of cognitive impairments in a variety of patient populations, in particular those with right hemisphere damage (RHD), traumatic brain injury (TBI), or dementia.

TREATMENT OF LINGUISTIC IMPAIRMENTS

Two general treatment approaches encompass the majority of behavioral procedures currently available for remediating the linguistic impairments of patients with neurogenic language disorders: the linguistic stimulation approach and the cognitive neuropsychological approach. The **stimulation approach** is the most widely used linguistic treatment approach in the United States, and, as Duffy and

Coelho (2001) conjectured, "may be thought to encompass all approaches to aphasia rehabilitation" (p. 341). Basically, **stimulation treatments** emphasize understanding what stimulus factors may impede or enhance patients' current linguistic abilities, and then expose patients to stimulus and task hierarchies that will "stimulate" functioning of compromised language functions and modalities. In contrast, in **cognitive neuropsychological treatments,** models of normal and/or disordered language are used to motivate treatment targets and procedures (Mitchum & Berndt, 1995; see also Chapter 1). Following a comprehensive assessment designed to delineate which specific linguistic processes (e.g., phoneme-to-grapheme conversion; phonological output lexicon) have been compromised (for further description of cognitive neuropsychological assessment procedures, see Chapter 4), the focus of cognitive neuropsychological treatments is to improve the disrupted processes or to capitalize on more intact processes, and then to evaluate how therapy effected change in trained as well as untrained linguistic stimuli, functions, and modalities. It is important to note that although the therapy procedures used when adhering to a cognitive neuropsychological treatment approach are often similar to those developed out of the stimulation approach, the rationale for these procedures is not. The following section of this chapter will review stimulation and cognitive neuropsychological treatments that have been developed to address linguistic impairments at the ICF level of body function.

Side Bar

Treatment Selection and Justification: Going Beyond "Because it Works!"

How important is it to understand the theoretical framework behind a treatment? If a treatment works, why not just use it? There are at least two good reasons for clinicians to understand the philosophy guiding a given intervention strategy. The first reason is that clinicians should be able to explain to patients, their families, or both the purpose of a treatment activity. Patients who understand how the treatment is intended to help them will be more motivated to participate in treatment and devote energy to the tasks and strategies. Further, caregivers are more likely to follow through with carryover activities if they understand their purpose. The second reason clinicians should understand the theory driving the intervention strategy is to provide the basis on which the therapy tasks can be modified to meet the needs of individual patients. To illustrate this concept, consider a treatment activity where the patient is attempting to name pictures of common nouns. In a stimulation-based treatment (described later in this chapter), the clinician provides various semantic, phonologic, or other cues based on which cues elicit the appropriate response. Thus, within this framework, the clinician modifies the intervention task based on how the patient responds to various cues. In contrast, in the cognitive neuropsychologically based treatment of semantic feature analysis (also described later in this chapter), "cues" are limited to semantic features. Thus, although the clinician might modify which semantic features are targeted, all identified

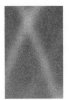

(continued)

features would be reviewed even if some features were not particularly helpful to the patient in generating the target name. Although these two treatment strategies may look very similar to a naïve observer, the informed clinician will understand how their purposes differ, as well as how each can be modified to meet the needs of individual patients.

PHONOLOGICAL AND ORTHOGRAPHIC TREATMENTS

As discussed in Chapter 5, assessment and consequently treatment of phonological and orthographic processes is most common when dealing with patients with aphasia. In contrast, patients with other types of neurogenic disorders do not frequently exhibit impairments at this language processing level, and when such impairments are present, they are typically not a rehabilitation priority. Accordingly, most treatment procedures reviewed in this section were developed for, and thus are most suitable for, patients with aphasia.

Phonological Treatments

Although deficits of segmental and suprasegmental aspects of phonology are possible in patients with neurogenic language disorders, there are currently limited treatment options available for remediating these types of language impairments. That is, most research to date has focused on qualifying and quantifying phonological impairments, rather than developing and validating treatment procedures. Accordingly, many of the therapy approaches and activities described below should be considered experimental.

Treatment of Segmental Impairments

Difficulties with discriminating or perceiving segmental aspects of phonology have been hypothesized to underlie the spoken and written word comprehension deficits of many patients with aphasia. Despite the possible prevalence of impairments at this level of language processing, few treatments have been described or evaluated in the research literature. An exception is a case study by Morris and colleagues (1996) in which a patient with global aphasia and significant speech perception problems was provided a set of treatment activities designed to improve his discrimination of auditory speech stimuli. Treatment tasks included: (1) phoneme-grapheme matching—choosing which of three letters matched a spoken stimulus; (2) phoneme discrimination—deciding if a pair of spoken syllables was the same or different; (3) auditory word-picture matching—choosing which of three pictures matched a spoken word; (4) written word-auditory word matching—selecting which of three written words matched a spoken word, (5) correct/incorrect judgment—deciding if a spoken word matched a written word or picture; and (6) nonword syllable same or different judgment—deciding if pairs of spoken consonant-vowel syllables were the same or different. Treatment stimuli were selected so that initially the patient practiced discriminating spoken stimuli that significantly differed, with respect to phoneme characteristics such as the distinctive features of voice, place, and manner of articulation (e.g., "cot" vs. "lock"); as he progressed, the stimuli more closely approximated each other (e.g., "cot" vs. "pot"). Following 12 therapy sessions, the patient's phoneme discrimination and repetition of untrained stimuli significantly improved; positive but nonsignificant changes on auditory lexical decision and synonym judgment tasks also were observed. Clearly these findings are encouraging and should motivate further investigation of treatments for auditory discrimination deficits.

In another case study, the commercially available Auditory Discrimination in Depth (ADD; Lindamood & Lindamood, 1975) was used to improve not only the phonological awareness but also reading and spelling abilities of a patient with mild, acquired alexia and agraphia (Conway et al., 1998). As shown in Table 9-1, initial ADD treatment sessions focus on increasing patients' awareness of how phonemes are produced. Next, treatment targets patients' ability to break down and, consequently, read and spell short nonword syllables into their component speech sounds. The final stages of the ADD program involve increasing the complexity and length of the spoken stimuli. Following intensive daily treatment (i.e., 2–4 hours per day for a total of over 100 hours), the patient of Conway and colleagues demonstrated improvements in reading aloud and spelling nonwords and regularly spelled words, in word and passage reading comprehension, and in reading rate. Relatedly, Yampolsky and Waters (2002) based their treatment on a different commercially available program, the Wilson Reading System (Wilson, 1996), which also focuses on phonological awareness, and found similar positive outcomes in terms of their patients' oral reading skills.

Because problems producing segmental aspects of phonology are often attributed, at least in part, to motor planning (i.e., apraxia of speech) or production (i.e., dysarthria) deficits, treatments for these output difficulties typically focus on motor speech skills and follow language treatments that assure patients have a sufficient linguistic base upon which they can practice motor speech skills. When treating patients with neurogenic language disorders who have concomitant apraxia, dysarthria, or both, clinicians should consult textbooks, such as that of Yorkston and colleagues (1999), for ideas regarding motor speech therapy approaches and activities.

Treatment of Suprasegmental Impairments

For a limited number of patients with RHD or TBI, treatment of suprasegmental phonology skills (i.e., production and comprehension of prosody) may be neces-

Table 9-1. Stages of the Auditory Discrimination in Depth Program (Lindamood & Lindamood, 1975)

STAGE	PURPOSE AND DESCRIPTION
Oral awareness training	Increase awareness of how individual phonemes are produced by providing visual (i.e., use of a mirror during phoneme production, drawings of articulators' positions) and verbal cues (i.e., provide names for particular articulator movements and voicing, such as "noisy lip-popper" for the phoneme /b/). Patients also are instructed to attend to tactile and kinesthetic feedback when producing individual phonemes (e.g., feel how and where the tongue touches the roof of the mouth when producing the /t/ sound).
Simple nonword training	Improve the ability to parse simple nonword syllables into individual phonemes by using visual cues and the oral awareness skills trained in the first treatment stage. Patients must determine how many phonemes are in a target stimulus, the order of these phonemes, and over time, similarities and differences between two target stimuli. At this stage, the ability to read and spell nonword syllables also is trained. Initially, patients point to drawings of articulators' positions to indicate the phonemic composition of target stimuli. As treatment progresses, the drawings are replaced by colored blocks (e.g., after hearing /ipi/, the patient points to a green block, a red block, and then another green block), letter tiles, and lastly, handwritten letters.
Complex nonword-word training	Train parsing, reading, and spelling of longer nonword and word mono syllabic stimuli using the methods described for Simple Nonword Training. Training of some common grapheme-to-phoneme conversion rules also is introduced (e.g., "qu" =/kw/).
Mutisyllable nonword-word training	Train parsing, reading, and spelling of longer nonword and word multi-syllabic stimuli using the methods described for Simple Nonword Training. Passage reading and training of common affixes also are introduced.

sary. We emphasize that improving suprasegmental processing will only infrequently be an appropriate treatment goal because in most patients: (1) other deficits underlie their apparent difficulties with this aspect of language (e.g., dysarthria may cause impaired production of prosody or stress; attention deficits may limit suprasegmental comprehension; Ryalls et al., 1987), and consequently treatment should be directed toward these other deficits; and/or (2) treating other linguistic and cognitive deficits, even those unrelated to their suprasegmental difficulties, will often have a greater impact on their recovery and return to daily activities and communicative interactions. Additionally, although several treatment procedures are briefly described below, none of these has been subjected to empirical study with any neurogenic patient population, and thus their efficacy has yet to be established (Tompkins, 1995; Wymer, Lindman, & Booksh, 2002).

If comprehension of suprasegmental aspects of language is deemed to affect significantly a given patient's daily communication interactions and thus is considered a suitable treatment target, clinicians might exploit one or more of the following tasks depending on the exact nature of the patient's impairment:

1. Present sentence stimuli that vary in terms of stress and intonational cues and have the patient explain or identify the correct interpretation of the stimuli. For example, the patient might be asked to contrast the meanings of "**You** went where?" versus "You went **where**?" in which the bold font indicates the most stressed word in the question;

2. Present pairs of stimuli, such as short phrases or sentences that slightly to substantially differ in terms of durational, intensity, and/or fundamental frequency cues and have the patient discriminate whether the two stimuli are the same or different and, if different, explain how they are different;

3. Present a pictured scene and a spoken sentence and ask the patient to identify the mood or attitude being communicated; and

4. Present a short story and have the patient determine if there was a discrepancy between the linguistic content of any sentences in the story and the stress and/or intonation with which the sentences were spoken.

For the above or other prosody comprehension tasks, clinicians should consider using audiotaped stimuli to assure that stimulus presentation is reliable across different sessions or within a session when the patient requests a repetition. Furthermore, audiotaped stimuli allow the clinician to pilot the stimuli on adults with no brain damage to assure that the target prosody cues are apparent (i.e., listeners without brain damage should be able to discriminate or explain the prosodic cues).

In terms of prosody production, our clinical experiences indicate that only patients who rely upon their speech as a source of income (e.g., radio announcer, actor) are typically interested in working on this aspect of language. In these cases, clinicians might consider treatment procedures such as contrastive stress exercises that were developed for dysarthria (e.g., Yorkston, Beukelman, Strand, & Bell, 1999) (see Table 9-2). Alternate therapy activities include: (1) provide patients with a set of spoken or written linguistic stimuli (e.g., word, phrase, or complete sentence), and require them to say each stimulus with a prescribed linguistic (e.g., declarative sentence vs. question intonation) or emotional prosody (e.g., nervous vs. angry); (2) show patients pictured scenes and have them generate a sentence that one of the characters in the scene might be saying with linguistic and/or emotional prosody that is appropriate to the picture's context; and (3) require patients to read short scenarios and then read aloud or generate a final quotation for one of the story characters with appropriate linguistic and/or emotional prosody. Some support for the use of these activities comes from Stringer (1996), who provided two months of "affective communication treatment" to a patient with prosodic production problems subsequent to a TBI. The treatment included providing visual feedback from a computerized pitch

Table 9-2. Contrastive Stress Procedures for Treating Prosody Production

STEPS	EXAMPLE
1. Present the patient with a sentence stimulus.	Clinician: "Dylan and Dennis played tennis yesterday."
2. Ask the patient a series of questions about the sentence, and require the patient to answer by restating the sentence with stress or emphasis on the appropriate word or words.	Clinician: "When did Dylan and Dennis play tennis?" Patient: "Dylan and Dennis played tennis **yesterday**." Clinician: "What did Dylan and Dennis play yesterday?" Patient: "Dylan and Dennis played **tennis** yesterday."
3. Provide the patient with feedback regarding the adequacy of his/her response. Cues to elicit the appropriate response include: (a) describe ways in which speech rate or vocal loudness or pitch can be used to indicate stress or emphasis (b) provide the sentence stimulus in both spoken and written formats to reduce memory demands, and have the patient identify the word or words to be stressed on the written stimulus before attempting a verbal production (c) tape record the patient's responses so that the patient can make off-line judgments regarding the adequacy of his/her responses (d) utilize software such as Visipitch or SpeechViewer or equipment such as a sound level meter to provide visual feedback concerning the adequacy of the patient's responses	

Note. Words in bold font are those that should be emphasized or stressed by the patient.

analysis system, as well as modeling and generating different emotional intonations and facial expressions. Although improvements were observed and maintained for at least two months following treatment termination, it is important to keep in mind that this was a case study, and thus lacked the experimental controls necessary to validate the effectiveness of these treatment procedures.

Orthographic Treatments

Treatments that target orthographic processing are designed to improve reading by enhancing letter recognition, grapheme-to-phoneme conversion, or both. They also may be used to improve spelling by training letter production, phoneme-to-grapheme conversion, or both. Because many of the following treatments for orthographic difficulties were designed for and evaluated on patients with relatively pure alexias or agraphias, further exploration of whether these programs are equally effective for patients demonstrating a broader spectrum of linguistic and cognitive symptoms is still needed.

Orthographic Treatments for Reading Problems

Several approaches have been used to remediate problems recognizing or decoding orthographic symbols. When problems recognizing individual letters appear to underlie patients' reading difficulties (e.g., patients can orally spell words but not read written versions of these words), a tactile-kinesthetic treatment may be utilized (Greenwald & Gonzalez-Rothi, 1998; Lott & Friedman, 1999; Maher, Clayton, Barrett, Schober-Peterson, & Rothi, 1998). The premise of this therapy is that although some patients may have limited access to orthographic information via the visual modality, this access can be facilitated through other modalities like touch or movement. The initial focus of treatment is naming of individual letters. If patients are unable to name the letter shown to them on a computer screen or index card, they are required to trace or copy the letter and then asked to name it. The tracing or copying process elicits kinesthetic stimulation, and if this is done on the patient's hand, then tactile stimulation also is achieved. Once patients' letter recognition has improved, word- and subsequently sentence-level stimuli are introduced. Positive outcomes in terms of improved letter and word recognition and reading rate have been reported (Lott & Friedman, 1999; Maher et al., 1998), even when patients have linguistic deficits beyond the orthographic level (e.g., Greenwald & Gonzalez-Rothi, 1998).

Other treatments address reading problems stemming from the inability to decode individual letters and letter combinations into their corresponding phonemic representations (i.e., grapheme-to-phoneme conversion deficits). For instance, in one approach, patients are taught to associate a key word with each grapheme (de Partz, 1986); for example, the word "baby" might be paired with the letter "b." Not only should the key words be personally relevant to the patient (e.g., a spouse's name serves as a key word for a certain grapheme), but they also should be words that the patient can consistently retrieve and say. During initial treatment sessions, patients are shown a letter and asked to provide the key word for that letter; once they say the key word, they are then asked to say just the first phoneme that corresponds to the sound of the target letter. As patients progress, they are encouraged to still think of the key word, but only say the sound. In the final stages, patients practice reading aloud, first nonwords (so that they don't use a whole-word reading strategy during therapy) and then real words using this key word technique for each letter in the stimulus. Additionally, patients are explicitly taught at least a small number of grapheme-to-phoneme conversion rules (e.g., a "c" followed by an "a," "o," or "u" is pronounced /k/; in remaining contexts it is pronounced /s/). Although the findings from several studies indicate that patients can learn which phonemes go with which graphemes using this treatment approach (de Partz, 1986; Hillis, 1993; Mitchum & Berndt, 1991), a few researchers found that their patients had difficulty learning how to blend phonemes once treatment progressed to the word level (e.g., Mitchum & Berndt, 1991). Accordingly, further research is needed to delineate which patient profiles are most suitable for this treatment approach.

Orthographic Treatments for Spelling Problems

A limited number of spelling treatments have been developed to address problems at the orthographic level. Many of these treatments are similar to those described in the previous section on orthographic treatments for reading problems. For example, the key word approach has been successfully used to remediate phoneme-to-grapheme conversion problems in several patients (Hillis Trupe, 1986; Hillis & Caramazza, 1994; Carlomagno, Iavarone, & Colombo, 1994). In this treatment, key words that the patients can spell are linked to target graphemes (e.g., "Robert" for the letter "r"). Patients are then taught how to use the initial sounds of their key words to write single graphemes and, as they progress, to use these key words covertly to help them sound out and spell nonwords and eventually real words. Specific phoneme-to-grapheme conversion rules also may be explicitly taught by first explaining the rule to patients and then having them practice using the rule during a variety of writing tasks, such as writing to dictation and completing written sentence closure tasks (de Partz, Seron, & Van der Linden, 1992). Most frequently these spelling treatments produce improvements on trained nonwords and words as well as untrained regularly spelled words. Because irregularly spelled words violate common phoneme-to-grapheme correspondences and conversion rules, lexical-semantic treatment approaches are more appropriate when patients have problems spelling these types of words (for information on lexical-semantic treatments, see the following section of this chapter).

For some patients, spelling problems stem from deficits of what Beeson and Rapcsak (2002) referred to as peripheral processes. These patients can often spell aloud nonwords and words, but display difficulty when required to write spontaneously and, in some cases, copy written stimuli. More specifically, peripheral deficits include problems recalling the visual and/or physical characteristics of individual letters (i.e., allographic conversion deficit), completing the visuomotor plan and requirements needed to write letters (e.g., apraxia, hemiparesis, visuoperceptual deficit), and attending to the writing process (i.e., visual neglect). For patients with allographic conversion impairments, two treatment approaches have been suggested. One involves teaching compensatory strategies, such as using an alphabet card when handwriting as a reminder of letter shapes (Ramage, Beeson, & Rapcsak, 1998), or typing on a typewriter or computer (Black, Behrmann, Bass,

& Hacker, 1989). The second approach capitalizes upon these patients' typically preserved oral spelling abilities by requiring them to self-dictate words before they write them. That is, patients dictate to themselves one letter at a time to help them write out words, checking after each letter for mistakes. Whereas this technique proved effective in two case studies (Pound, 1996; Ramage et al., 1998), less successful results were reported by Lesser (1990), indicating that further investigations are needed to specify which patients will benefit from this self-dictation procedure.

Several treatment strategies may be appropriate when motor, visuoconstruction, or attention problems underlie writing difficulties. For example, Beeson and Rapscak (2002) recommended intensive immediate and delayed copying tasks to help restore and automate motor plans in patients with apraxic deficits. Empirical support for this recommendation is lacking, however, given that currently there are no published studies on treating apraxic writing problems. Treatments for other motor- and attention-based writing difficulties, however, have been described in the research literature. As shown in Table 9-3, all of these are primarily compensatory in nature and require further investigation to substantiate their effectiveness.

LEXICAL-SEMANTIC TREATMENTS

Of the various linguistic symptoms associated with neurogenic language disorders, lexical-semantic processing deficits have without question been the focus of the

Table 9-3. Compensatory Strategies for Addressing Peripheral Writing Difficulties

COMPENSATORY STRATEGY	TARGET DEFICIT	AUTHOR(S)
Lined paper	letter size and spacing problems due to micrographia, letter/word spacing problems and upward slant due to visual neglect	Oliveira et al. (1997) Tompkins (1995)
Verbal reminders (e.g., "write big," "look left")	micrographia, visual neglect	Oliveira et al. (1997) Tompkins (1995)
Writing prosthesis (e.g., large grip pen, forearm skateboard)	dominant hand/arm hemiparesis	Brown et al., (1983) Leischner (1996) Whurr & Lorch (1991)
Typewriter or computer keyboard	allographic conversion deficit, apraxia	Beeson & Rapscak (2002) Black et al. (1989)

greatest number of treatment studies. Although these deficits are possible following the onset of any type of neurogenic language disorder (e.g., aphasia, dementia, cognitive-communicative disorders associated with TBI or RHD), the majority of procedures described below were designed for and evaluated on patients with aphasia. Therefore, when used with other patient populations, these treatments may need to be modified to circumvent or address a given patient's specific symptom profile (e.g., concomitant neglect or memory deficits). Furthermore, empirical investigations are still needed to examine the appropriateness and, consequently, effectiveness of these treatments for lexical-semantic problems associated with RHD, TBI, or dementia.

The Linguistic Stimulation Approach to Treating Lexical-Semantic Deficits

Many traditional lexical-semantic treatments are based upon a stimulation therapy model, and focus on identifying, providing, and ultimately fading cues to facilitate patients' lexical-semantic comprehension or production abilities. Additionally, therapy stimuli and activities in these traditional treatments usually are ordered such that those that are more difficult for patients are introduced later in the treatment process. Specific cues, stimuli, and activities should be selected on the basis of factors such as semantic category, stimulus length, or part of speech found to influence the patient's lexical-semantic abilities during the linguistic assessment (for a list of possible influential factors, see Table 5-4). Below we review some specific stimulation treatments that have been used successfully to target the spoken and/or written lexical-semantic processing abilities of patients with aphasia.

Stimulation Treatment for Lexical-Semantic Comprehension Deficits

One basic form of stimulation treatment has been traditionally used to remediate lexical-semantic comprehension deficits. This standard approach involves distinguishing one or more modalities through which a patient can access lexical-semantic information and then presenting treatment stimuli via these modalities to prime or "deblock" the impaired modality (Duffy & Coelho, 2001; Weigl, 1981). For example, if a patient has difficulty understanding spoken language, initial treatment activities might involve presenting written, gestural, *and* spoken forms of the target stimuli and having the patient select the correct pictures or objects that correspond to the target. As the patient progresses on this task, the written and gestural cues could be faded so that eventually the patient is completing a spoken word-to-picture matching task. The final stages of this treatment would focus on gradually increasing the complexity of the stimuli (e.g., decrease vocabulary familiarity, increase stimulus length to phrases or sentences, introduce various parts of speech) and the task demands (e.g., complete the task after a delay to increase memory demands, complete the task in a noisy environment to increase attention demands, increase the number and similarity of distracter items). Table 9-4 lists other therapy activities that might be used in stimulation treatments for lexical-semantic comprehension problems. Note that most of these activities can easily be adapted to target lexical-semantic production as well. Stimulation treatment has been used successfully, even with patients with severe comprehension deficits. For instance, Ulatowska and Richardson (1974) designed a series of deblocking activities that progressed from reading comprehension (e.g., arranging written words into phrases) to auditory comprehension tasks (e.g., matching spoken phrases to the written phrases used in previous activities) and found that following this treatment, their patient with Wernicke's aphasia showed substantial improvements in his written and spoken comprehension skills. Similarly, Helm-Estabrooks and

Table 9-4. Therapy Activities for Addressing Lexical-Semantic Comprehension Deficits

ACTIVITY	EXAMPLES
Pointing Tasks	Point to the picture or object that represents the spoken, written, and/or gestured word stimulus
	Point to the written word that represents the spoken, written, and/or gestured word stimulus
	Point to the picture, object, or written word that represents the spoken and/or written definition (e.g., "Point to the color of bananas.")
	Point to the picture, object, or written word that completes a spoken and/or written phrase or sentence (e.g., "The housekeeper _____ the floor.")
	Point to the pictured scene that represents the spoken and/or written description
Following Directions	Point to pictures or objects in the sequence specified by a spoken and/or written command (e.g., "Point to the girl in the pants and then to the boy in the hat.")
	Manipulate an object or set of objects in the manner and sequence specified by a spoken and/or written command (e.g., "Sign your name and then fold the paper in half.")
Answering Questions	Answer spoken and/or written yes/no questions about general information (e.g., "Is Canada south of the United States?")
	Answer spoken and/or written yes/no questions about pictured scenes or spoken and/or written stories or scenarios
	Answer spoken and/or written multiple-choice questions[1] about pictured scenes or spoken and/or written stories or scenarios
Sentence Verification	Determine if a spoken and/or written sentence makes sense (e.g., "The dairy farmer kept the cows in the garage.")

[1]Clinicians must keep in mind the increased memory demands involved in answering multiple-choice questions, particularly those presented verbally, compared to the other activities listed above.

Albert (2004) have described a treatment program called Treatment for Wernicke's Aphasia (TWA), which is designed to improve auditory comprehension by capitalizing on patients' more intact reading and repetition skills. Helm-Estabrooks and Albert recommended that TWA is most appropriate for patients with relatively preserved reading comprehension, at least at the single word level on an aphasia test. Steps of this treatment program include:

1. Patients complete written word-to-picture matching tasks to enhance their reading comprehension skills;

2. Auditory comprehension is stimulated through a process called **reauditorization,** in which patients are often better able to understand a word if they can say the word. More specifically, patients are required first to read aloud the items trained in the reading comprehension step, and then to repeat aloud these items when provided with a spoken model and a picture stimulus.

3. Patients complete spoken word-to-picture matching tasks.

Although no formal evaluation of TWA has yet been completed, the authors summarized a successful case and additionally provided sufficient description of procedural details so that their program could be easily applied in future clinical practice or research endeavors.

In summary, the stimulation approach to treating lexical-semantic comprehension deficits is widely used clinically. Because of an inordinate research focus on treatments for lexical-semantic production versus comprehension problems, however, only nominal empirical support for this treatment technique has accumulated thus far (e.g., Hough, 1993; Marshall & Neuburger, 1984; Ulatowska & Richardson, 1974). Although the studies that have been completed consistently reported that patients acquired comprehension of trained items following stimulation treatment, generalization effects to untrained items and modalities were variable. Accordingly, more research is necessary to determine the validity of these commonly used therapy procedures, particularly in terms of whether or not treatments evoke improvements in patients' understanding during their daily communication interactions and activities.

Stimulation Treatment for Lexical-Semantic Production Deficits

Numerous stimulation treatments described in the literature aim to remediate spoken or written lexical-semantic production problems. The most basic of these treatments requires patients to practice intensively repeating or copying a set of target items so that eventually they can produce these items without a verbal or written model. For example, Beeson and colleagues (Beeson, 1999; Beeson, Rising, & Volk, 2003) developed a writing program called Copy and Recall Treatment (CART) that consists of having patients practice repeatedly copying written words (that are presented in concert with their pictured representations), followed by written picture naming (i.e., only the pictures are presented). These researchers found that patients with severe writing deficits have been able to acquire and maintain production of trained vocabulary when this simple treatment was provided in either one-on-one therapy sessions or as a homework program. In their most recent study, Beeson et al. (2003) noted that patients who fail to complete their assigned writing homework consistently and accurately, and who have significant concomitant semantic and cognitive impairments, are less likely to benefit from CART.

Perhaps one of the most frequently used stimulation techniques entails developing and applying a **cueing hierarchy** to facilitate patients' lexical-semantic production abilities. The first step to cueing treatments involves determining what cues facilitate the individual patient's word retrieval skills (see Table 9-5 for a list of possible cues). These cues are then arranged into a hierarchy. Cues at the top of the hierarchy are those that provide the least amount of external support, and thus are expected to help the patient the least. In contrast, cues falling at the bottom of the hierarchy are those that provide greater amounts of external support, and thus are expected to help the patient the most. Although the relative strength of the cues shown in Table 9-5 can vary across individual patients, initial phoneme and semantic cues such as sentence completion are frequently the most potent (e.g., Pease & Goodglass, 1978). Recent studies by Marshall, Freed, and colleagues (Freed, Celery, & Marshall, 2004; Marshall, Karow, Freed, & Babcock, 2002) have shown that personalized cues also may be particularly potent for patients with aphasia. Personalized cues are ones that patients with aphasia create on their own to help them retrieve specific words. For example, a patient might come up with the cue "birthday" to help him retrieve the target word, "chocolate," because he always has chocolate cake for his birthday. Importantly, Marshall, Freed, and colleagues have found that compared to phonological cues, personalized cues can result in greater and more enduring word retrieval improvements.

Once the hierarchy has been created, it is used to facilitate the patient's lexical-semantic production abilities while completing word retrieval tasks. That is, when the patient cannot correctly complete an item, the clinician provides the first cue at the top of the hierarchy; if, following that cue, the patient still cannot complete the item correctly, the next cue is provided, with the clinician continuing to provide prompts until the patient is able to complete the target item correctly. Once the patient has provided a correct response, the patient can be required to work back up through the hierarchy to provide additional practice of the erred item, or alternately a new target item may be introduced. Figure 9-1 provides an example of a cueing hierarchy that might be used to target written naming.

Numerous studies have documented that cueing hierarchies can improve the spoken (McNeil, Small, Masterson, & Fossett, 1995; Wambaugh, Doyle, Martinez, & Kalinyak-Fliszar, 2002) and written (Beeson, 1999; Hillis, 1989; Murray & Karcher, 2000) lexical retrieval abilities of patients with aphasia when implemented via direct therapy, computer-based treatments, homework activities, or some combination

Table 9-5. **Cues that may be Used to Facilitate Spoken and/or Written Lexical-Semantic Production**

CUE TYPE	CUE EXAMPLE FOR THE TARGET "HORSE"
Semantically Based	
Superordinate	"It's an *animal*."
Coordinate	"It's like a *cow*."
Associate	"It eats *hay*."
Function	"You can *ride* it."
Phrase or sentence completion	"The jockey fell off of the _____."
Definition or description	"This is an animal that you can find on a farm or a ranch. You can ride or race them. You can see them at a rodeo. . ."
Antonym	n/a
Phonologically Based	
Initial phoneme or syllable	"It's a /h/. . ."
Number of syllables	"It has one syllable."
Real word or nonword rhyme	"It rhymes with *course*." "It rhymes with *gorce*."
Repetition	"It's a horse. Say *horse*."
Unison speech or singing	"It's a horse. Now say that word with me—*horse*."
Orthographically Based	
Initial grapheme	"It starts with an h."
Number of letters	"It has five letters."
Word shape	
Letter anagrams	o s h e r
Copying	"It's this word. Copy this word."
Reading aloud	"Here's the word. Read it aloud."
Others	
Sound effects	"neigh," "clip-clop"
Tactile	n/a
Gesture	Pretend to hold the reins and ride a horse.
Drawing	Clinician and/or patient draw a picture of a horse and then the patient tries to name it while drawing it.
Time delay	"Wait 5 seconds before telling me what this is."

of these therapy formats. Although cueing treatments invariably lead to acquisition of trained items, generalization to untrained items and/or language modalities and maintenance of treatment effects will depend on one or more of the following: (1) the nature of the patients' lexical-semantic deficit (e.g., semantic/conceptual vs.

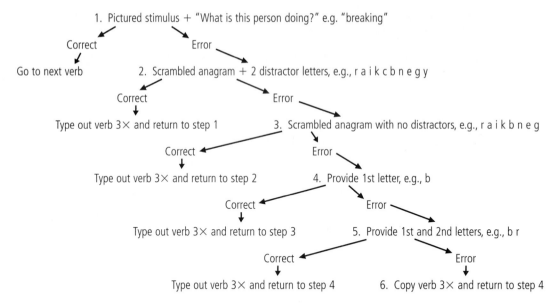

Figure 9-1. Example of a Cueing Hierarchy (Adapted from Hillis, 1989 and Murray & Karcher, 2000) for Training Written Naming of Verbs.

phonological access), (2) whether or not the patients have concomitant cognitive or motoric problems (e.g., generalization of a writing treatment to verbal skills would be unlikely in a patient with concomitant apraxia of speech), (3) whether or not patients continue to practice or use the trained vocabulary, and (4) whether or not patients learn to generate these cues independently (i.e., acquire a word retrieval strategy; DeDe, Parris, & Waters, 2003).

A few stimulation programs have been developed for specific patient populations. For example, **Voluntary Control of Involuntary Utterances** (VCIU; Helm-Estabrooks & Albert, 2004) was designed to stimulate propositional (i.e., voluntary) verbal output in patients whose current spoken language abilities are restricted to involuntary production of a small set of real words (e.g., stereotypical utterances such as "that's good."). Basic steps to the VCIU program include:

1. Make a list of all real words the patient has been reported to produce spontaneously.

2. Write one of these words on a card and require the patient to read it aloud. If the patient correctly reads the word aloud, it becomes a target stimulus for homework and future therapy sessions. If the patient is unable to read the word aloud, it is discarded and the next word on the patient's list is written on a card. This step is repeated until the clinician has attempted to elicit reading aloud of all words on the patient's list.

3. Pictures of the words that the patient was able to read aloud are then presented and the patient is required to name these pictures. If the patient is unable to complete confrontation naming of an item, he/she is shown the written word and asked to read it aloud. Note that if the patient produces an incorrect, real word while attempting to read aloud or name target stimuli, that incorrect word should be added to the patient's list, and thus should itself be evaluated to determine if it too may become a target stimulus.

Only one study to date has evaluated the effects of VCIU. In 1980, Helm and Barresi provided three to six months of VCIU to three patients with severely non-fluent output and mild to moderately impaired auditory comprehension abilities. Following treatment, all patients had acquired a spoken vocabulary of at least 250 words, and showed improved scores on responsive naming, confrontation naming, and animal naming subtests of the *Boston Diagnostic Aphasia Examination*. Little change, however, was observed in their performance of oral reading subtests. Whereas these findings and the anecdotal case reported by Helm-Estabrooks and Albert (2004) indicate encouraging outcomes, further studies with appropriate research design controls (e.g., larger sample size, assurance that all patients are beyond the spontaneous recovery period, inclusion of a control measure) remain needed to validate VCIU treatment effects.

Another stimulation program created for a specific patient group is **Response Elaboration Training** (RET; Kearns, 1985; Kearns & Scher, 1989). RET is designed to affect positively utterance length and information content in the verbal output of patients with nonfluent aphasia. It is considered a "loose training" program that involves incidental learning, reinforcement of patient-initiated output, and emphasis on utterance content (including lexical-semantic accuracy) versus form. A typical RET session includes the following:

1. the patient is asked to comment on a picture scene, making sure to discourage naming or concrete description;

2. the clinician models and reinforces the patient's initial utterance. For example, if the patient says "Man gun bad." in response to a newspaper picture of a war scene, the clinician might model "I agree, the soldier with the gun looks very mean or angry.";

3. the clinician utilizes wh-questions to elicit further responses and to encourage the patient to elaborate on earlier responses. For example, the clinician asks, "Why do you think the soldier is angry?" and the patient responds, "Guy.";

4. the clinician provides a model that combines the patient's previous responses. For example, the clinician responds, "I see, the soldier with the gun is mad at the prisoner.";

5. the patient is asked to repeat the clinician's model. For example, the clinician says, "Now you try to say this whole sentence.. . The soldier with the gun is mad at the prisoner."; and

6. the clinician reinforces the patient's response and models the sentence again. For instance, the clinician states, "Great job. The soldier with the gun is mad at the prisoner."

Note that at no time does the clinician directly correct the patient's spontaneous utterances, but rather only provides indirect feedback via conversational modeling.

Several studies have shown that RET is an effective means by which to increase the informational content of patients with nonfluent aphasia and mild to moderate apraxia of speech (Gaddie, Kearns, & Yedor, 1991; Kearns, 1985; Kearns & Scher, 1989), as well as those with nonfluent aphasia and severe apraxia of speech (Wambaugh & Martinez, 2000; Wambaugh et al., 2001). That is, following treatment, patients have been found to produce an increased number and variety of content words (particularly nouns) and slightly longer utterances while conversing about trained stimuli; additionally, patients show similar degrees of improvement with novel stimuli, conversational partners, and communicative settings and are able to maintain these gains over time. Marshall (2001) also presented a case in which a patient with Wernicke's aphasia successfully responded to this treatment approach, although clearly further research investigating the appropriateness of RET for patients representing a variety of language profiles is still needed.

Side Bar

To Modify or Not To Modify. . . That is the Question

Programmatic intervention strategies such as RET, Melodic Intonation Therapy (see below), and SFA are often appealing to clinicians, particularly those new to managing neurogenic language disorders, because procedures for these treatments are usually clearly described. Clinicians may wonder, however, whether it is appropriate to deviate from the treatment protocols specified in these programs. Several issues are relevant when considering this question. First, arguably the most important advantage of detailed treatment protocols is that they allow other clinicians and researchers to replicate the methods implemented by the original researchers. Careful review of groups of studies examining the same program, nevertheless, often reveal that program modifications are made to address the needs of the patients described in each study (e.g., Beeson, 1998 vs. Mayer & Murray, 2002). Second, it is common for the literature to include reports of treatment outcomes for only a small number of patients, perhaps none of whom exhibit precisely the same clinical presentation as the patient for whom the clinician is considering implementing the treatment. Thus, there are likely to be occasions when clinicians find it necessary to modify treatment procedures. Clinicians are encouraged, however, to be mindful of the theoretical framework driving the treatment program, and to develop modifications accordingly.

Melodic Intonation Therapy (MIT; Helm-Estabrooks & Albert, 2004; Sparks, 2001) is a stimulation treatment developed to alleviate the spoken language problems of patients with severe nonfluent aphasia. The impetus for its design was the clinical observation that patients with aphasia who have severely restricted verbal output often are able to retrieve and produce words correctly while singing. Accordingly, Albert and colleagues (1973) created the structured, hierarchical MIT program in which patients move from initially producing words and phrases in an intoned and rhythmic manner (like singing) to eventually saying these words with natural prosody. The summary of MIT procedures listed in Table 9-6 provides an overview of the treatment program. More detailed descriptions of MIT can be found in Helm-Estabrooks and Albert (2004) or in the commercially available MIT kit (Helm-Estabrooks, Nicholas, & Morgan, 1989), which includes specific therapy instructions, picture stimuli, scoring sheets, and videotaped examples. The results of several investigations indicate that MIT can improve production of trained words and phrases in patients representing a variety of aphasia profiles (Baker, 2000; Bonakdarpour, Eftekharzadeh, & Ashayeri, 2003; Goldfarb & Bader, 1979). Generalization in terms of increased phrase lengths, higher informational content, and improved lexical retrieval on untrained speech tasks and stimuli is most likely, however, only in patients with nonfluent aphasia whose lesions spare the temporal lobe, and who relatedly have relatively good auditory comprehension (Bonakdarpour et al., 2003; Naeser & Helm-Estabrooks, 1985; Sparks, Helm, & Albert, 1974). MIT also has been shown effective when: (1) caregivers were trained to administer the treatment protocol (Goldfarb & Bader, 1979), (2) it was adapted for other languages (Bonakdarpour et al., 2003; Popovici, Mihailescu, & Voinescu, 1992), and (3) it was modified by a music therapist for patients with profound verbal output impairments who did not benefit from the more traditional MIT format (Baker, 2000). Whether the verbal output improvements associated with MIT are a product of enhanced lexical-semantic access or motor speech recovery continues to be examined (Square, Martin, & Bose, 2001).

Cognitive Neuropsychological Approaches to Treating Lexical-Semantic Deficits

The most recent trend in treating lexical-semantic deficits has been to utilize therapies based upon cognitive neuropsychological models of language processing (see Chapter 1). Two general categories of model-based treatments have thus far been developed and evaluated: semantic-based treatments, which aim to remediate problems related to the integrity of or access to semantic or conceptual representations, and phonological-based treatments, which focus on deficits related to breakdowns within or in accessing phonological representations. Both of these approaches are described below in terms of specific therapy activities and current empirical support.

Table 9-6. Levels and Steps to Administering Melodic Intonation Therapy

LEVEL	STEP	BRIEF DESCRIPTION
1	1 – Humming	The clinician hums a tonal pattern for the target word or phrase while pointing to a picture or other cue related to the target. While the clinician hums the tonal pattern, he/she also taps the patient's left hand once for each syllable. No patient response is required at this level.
	2 – Unison singing	The clinician and patient hum or intone the target word or phrase together while the clinician taps the patient's hand.
	3 – Unison singing with fading	Same as previous step except halfway through the word or phrase the clinician stops intoning.
	4 – Immediate repetition	The patient repeats the clinician's model of the intoned and tapped word or phrase. During the patient's production the clinician still taps the patient's hand.
	5 – Response to a probe question	After the patient successfully repeats the intoned word or phrase, the clinician asks the patient an intoned question pertaining to the word or phrase (e.g., "What did you ask for?" for the target "Coffee, please."). The clinician may still tap the patient's hand when the patient answers the question with the intoned target.
2	1 – Introduce the target	Same as Step 1 of Level 1.
	2 – Unison with fading	Same as Step 3 of Level 1.
	3 – Delayed repetition	The patient repeats the clinician's model of the intoned and tapped word or phrase after a delay of approximately 6 seconds. During the patient's production, the clinician still taps the patient's hand.
	4 – Response to a probe question	Approximately 6 seconds after the patient successfully completes Step 3, the clinician intones a probe question to elicit another production of the intoned target by the patient.
3	1 – Delayed repetition	Same as Step 3 of Level 2.
	2 – Introduce sprechgesang	The clinician models the target word or phrase in sprechgesang (speaking with accentuated rhythm and stress, but normal intonation or pitch) and taps the patient's hand. No patient response is required at this level.
	3 – Sprechgesang with fading	Like Step 2 of Level 2, except sprechgesang rather than intoning is used.
	4 – Delayed spoken repetition	The patient repeats with normal speech prosody the clinician's spoken model of the target word or phrase after a delay of approximately 6 seconds. No hand-tapping cue is provided.
	5 – Response to a probe question	Like Step 4 of Level 2, except both the clinician's question and the patient's response should be produced with normal speech prosody.

Semantic Treatment Approaches

Several treatments for spoken or written word processing difficulties have been developed to strengthen semantic representations, access to or from semantic representations, or both. Semantic-level treatments should theoretically evoke improvements in *both* comprehension and production (Rapp & Caramazza, 1998). That is, according to many cognitive neuropsychological models of language, only one set of semantic representations is proposed to support comprehension and production of both spoken and written language. Thus, strengthening semantic representations, the organization of these representations, or both should positively affect both comprehension and production abilities. Specific tasks that are frequently used to target semantic processing skills include:

1. sorting or matching picture or word cards by semantic categories or associations;

2. spoken or written word-to-picture matching tasks in which distracter items are semantically related to the target items (e.g., for the target "hamburger," distracters might include "hot dog," "sandwich," and "ketchup");

3. spoken or written naming tasks in which one or more semantic cues such as the superordinate category, function, attributes, or semantic associates of the target item are provided to elicit the correct response (for a list of semantic cues, see Table 9-5);

4. spoken or written phrase or sentence completion tasks;

5. answering spoken or written semantically based questions about the target items (e.g., for the target "hamburger," questions might be "Do you eat hamburgers for breakfast?" or "Do you boil hamburgers?");

6. matching pictures or written words to spoken definitions; and

7. completing odd-one-out tasks in which the picture or written word that does not belong with the other pictures or words must be identified.

Few studies have examined whether these types of semantic tasks can help address auditory comprehension problems related to lexical-semantic processing deficits. Furthermore, the investigations that have been completed thus far have produced mixed results. For example, Jacobs and Thompson(1992) provided a series of semantic comprehension tasks to a patient with global aphasia and found only nominal improvements in his ability to identify spoken words and sort pictures of items from trained semantic categories; their patient also displayed little generalization to untrained comprehension or production tasks. In contrast, two other studies reported remarkable improvements in auditory comprehension when similar semantic-based tasks were used (Behrmann & Lieberthal, 1989; Grayson, Hilton, & Franklin, 1997). The patients in these investigations, however, appeared to have less severe and more circumscribed deficits compared to those of Jacobs and Thompson's (1992) patient. Therefore, further research is needed to resolve these inconsistent findings pertaining to the effects of semantic treatments on auditory, lexical-semantic comprehension deficits.

In terms of reading comprehension, a few semantic-based treatment approaches have been developed to increase patients' reliance on whole-word reading, which is also referred to as the lexical-semantic route for reading comprehension (Rothi & Moss, 1992; Friedman & Lott, 2000). In one treatment, patients, particularly those who solely rely on a slow and thus inefficient letter-by-letter reading strategy, are briefly (e.g., 50 ms) shown a written word, typically on a computer screen, and then asked to do one or more of the following: (1) read the word aloud, (2) determine if the word belongs to a target semantic category, (3) decide if the stimulus was a real or made-up word, or (4) determine if the word was part of an orally presented sentence. Improvements such as increased reading rates, improved recognition of trained words, and improved oral reading of trained and untrained words have been reported. Because less positive outcomes also have been reported (e.g., Maher et al., 1998), further research is necessary to identify which patients are most likely to benefit from this type of reading treatment.

Multiple Oral Rereading (MOR; Beeson, 1998; Beeson & Insalaco, 1998) is another treatment designed to increase use of whole-word reading in patients who rely on letter-by-letter reading. In MOR, patients read aloud repeatedly a preselected text to increase their reading rate. It is hypothesized that because repeated readings will allow increased familiarity with the content and syntactic structure of the text, patients will be able to shift over time to the more efficient whole-word reading strategy. Whereas patients have achieved faster text-reading rates following MOR (Beeson, 1998; Beeson & Insalaco, 1998), whether or not their reading comprehension was enhanced was not examined. Accordingly, Mayer and Murray (2002) developed a modified version of MOR to encourage text comprehension by having their patient answer a set of questions following each reading aloud of target passages. Despite the addition of these comprehension questions, their patient demonstrated improvements only in reading rate. These researchers identified several factors that may have limited their ability to identify or elicit comprehension improvements, including the low intensity of their treatment schedule and the use of inordinately difficult reading probe passages (i.e., probes were at a Grade 15 level, whereas treatment passages were near a Grade 9 level). Therefore, although MOR has consistently been found to improve reading rate in patients with a variety of symptom profiles, further investigations are needed to delineate the effects of this treatment on reading comprehension and to determine whether or not MOR is any more effective than simply practicing reading on a regular basis.

In contrast to the limited database pertaining to the effects of semantic treatments on spoken or written lexical-semantic comprehension, numerous studies have examined whether these treatments can ameliorate lexical-semantic production deficits, particularly spoken naming impairments (Doesborgh et al., 2004; Drew & Thompson, 1999; Ennis, 2001; Le Dorze, Boulay, Gaudreau, & Brassard,

1994; Wambaugh, 2003; Wambaugh et al., 2001, 2002). In these investigations, patients were provided one or more of the previously described semantic-based therapy activities, such as grouping pictures into semantic categories, answering semantic judgment questions, or completing naming tasks with the provision of semantic prompts (e.g., superordinate or attribute cue). Collectively, the results of these studies indicate that semantic treatments can evoke positive gains in the spoken word retrieval of patients with aphasia, regardless of what processing deficits (i.e., semantic, phonological, or both) underlie their naming impairments. Whereas initial research suggested that semantic therapies are superior to phonological therapies in terms of the durability of treatment effects on spoken naming abilities (Nickels & Best, 1996), more recent data do not support this contention (Doesborgh et al., 2004; Ennis, 2001; Wambaugh, 2003).

One specific semantic treatment that has been the subject of a growing number of studies is **Semantic Feature Analysis** (SFA; Boyle, 2001; Coelho, McHugh, & Boyle, 2000; Lowell, Beeson, & Holland, 1995). In SFA, a chart such as that shown in Figure 9-2 is used to help patients generate words that are semantically related to the target item. More specifically, patients are shown a picture and asked to name that picture. Regardless of their response accuracy, they are asked to come up with words that will fill each bubble on the chart, and these words in turn are written onto the chart either by the clinician or the patients themselves. If patients have difficulty generating these semantic features, the clinician provides them and adds them to the chart. Once the chart has been completed, patients are again asked to name the target item; if they still are unable to name the item, the clinician models the appropriate label. The goal of the SFA is to activate the semantic network (via elicitation of semantic features) to which the target item belongs, and this activation in turn should facilitate access to, and thus production of, the target item. Additionally, it is hoped that patients will begin to generate independently semantic features to self-cue themselves in communicative activities outside of the therapy room.

With SFA, patients with aphasia (Boyle, 2001; Conley & Coelho, 2003; Lowell et al., 1995), as well as those with naming difficulties subsequent to TBI (Coelho et al., 2000; Massaro & Tompkins, 1992), have shown improved spoken naming of trained and untrained items with good maintenance of these improvements. Some generalization to discourse also has been reported (Coelho et al., 2000). Comparable positive outcomes have been observed when a semantic specification treatment similar to SFA was applied to improve written naming in a patient with semantic-level deficits (Hillis, 1991). That is, this patient demonstrated improved written naming of trained items, and generalization to written naming of untrained exemplars of trained categories and to spoken naming and auditory comprehension of trained and untrained exemplars of trained categories. Because varying degrees of improvement and generalization were reported in previous SFA studies, further investigations are needed to identify which patient (e.g., aphasia severity, aphasia type, etiology) and procedural factors (e.g., treatment length) are most influential on SFA outcomes.

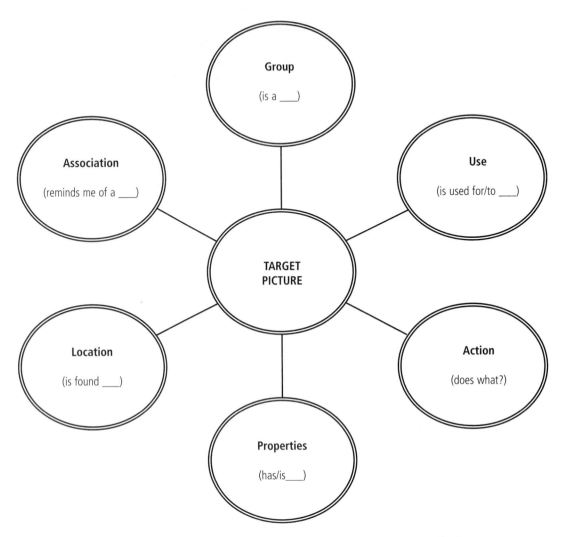

Figure 9-2. Example of a chart that may be used during Semantic Feature Analysis treatment.

How to maximize generalization effects associated with semantic treatments recently has been explored by Kiran and Thompson (2003). These researchers proposed that generalization could be enhanced by attending to the complexity of the trained stimuli. That is, given that training more "complex" syntactic structures (e.g., Thompson et al., 2003) and phonological forms (e.g., Gierut, 2001) has been shown to evoke improvements in untrained, simpler syntactic structures and phonological forms, respectively, Kiran and Thompson (2003) hypothesized that training atypical (i.e., more complex) category exemplars should result in improved naming of untrained, typical (i.e., less complex) category exemplars. These researchers provided four patients with moderately severe aphasia a semantic-based naming treatment that involved both comprehension and production activities (e.g., picture sorting, semantic judgment questions). They found that when atypical items of a target category were trained, generalization to untrained typical and intermediate exemplars of that treated category occurred. In contrast, nominal generalization was observed when typical items were trained. More recently, Mayer and colleagues (2004) attempted to elicit these complexity effects in three patients with severe to profound aphasia. In contrast to Kiran and Thompson, Mayer et al. found only item-specific training effects with no generalization to untrained exemplars, regardless of whether atypical or typical exemplars were treated. It is important to note, however, that Mayer and colleagues utilized a more traditional cueing hierarchy treatment because the semantic judgment questions used by Kiran and Thompson were beyond the comprehension capabilities of Mayer and colleagues' patients. Accordingly, further research is needed to determine if: (1) training complex stimuli evokes generalization in only certain patient populations, or, (2) the combination of a semantic-based treatment *and* training complex stimuli is necessary to evoke generalization.

Side Bar

Should clinicians focus only on one treatment strategy?

Describing intervention strategies individually can be misleading because of the potential implication that there is a single treatment that is "best" for each patient. Instead, clinical experience shows us that most patients with neurogenic language disorders exhibit impairments of many linguistic processes that are most effectively addressed with different intervention strategies. Consider Helen, a 45-year old woman who had experienced a stroke resulting in moderate anomia, alexia, and agraphia. During assessment it was revealed that Helen exhibited impairments both in semantic and phonological domains. Further, she displayed mild right-sided inattention. Helen's goal was to return to her former position as a volunteer receptionist for a local nonprofit agency. Treatment therefore emphasized the skills pertinent to this position (e.g., answering the telephone, writing down phone numbers). Because Helen's word-finding was facilitated by visual and/or kinesthetic cueing (i.e., writing the word with a pencil or spelling the word in the air), treatment initially targeted developing this compensatory strategy as a means of facilitating verbal expression as well as addressing some of the skills relevant to her vocational goals. Unfortunately, it soon became apparent that Helen also experienced difficulty with grapheme-to-phoneme conversion. Thus, even while the physical act of attempting to write the word facilitated her verbal expression, her written production of the target word was often spelled incorrectly. Moreover, her attempts to read back what she had written were limited by her right-sided inattention. Ultimately, Helen devised separate strategies for spoken and written expression. To facilitate accurate recording of telephone messages, Helen asked speakers to spell names letter-by-letter, which she would then read back letter-by-letter. She used a similar strategy for phone numbers.

Phonological Treatment Approaches

Phonological treatments are designed to strengthen the integrity of or facilitate access to phonological representations. When comprehension is being trained, spoken word-to-picture or object matching and/or spoken word-to-written word matching might be used. To stress phonological processing skills, distracter items for these tasks should be phonologically related to the target stimuli. For example, for the target "phone," distracter items might be "cone," "fawn," and "fin." Additional tasks include answering phonological judgment questions (e.g., for the target "phone," "Does this word rhyme with moan?" "Does this word have one syllable?"), or completing phonemic perception and discrimination tasks (see Treatment of Segmental Impairments section of this chapter). Although these treatment activities are commonly used in daily clinical practice, there is a dearth of research regarding their potential effects on patients' lexical-semantic comprehension abilities. When these tasks have been used in formal investigations, they were typically administered in concert with or subsequent to semantically based comprehension activities (e.g., Ennis, 2001; Grayson et al., 1997). Accordingly, the effects of phonological tasks by themselves on lexical-semantic comprehension, including to what extent they can evoke generalization to untrained stimuli and activities, remains to be proven.

In contrast, many researchers have used phonologically based treatments to remediate lexical-semantic production in patients with aphasia. When production is being trained, one or more of the following tasks might be utilized: (1) repeating, (2) reading aloud, (3) making phonological judgments, and (4) naming following or in concert with the provision of one or a hierarchy of phonologically based cues (see Table 9-5). Extensive research indicates that phonological treatments can facilitate spoken word retrieval in patients whose naming deficits have been traced to problems at primarily phonological output levels (DeDe et al., 2003; Murray & Kim, 2005), those with predominately semantic-level problems (Raymer, Thompson, Jacobs, & Le Grand, 1993; Wambaugh, 2003), and as those with problems with the connection between semantic and phonological levels (Hickin, Best, Herbert, Howard, & Osborne, 2002; Robson, Marshall, Pring, & Chiat, 1998a). Inconsistent findings, however, have been reported concerning whether phonological treatment effects are maintained over time (e.g., Nickels & Best, 1996 vs. Wambaugh et al., 2001) or generalize to untrained items and modalities (e.g., DeDe et al., 2003 vs. Raymer et al., 1993). Factors that may influence the degree and persistence of improvements following phonological treatment include the part of speech being trained (e.g., noun vs. verb; Wambaugh et al., 2002), and the degree to which patients actively participate in choosing or self-generating the cue (DeDe et al., 2003; Hickin et al., 2002).

Combined Semantic and Phonological Treatment Approaches

Review of the effects of semantic- versus phonological-based treatments indicates that there does not appear to be a direct relationship between type of lexical-semantic deficit (i.e., semantic level vs. phonological level vs. both) and the most effective or efficient treatment approach. For example, investigators have found that patients with phonological-level deficits are not the only ones to benefit from phonological-based treatment (e.g., Raymer et al., 1993). Accordingly, for many patients a therapy program that combines semantic and phonological protocols will be most efficient. Indeed, in the research literature, the most remarkable improvements in lexical-semantic comprehension, production, or both were often observed when patients received both semantic- and phonological-based activities (e.g., Grayson et al., 1997; Le Dorze et al., 1994).

MORPHOSYNTACTIC TREATMENTS

Whereas substantial research has aimed at qualifying and quantifying morphosyntactic processing deficits associated with aphasia (e.g., Bastiaanse & Edwards, 2001; Caplan & Hanna, 1998), a more limited literature has examined treatments for these deficits. Because there is a dearth of research pertaining to the integrity of morphosyntactic processing following TBI, RHD, or onset of dementia as well as treatments for these possible deficits, our discussion will focus on morphosyntactic procedures developed for patients with aphasia; whether these procedures can or should be used with other neurogenic patient populations remains to be proven.

The Linguistic Stimulation Approach to Treating Morphosyntactic Deficits

Stimulation treatments for morphosyntactic deficits often involve determining a hierarchy of difficulty for comprehending and producing morphosyntactic structures, and then, in treatment, progressing through that hierarchy from the easiest to the most complex structures. Morphosyntactic production deficits are typically remediated by having patients practice producing sentences that include the target morphosyntactic structure. Morphosyntactic comprehension deficits may be addressed through activities that require patients to identify the target morphosyntactic structures, such as pointing to the picture that corresponds to the target sentence or manipulating objects so as to act out the target sentence.

Although stimulation activities to target morphosyntactic production or comprehension are frequently described in textbooks and therapy workbooks (e.g., Duffy & Coelho, 2001), empirical investigation of the efficacy of these tasks has almost exclusively focused on production treatments. For example, one of the more popular morphosyntactic stimulation approaches described in the research literature is the Helm Elicited Program for Syntax Stimulation (HELPSS; Helm-Estabrooks, 1981; Helm-Estabrooks & Albert, 1991). Based upon earlier research by Gleason and colleagues (1975), the HELPSS trains production of the hierarchy of sentence constructions shown in Table 9-7. Each sentence construction is practiced

Table 9-7. Hierarchies of Syntactic Constructions for the Helm Elicited Program for Syntax Stimulation (HELPSS) and the Sentence Production Program for Aphasia (SPPA)

SENTENCE CONSTRUCTION TYPE (FROM EASIEST TO MOST COMPLEX)	EXAMPLES
Imperative intransitive	"Lie down." "Wake up."
Imperative transitive	"Wash the dishes." "Drink your milk."
Wh-interrogative	"What are you writing?" "Where are my shoes?"
Wh- interrogative: what and who (SPPA only)	"Who is coming?" "What are you watching?"
Wh- interrogative: where and when (SPPA only)	"Where is the hospital?" "When are we landing?"
Declarative transitive	"She cleans teeth." "He teaches school."
Declarative intransitive	"She skates." "He swims."
Comparative	"They are funnier." "She is taller."
Passive	"The suitcases were lost." "The car was towed."
Yes/no questions	"Did you buy the paper?" "Is it sad?"
Direct and indirect object	"They give Pat a cake." "He reads his grandchild a story."
Embedded sentences	"She wanted him to be healthy." "She wanted him to be rich."
Future	"He will hike." "He will sleep."

Note. Only those sentence constructions in bold font are trained as part of SPPA. HELPSS trains those in bold and regular font, unless otherwise noted.

at two levels: Level A, which elicits delayed imitation, and Level B, which elicits a spontaneous response via story completion cues. At both Level A and Level B the patient is read a short story and shown a picture depicting that story. For example, to elicit the Direct and Indirect Object sentence "They give Pat a cake" at Level A, the clinician would read the following: "It's Pat's birthday. Her friends want to celebrate, so they give Pat a cake. What do they do?" (Helm-Estabrooks & Albert, 1991, p. 226). To elicit that same sentence at Level B, the clinician would read "It's Pat's birthday and her friends want to celebrate, so what do they do?" (Helm-

Estabrooks & Albert, 1991, p. 226). Treatment proceeds by first training at Level A the simplest sentence construction that the patient has difficulty producing. Once the patient completes Level A probes for that sentence construction with 90% accuracy, Level B probes for that sentence construction are introduced. When the patient can complete Level B probes with 90% accuracy, Level A probes for the next most difficult sentence construction in the hierarchy are trained. Treatment continues until the patient has progressed through the hierarchy of sentence types. More recently, Helm-Estabrooks and Nicholas (2000) published a revised version of HELPSS, referred to as Sentence Production Program for Aphasia (SPPA). Differences between HELPSS and SPPA include: (1) SPPA targets only eight sentence constructions (see Table 9-7) by excluding HELPSS sentence constructions such as passives and embedded clauses that are viewed as less applicable in daily communication interactions and that are particularly challenging for patients with aphasia; (2) SPPA includes a similar number of exemplars for each sentence construction; and (3) SPPA stimuli revolve around a restricted set of characters who represent a range of ages and ethnicities.

There is some empirical support for using HELPSS to improve the morphosyntactic production abilities of patients with aphasia, at least those with nonfluent language profiles. For example, researchers have reported that patients with chronic Broca's aphasia demonstrate increased phrase length and sentence grammaticality in their spoken discourse following HELPSS (Fink et al., 1995; Helm-Estabrooks, Fitzpatrick, & Barresi, 1981; Helm-Estabrooks & Ramsberger, 1986b; Murray & Ray, 2001). These improvements have even been reported when HELPSS was provided over the telephone to patients who were unable to attend clinic sessions (Helm-Estabrooks & Ramsberger, 1986a). Generalization of treatment effects, however, has most frequently been limited to untrained exemplars of trained sentence constructions, rather than extending to untrained sentence constructions (e.g., Doyle, Goldstein, & Bourgeois, 1987; Fink et al., 1995). Currently, there are no published studies evaluating the efficacy of SPPA. Likewise, researchers have yet to explore whether or not HELPSS or SPPA are appropriate for patients with fluent language profiles or for written morphosyntactic deficits. Finally, given that most research has focused on stimulation treatments for morphosyntactic production impairments, the development and examination of stimulation activities that target morphosyntactic comprehension abilities are still needed.

Linguistic Theory Motivated Approaches to Treating Morphosyntactic Deficits

In contrast to stimulation morphosyntactic treatments, which tend to target sentence structures on the basis of overt impairment rather than theory, other treatment procedures have been developed to reflect current linguistic models of morphosyntactic processing in adults with or without aphasia. In particular, two theoretically motivated approaches, **mapping therapy** and **Treatment of Underlying Forms** (TUFF), have been created to treat deficits of grammatical production, comprehension, or both, and to date have proven effective for at least some patients with aphasia.

The theoretical impetus of mapping therapy is Garrett's model (1988) of sentence production. According to Garrett, there are two levels of representation that contribute to the final production or comprehension of a sentence: (1) the Functional or semantic level at which words are assigned a thematic role (e.g., agent or who is doing the action), and (2) the Positional level at which words and morphemes are arranged into syntactic frames and assigned phonological forms. Advocates of mapping therapy propose that patients with agrammatism experience problems "mapping relations between the abstract functional level and surface syntax at the positional level" (Rochon & Reichman, 2003, p. 203). These difficulties in turn result in problems processing sentences like those shown below. Sentence (1) is noncanonical (i.e., the second vs. first noun is the agent or action "doer"), and sentence (2) is reversible (i.e., either noun might be the agent). Most difficult would be noncanonical, reversible sentences like that shown in sentence (3).

1. passive sentence with noncanonical order: The guitar was played by Dylan.
2. reversible sentence: Dylan was chasing the dog.
3. noncanonical, reversible sentence: Dylan was chased by the dog.

The overall goal of mapping therapy, therefore, is to improve patients' ability to map or understand the connection between the Positional and Functional levels of sentences such as those exemplified above (i.e., noncanonical and/or reversible), which in turn is expected to alleviate their grammatical comprehension and/or production impairments (Byng, 1988; Fink et al., 1998; Rochon & Reichman, 2003, 2004; Schwartz, Saffran, Fink, Myers, & Martin, 1994). Although there has been some divergence in the activities and language behaviors targeted during treatment (e.g., target sentence structure, comprehension vs. production), most mapping therapies have utilized a sentence query procedure to increase patients' awareness of the relationship between words' thematic roles and their location within a sentence. For example, steps for a mapping therapy session might include the following:

1. Present a pictured scene and/or a spoken or written model of the target sentence structure (e.g., "The nurse was greeted by the doctor."), and ask the patient to identify the action (i.e., verb) by manipulating objects to demonstrate the action and/or underlining or saying the appropriate word in the sentence stimulus;
2. Next, require the patient to identify who was doing the action (i.e., agent) by pointing to the correct object/figure and/or underlining or saying the appropriate word in the sentence stimulus;

3. Instruct the patient to identify who the action was done to (i.e., theme) by pointing to the correct object/figure and/or underlining or saying the appropriate word in the sentence stimulus;

4. If sentence production is being targeted, the final step would be to have the patient produce the correct sentence structure in response to the picture stimulus.

The results of several treatment studies indicate that mapping therapy can positively affect the sentence processing abilities of patients with nonfluent (Byng, 1988; Fink, Schwartz, & Myers, 1998; Schwartz et al., 1994) or mixed (Rochon & Reichman, 2003; 2004) aphasia profiles. That is, patients have been found to improve on trained sentence structures (i.e., primarily passives and/or object clefts) with generalization to untrained exemplars of the trained structures. Additionally, when sentence comprehension abilities have been trained, some generalization to production at the sentence or discourse level has been observed (Byng, 1988; Rochon & Reichman, 2004; Schwartz et al., 1994). In contrast, studies have not demonstrated clearly that sentence production training improves sentence comprehension or that either sentence production or comprehension training generalizes to untrained sentence structures (Rochon & Reichman, 2003).

TUFF, previously referred to as Linguistic Specific Treatment, is based upon Chomsky's government binding theory (for a review, see Shapiro, 1997) and the proposition that patients with agrammatism have difficulty processing grammatically complex sentences in which there has been phrase movement (e.g., passives, sentences with embedding) (Ballard & Thompson, 1999; Jacobs & Thompson, 2000; Thompson et al., 1998, 2003). An additional tenet of TUFF is that targeting syntactically complex sentence types, in particular those with noncanonical order (i.e., phrase movement), should effect generalization to syntactically related, but less complex sentence types. For example, treating sentences with wh-movement such as that shown in sentence (1) below should result in improved processing of other less complex wh-movement sentence forms, such as that shown in sentence (2), but evoke no change in processing sentences with other, unrelated forms of movement, such as that shown in sentence (3).

1. More complex wh-movement structure: $[_{IP}I$ know $[_{CP}$who$_i$ $[_{IP}$Dylan kissed *trace$_i$*$]]]$

2. Less complex wh-movement structure: $[_{CP}$Who$_i$ has $[_{IP}$Dylan kissed *trace$_i$*$]]$

3. Unrelated, noun phrase movement structure: $[_{IP}$The *girl$_i$* was kissed *trace$_i$* by Dylan$]$

The overall goal of TUFF, therefore, is to remediate patients' ability to process phrase movement by increasing their awareness and understanding of verbs, verb argument structure, and how certain sentence constituents move to form noncanonical sentence types, and by requiring them to practice producing noncanonical sentence types. Specific treatment steps include the following:

1. Provide a spoken model of the target sentence structure (e.g., "I know who the girl splashed."), and require the patient to produce a similar sentence with the same sentence form that corresponds to a picture stimulus (e.g., "I know who the boy splashed.");

2. Regardless of the patient's accuracy in step (a), present a set of written word/phrase cards that make up the canonical (i.e., active form) sentence (e.g., "The boy splashed the girl."), and have the patient identify the verb, the agent (e.g., "the boy"), and the theme (e.g., "the girl");

3. Provide the additional written word/phrase cards necessary to complete the target sentence structure, and model how to arrange all the cards to form the target sentence structure (e.g., "I know who the boy splashed."). Require the patient to read this target sentence aloud and then identify which words within it represent the verb, agent, and theme;

4. Shuffle the word/phrase cards, and then have the patient form and read aloud the target sentence structure;

5. Remove the word/phrase cards, and have the patient provide the target sentence structure.

Several investigations have been conducted to determine the effects of TUFF on the grammatical production abilities of patients with Broca's or nonfluent aphasia profiles (Ballard & Thompson, 1999; Jacobs, 2001; Jacobs & Thompson, 2000; Thompson et al., 1998, 2003). Data from these studies indicate that TUFF can evoke improvements in these patients' production of trained and linguistically related, untrained sentence structures. Modest generalization to untrained production tasks (i.e., narrative discourse) and output modalities (i.e., writing) also has been reported. Notably, less impressive findings were obtained when patients with fluent or mixed aphasia profiles and, in a few cases, with concomitant cognitive deficits were provided TUFF (Murray, Ballard, & Karcher, 2004); whereas these patients did acquire the trained complex sentence structures, they demonstrated nominal or erratic generalization effects. These results suggest that patients with more isolated grammatical difficulties may be the best candidates for TUFF.

The above review indicates that morphosyntactic treatments that are motivated by linguistic theory can be effective in improving the deficits of sentence comprehension, production, or both associated with chronic aphasia. With few exceptions (e.g., Rochon & Reichman, 2004; Murray et al., 2004), however, the effects of these treatments have been explored with only patients who have Broca's or nonfluent aphasia. Consequently, further research is clearly necessary to determine if these treatments are equally effective for patients with other language profiles, to identify what treatment adaptations may be necessary when working with these patients, or both.

PRAGMATICS AND DISCOURSE TREATMENTS

Although a rich literature describes the nature of pragmatic impairments common in patients with neurogenic language disorders (see Chapter 2), and a number of tools are available to aid in identifying such impairments (see Chapter 5), comparatively fewer data exist to guide treating pragmatic impairments. Nonetheless, clinicians can refer to a number of theory-driven intervention approaches that have been described (Adams, Lloyd, Aldred, & Baxendale, 2003; Braunling-McMorrow, Lloyd, & Fralish, 1986; Ducharme, 1999; Halper, Cherney, & Burns, 1996; Johnson, Simpson, & O' Connell, 2003; Myers, 1999; Sohlberg & Mateer, 2001a; Tompkins, 1995; Wiseman-Hakes, Stewart, Wasserman, & Schuller, 1998), as well as develop individualized interventions based on current theoretical models of pragmatics.

Pragmatic aspects of communication are highly context-dependent and are further influenced by cultural norms and individual subjectivity (McGann & Werven, 1999). These features of pragmatic behaviors have several implications for planning treatment activities. First, clinicians should be mindful of subjectivity and cultural variations when selecting treatment goals, stimuli, and activities. For example, cultures can vary in terms of which discourse genres are more highly valued, encountered, or both, and thus the patient's culture must be considered when choosing what genre will be targeted in treatment. Likewise, pragmatic conventions of some cultures are particularly sensitive to age or class differences between communication participants, whereas other cultures may be more or less accepting of irony or sarcasm as acceptable communication styles. The nature of prosodic markings also differs across cultures and dialects. Accordingly, if the clinician does not share the culture, dialect, or both of the patient, or if the clinician has idiosyncratic pragmatic behaviors, it may be helpful to utilize standardized treatment materials appropriate to the patient. Recorded stimuli (e.g., Tompkins, 1995) and standardized scenarios (e.g., Bayles & Tomoeda, 1993; Nicholas & Brookshire, 1993) may be used, or if such materials are inappropriate, the clinician may choose to invite other individuals whose communication behaviors share the same pragmatic conventions as the patient to participate in treatment activities (e.g., Wiseman-Hakes, Stewart, Wasserman, & Schuller, 1998).

Second, because pragmatic aspects of communication are highly influenced by context, clinicians may find it difficult to address pragmatic skills in relatively context-free activities such as stimulus-response drills (Cherney & Halper, 2000). Instead, clinicians will find that treatment activities, such as role-playing, perspective-taking, and group treatment, that incorporate rich contextual cues are particularly useful in this area of treatment (Holland & Hinckley, 2002; Hopper & Holland, 1998; Sohlberg & Mateer, 2001a). In fact, some texts incorporate treatment of pragmatics into the discussion of treatment at the ICF levels of activity and participation (see Chapter 11), particularly when addressing pragmatic aspects of communication for patients with aphasia (Holland, 1996; Holland & Hinckley, 2002; Wright & Newhoff, 2005).

Finally, it is helpful to remember that many pragmatic conventions are learned implicitly, that is, without conscious awareness. Although many adults experienced direct instruction in phonics, reading, writing, and grammar, it is unlikely that they had school coursework on appropriate loudness levels, how to alter intonation to change sentence meaning, how close to stand to individuals when speaking (i.e., proxemics), or other pragmatic behaviors. Thus, developing metalinguistic awareness of these aspects of communication may be the first step in addressing specific pragmatic skills (Sohlberg & Mateer, 2001a; Tompkins, 1995). Clinicians should also consider that given the automatic nature of many pragmatic processes, metalinguistic tasks, like those used to evaluate and remediate pragmatic problems, may mask underlying pragmatic competence (Tompkins, 1995). Detailed discussion of these issues and the implication for assessment and treatment can be found in Tompkins (1991) and Tompkins, Bloise, Timko, and Baumgaertner (1994).

The following sections of this chapter discuss strategies for addressing various aspects of pragmatic comprehension and production. Although the discussion is organized with respect to specific pragmatic skills, many skill areas overlap; consequently, several treatment strategies are appropriate for addressing a variety of pragmatic symptoms. Because disruptions in pragmatic behaviors are most apparent in individuals with RHD and TBI, clinicians also may wish to consult the more detailed discussions of pragmatic treatment included in texts that exclusively focus on these populations (e.g., Halper et al., 1996; Myers, 1999; Sohlberg & Mateer, 2001a; Tompkins, 1995).

Figurative Language and Alternative Meanings Treatments

Many linguistic messages are ambiguous or have two or more alternative interpretations, depending on the communicative context. Lexical-semantic ambiguity results when single words have more than one meaning. For example, the homograph "block" can be used to denote a child's toy, a city division, or a strategic movement in the game of football. Similarly, the homophones "hair" and "hare" have different meanings. Linguistic ambiguity may be most apparent in the case of figurative language, which includes metaphors (e.g., "He's a snake.") and idioms (e.g., "She has her hands full."). When linguistic ambiguity is present, the task for the listener is to determine which possible meaning is most appropriate to the communicative context, keeping in mind that the communicative context includes information pertaining to: (1) the current physical environment (e.g., location of current communicative interaction, number of communicative partners, time of day), (2) the social and cognitive environment (e.g., social status of communicative partners, amount of knowledge shared among the communicative partners, emotional status of communicative partners), and (3) the verbal and nonverbal environment (e.g., colloquial vs. formal vocabulary, body language and/or facial expressions of communicative partners).

An essential first step to remediating difficulties with figurative language and other forms of alternate meanings is to assure appropriate awareness of linguistic ambiguity. The clinician can identify examples of homographs, idioms, and metaphors to prompt discussion of alternative interpretations, including consideration of the contexts in which each meaning is most likely to apply. As Myers (1999) noted, however, many patients who show apparent deficits in interpreting idioms during structured clinical tasks demonstrate greater competence when figurative language is used in conversation. For these patients, targeting awareness of lexical ambiguity may not be necessary. Instead, if it is clear the patient understands the concept of ambiguity, the clinician can devise scenarios and have the patient determine the most appropriate interpretation of messages within a given context. If necessary, the clinician can assist the patient in identifying the most important contextual features to assist in determining the meaning of ambiguous messages (Penn et al., 1997; Tompkins, 1995). Myers (1999) described a variety of activities for targeting activation of alternative meanings (e.g., developing semantic associations for homographs: stand/sit, stand/platform), as well as suppression of inappropriate interpretations (e.g., selecting the appropriate interpretation when several possible alternatives have been identified).

Although patients with neurogenic language disorders may exhibit reduced use of figurative language, this characteristic may interfere minimally with communication because explicit language is generally easily understood by communication partners. However, if it is deemed appropriate, clinicians may target production by devising scenarios in which the use of idioms, metaphors, and other forms of figurative language is appropriate. Treatment might begin with forced choice, in which the patient identifies the expression that best matches a presented context. For example, presented with an illustration of a man with money overflowing from his wallet, the patient selects the most appropriate metaphor from the choices, "He's loaded," "He's a gas," or "He's coldhearted." Eventually, the patient is responsible for generating independently appropriate metaphors/idioms for pictured, written, or live-action stimuli and scenarios.

Training alternative meanings also may be necessary to help patients apply newly acquired language skills or strategies to a variety of communicative settings. For example, Robson and colleagues (1998b; 2001) found that although their patients with severe aphasia and jargon were able to acquire a small written vocabulary via a writing treatment program, few of these patients used their written vocabulary during daily communicative activities. Therefore, these researchers added a "message therapy" to their writing treatment protocol that included: (1) tasks to show explicitly how patients could use their "new" words to represent more complex messages (e.g., "shoe" might not only be used to label the object, but also to ask for help finding one's shoes, to indicate that one wants to go for a walk, to indicate that one's feet are cold, etc.), and (2) tasks to practice communicating these more complex messages to their daily communicative partners. Following the inclusion of these tasks that directly targeted the communicative uses (or alternative meanings) of trained written vocabulary, Robson et al. found remarkable improvements in the functional communication abilities of their patients with severe aphasia.

Discourse Treatment

As illustrated in Chapters 1 and 7, the term "discourse" covers a broad spectrum of communication behaviors. Although treatment activities addressing discourse comprehension and/or production may target a number of specific skills, the basic strategies are quite similar across skill areas. In particular, discourse treatments by necessity incorporate extended text, messages, and/or exchanges and emphasize the construction, integration, or both of meaning beyond the sentence level. Clinicians may find that many of the treatment activities described in this section lend themselves well to targeting several discourse skills simultaneously.

Topic Coherence and Cohesion

Topic coherence and cohesion skills are vital to effective discourse production. Because these skills rely on lexical-semantic and grammatical markers, it may be helpful to target deficits in lexical-semantics, morphosyntax, or both prior to or concurrently with discourse targets. Many patients with discourse deficits will benefit from treatment activities that facilitate awareness of their coherence and cohesion errors (e.g., abrupt topic shift, inappropriate use of ellipsis or vague reference), as well as their understanding of strategies to enhance their coherence (e.g., use of disjunctive markers), cohesion (e.g., use of synonyms instead of exact repetition), or both. Barrier games and story-retelling (see also Chapter 11) may provide a context not only for error detection, but also discourse production practice and self-monitoring (Busch, Brookshire, & Nicholas, 1988; Tompkins, 1995).

Because **barrier games** are particularly helpful for addressing a variety of pragmatic and discourse goals, it is appropriate to provide a more detailed description of how to set up this type of activity. The basic premise of a barrier activity is to place a solid barrier such as a game board or a large book standing on its side between the patient and the clinician or other communication partner so as to create a more "natural" communication context. For example, the barrier can create the communicative need for communication partners to establish a conversational topic, provide accurate and specific referents, and so forth. Typically, similar sets of treatment stimuli or materials are placed on the patient's and the clinician's sides of the barrier, and activities such as describing a specific stimulus (e.g., a specific person in a group photograph), giving instructions (e.g., "First, put the family reunion photo above the summer vacation photo. Second, put the graduation photo below the summer vacation photo."), or asking questions about the materials (e.g., "Do you have a picture of a short woman wearing a black hat?") are completed. Because each communication partner cannot see or, more ideally, does not know to what materials the other communication partner has access, successful communicative exchanges during barrier activities will require each partner not only to utilize specific and efficient language output, but also to pay close attention to the other partner's verbal output, as many nonverbal cues have been eliminated. Examples of the numerous discourse and pragmatic behaviors that can be practiced via barrier games include production of indirect requests, reduction of tangential comments, and use of specific vocabulary or referents (vs. nonspecific pronouns or content words).

Two aspects of topic coherence that are easily targeted in barrier games or other discourse activities are topic introduction and maintenance. Early treatment activities may be relatively didactic, with the clinician asking patients to simply identify the topic and/or main idea of a spoken or written discourse sample such as a brief story or narrative. Next, this activity may be elaborated to include sequential or concurrent stimuli for which patients must identify when new information is available, as well as when content is repeated (Tompkins, 1995). Finally, patients can practice identifying or utilizing discourse markers that indicate when new information is consistent with (e.g., "In addition. . .") , related to (e.g., "Similarly. . ."), or inconsistent/unrelated (e.g., "In contrast. . .") to the previous or current content or topic (Wiseman-Hakes et al., 1998). Early in treatment, the clinician may choose to alert the patient to coherence breakdowns in an online manner. As the discourse sequences become longer or as the patient gains skill in topic maintenance, however, video and other recordings, including dictation or written discourse, may facilitate development of online, self-evaluation skills.

To address reading comprehension deficits at the discourse level, clinicians might utilize or adapt one of the techniques used in the education literature (e.g., Penn et al., 1997; Winograd & Hare, 1988). For example, patients who have difficulty identifying relevant information or integrating information across a text could be taught to complete the following steps when reading: (1) preview headings and subheadings to identify the main ideas, (2) write down questions about those main ideas, (3) read the text so that those questions can be answered, (4) paraphrase or summarize what has been read, and (5) review the text again to assure understanding of the text and that questions were answered correctly.

Treatment of topic cohesion entails more sophisticated metalinguistics than are necessary for activities targeting topic maintenance or coherence. Effective topic cohesion requires speakers to be aware of not only the information that has been communicated, but also the specific lexical and morphosyntactic structures used to communicate the information. For example, effective use of pronouns (e.g., it, those, his) requires that the appropriate referents have been specified earlier in the discourse (e.g., referent and pronoun agree in number and gender). Likewise, an elliptical statement such as "They did." is appropriate only following a syntactically elaborated preface such as "I thought Sarah and Lucy said they'd meet us here." Although topic cohesion may be a more subtle skill than topic coherence, many of the treatment strategies discussed with respect to coherence also are appropriate for cohesion. For example, given a context-rich stimulus, the clinician can prompt the patient to identify first the topic and then to formulate one or two sentences summarizing the main ideas. As the patient elaborates the discourse sequence, specific cohesion strategies (e.g., pronouns, synonymy, ellipsis) can be targeted.

Inferencing

Inferencing, or "gleaning information that is not specifically provided" (Tompkins, 1995, p. 254), is a communicative skill frequently enlisted in discourse. Treating inferencing involves first helping the patient become aware of implied meanings. This process is very similar to what was described in earlier sections addressing awareness of ambiguity. Specifically, using picture description or story-retelling, the patient, with or without assistance from the clinician, can identify stated or explicit information. The clinician can then propose additional implied meanings or information, discussing the cues that led to each inference (Penn et al., 1997). A number of activities can provide patients with practice identifying cues leading to inference, including describing relationships among stimuli (e.g., categorizing), speculating about characters' motives, and identifying incongruities and absurdities. Ultimately, patients can be asked to draw inferences from larger discourse texts and to develop text from which listeners or readers must draw inferences.

Conversational Skills

Conversational skills are frequently considered an aspect of discourse, particularly given that effective conversations are characterized by coherence and cohesion, and may include the use of implied meanings. However, effective conversation also depends on appropriate use and comprehension of prosodic and nonverbal cues and figurative language, as well as adherence to social convention. Thus, treatment targeting conversational skills may incorporate the activities addressing these related linguistic abilities that are discussed in other sections of this chapter. In addition to these skills, turn-taking is a key conversational skill.

To increase patients' awareness of turn-taking behaviors, the clinician may first describe behaviors that signal the beginning or end of a conversational turn (e.g., significant pause, direct questions) (Tompkins, 1995; Wiseman-Hakes et al., 1998). The clinician and patient can then review audio or video recordings of conversations, identifying where specific turn-taking cues were used and whether or not the cues were effective. Similar activities can be used to address other aspects of turn taking, such as length of turn, signaling the desire to have a turn, and inappropriate interrupting (Snow & Douglas, 2000). As suggested previously for treating pragmatic targets, conversational skills may be effectively addressed during group treatment, affording patients an opportunity to evaluate and provide feedback about other participants' conversational skills while at the same time practicing their own. Reviewing videotapes or transcripts of the patient's conversations, including those occurring during group treatment, may also be helpful.

It also is important to keep in mind that as patients progress in the treatments previously described to target specific phonological, lexical-semantic, or morphosyntactic deficits, practice of trained behaviors at a conversational level should also be included. That is, many previously reviewed treatments primarily focus on training production or comprehension of language targets at the word or sentence level, with the assumption that if patients become competent at word or sentence levels, their ability to apply trained behaviors to discourse and conversation should also improve. Findings from some recent studies, however, indicate that meaningful improvements at the discourse and conversational levels are more likely when treatment specifically includes activities at these language levels (e.g., Herbert, Best, Hickin, Howard, & Osborne, 2003; Peach & Wong, 2004).

Social Conventions Treatments

Patients with TBI and certain forms of dementia (e.g., Pick's disease) are particularly prone to deficits in the social aspects of communication (see Chapter 2), although these deficits may also be observed in patients with RHD or other types of dementia (e.g., Alzheimer's disease), and less frequently in those with aphasia. Social communication incorporates behaviors related to prosody and nonverbal communication as well as discourse skills. Thus, the strategies for addressing those aspects of social skills are the same as those described in earlier sections.

A key social skill influencing the effectiveness of communication is sensitivity to the listener and to the environment (Tompkins, 1995). Typical communication exchanges, including what information is exchanged, in what detail, and with which words and grammatical structures, are strongly influenced by what each participant presupposes about the listeners, as well as by the communication context. As is true for many pragmatic behaviors, sensitivity to listener needs and contextual influences occurs relatively automatically. Patients with neurogenic language disorders, however, may need to develop greater conscious awareness of these issues, as well as explicit knowledge of how communication behaviors must be modified once listener or environmental cues are identified. The clinician may devise scenarios in which the patient must anticipate a listener's prior knowledge about a potential conversation topic (e.g., talking to a spouse about work, talking to a vocational rehabilitation agent regarding accommodation needs). The clinician and patient may then discuss or role-play communication interactions related to the different scenarios. Video recordings or transcripts of simulated or real interactions may assist the patient in identifying mismatches in communication style and listener needs/environmental context.

Communication: A Focus of Study and Service in Disciplines Other Than Speech-Language Pathology

The nature of communication exchanges among normal adults is in itself an entire field of study. University communication departments typically offer courses in topics such as organizational communication, small group communication, interpersonal communication, and nonverbal communication, recognizing that each of these communication contexts has unique characteristics and influences. Clinicians are encouraged to explore the wealth of information available regarding normal adult communication to assist in both assessment and remediation of higher-level communication deficits.

Another aspect of social communication that may be targeted for intervention is humor (Parenté & Herrmann, 2003). "Sense of humor" is a highly personal characteristic, and varies considerably, even among individuals without neurogenic language disorders. Tompkins (1995) argued that distressing changes in sense of humor accompanying neurogenic language disorders likely reflect difficulties in one or more of the following: interpreting nonverbal cues, making inferences, or comprehending intentional use of alternate meanings of words and phrases. The treatment activities for addressing each of these skills suggested earlier in this chapter can easily be modified to incorporate stimuli with humorous content, such as riddles that use plays on words or comic strips depicting characters using facial expressions.

The social conventions of compliments, politeness, criticism, social confrontation, and questions/answers are also appropriate targets for pragmatic treatment. In a study examining the benefit of group social skills treatment for patients with TBI, Braunling-McMorrow et al. (1986) described a variation of the "Sorry" board game in which the standard game cards were replaced with cards describing social situations, along with a prompt to elicit appropriate communicative responses to the scenario. During the game, each patient developed a response to the prompt on the card drawn during his or her turn. If the response was judged by the clinician to be appropriate, the patient moved a game piece forward on the board. Feedback was provided following inappropriate responses. The authors reported that their patients with TBI demonstrated increased frequency of appropriate social responses both during the treatment activity and on generalization measures obtained outside of treatment.

Although not specifically described in the study, this game could easily be modified so that group participants are responsible for judging the appropriateness of a response, providing feedback about how to improve the response, or both.

In summary, although a variety of treatment activity options are available, particularly to the creative clinician, to address the pragmatic impairments and disabilities of patients with neurogenic language disorders, empirical verification of the effectiveness of these activities is sadly lacking. A few areas in need of further research include determining which patient populations respond best to which treatment approach (e.g., TBI vs. RHD; patients with poor vs. good awareness of deficits; mild vs. severe linguistic and/or cognitive impairments), examining whether treatment effects are maintained following treatment termination, and documenting which treatment protocols result in generalization to untrained stimuli, tasks, and contexts.

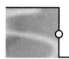

TREATMENT OF COGNITIVE IMPAIRMENTS AND DISABILITIES

Generally, two treatment approaches have been exploited to remediate cognitive impairments associated with neurogenic language disorders: behavioral or cognitive rehabilitation and pharmacotherapy (see Chapter 10). In terms of cognitive rehabilitation, most programs, particularly those that were first developed, are similar to stimulation language therapies. For example, these programs provide extensive practice at responding to stimuli and activities that gradually increase in complexity in order to facilitate functioning of the impaired cognitive process or processes. Unfortunately, few of these traditional therapies have produced remarkable generalization to untrained stimuli and daily activities. More recently developed programs, however, extend beyond stimulating the impaired cognitive function and additionally incorporate training compensatory strategies, practicing with stimuli and tasks that are encountered in the patients' daily routines, or both. This section of the chapter provides examples of these varied forms of cognitive rehabilitation that have been used to address the concomitant attention, memory, and executive function impairments of patients representing a variety of neurogenic language disorders.

ATTENTION TREATMENTS

Given that attention impairments are perhaps the most frequently occurring symptom following brain damage of any form or severity and that they can have dire consequences on rehabilitation and functional outcomes, it is not surprising that numerous treatment protocols have been developed to address this pervasive cognitive problem. The majority of these protocols attempt to retrain directly one or more attention functions through a structured hierarchy of paper-and-pencil or computerized attention tasks (e.g., Bracy, 1983; Parenté & Anderson-Parenté, 1991; Sturmes et al., 1997). That is, patients are given intensive and repetitive practice at completing sets of tasks, which are organized not only in terms of general difficulty or complexity, but also in terms of what specific attention function they target (e.g., sustained attention, attention switching, divided attention). As the patients progress on the simpler tasks that target less complex attention functions (e.g., sustained attention), new tasks that are more difficult and target the same attention function or a more complex attention function (e.g., selective attention) are introduced.

Sohlberg, Mateer, and colleagues have developed two structured programs, Attention Process Training (APT; Sohlberg & Mateer, 1986) and Attention Process Training–II (APT-II; Sohlberg, Johnson, Paul, Raskin, & Mateer, 2001), that are good examples of attention retraining protocols. Both programs consist of tasks that are graded in difficulty and target sustained, selective, alternating, and divided attention in auditory and/or visual modalities (for examples, see Table 9-8). APT was designed for patients with TBI with moderate to severe attention problems, and because APT-II contains more complex and demanding attention tasks, it is recommended for patients with TBI who have mild attention problems. Although researchers have found that patients with TBI (Palmese & Raskin, 2000; Park, Moscovitch, & Robertson, 1999; Sohlberg, McLaughlin, Pavese, Heidrick, & Posner, 2000) or aphasia (Murray, Keeton, & Karcher, in press) show improved

Table 9-8. **Examples of Activities from the Attention Process Training—II Program (Sohlberg et al., 2001)**

ATTENTION FUNCTION	EXAMPLE ACTIVITY	PERFORMANCE MEASURES
Sustained Attention	Respond to a target number embedded in an audiotaped sequence of numbers.	Accuracy, omissions, false positives
Selective Attention	Respond to a target number embedded in an audiotaped sequence of numbers recorded in the presence of distracting noise.	Accuracy, omissions, false positives
Alternating Attention	Cancellation task, initiating with the cancellation of odd numbers, and then switching to canceling even numbers when prompted by the clinician.	Accuracy, switching errors
Divided Attention	Card sorting by suit while selecting those cards that have the letter "e" in their name.	Accuracy, time to completion

performance of trained tasks after receiving APT or APT-II, conflicting results have emerged with respect to generalization to untrained attention tasks or measures of other cognitive abilities. For example, whereas Sohlberg, Mateer, and colleagues (2000) reported improvements in memory, learning, executive functioning, and functional independence following APT, Park and colleagues (1999) found nominal change in their patients' performance of a memory test after receiving APT. In an attempt to resolve these and other discrepancies in the attention retraining literature, particularly with respect to generalization effects, several comprehensive review papers have been written (Cicerone et al., 2000; Park & Ingles, 2001; Sohlberg et al., 2003). Collectively, the authors of these reviews have concluded that optimal improvements are more likely if: (1) the structured, attention retraining tasks are combined with strategy training (see below for a description of strategy training treatments); (2) intensive training is provided with an optimal session length of 60 minutes; (3) complex (e.g., divided attention) rather than simple attention functions (e.g., sustained attention) are trained; and (4) only tasks that target the specific needs and deficits of a given patient are utilized, rather than progressing through standard programs in their entirety.

More recently, researchers have explored the utility of treatments in which patients are taught strategies to help manage or monitor their attention (Butler & Copeland, 2002; Cicerone, 2002). Typically in these treatments, patients are trained to use their strategies while completing tasks like those found in the attention retraining programs described in the previous paragraph. For instance, Cicerone (2002) gave four patients with TBI his "working attention" treatment, and compared their pre- and post-treatment test performances to those of four patients with TBI who had been referred for treatment but could not attend. Cicerone's treatment consisted of two components. For the first half of each therapy session, patients completed a working memory task under different attention conditions. For the working memory task, patients worked through a stack of playing cards by recalling the number on the card that was one, two, or three back from the card currently being viewed. In more complex, divided attention conditions, patients completed this task while (1) sorting the cards according to suit, (2) completing a verbal fluency task, or (3) completing a secondary task similar to one of their daily activities (e.g., a patient who previously made a lot of conference calls shadowed audiotaped lectures while completing the working memory task). During the latter half of each session, patients were (1) counseled regarding their performance of treatment tasks, (2) assisted with identifying task and emotional variables that influenced their performance, and (3) taught strategies to aid their performance, including use of verbal mediation, rehearsal, self-pacing, task demands estimation, and positive self-statements. Patients also completed emphasis change training, which involved practicing to shift attentional priority during the divided attention activities. Cicerone reported that patients receiving his working attention treatment achieved better attention test scores and reported fewer attentional difficulties during daily tasks than those patients who could not attend treatment.

Additionally, whereas all treated patients returned to work, none of the control group did so. Cicerone's findings, as well as those from other strategy-training treatment studies (e.g., Butler & Copeland, 2002), are encouraging and indicate a need to further explore strategy training to delineate which patients and what type of attention problems might be best served by this form of attention treatment.

Side Bar

Who Wants to Treat Attention Disorders—Anyone or Everyone?

As discussed in Chapters 3 and 4, disciplines other than speech-language pathology often address the attention impairments that may accompany neurogenic language disorders. In particular, rehabilitative neuropsychologists may target various aspects of attention in their treatment. Occupational therapists often target neglect as a component of a treatment plan addressing bathing, grooming, feeding, and other activities of daily living. Accordingly, clinicians may find it helpful to collaborate with these other rehabilitation disciplines when developing treatment goals, designing specific intervention activities, or both to assure that services aren't being duplicated across disciplines or, alternatively, that services are not overlooked because each therapist incorrectly assumed that another discipline would take responsibility.

Another approach that has produced positive outcomes involves incorporating functional attention tasks that resemble patients' everyday communicative and cognitive activities into treatment. For example, the attention treatment program developed by Wilson and Robertson (1992) evolved from the complaint of their patient with TBI of frequent attention slips while reading. Each day, the patient completed short homework sessions during which he read a novel and kept track of how long he read before experiencing an attention slip. Additionally, prior to reading, the patient completed relaxation exercises such as controlled breathing to help alleviate negative thoughts or emotions that might interrupt his concentration and reading. By the end of treatment, the patient had progressed from one and a half minutes of reading without an attention slip in a quiet environment to five minutes of reading without an attention slip in the presence of distraction (i.e., talk radio programs). The patient also showed improvements in reading untrained text, and reported that following treatment, he had resumed reading for pleasure. Importantly, attention retraining programs have begun to acknowledge the importance of integrating into therapy more functional versus contrived tasks (e.g., scanning the financial section of a newspaper for a certain stock vs. scanning a worksheet to circle a certain abstract design). For example, in their APT-II program, Sohlberg and colleagues (2001) recommended identifying and utilizing daily activities that involve the same attention functions being targeted by APT-II tasks in order to maximize generalization of retrained attention skills to patients' everyday functioning.

In summary, a growing literature indicates that cognitive rehabilitation can positively affect the attention abilities of patients with TBI. Those programs that incorporate strategy training and functional daily activities are more likely to encourage generalization to untrained, real-world stimuli, tasks, and environments than protocols that rely solely on retraining attention via structured and controlled, but artificial exercises. To further our understanding of how best to remediate attention disorders, future studies should explore the effects of existing treatment protocols on a broader range of patient populations (e.g., RHD, dementia, aphasia). Additionally, research is needed to specify when we should be treating which attention functions (e.g., acute vs. chronic stages of recovery), whether certain attention functions respond better to certain therapy approaches, and how much training is necessary to optimize treatment and generalization effects.

Treatment of Neglect

Currently, several therapy approaches have been developed to address the attentional problem of neglect. These approaches vary from environmental modifications to attempting to remediate cognitive deficits contributing to neglect. Whereas there is some evidence to indicate that provision of one or several of these neglect treatments may result in greater neglect recovery than when a general cognitive retraining program is used (Paolucci et al., 1996), few neglect treatments have yet proven effective in producing gains that persist beyond treatment termination or that generalize to daily living activities (Gordon et al., 1985). Accordingly, unless otherwise stated, clinicians should primarily expect task-specific gains when applying one or more of the neglect treatments described in this chapter.

Environmental and task modifications such as drawing a red line down the neglected side of a page to assist reading, placing a brightly colored bracelet or sweatband on the patient's neglected wrist to encourage visual attention to that side of the body, or putting brightly colored clothes or a flashing light on the neglected side of a clothes closet can help reduce the negative consequences of neglect, particularly in patients who have little awareness of their neglect (see Chapter 11 for further examples). Additionally, the following are examples of devices and procedures that provide patients the impression that their environment has been shifted toward their neglected side, and thus can reduce the effects of neglect, at least in some patients, while or immediately after they utilize the device or receive the stimulation:

1. monocular eye patching, in which the lens of the non-neglected side is blocked or shaded on a pair of glasses (Walker, Young, & Lincoln, 1996);

2. hemispatial sunglasses, in which the non-neglected hemifield of each lens is shaded (Beis, Andre, Baumgarten, & Challier, 1999);

3. prism lenses, which after wearing cause a natural adjustment of the eyes in which visual focus shifts toward the neglected side (Rossetti et al., 1998; Frassinetti, Angeli, Menghello, Avanzi, & Ladavas, 2002); and,

4. exciting vestibular organs on the neglected side via ear irrigation (Rode, Tiliket, Charlopain, & Boisson, 1998), visual motion stimulation (e.g., stimuli are shown on a computer or video monitor moving from the neglected to the non-neglected side; Kerkhoff, 2000), or neck vibrotactile stimulation (Karnath, 1994).

Typically, neglect improvement dissipates after these devices or vestibular stimulation are removed, unless the patients have had intensive and prolonged exposure to the device or stimulation (Beis et al., 1999; Frassinetti et al., 2002). Generalization should not necessarily be expected, given that the above adaptations do not necessarily attempt to fix the patient's neglect but rather focus on changing variables in the environment, modifying task demands, or altering visual or vestibular input. Furthermore, in some patients, eye patching has been shown to aggravate rather than alleviate neglect (Barrett, Crucian, Beversdorf, & Heilman, 2001). Accordingly, environmental modifications appear most appropriate for patients who do not respond to other treatment approaches, or whose severe deficits in other areas of cognition make them inappropriate candidates for other treatments. Environmental adaptations also may be useful when other cognitive or linguistic impairments are being treated by reducing the probability that neglect will interfere with the patient's performance of therapy activities.

Another approach to treating neglect focuses on remediating cognitive problems that contribute to neglect. For instance, because patients with neglect inadequately move their eyes, head, or body to attend to stimuli or activities on their neglected side, treatment aims to increase their active attention to the neglected side. In therapy, patients practice activities in which they demonstrate neglect, and during the practice clinicians provide one or several cues to encourage patients to attend to their neglected side. These cues might be verbal, such as "Don't forget to look all the way to left side of the page"; visual, such as flashing a light on the neglected side or placing a visual "anchor" such as a red line on the neglected side; auditory, such as presenting a tone burst on the neglected side; or tactile, such as tapping the neglected hand. Over time, clinician cueing should be faded as patients' performances improve. Most frequently, clinicians require patients to practice repetitively visual scanning, figure copying, and cancellation tasks similar to those used to diagnose neglect (see Chapter 6). These might be completed with real objects or paper and pencil, or as a computerized activity. Even though these tasks are popular and, with practice, patients can indeed improve their performance of these tasks (or tasks that are similar to practiced tasks), there is little empirical support for their use given that they fail to evoke generalization to more functional, real-world activities (Hajek, Kates, Donnelly, & McGree, 1993; Manly, 2002). Accordingly, if this approach to neglect treatment is adopted, clinicians must incorporate functional activities such as dressing, writing, or cooking, rather than contrived tasks such as line bisection or canceling out target letters or symbols.

A related approach is to teach patients to cue themselves. This approach may result in generalization as long as patients are sufficiently aware of their neglect and the possible consequences of that neglect (Golisz, 1998; Manly, 2002). For instance, Niemeier (1998) taught a group of stroke patients with neglect a "lighthouse" imagery strategy in which they were asked to imagine that their eyes were like the light in a lighthouse sweeping all the way from the left to the right. While completing a variety of tasks (e.g., computer activities, locating items in the room), patients were initially cued by their clinicians to use the strategy; family and other health care team members also were educated about the strategy and encouraged to remind patients about its use. Over time, cues were faded as patients' performances improved and they began to apply the strategy independently. Following treatment, patients not only demonstrated significant improvements on tests of neglect and attention, but also performed these tests better than a group of patients who did not receive the imagery training. Additionally, the subjective reports of the family and caregivers suggested reductions in neglect when patients completed activities in settings outside of the rehabilitation facility.

Limb activation represents another effective technique that patients can learn as a self-cue or strategy to help alleviate neglect symptoms. This technique involves training patients to move some part of the neglected side of their body in the neglected hemispace while they complete daily activities that might be negatively affected by their neglect (Robertson et al., 1992, 1998). For example, a patient with left neglect might be trained to tap the fingers of his left hand on his left knee during reading tasks. This limb movement is proposed to decrease neglect symptoms by increasing activation within neural areas of the damaged hemisphere that contribute to attention. As in other cueing approaches, training proceeds with the clinician initially reminding patients to use limb activation while they complete therapy activities; as the patients' performances improve, clinician cueing is faded so that patients become responsible for remembering to utilize the strategy. For patients who have difficulty remembering to use the strategy, Robertson and colleagues (1992) created a small "neglect alert device." The device has a hand-held button that has to be pressed on a regular basis (e.g., once every five seconds) to avoid setting off a buzzer. Several studies have shown that limb activation training with or without the use of this device can alleviate neglect symptoms, regardless of whether the movement of the neglected limb is part of the target activity (Robertson et al., 1992; Samuel et al., 2000; Wilson et al., 2000). Not all patients, however, benefit from this technique (Manly, 2002), and obviously, it is inappropriate for patients with dense hemiplegia. Furthermore, variable degrees of generalization and maintenance of treatment effects have been reported (e.g., Maddicks, Marzillier, & Parker, 2003 vs. Samuel et al., 2000), which may be, at least in part, related to procedural differences among previous investigations. For example, some studies examined upper limb activation whereas others examined lower limb activation, some studies included patients who were in the acute stages of recovery whereas more chronic patients were used in other studies, and some studies evaluated limb activation by itself whereas others evaluated limb activation in combination with other neglect treatment procedures. Accordingly, further research is needed to help delineate when and to whom this treatment should be taught.

Review of the neglect treatment literature indicates that few treatments evoke remarkable generalization to untrained, everyday tasks. More positive findings, however, are beginning to accrue when two or more of these treatments are used in concert. For example, Schindler and colleagues (2002) found that compared to visual exploration/scanning activities by themselves, providing neck stimulation along with visual exploration/scanning activities resulted in greater improvements in activities of daily living and untrained visual and tactile search tasks. Therefore, researchers should focus future efforts on evaluating the effects of other neglect treatment combinations, particularly in terms of carryover to untrained, functional tasks.

MEMORY TREATMENTS

Whereas some memory therapy approaches have been designed to treat overall memory functioning, others focus on remediating only certain memory functions (e.g., prospective memory) or on exploiting intact memory functions to support impaired ones. Those programs that attempt to restore general memory abilities typically involve structured and repetitive drills such as digit or word span tasks or list-learning activities (Berg, Koning-Haanstra, & Deelmman, 1991; Sohlberg & Mateer, 2001a). During these activities, patients are presented with novel information, and then asked to recall that information at a later time, following a filled or unfilled delay. By manipulating one or more of the variables listed in Table 9-9, clinicians may make memory activities more difficult or easier (Bayles & Kim, 2003). Given the abundance of workbooks and computer software programs that contain these types of tasks, this approach to treating memory continues to appear quite popular. Numerous studies, however, have shown that even though these treatments may result in improved recall of trained stimuli, generalization to untrained stimuli and novel contexts is unlikely (Mateer et al. 1999; Tate, 1997). Nevertheless, in certain cases, retention of only trained material may still represent clinical success and have positive effects on patients' everyday functioning, particularly when the trained material is functional. For example, Arkin (1991; 1998) provided patients in the early and middle stages of Alzheimer's disease with audio- or videotaped narratives about their own autobiographical or factual information. After the narrative was presented, the patients completed a quiz about facts within the narrative (with the correct answers provided on the tape). Arkin found that indeed these patients could learn and retain the material for periods as long as one month following their last supervised practice session. These improvements in recalling

Table 9-9. Variables for Manipulating the Difficulty of Memory Activities

VARIABLE	POORER RECALL IF. . .
Amount of to-be-remembered information	more information
Type of to-be-remembered information: 　Syntactic complexity 　Emotional valence 　Self- vs. clinician-generated 　Modality	 more complex syntax lower emotional content clinician-generated material or cues dependent on other concomitant deficits (e.g., for certain aphasia and dementia patient populations, spoken language may be more difficult to remember than written language) and premorbid learning preferences (e.g., prior to his stroke, the patient was better at learning and recalling material presented visually vs. an auditory format)
Similarity of encoding and retrieval conditions	dissimilar encoding and retrieval conditions
Encoding strategy	shallow strategy (e.g., rote rehearsal vs. semantic elaboration)
Type of recall task	free recall (vs. recognition or cued recall)

the trained information also resulted in more positive views of the patients' abilities, not only by the caregivers but also by the patients themselves.

Patients also might be trained to use internal **mnemonic strategies** to enhance memory encoding (or storing) and retrieval (Tate, 1997). Examples of internal mnemonic strategies include the following: (1) visual imagery, which includes the method of loci in which patients imagine key words in the to-be-recalled information linked to specific locations, such as along a familiar route or on their body; (2) semantic elaboration, in which, when presented with a to-be-recalled object, patients think about a number of the object's semantic features, such as its use, location, or composition; and (3) verbal organization, in which patients create acronyms or paired associations to encode and recall information or use alphabet search to prompt recall of a person's name or other to-be-recalled information. Within sessions, patients are first provided with a description and examples of the target mnemonic strategy. Next, they are instructed to utilize one or more of these strategies when presented with to-be-recalled information, and may also be cued to apply these strategies when attempting to recall the information. Research indicates that although patients with a variety of forms of brain damage (e.g., stroke,

TBI, infection) may improve their recall of trained material using internal strategies, few, particularly those with moderate or severe memory problems, demonstrate spontaneous, independent use of these strategies outside of therapy (Cicerone et al., 2000; Miller, 1992; Oberg & Turkstra, 1998; Wilson, 1982). Given that executive functions such as initiation, self-regulation, and problem solving help support autonomous use of internal mnemonic strategies, and that many patients with memory disorders have concomitant executive functioning deficits, it is not surprising that only patients with mild and relatively isolated memory impairments are able to apply these strategies independently in real-life contexts (Kaschel et al., 2002). Again, however, if only treatment-specific gains are wanted, training use of one or more of these strategies may be appropriate. For example, Oberg and Turkstra (1998) taught two adolescent patients with TBI an elaboration strategy that resulted in their acquisition of vocabulary needed for school. Although these patients continued to require clinician assistance to apply the strategy, they were able to learn and retain the trained material that they needed for their current school activities. In this case, even though generalization was not achieved, the domain-specific effects still resulted in functional gains for the patients.

Another treatment approach involves training specific memory functions. For example, Sohlberg and colleagues (1985; 1992) developed a treatment protocol to address problems with **prospective memory,** or the ability to recall and carry out future intentions. Prospective memory can be time-based, such as remembering when to take your medication or to turn off the lawn sprinkler, or event-based, such as remembering to give a note to a teacher the next time you see him (Groot, Wilson, Evans, & Watson, 2002); typically, time-based prospective recall is more demanding in terms of both memory and executive functioning. The goal of Sohlberg et al.'s Prospective Memory Process Training (PROMPT) program is to extend the amount of time a patient is able to remember to carry out specified tasks at specified times. Thus, PROMPT's focus is on the more complex, time-based prospective memory skills. In its most basic form, patients are instructed to complete a task after a set time interval. If patients complete the task at the correct time, the time interval is increased; if they are unable to complete the task without cueing, the time interval is decreased. In addition to varying the length of the time delay, the following variables can be manipulated to make PROMPT easier or more difficult: (1) difficulty of the prospective task (e.g., simple motor task vs. complex multimodality task), (2) presence or absence of a distracter during the time delay (e.g., sitting with no distraction vs. completing another task during the delay), and (3) presence or absence of prompts (e.g., allow the use of a watch alarm vs. independent recall of when to complete the task). Only one variable at a time should be manipulated so that the effects of that variable on the patient's performance can be examined. Clinicians can purchase Prospective Memory Screening/Training materials (Sohlberg & Mateer, 2001b), which include a test for screening prospective memory abilities as well as detailed instructions and record sheets for administering PROMPT.

Data from a limited number of studies conducted by the authors of PROMPT and their colleagues (Raskin & Sohlberg, 1996; Sohlberg, White, Evans, & Mateer, 1992) indicate that patients with prospective memory problems subsequent to TBI and stroke improve on trained tasks, and may, at least in some cases, display improved recall and completion of untrained, real-world tasks such as completing routine chores at home. Further research is necessary, however, given the weak design of the existing studies (e.g., lack of control groups, inclusion of subjective measures or measures with poor test-retest reliability) (Deelman, 2001).

Spaced retrieval is a memory treatment closely related to PROMPT. This technique, like PROMPT, involves patients practicing to recall information or to use a strategy over progressively longer time intervals (Brush & Camp, 1998a, 1998b). Unlike PROMPT, however, in spaced retrieval, cues are provided to the patient (see Table 9-10). For instance, during a session, the patient is asked to recall a piece of information, such as the clinician's name, after a set amount of time (e.g., 30 seconds). If the patient recalls accurately, the time interval is doubled (e.g., 60 seconds); if the patient errs, the clinician provides the correct answer, asks the patient to repeat it, and then reduces the time interval (e.g., 15 seconds). The period during the time delay may remain free from distraction or be filled with related or unrelated activities (e.g., games, conversation). If the patient makes a lot of errors, time intervals may be increased more gradually (vs. doubling the time interval), as ideally the patient should be error-free during training sessions (further information about Errorless Learning is provided later in this chapter). Spaced retrieval is proposed to facilitate learning and recall by exploiting automatic, implicit memory functions; that is, through this technique's shaping procedures, patients can acquire and subsequently recall trained material or tasks with little effort and, in some cases, little awareness. No generalization to untrained material or tasks is expected.

Numerous studies have found that spaced retrieval is an effective means by which to teach recall of a variety of new or previously known materials (e.g., caregivers' names, the patient's room number and location, stories) and activities (e.g., compensatory swallowing techniques, use of external memory aids) to patients with various degrees of memory impairment related to TBI, infection, stroke, or dementia (Bourgeois et al., 2003; Bourgeois & Melton, 2004; Brush & Camp, 1998a, 1998b; Hopper, 2004; Mahendra & Arkin, 2003). Notably, even patients with progressive forms of dementia are able to maintain their recall of trained materials or tasks for extended periods (e.g., several months) following treatment termination. Furthermore, research indicates that caregivers can easily be trained to implement spaced retrieval at home to help address memory issues encountered in the patients' daily environment (Arkin, 1991; McKitrick & Camp, 1993).

Like spaced retrieval, several additional memory treatment approaches exploit implicit or procedural memory skills to facilitate learning and recall of new or previously known information and skills. That is, in many neurogenic patient populations (e.g., TBI, certain dementing illnesses such as Alzheimer's disease),

Table 9-10. Steps for Administering Spaced Retrieval Treatment

STEP	EXAMPLE
1. Inform patient that treatment will focus on practicing to remember information/activity. Provide the to-be-remembered information or demonstrate the to-be-remembered activity.	"We're going to work on helping you to remember your room number. Your room number is 183. What is your room number? Good, you remembered it."
2. Pause and take a brief break, and then ask the patient to recall the information/activity.	After five seconds, "Let's try that again. What is your room number?"
3. If the patient correctly recalls the information/activity, move to Step 4. If the patient is unable to recall the information/activity correctly, provide the correct response and have the patient repeat the correct response. Then repeat Step 2. If, after three tries, the patient cannot complete Step 2 accurately, stop the spaced retrieval session and try at a later date.	
4. Increase the time interval, and fill the pause time with conversation that is or is not related to the therapy activity.	During the 10-second break, "That's right. Now we're going to practice remembering your room number several more times so that it will be easy for you to remember where you live in this building. Let's try it again. What is your room number?"
5. If the patient correctly recalls the information/activity, move to Step 6. If the patient is unable to recall the information/activity correctly, provide the correct response and have the patient repeat the correct response. Then return to Step 2.	
6. Increase the time interval again and fill the pause time with conversation that is or is not related to the therapy activity.	During the 20-second break, "You are doing an excellent job of remembering your room number. You are getting it correct and you are remembering it for a longer time. The goal of this practice is to help you remember information for longer and longer periods of time so that hopefully, you will always remember it. To make sure you remember your room number, we're going to keep on practicing for a while longer today. So, can you tell me what is your room number?"
7. If the patient correctly recalls the information/activity, move to Step 8. If the patient is unable to recall the information/activity correctly, provide the correct response and have the patient repeat the correct response. Then return to the last time interval at which the patient successfully recalled the information/activity.	
8. Continue to ask the patient to recall the information/activity after increasingly longer breaks.	

implicit or procedural memory appears relatively intact compared to other declarative memory functions and explicit or effortful learning and recall mechanisms (e.g., use of volitional rehearsal, chunking, or other encoding strategies) (Mateer et al., 1999). Accordingly, Glisky and colleagues (Glisky, 1992; Glisky & Schacter, 1989; Glisky et al., 1986) developed a "vanishing cues" training approach, sometimes referred to as backward chaining, in which patients, particularly during initial sessions, are provided with a level of cueing that will assure they recall accurately. As patients progress, the extent of cueing is gradually faded until they can recall the information or task without any cueing. Glisky (Glisky, 1992; Glisky & Schacter, 1989) and other researchers (van der Linden, Meulemans, & Lorrain, 1994) have shown that this technique is effective in teaching vocabulary and a variety of skills, such as the use of a word processing program, to patients with memory disorders related to TBI or other acquired neurological disorders including encephalitis, stroke, and Korsakoff's disease. Although vanishing cues has proven successful with some patients, even those who are unable to recall participating in therapy, clinicians must keep in mind that learning achieved via this method is typically slow and task or material specific.

Another approach based upon implicit learning mechanisms is "errorless learning." Advocates of this approach propose that patients who must depend on implicit learning will have difficulty dealing with error responses because if they make a lot of errors, incorrect as well as correct responses will be automatically reinforced over time (Wilson & Evans, 1996; Wilson, Baddeley, Evans, & Shiel, 1994). Therefore, if patients are prevented from making errors during the initial stages of learning, they should acquire the new information or skill more quickly. Accordingly, as the name implies, in **errorless learning,** patients are not allowed to make errors. For example, if they have been asked to recall the name of a person, they will be instructed to give that name only if they are absolutely positive they are correct. If they are not completely confident in their answer, they are given a letter cue, and again asked to respond only if they are positive they are correct. Cues are provided until patients are certain they can answer accurately. As therapy progresses, patients should require fewer cues and eventually no cues before they can confidently recall the correct information or carry out the action correctly.

Studies involving patients with TBI, stroke, and dementia indicate that errorless learning is an effective means by which to train learning and recall of specific vocabulary (e.g., names of people or objects) or skills (e.g., compensatory strategy use, daily hygiene behaviors) (Clare et al., 2000; Hunkin, Squires, Aldrich, & Parkin, 1998; Squires, Hunkin, & Parkin, 1996; Wilson & Manly, 2003). More recent research indicates, however, that only when training recall of certain types of information is errorless learning more effectual than errorful learning, in which patients are allowed to make guesses even if they are unsure of their response accuracy. For example, Evans et al. (2000) compared the effects of errorless and errorful learning approaches on the memory abilities of patients with neurogenic disorders and found that errorless learning was more effective for teaching face-name associations, but in more functional tasks such as programming a Palm Pilot, errorful learning appeared more useful. Kalla and colleagues (2001) also found a slight advantage for errorless over errorful learning in training face-name associations to memory-impaired patients. Because previous errorless learning investigations have varied in terms of the types and complexity of information and tasks trained, the intensity of training provided, and the duration of follow-up, further research is needed to delineate specific errorless learning treatment procedures for specific patient populations.

The above review of direct memory training approaches indicates that clinicians should expect only domain-specific treatment effects (i.e., nominal generalization to untrained stimuli or tasks) and that protocols such as spaced retrieval and vanishing cues that capitalize on implicit memory functioning can evoke positive outcomes, even in patients with severe or progressive memory deficits. Additionally, although these various direct treatment approaches were described separately, this does not mean that they cannot be combined in daily clinical practice. On the contrary, findings from several studies support integrating procedures (Clare et al., 2000; Mahendra & Arkin, 2003; Wilson & Manly, 2003). For example, Hunkin and colleagues (1998) demonstrated that combining aspects of spaced retrieval, errorless learning, and vanishing cues treatments resulted in the successful acquisition of a set of computer skills in their patient with severe memory impairment. Finally, it should be noted that in addition to the memory treatments reviewed above, other approaches have proven effective for addressing memory impairments associated with neurogenic language disorders. These approaches, however, are described elsewhere because they focus on either teaching the use of external aids (see Chapter 11) or addressing executive function deficits such as poor deficit awareness or impaired self-monitoring, which can compromise memory functioning (see the following section of this chapter).

EXECUTIVE FUNCTION TREATMENTS

Of the various cognitive problems with which patients with neurogenic language disorders may present, treatment of executive function deficits has received the least systematic investigation, despite the dire consequences of such deficits upon patients' ability to function independently. Effective executive function treatments are also needed, given that progress in other cognitive and linguistic domains will depend upon recovery of executive abilities such as error monitoring (e.g., to determine if the correct word was retrieved and produced), inhibition (e.g., to avoid perseveration), and problem solving (e.g., to determine when a compensatory strategy will need to be utilized). The following section of this chapter describes two general approaches for addressing executive function impairments. First, we briefly review a number of environmental adaptations that can be introduced to help support patients' executive functioning (see also Chapter 11). Second, we describe in greater detail treatment techniques that have been developed for specific executive function abilities (e.g., awareness, problem solving).

Environmental Adaptation Approaches

Clinicians may opt to introduce environmental modifications when patients' cognitive impairments are so broad and severe that direct remediation approaches are unlikely to be successful, or when patients are in the earliest stages of recovery, such as the post-traumatic amnesia phase of TBI, when direct remediation is often inappropriate. Additionally, environmental adaptations can be used effectively to supplement direct remediation approaches.

One frequent environmental modification is to reduce task demands (Mateer, 1999). For example, to reduce the executive demands of therapy tasks or daily activities, clinicians might: (1) simplify tasks by breaking them down into a series of steps, (2) give patients longer to complete tasks, (3) remove or minimize stimuli that elicit inappropriate behavior (e.g., avoid conversational topics that elicit disinhibited arguing and aggressive outbursts), (4) provide breaks to minimize frustration and fatigue, or (5) reduce or eliminate environmental distractions such as noise or visual clutter.

Another approach is to provide external support via cueing or prompting. For example, many patients demonstrate adequate knowledge of what steps or skills are needed to complete complex executive tasks, but fail to apply this knowledge online. When these patients are provided cues in the form of verbal reminders, alarm systems, or even nonspecific, periodic tones, however, improvements in a variety of executive behaviors, including initiation (Sohlberg, Sprunk, & Metzelaar, 1988) and goal management (Manly et al., 2002; 2004), have been observed. Further research is needed to evaluate if these types of external modifications can provide long-term support and to determine how these modifications might best be combined with direct, behavioral interventions such as those described below.

Treatments for Specific Executive Functions

In addition to or instead of altering the patients' environment, a number of treatments have been developed to address specific executive function impairments by teaching strategies or practicing tasks designed to restore underlying executive abilities. For the most part, these treatment protocols are in the preliminary stages of development, given that further research is still needed to document the reliability of treatment effects, to determine generalization and maintenance of treatment effects, and to delineate which patients are most likely to benefit from the treatment.

Awareness Training

Awareness training targets not only patients' understanding of their current strengths and weaknesses, but also their ability to monitor their performance online. If patients are unaware of certain linguistic or cognitive impairments, awareness training should be the first treatment priority, even before those linguistic or cognitive impairments are treated. Obviously, patients with poor deficit awareness will neither understand nor see the need for treatment, and consequently, even if they can be convinced to attend treatment sessions, they will certainly not be motivated to benefit from treatment. Unfortunately, although researchers agree on the importance of addressing awareness deficits (e.g., Prigatano, 1991; Tompkins, 1995), few awareness treatments have been developed or submitted to empirical investigation. Therefore, without exception, the following approaches require further study to validate treatment effects.

One approach to addressing poor deficit awareness is to educate patients about the nature and implications of their linguistic and/or cognitive impairments. One or more of the following treatment tasks might be used (Sohlberg & Mateer, 2001a; Tompkins, 1995; Ylvisaker, Szekeres, & Feeney, 1998): (1) provide in spoken, written, or videotape form a description of their neurological disorder and resulting cognitive and/or linguistic symptoms (e.g., brochures, medical records), being sure to accommodate for the patients' deficits (e.g., use simple and short sentences for patients with comprehension deficits); (2) have patients educate or describe to others (e.g., family, co-workers, health care workers, other patients) their neurological disorders and cognitive and/or linguistic symptoms through activities such as giving a presentation, writing a narrative or educational brochure, or creating a self-advocacy videotape (see Table 9-11); (3) compare patients' ratings of their current abilities to those of their family, friends, and/or health care team to identify and discuss areas of agreement and discrepancy; (4) have patients view, judge, describe, and discuss videotaped, written, or audiotaped samples of other patients who display similar cognitive and/or linguistic symptom profiles; and (5) utilize a game format such as the Road to Awareness board game of Chittum, Johnson, Chittum, Guercio, and McMorrow (1996) to have patients ask and answer questions about their neurological disorder and resulting symptoms.

Another option is to engage patients in activities that help them experience alterations in their abilities and behaviors since the onset of their neurological disorder (Cicerone & Giacino, 1992; Schlund, 1999; Stuss, 1991). For example, patients might be required to complete tasks that are likely to elicit negative and positive behaviors, but, prior to completing the tasks, also asked to predict their performance. Relatedly, patients might be asked to rate, tally, or track their performance while completing activities. Following task completion, patients compare their predictions or ratings with their actual performance to identify and discuss discrepancies and agreements. Another possible activity is role-playing, in which patients act out one or more of the following: (1) negative symptoms, (2) strategies

Table 9-11. Goals and Procedures for Making Transitional or Self-Advocacy Videotapes (Adapted from Ylvisaker et al., 1998)

Goals

1. Enhance patients' self-esteem and sense of control
2. Increase patients' awareness of their cognitive and/or linguistic strengths and weaknesses
3. Encourage patients' active involvement in their rehabilitation program
4. Educate family and caregivers about patients' cognitive and/or linguistic strengths and weaknesses
5. Encourage interdisciplinary collaboration

Procedures

1. Decide what content the videotape should contain. Regardless of which of the following content areas are included, clinicians must assure that strengths as well as weaknesses are emphasized.
   a. Motoric strengths, weaknesses, and rehabilitation issues (e.g., necessary prostheses, types and frequency of cues needed)
   b. Cognitive strengths, weaknesses, and rehabilitation issues (e.g., types of compensatory behavioral strategies being used, types of external devices being used, helpful environmental modifications, types and frequency of cues needed)
   c. Linguistic strengths, weaknesses, and rehabilitation issues (e.g., types of behavioral compensatory strategies being used, types of external devices being used, helpful environmental modifications, types and frequency of cues needed)
   d. Other strengths, weaknesses, and rehabilitation issues (e.g., behavioral problems and modification procedures, emotional well-being, social issues)
2. Determine how the content will be communicated or demonstrated on the videotape. Possible options include segments with:
   a. Role-playing strengths, weaknesses, and/or rehabilitation strategies or procedures
   b. Samples of actual treatment sessions to demonstrate strengths, weaknesses, and/or rehabilitation strategies or procedures, or to document improvements over time
   c. Samples of the patient in natural contexts to demonstrate strengths, weaknesses, and/or rehabilitation strategies or procedures, or to document improvements over time
   d. Patient and clinician conversing about the patient's strengths, weaknesses, and/or rehabilitation strategies or procedures
   e. Creating a written script or story that the patient will read to describe his or her strengths, weaknesses, and/or rehabilitation strategies or procedures
   f. Family, caregivers, and/or other healthcare team members giving their accounts of the patient's strengths, weaknesses, and/or rehabilitation strategies or procedures
3. Decide who will do the videotaping and editing
4. Assure that appropriate videotaping release forms have been signed

to avoid or compensate for negative symptoms, or (3) consequences of negative symptoms (e.g., the social reaction of peers when inappropriate language is used). When completing these and other educational tasks, clinicians must be cognizant to avoid excessive confrontation that might cause a defensive reaction or loss of self-worth in the patient. This can be avoided, at least in part, not only by assuring that awareness training activities focus on increasing awareness of deficits, but also by increasing awareness and appreciation of patients' areas of strength; for instance, clinicians should assure that in addition to being able to identify their errors, patients can accurately judge when they have correctly completed a task. It also is important to note that this educational approach is unlikely to be successful with patients who have profound global unawareness and severe concomitant cognitive deficits (Sohlberg & Mateer, 2001a). In these cases, treatment efforts will be more productive if aimed at caregiver education and training (see Chapter 11).

Once patients have a better sense of the presence and nature of their deficits, treatment can focus on addressing difficulties with self-monitoring and, relatedly, strategy decision-making (e.g., knowing when and how to implement trained linguistic or cognitive strategies). Generally, treatment involves teaching patients: (1) to review tasks prior to completing them so that, given their impairments, they can make a prediction regarding task difficulty; (2) based on that review, to make decisions regarding which strategies if any are most appropriate; (3) to apply the strategies; and (4) to monitor the outcome of their strategy use. Examples of specific procedures that have been used include (Avery & Kennedy, 2002; Golisz, 1998; Sohlberg & Mateer, 2001a; Ylvisaker et al., 1998):

1. Requiring patients to predict their performance prior to completing treatment tasks (which may include an identification of factors that may or may not make the task difficult), and comparing this prediction to their actual performance;

2. Requiring patients to estimate or rate how well they did following completion of treatment tasks, particularly after a delay versus immediately after task completion, and comparing this estimation to their actual performance;

3. Encouraging patients to use verbal mediation or self-questions prior to or while completing treatment tasks (e.g., Will I need to take notes during this listening task to help my understanding? Did I check that the oven was turned off?);

4. Using video- or audiotape feedback following completion of treatment tasks so that patients can make off-line judgments about task difficulty, their strategy use, and their task performance; and

5. Identifying situations or materials for which trained strategies or behaviors will and will not be appropriate.

These types of activities have been found to help improve patients' understanding of and use of strategies for their memory (Lawson & Rice, 1989; Schlund, 1999), attention (Fasotti, Kovacs, Eling, & Brouwer, 2000; Tham & Tegner, 1997), or executive functioning abilities (Stuss, 1991). Most previous research, however, has been conducted with patients whose cognitive problems are a product of TBI. Consequently, further study of how other patient populations respond to these treatment activities, and whether these activities are similarly effective for addressing impaired monitoring and application of strategies for linguistic deficits, is needed.

Treatment of Perseveration

Although perseveration commonly accompanies a variety of neurogenic language disorders, few formal treatments have been developed to ameliorate the linguistic and cognitive problems that may result from this executive function deficit. An exception is Treatment for Aphasic Perseveration (TAP; Helm-Estabrooks et al., 1987; Helm-Estabrooks & Albert, 2004). As the name indicates, TAP aims to reduce verbal perseveration in patients with aphasia so as to increase their spoken lexical-retrieval accuracy and fluency. The first step to TAP is to determine if it is appropriate for a given patient by calculating that patient's perseveration severity rating. This rating is computed by having the patient complete the Confrontation Naming subtest of the *Boston Diagnostic Aphasia Examination* (BDAE), and then analyzing the percentage of items on which the patient perseverated: Patients who perseverate on 20% or more of the items are considered appropriate TAP candidates. Next, a stimulus hierarchy is developed so that easier semantic categories and stimuli are presented at the beginning of each therapy session, and more difficult ones are presented later. Categories and items are generated directly from the BDEA Confrontation Naming subtest. For example, if during testing the patient showed the least perseveration and best accuracy while naming body parts, body parts are targeted first within a TAP session; if most perseveration and least accurate naming occurred while the patient was naming letters, letter naming would not be trained until later in the TAP program. The final steps of TAP involve carrying out the actual therapy sessions. First, patients are educated about perseveration and why TAP is being administered. Next, sessions focus on training confrontation naming by stimulating spoken lexical-semantic retrieval via semantic, phonological, orthographic, or other cues (for cue options, see Table 9-5), by increasing the patient's awareness of their perseveration, and by teaching strategies to minimize perseverations. That is, if the patient cannot name an item, up to three cues are provided to facilitate retrieval of the spoken label. If the patient perseverates while attempting to name the item, the clinician points out the perseverative response to the patient (e.g., write the perseveration on a piece of paper and then rip up the paper and leave the pieces as a reminder in case the patient makes the same perseverative error again), and then slows the stimulus presentation rate or provides an overt break before presenting the next stimulus (e.g., introduce that a new item is being given; have the patient complete a distracter task between items). Additionally, patients are taught to try to avoid perseveration by waiting before answering or, when they feel like they might perseverate, by not responding and instead asking for help.

Currently, only one empirical investigation of TAP has been completed (Helm-Estabrooks, Emery, & Albert, 1987). In this study, the effects of TAP were compared to those of other traditional language treatments (e.g., auditory comprehension or stimulation therapy, VCIU) in three patients with varying aphasia types. Whereas all patients showed greater decreases in perseveration following TAP versus the alternative treatment, generalization to untrained tasks, stimuli, or language modalities was not explored, leaving the need for additional examination of this treatment approach.

Treatment of Disinhibition

Difficulty inhibiting impulsive or inappropriate behavior can have dire consequences on social functioning and completion of daily activities. Only a limited number of treatment approaches, however, have been described to address this type of executive dysfunction. Blake and colleagues (as cited by Mateer, 1999) developed a protocol to treat their patient's impaired inhibition of interruptive behavior. In this treatment, the patient was first taught those individuals with whom he was allowed to interact and those he was not. To aid his discrimination of appropriate and inappropriate conversational partners, staff members he was allowed to approach wore large green squares and those he was not to approach wore large red squares. Appropriate discrimination (i.e., approaching only staff with green squares) was rewarded with extended conversation, whereas inappropriate discrimination (i.e., approaching staff with red squares) was addressed by ignoring the patient. As the patient's inappropriate interruptive behavior began to decrease, the saliency of the external cues was reduced by shrinking the size of the staff's badges. Eventually, staff reported nominal disruption by this patient while on the rehabilitation unit, even when the visual cues had been completely faded.

Alderman and colleagues (Alderman, 1996; Alderman, Fry, & Youngson, 1995) have similarly shown that other behavioral modification approaches, in particular response cost programs, may be effective in increasing inhibitory control. In response cost paradigms, patients are given a set number of tokens, which after a certain period of time can be exchanged for a reward. Each time they display a targeted negative behavior, however, one or more of their tokens are taken away, and they are reminded why they are losing the tokens; consequently, having fewer tokens results in a smaller number or variety of rewards when tokens are eventually exchanged. Alderman et al. (1995) found that this behavioral approach was effective in reducing improper verbalizations in a patient with brain damage related to encephalitis. Whereas the patient displayed improved inhibitory control in a variety of contexts on her rehabilitation unit following the response cost treatment, generalization to settings outside of her rehabilitation environment did not occur. Accordingly, primarily context-specific training effects should be expected with this type of behavioral technique.

Treatment of Goal Setting and Problem Solving Impairments

Disorganized behavior is a frequent executive function deficit subsequent to TBI and other forms of brain damage that compromise frontal lobe functioning (Levine et al., 1998). This disorganization has been linked to problems implementing and maintaining goal-directed behavior, and is known to negatively affect occupational outcomes. Accordingly, treatment protocols have been developed to teach systematic goal setting and problem solving to patients with executive problems, primarily subsequent to TBI.

One approach involves teaching task-specific routines (Martelli, 1999; Sohlberg & Mateer, 2001a). That is, complex daily behaviors such as maintaining personal hygiene, getting to work, shopping, household cleaning, and operating household appliances or electronic equipment, which patients are unable to complete independently, are taught via the following therapy procedures: (1) the behavior or routine is analyzed and divided into a series of simple steps; (2) a checklist is developed and reviewed with patients so they can see what steps need to be completed, in what order the steps should be completed, and how to record what steps have been completed; (3) extensive practice is provided to help automate checklist use and completion of the complex behavior or routine; and (4) even after the target behavior appears habitual, periodic "retraining" sessions may be necessary, particularly if there are alterations in patients' daily environments or schedules. In selecting which behavior or behaviors to target, clinicians should consider the functional impact of training the patient's independent completion of the routine, which behavior caregivers recommend training, and, perhaps most importantly, which behavior the patient recommends training to maximize his or her motivation during the exhaustive training sessions that are often needed to habituate the behavior (Ylvisaker et al., 1998). Additionally, because generalization is not expected with this type of treatment, training should be conducted in the same context in which the routine will take place (Sohlberg & Mateer, 2001a). Despite limited generalization, this approach to remediating executive problems is recommended for patients with severe memory and/or awareness deficits, or who do not benefit from other self-instructional techniques such as those described in the following paragraph.

Other treatment approaches are similar to teaching task-specific routines in that they focus on breaking down complex behaviors into sequences of simpler steps. They differ, however, in that they also train patients to adopt a strategy that may help them complete a variety of complex behaviors. For example, Robertson (1996) developed the five-stage Goal Management Training (GMT) program depicted in Figure 9-3. Initial sessions teach patients about each stage by describing what the stage is, giving examples of what happens when there is a breakdown at that stage, and demonstrating appropriate completion of the stage using examples from everyday tasks. The patients then practice applying these steps while completing a series of paper-and-pencil versions of everyday, complex tasks (e.g.,

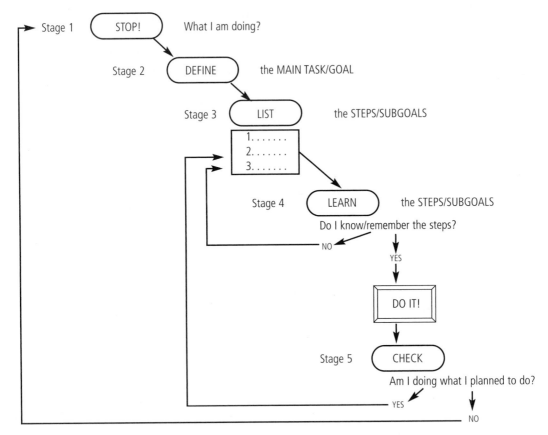

Figure 9-3. The Five Stages of Robertson's (1996) Goal Management Training.

proofreading, how to deal with a power outage). Final sessions of the program involve using the steps, with a visual reminder or flowchart of the steps if necessary, to complete real-life activities (e.g., setting up an answering machine). Levine et al. (2000) found that even following a single hour of GMT, a group of patients with TBI completed a set of everyday tasks significantly more accurately and more slowly, indicating more attention to task completion. These researchers also provided a more comprehensive GMT program to a postencephalitic patient to address her difficulties with daily meal preparation. Following five GMT sessions, which included specific instructions and a checklist regarding how to apply GMT steps to meal preparation, the patient achieved and maintained improved performance of everyday paper-and-pencil tasks, and reductions in problem behaviors that impeded her ability to complete meal preparation. She also reported fewer difficulties with meal preparation following treatment, as quantified by her entries into the self-report diary she was required to keep during the study. Other researchers also have reported positive outcomes when treatments similar to GMT were utilized to address problems in completing other real-world activities (e.g., math assignments, use of memory diary) in both individual (Crowley & Miles, 1991; Ownsworth & McFarland, 1999; von Cramon & Mattes-von Cramon, 1992) and group (Rath, Simon, Langenbahn, Sherr, & Diller, 2003) therapy settings. These initial, promising results deserve follow-up to examine further the generalization potential of GMT and other similar therapy protocols.

COGNITIVE APPROACHES TO TREATING LINGUISTIC IMPAIRMENTS AND DISABILITIES

Recently, researchers have begun to explore whether directly treating cognition or utilizing cognitive treatment approaches such as errorless learning will positively affect the linguistic abilities of patients with neurogenic language disorders. For example, a limited number of studies have examined the effects of direct attention, memory, or executive function training on the linguistic abilities of patients with aphasia (Francis et al., 2003; Helm-Estabrooks, Connor, & Albert, 2000; Mayer & Murray, 2002; Murray et al., in press) or dementia (Brush & Camp, 1999; Mahendra & Arkin, 2003). Whereas in all of these investigations, patients demonstrated improvements on trained cognitive tasks, the degree of generalization to untrained language skills has been variable. For instance, Helm-Estabrooks and colleagues (2000) reported that their two patients with aphasia achieved improved scores on auditory comprehension tests following a nonlinguistic treatment that included a variety of attention and problem-solving tasks (for a detailed description of this treatment protocol, see Helm-Estabrooks & Albert, 2004); likewise, Mayer and Murray (2003) found that their patient with aphasia displayed similar gains in reading when provided a working memory treatment, as when given a version of the Multiple Oral Rereading program. In contrast, Murray and colleagues (in press) observed negligible improvements in the auditory comprehension abilities of their patient with aphasia after the patient was provided Attention Process Training-II. Clearly, further research is indicated to determine which patients or linguistic symptoms might benefit from which, if any, direct cognitive training program.

Researchers also have explored adapting cognitive treatment approaches to train linguistic skills directly. For instance, Abel, Schultz, Radermacher, Willmes, and Huber (2003) reported that both a vanishing cues and a traditional cueing hierarchy approach were effective in improving confrontation naming in a group of patients with aphasia. Although none of their patients appeared to profit from just the vanishing cues approach, and several only improved with the traditional approach, these researchers noted that their alternating treatment design may have interfered with implicit learning, upon which the vanishing cues approach is based. Similarly, in their review of anomia treatments, Fillingham and colleagues (2003) found similar rates of naming improvement in studies utilizing errorless versus errorful learning. These researchers recommended further investigation of errorless learning treatments for naming impairments, as currently, relatively few studies have employed errorless learning procedures. Furthermore, those that have been completed have tended to include only patients with fluent aphasia, failed to provide sufficient information regarding maintenance or generalization of treatment effects, and did not establish whether errorless learning rates are faster and outcomes more enduring compared to those associated with the errorful learning procedures of most traditional aphasia treatments.

Another cognitive approach is based upon a strategy used to alleviate neglect, that is, limb activation. Richards and colleagues (2002; 2003; Wierenga et al., 2003) required patients with nonfluent aphasia to perform either complex left limb movements designed to encourage activation of right hemisphere areas dedicated to response initiation or intention, or a head turn toward their left side that was designed to promote more general attention mechanisms within the right hemisphere during traditional phonological naming treatment. They found that both the limb and head movements produced positive outcomes, with a trend toward better improvement with the intention treatment (i.e., left limb activation). Further research is necessary to resolve inconsistent generalization effects (e.g., Richards et al., 2003 vs. Richards et al., 2002), and to determine whether improvements associated with the intention or attention treatment should be attributed to the additional limb or head movement, respectively, or simply to phonological stimulation, given that a direct comparison of intention/attention treatment outcomes to traditional naming treatment outcomes has not yet been completed.

The above cognitive approaches to treating linguistic impairments appear to hold promise. Recommendations regarding which cognitive treatment protocols are most effective, which patients (e.g., acute vs. chronic) are most likely to benefit from cognitive treatment, or which linguistic symptoms (e.g., lexical-semantic retrieval vs. syntactic processing) are most amenable to a cognitive approach cannot be forwarded until the completion of further empirical investigation.

USE OF COMMERCIALLY AVAILABLE WORKBOOKS AND COMPUTER SOFTWARE FOR TREATING LINGUISTIC OR COGNITIVE IMPAIRMENTS AND DISABILITIES

To allow quick identification of treatment stimuli and activities, numerous commercially available workbooks and computer software programs have been developed. As shown in Table 9-12, some workbooks and software programs provide activities for a broad range of linguistic and/or cognitive deficits (e.g., *Workbook of activities for language and cognition*; Tomlin, 2002), whereas others focus on a narrower range of impairments (e.g., *Left visual inattention workbook*; Knauss, 1998). The functionality of these workbook and software program tasks also varies, from contrived (e.g., canceling out filled-in circles to target visual scanning) to more

Table 9-12. Examples of Workbooks and Software Programs for Treating Linguistic and/or Cognitive Impairments and Disabilities

	PRIMARY TARGET AREA(S)	AUTHOR(S)
Workbooks		
Attention Workbook Volume 1	Attention	Evanofski (1997)
Behavior: Functional Rehabilitation Activity Manual	Pragmatics	Messenger & Ziarnek (2004)
Cognition: Functional Rehabilitation Activity Manual	Various cognitive skills	Messenger & Ziarnek (2004)
Cognitive Linguistic Task Book	Various cognitive and linguistic skills	Helm-Estabrooks (1995)
Critical Thinking for Activities of Daily Living and Communication	Pragmatics and executive functioning	Daly & Fouche (1999)
Left Visual Inattention Workbook	Visual neglect	Knauss (1998)
The Brain Injury Workbook	Various cognitive skills	Powell & Malia (2003)
The Source for Aphasia Therapy	Various linguistic skills	Arnold (1999)
Therapy Guide for Language and Speech Disorders: Reading Comprehension Materials	Reading and attention (neglect)	Kilpatrick (1977)
Workbook of Activities for Language and Cognition	Various cognitive and linguistic skills	Tomlin (2002)
Software		
Aphasia Tutor	Various linguistic skills	Bungalow Software (2004)
Brainwave-Revised	Various cognitive skills	Malia et al. (1997)
Captain's Log	Various cognitive skills	BrainTrain (1985)
Cognitive Package	Various cognitive skills	Bungalow Software (2004)
MossTalk Words	Lexical-semantic retrieval	Fink et al. (2001, 2002)
Parrot Software	Various cognitive and linguistic skills	Parrot Software (1982–2003)
PSSCogRehab	Various cognitive skills	Bracy (1994)
Rosetta Stone Language Learning Programs	Various linguistic skills	Fairfield Language Technologies (2001)

applied and realistic activities (e.g., identifying important information on medicine prescriptions to target reading comprehension). Given the abundance of material choices and the range in quality of these materials, clinicians should carefully consider the following advantages and disadvantages associated with workbook or computerized activities.

There are a number of possible incentives to using workbooks, computer software programs, or both in linguistic or cognitive treatments. For example, these published products may improve the cost effectiveness of treatment by increasing the amount of time patients are involved in treatment tasks, while at the same time reducing the amount of direct clinician contact time necessary (Katz & Wertz, 1997; Wertz & Katz, 2004). Relatedly, they serve to provide additional at-home practice opportunities (Ruiz, 2000). Finally, and most importantly, a growing number of studies have reported positive and enduring improvements in a number of linguistic abilities, such as written and spoken lexical retrieval (Aftonomos, Appelbaum, & Steele, 1999; Deloche, Dordain, & Kremin, 1993; Fink et al., 2001, 2002), written spelling (Mortley, Enderby, & Petheram, 2001), production and comprehension of written syntax (Crerar, Ellis, & Dean, 1996), and reading (Aftonomos et al., 1999; Katz & Wertz, 1997), and cognitive skills such as attention (Chen, Thomas, Glueckauf, & Bracy, 1997; Niemann, Ruff, & Baser, 1990; Webster et al., 2001) and memory (Chen et al., 1997; Niemann et al., 1990), when computer-assisted therapy programs have been utilized, particularly when close supervision of a clinician was available.

Unfortunately, several problems also have emerged as clinicians have begun to exploit these treatment materials (Katz, 2000; Matthews, Harley, & Malec, 1992; Wertz & Katz, 2004). First, many workbooks and software programs consist of repetitive drills that lack the flexibility to adjust the stimuli, task procedures, or both to meet the needs of individual patients. Second, obtaining financial support to purchase computers or software is difficult. Third, many workbooks and programs lack construct validity in that there is no research to support that the linguistic or cognitive processes they purport to address are actually being addressed. Fourth, these types of published materials are limited in terms of what areas of language and cognition can be targeted. For example, because they focus on basic language abilities and have limited application to nonverbal communication (e.g., facial expressions, gestures, contextual cues) or spoken language skills (beyond naming), they are inadequate for addressing social communication or high-level language difficulties that are common among patients with neurogenic language disorders. Fifth, extensive time practicing workbook or software activities may lead to social isolation, which is already problematic in many patients with neurogenic language disorders. Finally, within the limited research literature examining the effectiveness of computerized programs, not all patients respond positively, and often there is nominal generalization to untrained stimuli or tasks (e.g., Fink et al., 2002; Katz & Wertz, 1997). We are unaware of any formal, well-designed studies evaluating the use of workbook activities in treatment.

The above review indicates that workbooks and computer software can foster improvements in the linguistic and cognitive abilities of at least some patients with neurogenic language disorders when clinicians take an active role in evaluating the appropriateness of the workbook or software activities for each individual patient. Because of limitations such as suspect validity and restricted usefulness for targeting certain linguistic and cognitive abilities (e.g., spoken discourse), most researchers concur that currently, the use of workbooks, computer software, or both should, at most, be considered "a component in an organized treatment program versus being improperly viewed as treatment itself" (Matthews et al., 1992, p. 122), and recommend further research to determine which patients are most likely to benefit from these treatment activities.

○ GENERALIZATION AND TRANSFER OF LEARNING

Regardless of which linguistic or cognitive ability is being targeted, or which treatment approach is being used, clinicians must incorporate treatment procedures to ensure that patients will carry over and transfer trained behaviors and strategies to daily activities and environments. Without conscious efforts to target generalization, patients will no doubt display task-specific improvements, which may still be a positive outcome, but not as positive an outcome. Research indicates that considering the following factors when selecting treatment stimuli, activities, and approaches will help ensure maximal generalization of treatment effects (Golisz, 1998; Lloyd & Cuvo, 1994; Sohlberg & Raskin, 1996; Wressle et al., 2002).

First, treatments that incorporate a variety of tasks, contexts, and stimuli produce greater success and generalization. For example, several pictures (e.g., photograph, line drawing, cartoon) of a word being trained as part of a word retrieval treatment should be used; likewise, text written in different font styles, colors, and sizes might be used during a reading treatment program. Training sessions might alternate between the therapy room, the patient's hospital room, and the clinic waiting room to vary the environmental context. These types of manipulations overtly teach the patient that the strategy or behavior being taught applies for general use and multiple contexts. Clinicians should keep in mind that this variability tends to reduce the rate of knowledge or skill acquisition, and thus should counsel patients and caregivers accordingly, emphasizing the long-term benefits (i.e., increased generalization) of such a treatment approach.

Second, training should include functional and personally relevant stimuli and strategies or, relatedly, should target linguistic or cognitive goals and functions that correspond to patients' daily needs and activities. Patients will find it easier to relate these types of stimuli and behaviors to their existing knowledge and experience base, be motivated to practice and utilize the skills being trained, and consequently be more likely to apply trained skills within their daily environments. Caregivers also will be more likely to reinforce patients' use of trained skills if they too can see the functional benefits of such skills.

A final factor to consider when planning treatments that will ensure or maximize the probability of generalization is the amount of practice or training provided (Basso & Caporali, 2001). With few exceptions, those treatment approaches previously described in this chapter that facilitated improvement to untrained stimuli, skills, or contexts provided patients with intensive and/or extensive practice. Even though in most health care settings funding or approval of direct treatment is typically restricted, clinicians can still assure sufficient opportunities for practice by developing detailed homework programs, training families or other caregivers to administer the treatment protocol, or both.

SUMMARY

Numerous treatment approaches and procedures have been developed to facilitate the linguistic and cognitive recovery of patients with neurogenic language disorders. As reviewed in this chapter, however, few treatments have been sufficiently investigated with respect to which patient populations might benefit from the approach (e.g., those with aphasia vs. TBI; those with acute vs. chronic deficits), how well treatment effects are maintained over time, and whether treatment effects generalize to real-world contexts and thus are truly compatible with patients' needs. Furthermore, despite the number of therapy options currently available, there remains a desperate need to develop and critically examine treatments for certain symptoms (e.g., severe auditory comprehension deficits) and, relatedly, certain patient populations (e.g., patients with RHD). Finally, the benefits of combining two or more of the linguistic and/or cognitive treatments described in this chapter or of coalescing therapy procedures mentioned in this chapter with those described in Chapters 10 and 11 have yet to be systematically explored. Despite these research needs, clinicians should be assured that sufficient empirical support has accumulated to justify providing treatment services to patients with neurogenic language disorders. By keeping abreast of research developments, clinicians will be able not only to advocate effectively for treatment services for their patients with neurogenic language disorders, but also to select and provide treatment procedures that are most suitable for each individual patient.

Chapter 10

Remediation of Function: Pharmacotherapy Approaches

LEARNING OBJECTIVES

After reading this chapter you should be able to:

- Identify pharmacotherapies that may be used to address linguistic disorders in patients with neurogenic language disorders.

- Identify pharmacotherapies that may be used to address cognitive disorders in patients with neurogenic language disorders.

- Discuss future research needs pertaining to pharmacotherapy for patients with neurogenic language disorders.

KEY TERMS

acetylcholine
agonists
amphetamine
antagonists
bromocriptine
catecholamine system

cholinergic system
donepezil
dopamine
methylphenidate
neurotransmitters
norepinephrine/ noradrenalin

pharmacotherapy
selective serotonin reuptake inhibitors

INTRODUCTION

In contrast to the behavioral treatments reviewed in Chapter 9 that require practice of target linguistic or cognitive behaviors or strategies, **pharmacotherapy,** or drug treatment, aims to replace or augment behavioral practice with medications. Pharmacotherapy focuses on direct remediation of physiological deficits (i.e., the ICF level of body structure), which in turn should result in resolution of problematic linguistic and/or cognitive behaviors at the ICF level of body function. Over the past few decades, extensive research funds have been spent on developing and evaluating medications that will prevent or remediate a variety of diseases and medical conditions known to cause neurogenic language disorders. Although researchers have most frequently examined the effects of these medications on the memory and attention abilities of patients with neurogenic language disorders related to Alzheimer's disease or traumatic brain injury, there is increasing interest in exploring drugs that will alleviate the linguistic and cognitive problems of other patient populations.

Whereas it is clearly beyond the purview of speech-language pathologists to prescribe medications (see Chapter 4 for a description of the various health care team members), they are responsible for identifying positive as well as negative changes in the linguistic and cognitive abilities of their patients who take these medications. That is, clinicians' observations are essential to helping health care teams monitor the effects of medications in terms of changes in target behaviors or the onset of negative side effects and, relatedly, whether patients should continue with a given medication or whether a new medication or dosage level is needed (Barrett, 2000). Accordingly, knowing what behavioral outcomes have been associated with specific medications will help clinicians direct their observational focus when providing services to patients receiving pharmacotherapy; this knowledge also will empower clinicians to make suggestions to the medical team regarding the prescription of certain medications as possible treatment options.

The purpose of this chapter is to review the variety of medications that have been effective or show promise for remediating linguistic and cognitive impairments associated with neurogenic language disorders. Before describing these drug treatments, however, it is important to have some basic understanding of how medications affect brain functioning. Therefore, this chapter begins with a brief discussion of neurotransmitters and their role in pharmacotherapy.

THE BASICS OF PHARMACOTHERAPY: NEUROTRANSMITTERS

Both static (e.g., stroke, head injury) and progressive forms (e.g., tumors, Parkinson's disease, Alzheimer's disease) of brain damage result in injury not only to brain tissue, but also to the **neurotransmitter** systems that underlie communication among neurons. More specifically, neurotransmitters are chemicals that facilitate message transmission among neurons. For example, in some cases, neurotransmitters may be excitatory and increase the activity of neurons; in other cases, neurotransmitters are inhibitory and decrease neuronal activity. Following the onset of brain damage or disease, the availability of certain neurotransmitters, the sensitivity of neurons to certain neurotransmitters, or both may be compromised. Impairment of two neurotransmitter systems, the **catecholamine** and **cholinergic** systems, have been posited to underlie many of the linguistic and cognitive symptoms associated with neurogenic language disorders. Consequently, the goal of most drug treatments for neurogenic language disorders is to restore these disrupted neurotransmitter systems, which in turn should facilitate linguistic and cognitive recovery in the case of static brain injury, or slow linguistic and cognitive deterioration in the case of progressive brain disorders.

Medications can affect neurotransmitter systems in two basic ways: They may facilitate the effects of one or more neurotransmitters, or they may inhibit the effects of one or more neurotransmitters. Drugs designed to increase the amount or efficiency of neurotransmitters are referred to as **agonists;** for example, a drug that increases levels of dopamine, a neurotransmitter essential to a variety of cognitive functions, would be called a dopamine agonist. In contrast, drugs that reduce the amount or efficiency of neurotransmitters are called **antagonists.** Therefore, dopamine antagonists decrease levels of dopamine. Information about specific agonists and antagonists used to manage neurogenic language disorders is provided in the following sections of this chapter.

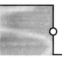

Side Bar

Finding the "Language Neurotransmitter:" A Possible or Impossible Challenge?

Without question, neuroscientists have determined that the neural areas that support linguistic and cognitive functioning utilize a certain set of neurotransmitters, including dopamine, acetylcholine, and noradrenalin. Have they, however, yet found that specific neurotransmitters uniquely support specific linguistic or cognitive functions? The answer is that currently there are no known exclusive relationships between a neurotransmitter and circumscribed linguistic or cognitive abilities. That is, as of yet, there is no "language neurotransmitter." Instead, the neurotransmitters that have been identified to underlie linguistic and cognitive functioning are known to sustain not only a variety of linguistic and cognitive abilities, but also a number of additional skills. For example, dopamine has been associated with verbal fluency, emotional functioning, and motor performance, as well as several cognitive functions, including attention and working memory. Likewise, other neurotransmitters such as noradrenalin and serotonin have also been associated with at least some of these linguistic, emotional, cognitive, and motor abilities. Therefore, when a patient is given a drug designed to increase levels of a certain neurotransmitter in the hopes that it will help resolve certain linguistic or cognitive symptoms, it is important to realize that other neurotransmitter levels may still need to be adjusted to resolve those symptoms and that other abilities may inadvertently be altered.

PHARMACOLOGICAL TREATMENT OF LINGUISTIC IMPAIRMENTS

To date, pharmacotherapy for linguistic impairments has focused primarily on remediating aphasic symptoms with drugs that increase activity within the catecholamine or cholinergic systems. These drugs also have been prescribed to patients with other neurogenic disorders, including those with traumatic brain injury (TBI), right hemisphere brain damage (RHD), or dementia; research and clinical focus with these patient populations, however, has been limited to these drugs' effects on cognitive, emotional, or behavioral outcomes rather than linguistic deficits (see Pharmacological Treatment of Cognitive Impairments section of this chapter). Consequently, because little is known about whether pharmacotherapy can address linguistic symptoms associated with these other neurogenic disorders, our review will concentrate on drug treatments that may facilitate linguistic recovery in patients with aphasia.

ENHANCING THE CATECHOLAMINE SYSTEM

The catecholamine system includes two neurotransmitters, **dopamine** and **norepinephrine,** which also is sometimes referred to as **noradrenalin.** Both of these neurotransmitters have been linked to a number of cognitive and linguistic functions (Tanaka & Bachman, 2000; Walker-Batson et al., 2001). Accordingly, researchers have explored whether dopamine and noradrenergic agonists positively affect language recovery in patients with aphasia when administered by themselves or in concert with behavioral treatments (see Table 10-1).

The effects of **bromocriptine,** a dopamine agonist, on the language abilities of patients with aphasia have been examined in a number of studies. A predominance of dopamine projections have been identified in the frontal cortex and left hemisphere; thus it has been proposed that certain language functions such as language initiation and verbal fluency, which are dependent upon functioning of left frontal regions, may be supported by this neurotransmitter (Gold, VanDam, & Silliman, 2000; Tanaka & Bachman, 2000). Whereas several investigations have obtained null or mixed findings (Gupta, Mlcoch, Scolaro, & Moritz, 1995; MacLennan et al., 1991; Ozeren, Sarica, Mavi, & Demirkiran, 1995; Sabe, Leiguarda, & Starkstein, 1992), a few have reported positive outcomes in terms of improved verbal fluency, word retrieval, or both (Albert, Bachman, Morgan, & Helm-Estabrooks, 1988; Bragoni et al., 2000; Gold et al., 2000; Gupta & Mlcoch, 1992). Unfortunately, the majority of these studies had methodological weaknesses, including inadequate control of placebo or practice effects (e.g., Albert et al., 1988) and a lack of a drug withdrawal phase (e.g., Gupta & Mlcoch, 1992). Furthermore, all studies utilizing bromocriptine have only involved patients with nonfluent aphasia profiles, and thus the effects of this drug on fluent aphasia profiles have yet to be explored. Finally, with the exception of Bragoni et al.'s work (2000), bromocriptine was prescribed in the absence of behavioral aphasia treatment. Accordingly, whether more substantial and enduring improvements can be obtained when this drug and behavioral treatment are provided in concert requires further exploration. Given the nominal improvements previously reported, the negative side effects that may develop with long-term use of this drug (e.g., movement disorders, nausea), and the poor design of prior investigations, prescription of bromocriptine for ameliorating chronic aphasia symptoms is not recommended until further research is conducted.

Table 10-1. Drugs Used to Treat Linguistic and Cognitive Deficits in Adults with Neurogenic Language Disorders

DRUG GROUP	GENERIC (AND COMMERICAL) DRUG NAMES	PHYSIOLOGICAL MECHANISM	POSITIVE BEHAVIORAL EFFECTS	TARGET NEUROGENIC DISORDER
Stimulants	Amphetamines (Dexedrin)	dopamine and noradrenergic agonist	↑ memory, language, attention	aphasia, traumatic brain injury
	Methylphenidate (Ritalin)	dopamine and noradrenergic agonist	↑ attention, language, initiation, memory; ↓ apathy, neglect, depression	aphasia, traumatic brain injury, right hemisphere stroke, multi-infarct dementia
	Amantadine (Symmetrel)	dopamine agonist	↑ attention, learning, alertness, information processing speed; ↓ fatigue, agitation, perseveration	traumatic brain injury, multiple sclerosis, Alzheimer's disease
	Bromocriptine (Parlodel)	dopamine agonist	↑ memory, motivation, executive functions, verbal fluency, reading; ↓ apathy, neglect	nonfluent aphasia, traumatic brain injury, right hemisphere stroke
	Selegiline (Eldepryl)	dopamine agonist	↑ memory, attention, learning, ADL	traumatic brain injury, Alzheimer's disease, HIV-associated dementia
	Carbidopa-Levodopa (Sinemet)	dopamine agonist	↑ attention, arousal	traumatic brain injury
	Bifemelane hydrocholoride	dopamine agonist cholinergic agonist	↑ auditory comprehension, naming, repetition, memory, reading, writing	aphasia, multi-infarct dementia
	Tacrine (Cognex)	cholinergic agonist	↑ memory, naming, general cognitive abilities	Alzheimer's disease, traumatic brain injury, Parkinson's disease
	Donepezil (Aricept)	cholinergic agonist	↑ memory, ADL, attention, auditory comprehension, verbal fluency; ↓ general cognitive decline, apathy	Alzheimer's disease, multi-infarct dementia, multiple sclerosis, traumatic brain injury, aphasia, Parkinson's disease, dementia with Lewy bodies
	Rivastigmine (Exelon)	cholinergic agonist	↑ memory, ADL, attention, general cognitive abilities	Alzheimer's disease, Parkinson's disease, dementia with Lewy bodies

(continues)

Table 10-1. *Continued.*

DRUG GROUP	GENERIC (AND COMMERICAL) DRUG NAMES	PHYSIOLOGICAL MECHANISM	POSITIVE BEHAVIORAL EFFECTS	TARGET NEUROGENIC DISORDER
Stimulants (continued)	Galantamine (Reminyl)	cholinergic agonist	↑ memory, ADL, naming, auditory comprehension, verbal fluency; ↓ behavioral symptoms	Alzheimer's disease, multi-infarct dementia, aphasia, Parkinson's disease
	Physostigmine	cholinergic agonist	↑ naming, attention, memory	Alzheimer's disease, aphasia, traumatic brain injury
	Modafinil (Provigil)	possible dopamine and/or glutamine agonist	↓ fatigue; ↑ attention	multiple sclerosis, stroke, Alzheimer's disease, Parkinson's disease, traumatic brain injury
SSRIs (Selective Serotonin Reuptake Inhibitors)	Sertraline (Zoloft)	serotonin agonist	↑ memory, attention; ↓ depression, perseveration, disinhibition	aphasia, traumatic brain injury, fronto-temporal dementia
Neuroleptics/ Antipsychotics	Haloperidol (Haldol)	dopamine antagonist	↓ irritability, agitation, hyperactivity, hostility; ↑ social interaction, alertness	dementia, traumatic brain injury
Nootropics	Piracetam	cholinergic agonist	↑ language, memory; ↓ general cognitive decline	aphasia, stroke, Alzheimer's disease, traumatic brain injury
Vasodilator	Nimodipine	calcium antagonist	↑ learning, memory	subcortical vascular dementia, traumatic brain injury, HIV-associated dementia

Note. ADL = activities of daily living.

Amphetamines also mediate the catecholamine system, particularly noradrenergic functioning, and have been administered to patients with various types and severities of aphasia. Both negative (Darley, Keith, & Sasanuma, 1977) and positive (McNeil et al., 1995; Walker-Batson et al., 1992; 1996; 2001) outcomes have been reported. Interestingly, significant improvements were noted only in studies in which amphetamines were used to complement behavioral aphasia treatments in the acute stages of patients' recovery (e.g., McNeil et al., 1995; Walker-Batson et al., 2001). Similar findings are reported for motor recovery in stroke patients when amphetamines are combined with physical therapy (Gladstone et al., 2004; Walker-Batson et al., 1995). The predominantly positive outcomes of these studies support conducting further research to explore the long-term effects of combining amphetamines and behavioral treatment, and to determine whether similar results can be obtained when patients have chronic language disorders.

ENHANCING THE CHOLINERGIC SYSTEM

The cholinergic system relies upon **acetylcholine,** a neurotransmitter that has been linked to several linguistic and cognitive functions (e.g., naming, attention, memory) and, when deficient, to certain neurogenic disorders (e.g., Alzheimer's disease) (Hughes, Jacobs, & Heilman, 2000; Jacobs et al., 1994; Tanaka & Bachman, 2000). Likewise, in healthy individuals, greater cholinergic activity has been observed in the left versus right temporal lobe, and acetylcholine has been posited to enhance signal-to-noise ratios within cortical regions. Accordingly, researchers have speculated that providing cholinergic agonists should facilitate language abilities such as naming or word-finding skills.

As predicted, improvements in general as well as specific language abilities, in particular naming, auditory comprehension, and repetition, have been reported when cholinergic agents such as galantamine, physostigmine, bifemelane hydrochloride, or piracetam have been administered to patients with dementia (Farlow et al., 1992) or acute or chronic aphasia (De Deyn, De Reuck, Orgogozo, Vlietinck, & Deberdt, 1997; Hughes et al., 2000; Jacobs et al., 1994; Kabasawa et al., 1994; Pashek & Bachman, 2003) (see Table 10-1). For example, in a few randomized double-blind, placebo-controlled investigations, patients with aphasia who received piracetam plus traditional language treatment displayed significantly greater improvements in their overall aphasia severity, compared to patients who received a placebo plus traditional language treatment (Enderby, Broeckx, Hospers, Schildermans, & Deberdt, 1994; Huber, Willmes, Poeck, Van Vleymen, & Deberdt, 1997; Kessler, Thiel, Karbe, & Heiss, 2000). More specifically, the piracetam group achieved higher gains in their naming, writing, auditory comprehension, repetition, and phonological, semantic, and syntactic aspects of their spontaneous verbal output compared to the placebo group. Further exploration of these positive outcomes are needed, however, as many of the above cited studies had weak designs;

that is, these studies failed to control for a number of confounds including spontaneous recovery, placebo, and practice effects, neglected to indicate whether or not the cholinergic agonist was provided by itself or in concert with behavioral language treatment, or both (e.g., Jacobs et al., 1994; Kabasawa et al., 1994; Pashek & Bachman, 2003; Tanaka, Miyazaki, & Albert, 1997).

SUMMARY OF PHARMACOTHERAPY FOR LINGUISTIC IMPAIRMENTS

The study of pharmacotherapy for linguistic impairments is only in its infancy. Not only have a limited number of investigations been completed, but those that have been completed often have produced disparate findings. These conflicting data can be attributed, at least in part, to one or more of the following methodology differences across the studies: (1) varying patient selection criteria, such as whether patients who had or did not have concomitant emotional disorders were included or whether patients were in the acute or chronic stage of aphasia recovery; (2) use of different study designs, such as a blind (i.e., test examiners did not know which patients were receiving the drug treatment) versus an open-label (i.e., test examiners are aware of which patients were receiving the drug treatment) design; and (3) inclusion of different outcome measures, such as using different aphasia tests or including versus excluding patient or caregiver feedback.

Although definitive conclusions regarding the efficacy of pharmacotherapy for linguistic impairments cannot yet be made, findings from the existing literature do suggest that drug treatments will not replace more traditional, linguistic treatments, but rather serve to enhance the extent of recovery achieved with these behavioral treatments. Numerous avenues of research remain to be explored, including determining: (1) optimal dosages to maximize positive effects and minimize negative side effects, (2) whether drugs directly affect language abilities or affect them indirectly via their influence on other cognitive functions (e.g., attention, working memory) or emotional status (e.g., depression, anxiety), (3) whether the linguistic impairments of patients with neurogenic language disorders other than aphasia (e.g., RHD, TBI) respond to pharmacotherapy, (4) if certain types and/or severities of linguistic deficits or particular sites and/or sizes of brain lesions are more or less ameliorable to pharmacotherapy, (5) long-term effects of drug treatments on linguistic abilities or response to behavioral language treatments once the drug has been discontinued, and (6) the effects of combination agonist therapies (e.g., dopaminergic + cholinergic agonist drug treatment).

PHARMACOLOGICAL TREATMENT OF COGNITIVE IMPAIRMENTS

There has been increasing research to explore whether certain drugs may help ameliorate cognitive deficits associated with a variety of acquired neurogenic disorders.

As with pharmacotherapy for linguistic deficits, drug treatments for cognitive impairments have been designed primarily to manipulate catecholamine and/or cholinergic neurotransmitter systems because of their documented involvement in a number of cognitive functions and their vulnerability in many neurological disorders (Ericksen, Cifu, & Burnett, 2001; Smith Doody, 2003).

ENHANCING THE CATECHOLAMINE SYSTEM

A number of dopaminergic and noradrenergic agonists have been used to treat a spectrum of cognitive problems associated with TBI, progressive neurological disorders such as Alzheimer's and Parkinson's diseases, and, to a lesser extent, stroke (see Table 10-1). For example, **methylphenidate,** more commonly known as Ritalin, has been the focus of numerous investigations with a variety of neurogenic patient populations. In patients with stroke, methylphenidate has been found useful in treating left neglect (Hurford, Stringer, & Jann, 1998) and apathy (Watanabe et al., 1995), but ineffective for memory problems (Tiberti et al., 1998). Whereas some studies report that this drug positively affects memory and attention in patients with TBI (Plenger et al., 1996; Whyte et al., 1997), others observed nominal effects, particularly when patients with TBI were in the more chronic stages of recovery (Speech, Rao, Osmon, & Sperry, 1993). These mixed findings have led researchers to conclude that in TBI, methylphenidate is most effective in assisting acute recovery of cognitive abilities (Kajs-Wyllie, 2002). Further studies are needed, however, to examine methylphenidate's long-term efficacy, and thus specify at what point this drug may no longer augment cognitive recovery subsequent to TBI.

Another dopaminergic agonist, amantadine, also has been shown to assist in the acute and chronic cognitive recovery of patients with TBI, including those in a vegetative or minimally conscious state (Kraus & Maki, 1997; Saniova, Drobny, Kneslova, & Minarik, 2004). It also has been found to enhance general cognitive functioning in patients with Alzheimer's disease, even those in the end stages of the disease (Erkulwater & Pillai, 1989). For example, Patrick et al. (2002) gave amantadine to 10 children who were minimally responsive due to TBI, stroke, or infection and found that compared to their baseline performances, the children scored significantly better on a test measuring attention, communication, and response to sensory stimulation following this drug treatment. Furthermore, their rates of test improvement were significantly greater while on the medication versus prior to receiving the medication, indicating that in these severely impaired patients, this dopamine agonist may accelerate recovery. Although initial findings suggest that dopamine agonists may be particularly useful in enhancing cognitive functions in acute or severely impaired neurogenic patient populations, further empirical investigation is necessary, as much of this research has been limited to case studies (e.g., Kraus & Maki, 1997).

Side
Bar

The Roles of Speech-Language Pathologists in Pharmacotherapy

At the beginning of this chapter, we mentioned two important ways that speech-language pathologists can contribute to the process of pharmacotherapy. First, if they keep abreast of pharmacotherapy research, they may make suggestions to the medical team about drugs that may prove to positively affect the linguistic and/or cognitive symptoms of their patient. Second, they can provide important observational data pertaining to the effects of prescribed medications on the linguistic and cognitive abilities of their patients. Another possible contribution can be providing behavioral treatments (see Chapter 9) or training compensatory strategies (see Chapter 11) that will help assure that patients take their medications on a regular basis in order to optimize pharmacotherapy effects. For example, the clinician might add the times at which a patient with TBI is to take his medication to that patient's memory book. Treatment might then focus on several of the following: (1) making sure the patient knew where he could find this medication information within his memory book, (2) training the patient to consult this section of his memory book on a regular basis, (3) training caregivers to cue the patient to consult this section of his memory book on a regular basis, and (d) monitoring how frequently the patient independently or with cueing took his medication at the right time.

ENHANCING THE CHOLINERGIC SYSTEM

Substantial research indicates that cholinergic agonists such as rivastigmine, physostigmine, galantamine, and tacrine can enhance cognitive recovery in a variety of neurogenic patient populations, in particular those with dementia or TBI (e.g., Aarsland, Hutchinson, & Larsen, 2003; Byrne, 2000) (see Table 10-1). Because of its longer-acting properties and lower risk of negative side effects compared to other cholinergic agents such as tacrine, **donepezil** has become one of the most frequently prescribed cognitive enhancing medications (Burn & McKeith, 2003; Griffin, van Reekum, & Masanic, 2003). For instance, in patients in the acute or chronic stages of TBI recovery, gains in short- and long-term verbal memory, visuoperception, alertness, social interaction, and activities of daily living have been reported following administration of donepezil (Griffin et al., 2003; Masanic, Bayley, & van Reekum, 2001). Likewise, patients ranging from the early to late stages of dementing diseases such as Alzheimer's disease, multi-infarct dementia, Parkinson's disease, and dementia with Lewy bodies have been found to display significant improvements in their general cognitive abilities, slowing in their rates of cognitive and functional decline, or both when taking donepezil, compared to those receiving placebo treatment (Burn & McKeith, 2003; Li et al., 2002; Smith Doody, 2003). Although further investigation of the long-term effects of cholinergic agonists is needed, the positive findings reported to date are particularly encouraging given the strong research designs of many previous studies.

OTHER PHARMACOLOGICAL APPROACHES

As shown in Table 10-1, a number of other drugs have been found to ameliorate the cognitive or emotional-behavioral problems that frequently coexist with neurogenic language disorders. For example, neuroleptic or antipsychotic medications, which affect brain functioning by reducing activity within dopaminergic systems (i.e., dopaminergic antagonists), have been successfully used to reduce negative behaviors such as agitation and to enhance alertness and responsiveness to rehabilitation in patients with dementia or TBI (Cardenas, 1987; Ericksen et al., 2001). Researchers also have begun to explore the effects of **selective serotonin reuptake inhibitors** (SSRIs) such as sertraline on a variety of cognitive disorders associated with acquired brain damage or disease (Ericksen et al., 2001; Meythaler, Depalma, Devivo, Guin-Renfroe, & Novack, 2001). Rationale for prescribing SSRIs includes: (1) serotonin levels are reduced in certain neurological disorders, (2) the serotonergic system affects functioning of neural areas crucial to a number of cognitive functions, including attention or arousal (i.e., reticular formation) and memory (i.e., hippocampus), and (3) SSRIs are commonly used to treat depression, which is a frequent concomitant symptom in neurogenic language disorders. Some initial SSRI studies have produced positive findings, including reduced perseveration in aphasia (Tanaka & Albert, 2003), improved attention and memory in TBI (Ericksen et al., 2001; Meythaler et al., 2001), and decreased disinhibition in frontotemporal dementia (Swartz et al., 1997). Another benefit of SSRIs is that they produce nominal negative side effects (Meythaler et al., 2001). Lastly, modafinil, a drug initially used to treat narcolepsy, is now being investigated regarding its potential to reduce fatigue and depression and, consequently, to enhance attention and other cognitive abilities in a spectrum of neurological disorders, including stroke, TBI, and Alzheimer's and Parkinson's diseases (Cochran, 2001; Kajs-Wyllie, 2002).

SUMMARY OF PHARMACOTHERAPY FOR COGNITIVE IMPAIRMENTS

As concluded in our review of pharmacological treatments for linguistic impairments, further investigation of the efficacy of pharmacotherapy for cognitive impairments is warranted to rectify the methodological weaknesses of some previous studies (e.g., reliance on subjective vs. objective measures; failure to control for placebo or practice effects), as well as to explore issues that have yet to be addressed. For example, nominal research has compared the effects of drug treatment alone to a combined drug and behavioral treatment approach. An exception is a study by Chapman and colleagues (2004). These investigators found slower rates of decline in emotional well-being, discourse production and comprehension, and completion of daily activities in patients with Alzheimer's disease who received donepezil *and* cognitive-linguistic treatment, compared to those who received only the drug treatment. Given these encouraging, albeit preliminary results and the positive outcomes associated with integrating drug and behavioral therapies to treat language impairments (e.g., Kessler et al., 2000), it is predicted that the combined treatment approach holds promise as an effective approach to managing cognitive problems associated with a spectrum neurogenic disorders.

Other research avenues to pursue in the area of pharmacotherapy for cognitive impairments include examining the effects of combination drug treatments such as prescribing cholinergic agonists in concert with SSRIs. Future studies should also include outcome measures that evaluate a broader range of cognitive abilities, in particular executive functions, and assure that more patients with aphasia or RHD are represented in the subject samples. Finally there remains a need to determine which patient characteristics (e.g., age, dementia severity, concomitant symptoms) can help health care teams predict which patients will most likely benefit from pharmacotherapy for cognitive impairments.

SUMMARY

A relatively new approach to resolving the linguistic and cognitive impairments associated with neurogenic language disorders involves prescribing medications. These medications are designed to remediate the alterations in neurotransmitter systems that occur subsequent to the onset of brain damage or disease. The majority of drugs that have been investigated to date affect the catecholamine or cholinergic neurotransmitter systems because these systems have been shown to have important ties to a number of linguistic and cognitive functions. Indeed, initial research indicates that pharmacotherapies that target these neurotransmitter systems can produce positive changes in the linguistic and/or cognitive functioning of patients with static (e.g., stroke, TBI) or progressive brain damage (e.g., Alzheimer's disease). Importantly, however, the most consistently positive findings have been reported when the drugs are used to supplement behavioral treatments. It is anticipated that adults with neurogenic language disorders will benefit greatly from future research designed to identify additional pharmacotherapy and behavioral treatment combinations, to specify which patients are most likely to respond positively to these treatment regimens, or both.

Chapter 11

Remediation of Activity and Participation

LEARNING OBJECTIVES

After reading this chapter you should be able to:

- Discuss the relationship between impairment and activity/participation remediation strategies.

- Identify a variety of compensatory strategies that may enhance the communication or cognitive functioning of patients with neurogenic language disorders.

- Describe treatment approaches that target the use of multiple modalities to enhance communication effectiveness.

- List external devices that may be used to help patients compensate for their linguistic and/or cognitive impairments.

- Describe training procedures for fostering patients' effective use of compensatory strategies or external devices.

KEY TERMS

acupuncture
augmentative communication
authentic context
biofeedback
complementary and alternative medicine

guided imagery
interaction
multimodal communication
progressive muscle relaxation
relaxation therapy

sensory stimulation
transaction
transcutaneous electrical nerve stimulation

- Discuss the benefits of group treatment and identify characteristics of effective group intervention strategies.

- Identify a variety of strategies for modifying the environment to enhance communication effectiveness and cognitive functioning.

- Describe how training caregivers and volunteers may facilitate the life participation of patients with neurogenic language disorders.

- Discuss the issues surrounding the chronicity of

neurogenic language disorders, including the role of speech-language pathologists in providing counseling and education, and identifying other community resources available to assist patients and their caregivers in participating fully in desired activities.

- Describe alternative treatment approaches that have been used to alleviate the effects of linguistic and/or cognitive deficits in patients with neurogenic language disorders.

INTRODUCTION

The impairment level treatment strategies discussed in Chapters 9 and 10 will often result in observable changes in communicative and cognitive activities and life participation. As the underlying impairments contributing to neurogenic language disorders are remediated, it is anticipated that patients will be more effective communicators in daily situations and will resume participation in many previously enjoyed personal, social, and professional activities, which is the ultimate goal of treatment. In addition to these impairment level strategies, however, clinicians also may select treatments that directly target communicative and cognitive effectiveness, participation, or both. Activity and participation level treatments may help facilitate carryover of improved linguistic and cognitive capabilities to functional communicative and cognitive effectiveness functioning (and thus be used in concert with procedures described in Chapters 9 and 10), may serve to "fill the gap" when underlying cognitive and/or linguistic functions are not completely restored, and can be implemented from the outset of treatment. Because these treatment activities tend to involve daily, functional communicative and cognitive behaviors, patients with neurogenic language disorders and their caregivers may find them more intrinsically reinforcing and thus help them stay motivated to participate actively in treatment (Manochiopinig, Reed, Sheard, & Choo, 1997). Finally, because activity and participation level treatments are not specific to underlying impairments, many of the strategies are appropriate for individuals affected by aphasia, dementia, and other cognitive-communicative disorders.

ACTIVITY-FOCUSED TREATMENTS

The first section of this chapter reviews a number of strategies for targeting the ICF level of activity. Most of these strategies emphasize modifying the patients' communicative or cognitive behaviors, whereas others aim to enhance their communicative and cognitive effectiveness by modifying their environment, training their communication partners and caregivers, or both.

COMPENSATORY STRATEGIES

Instruction in the use of compensatory strategies is a common component of intervention for many neurogenic language disorders. Compensatory strategies allow patients to communicate or to complete daily activities more effectively in spite of the presence of significant linguistic and/or cognitive impairments. In general, patients compensate by exploiting intact linguistic and cognitive skills to circumvent the limitations imposed by underlying impairments. Some strategies rely primarily on the patient utilizing readily available communication modalities (e.g., drawing, gesturing) or more deliberate cognitive functioning, whereas other strategies incorporate external devices that serve to cue or replace verbal output, or to support problematic cognitive functions.

Multimodality Communication Approaches

Although a hallmark of aphasia is language impairment evident across communication modalities (i.e., speaking, listening, reading, writing, gesturing), many patients experiencing neurogenic language disorders will demonstrate areas of relative strength in one or more modalities. As these strengths become apparent, clinicians can help patients exploit the stronger modalities to compensate for weaker ones.

Drawing

The use of drawing to compensate for linguistic impairment has intuitive appeal, as visuospatial skills often remain relatively intact following damage to the language-dominant hemisphere and most patients retain at least a basic ability to draw and interpret drawings. Anyone who has played the popular game Pictionary™, however, knows that communicating complex ideas graphically can be very difficult. Nonetheless, clinicians can help patients with neurogenic language disorders develop drawing as an effective mode of communication.

An obvious factor influencing the potential effectiveness of drawing as a communication modality is drawing ability, which may be compromised by motor impairments affecting limb movements (e.g., hemiparesis, limb apraxia). Moreover, many patients with aphasia will be forced to use their nondominant hand for drawing, which may have a significant impact on drawing speed, coordination, and legibility. Visual problems also may impede drawing legibility. Accordingly, clinicians must carefully assess the patient's drawing ability (see Chapters 5 and 6) with consideration of motoric and visuospatial limitations.

If drawing appears to have communicative potential, clinicians may consider "Back to the Drawing Board" (Morgan & Helm-Estabrooks, 1987) or its more recent revision, "Communicative Drawing Program" (CDP; Helm-Estabrooks & Albert, 2004), as treatment approaches to develop basic drawing skills for communicative purposes. CDP involves ten sequential steps, beginning with activities targeting foundational conceptual skills and progressing to drawing complete scenes (see Figure 11-1). The authors recommended that patients master each step (i.e., 100% accuracy) before proceeding to the next step in the program.

Once basic drawing ability has been established, patients must develop strategies for effectively using drawing as a communication modality; that is, they must be able to transfer basic drawing skills to daily communicative interactions. Clinicians may be pleasantly surprised to learn that the strategies used in Pictionary™ apply very well to graphic communication. Although a specific time limit is not generally imposed in typical communication interactions, communication is enhanced

Step One: Semantic-Conceptual Knowledge. Given a selection of ten pictured items, the individual must identify which five items belong together (share relevant semantic features). Although the clinician selects the pictures based on common superordinate categories, this information is not made available to the individual.

Step Two: Knowledge of Object Color Properties. The individual must select appropriate colored markers for nine line drawings of objects generally associated with specific colors (e.g., flag, witch's hat). He or she then colors in the line drawing with the selected marker.

Step Three: Outlining Pictures of Objects with Distinct Shape Properties. The individual uses a pen to outline (draw around the outside lines) line drawn pictures (e.g., church, apple).

Step Four: Copying Geometric Shapes. The individual copies geometric shapes from line drawings, with instruction to match the target with respect to size, shape, and three-dimensional properties.

Step Five: Completing Drawings with Missing Features. The individual identifies missing features from line drawings and then completes the drawings with his or her own pen.

Step Six: Drawing Characteristic Shapes from Memory. The individual is asked to study pictures of common objects (e.g., hammer) and then to draw the item from memory once the picture has been removed from view.

Step Seven: Drawing Objects from Stored Representations. The individual draws items that are presented verbally or by printed word, but without a picture or drawing.

Step Eight: Drawing Objects within Categories. The individual is presented with a verbal stimulus that is an exemplar (e.g., tulip) of a superordinate category (e.g., flower). The individual is then instructed to draw another exemplar of that category.

Step Nine: Generative Drawing of Animals and Modes of Transportation. The individual draws as many exemplars as possible from these two superordinate categories.

Step Ten: Drawing Cartooned Scenes. The individual is asked to study paneled cartoons and then draw the scene from memory. This step begins with single-paneled cartoons and progresses to multiple-paneled cartoons.

Figure 11-1. Communicative Drawing Program by Helm-Estabrooks and Albert (2004). Patients learn to use drawing as a primary or augmentative mode of communication.

when message exchange occurs at a reasonable pace. Accordingly, because drawing usually requires more time than is typically needed to speak a message, patients must learn to convey their drawn messages as efficiently as possible. Figure 11-2 lists several strategies for improving efficiency of graphic communication, and Figure 11-3 provides examples of efficient and inefficient drawings.

As with most communication modes, graphic communication will be enhanced if the drawer is sensitive to the receiver's comprehension and can employ repair strategies. These strategies may include adding detail to help receivers differentiate similar concepts (e.g., house vs. school vs. store), or drawing additional pictures if receivers overlook or need elaboration of a key concept (e.g., adding a

- Avoid producing one drawing for each word in a sentence. Use one or two drawings of the most relevant concepts to capture the "gist" of the message
- Use arrows and other icons to convey relationships among pictures
- Avoid unnecessary detail, and discontinue detailing a picture once it has been appropriately identified by the communication partner
- Point to previous drawings rather than redrawing pictures if a concept is repeated in subsequent messages
- Use color only if meaning is unclear without it

Figure 11-2. Strategies for facilitating efficiency of graphic communication. Whether incorporated into a formal or informal graphic communication training program, patients should be aware of strategies to enhance the efficiency of drawings.

car between pictures if the intent is to communicate a mode of transportation). Likewise, Lyon and Helm-Estabrooks (1987) recommended training communication partners to utilize certain spoken and graphic prompts that serve to elicit these types of drawing strategies and thus enhance successful communicative interactions. Also, clinicians should keep in mind that just as drawing can aid patients' message production, it can also aid their message comprehension, and thus caregivers in addition to patients might be trained on all of the above procedures.

Importantly, several case studies support the use of drawing programs with patients who have severe spoken and written language production deficits, including those with concomitant hemiparesis (e.g., Rao, 1995) or progressive disorders (e.g., Murray, 1998). Further investigations with stronger research designs are needed not only to replicate and validate previous findings, but also to specify further which patients are most likely to benefit from drawing therapy and which treatment procedures result in the greatest generalization of trained drawing skills to daily communicative interactions.

Gesturing

Unlike drawing, gesturing is a communication mode that is used regularly by many speakers for such purposes as clarifying meaning, adding emphasis, or even replacing speech (e.g., waving hello, pointing in response to "where" questions). Moreover, many gestures are universally recognized by communicators of a given language or dialect (e.g., the "OK" gesture, wiping the hand across the forehead to express relief). Because patients likely used gestures to enhance communication prior to the onset of their neurogenic language disorder, they often are willing to expand their use of gestures to further enhance communicative effectiveness. As with drawing and writing, however, it is important to keep in mind that many patients will be attempting to use this communication mode in the presence of motor deficits affecting one or both limbs.

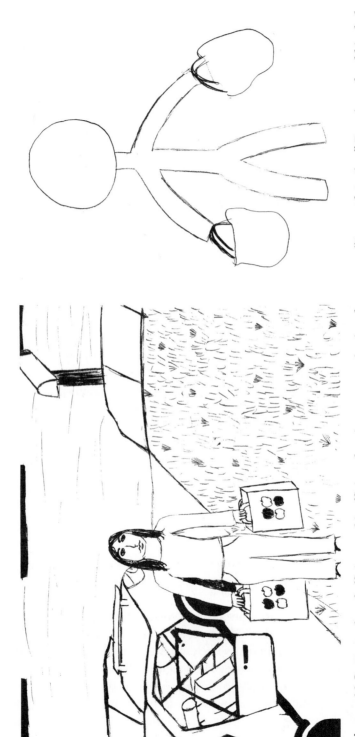

Figure 11-3. Examples of efficient and inefficient drawings communicating the message "I went shopping." Drawings should include enough detail to communicate the message without including details extraneous to the message.

Although many conventional gestures exist to communicate a great variety of meanings, most patients with neurogenic language disorders will need to develop a more elaborate gesture system to communicate the complex messages characteristic of adult life. Several gestural codes have been suggested as potentially effective communication modes for patients with neurogenic language disorders, in particular those with severe aphasia. Although highly developed sign systems are used by deaf cultures, these systems have several disadvantages for patients with aphasia. First, many sign languages, including American Sign Language (ASL), are unique languages with word forms and syntax dissimilar from English or other spoken languages. Accordingly, it is unreasonable to expect that patients with an impaired language system will learn an entirely new language such as this. Signed Exact English (SEE) partially addresses this problem by using ASL signs with standard English syntax. Both ASL and SEE utilize bimanual signs, however, that can be difficult for patients with hemiplegia or hemiparesis to produce. Moreover, the communicative effectiveness of ASL or SEE will be limited by the number of potential communication partners familiar with the language. A better choice, therefore, is Amer-Ind, a gestural code based on American Indian hand talk (Skelly, 1979). This system can be used with one hand and utilizes gestures that are relatively transparent (i.e., understandable to individuals unfamiliar with the code) (Campbell & Jackson, 1995; Daniloff, Fritelli, Buckingham, Hoffman, & Daniloff, 1986). Because of these features, Amer-Ind has been more widely recommended than any other gestural system for patients with aphasia, and indeed some research supports this contention. For instance, several studies have reported that patients with moderate, severe, and even progressive forms of aphasia have been able to acquire, use, and, in some cases, even sequence three or more Amer-Ind signs to improve their communication success (Dowden, Marshall, & Tompkins, 1981; Heilman, Rothi, Campanella, & Wolfson, 1979; Schneider, Thompson, & Luring, 1996).

For some patients with profound deficits of language, other aspects of cognition, or both, however, even relatively simple gestural systems such as Amer-Ind may be inappropriate (Coelho & Duffy, 1987). These patients may instead benefit from instruction in using **pantomime,** a form of gestural communication that involves a series of relatively transparent movements that are associated with a given activity or situation. For example, to pantomime pouring a glass of milk, an individual might pretend to hold a glass in one hand while holding the other hand in an open posture and tipping that hand toward the hand "holding the glass." To train pantomime use as a communication modality, clinicians may utilize Visual Action Therapy (VAT; Helm-Estabrooks, Fitzpatrick, & Baresi, 1982; Helm-Estabrooks & Albert, 2004). The steps in VAT are designed to help patients first comprehend how pantomimed movements represent ideas or concepts, and then to learn to produce a set of pantomimes (see Figure 11-4). The program begins with training pantomimes that involve proximal gestures (i.e., those using gross limb movements such as waving a flag), then progresses to pantomimes that involve distal gestures (e.g., dialing a telephone), and finally progresses to panto-

Step One: Matching Pictures and Objects. This step is further broken down into smaller steps of placing objects on pictures, placing pictures on objects, pointing to objects when presented with the picture, and pointing to pictures when presented with the object.

Step Two: Object Use Training. The individual must demonstrate the ability to use each object appropriately.

Step Three: Action Picture Demonstration. The clinician selects an object and then provides the individual with an action picture incorporating that object. Then the clinician manipulates the object in the manner that is depicted on an action picture.

Step Four: Following Action Picture Commands. The individual must select the appropriate object from a group of objects and manipulate it in the manner that is depicted on an action picture.

Step Five: Pantomimed Gesture Demonstration. The individual identifies missing features from line drawings and then completes the drawings with his or her own pen.

Step Six: Pantomimed Gesture Recognition. The individual must identify from a selection the object that corresponds to a pantomime produced by the clinician.

Step Seven: Pantomimed Gesture Production. The individual produces the appropriate pantomime when provided with the corresponding object.

Step Eight: Representation of Hidden Objects Demonstration. The clinician models pantomimes associated with objects that are known to the individual but are out of immediate view.

Step Nine: Production of Gestures for Hidden Objects. The individual produces pantomime to request an object that is known to both participants but is out of immediate view.

Figure 11-4. Visual Action Therapy. The use of pantomimes may serve as a helpful precursor to formal gesture communication systems or may serve as a primary mode of communication.

mimes that involve oral gestures (e.g., sipping from a straw). When all three phases are mastered, Helm-Estabrooks and colleagues have recommended expanding the gesture repertoire by incorporating Amer-Ind signs. Although preliminary studies conducted by the VAT developers have yielded positive outcomes (e.g., improved aphasia test battery scores) for patients with global aphasia (Helm-Estabrooks et al., 1982; Ramsberger & Helm-Estabrooks, 1989), further investigations with more rigorous research designs are needed not only to confirm these findings but also to examine how well, if at all, gesture use generalizes to daily communicative activities (Conlon & McNeil, 1991).

Augmentative Communication

Although both graphic and gestural communication are typically "augmentative" to spoken communication, the term **augmentative communication** is generally used to denote a communication system whereby the speaker points to or otherwise selects written words or pictured symbols to communicate meaning. It is important to keep in mind that augmentative communication devices can facilitate not only the expressive abilities of patients, but also their comprehension accuracy. For instance, communication partners might augment their speech by pointing to pictures on a patient's augmentative system to emphasize key points of their message. Augmentative communication systems range from the very simple (e.g., a single sheet of paper with the words "yes" and "no" in large print) to the very complex (e.g., computer-synthesized voice activated by eye-blink switches). Importantly, these devices can be used to facilitate not only "online" but also "off-line" communication (van de Sandt-Koenderman, 2004). That is, patients with neurogenic language disorders may be able to use these devices to prepare for future communication encounters (e.g., a repairman coming to fix a home appliance; a telephone call to make an appointment; a parent-teacher conference) by pre-selecting and/or preprogramming messages. The applications of augmentative communication range beyond neurogenic language disorders, and thus a thorough discussion of the principles guiding the development of augmentative systems is beyond the scope of this text (for an in-depth review, see Beukelman, Yorkston, & Reichle, 2000). It is, however, useful to explore the issues that must be considered when developing augmentative communication systems for patients with neurogenic language disorders.

The nature of neurogenic language disorders dictates that augmentative communication systems selected for these patients should not rely heavily on linguistic processing. For example, whereas some patients demonstrate adequate reading skills to use print (at least at the letter or word level), others may benefit from graphic symbols or photographs. Clinicians also must be sensitive to the presence of deficits of visuoperception, attention, or both that will influence the size and/or placement of items. For instance if a patient with aphasia has concomitant right neglect, items may need to be placed in a vertical rather than horizontal array so that the patient is able to view readily all item choices. Similarly, motor deficits such as hemiplegia or limb apraxia may limit access options, in that patients may need to access the system with their nondominant or a weak hand. Memory and executive function abilities also must be considered, particularly in terms of the amount and organization of information to be contained within the system, and in terms of the complexity of the operational skills that will be necessary for independent system use. For example, a patient with severe cognitive and motor speech deficits related to traumatic brain injury (TBI) may be able to select items on a high-tech, dynamic screen device when provided with clinician prompting, but without guidance be unable to find these same items because of memory limitations. Finally, clinicians should be diligent in selecting age-appropriate symbols and/or photographs and should consult with patients and their caregivers regarding which words and phrases should be included within the augmentative communication system.

Individualized augmentative communication systems may play an important role in maximizing communication effectiveness for patients with neurogenic language disorders. Additionally, many patients may benefit from impromptu augmentative communication systems. For example, patients with limited verbal expression may point to items on a menu to facilitate ordering in a restaurant. Store catalogs and newspaper inserts may be used to develop shopping lists and/or request assistance from store clerks. Importantly, all patients with aphasia, even those with mild linguistic deficits, should carry a small card listing important personal information and providing a brief description of aphasia so that if they find themselves in an emergency, this card can be used to augment their spoken output, which will no doubt be affected negatively by the stress of the situation. Conveniently, these types of cards can be obtained for free from the National Aphasia Association (go to www.naa.org for further information). Creative clinicians will be on the alert for other readily available and low-cost products and materials that can augment the communication abilities of the adult with a neurogenic language disorder.

Despite the inherent benefits of augmentative communication devices and advances in technology that have led to more portable and generative devices, clinicians often have limited awareness or understanding of augmentative device options and training procedures (van de Sandt-Koenderman, 2004). There also has been limited empirical examination of augmentative device use by patients with neurogenic language disorders. The results of initial investigations, however, are encouraging. For example, findings from several studies indicate that patients with moderate to severe forms of nonfluent aphasia can improve their lexical-retrieval and syntax formulation abilities via the Computer-Assisted Visual Communication system (C-VIC; Shelton et al., 1996) or devices similar to it (e.g., Lingraphica or C-Speak Aphasia; Aftonomos et al., 1999, Nicholas & Elliott, 1999, respectively). These devices run on Macintosh or Windows-based computers, and require patients to select and sequence icons that represent various lexical items (e.g., nouns, verbs, conjunctions) to compose messages. Such systems are relatively portable if installed on laptop computers. Even this solution, however, is only feasible primarily for patients who might attach the computer to a wheelchair.

A new system, which appears to have greater potential for functional use, is the Personal Communication Assistant for Dysphasic People (PCAD; van de Sandt-Koenderman, 2004). This system runs on a palmtop computer and can be adapted for individual patients by loading only certain software modules on the computer. Example modules include: (1) hierarchically represented vocabulary, (2) digitized or synthesized speech output, (3) options in which the patient can draw or type information into the device, and (4) phonemic cueing, in which the initial sound of a word or phrase is generated by the device. The findings of a multiple-case study, as summarized by van de Sandt-Koenderman, indicated that: (1) all 22 patients with aphasia involved in the study learned to operate PCAD, (2) 17 patients were able to employ the device in daily communicative settings and activities, and (3) of the six patients who were followed after training terminated, four were still using the device in daily contexts when interviewed nine months post-treatment, and one, who was followed for an even longer period, reported using it on a regular basis two years post-treatment. These results indicate that further investigation of PCAD as well as other recently developed technologies (e.g., ReadingPen, Dragon NaturallySpeaking® voice-recognition software, word prediction software) is certainly warranted.

Additional Issues

Whereas drawing, gesturing, or the use of augmentative communication may serve as the principal communication mode for some patients with neurogenic language disorders, even patients whose primary output modality is speech may effectively exploit these other modalities. In fact, there is evidence that pairing another modality with speech may actually enhance verbal output (e.g., Hanlon, Brown, & Gerstman, 1990; Lyon & Helm-Estabrooks, 1987). Nonetheless, clinicians should be sensitive to the fact that some patients, their caregivers, or both may be reluctant to adopt multimodality and/or augmentative communication strategies. Some may perceive drawing or gesturing to be juvenile or judge their own drawing ability to be inadequate. Others may be embarrassed by their need for gesturing or pointing to pictures to assist their comprehension or expression abilities, whereas others may perceive that accepting use of augmentative communication is the same as accepting that the patient will never talk. In these situations, clinicians must help patients and caregivers appreciate that the benefits of enhanced communication usually outweigh the potential disadvantages.

A valuable feature of multimodality approaches is that they can be introduced at nearly any point in recovery. Many patients may benefit from using gestures or augmentative communication very early post onset, when deficits tend to be most severe. Acceptance of multiple modalities at this stage may be enhanced because patients and their family members may perceive the alternate modality as a temporary strategy that will be discontinued when patients regain their ability to understand and/or use verbal communication. During the chronic stage of the neurogenic language disorder is another time when patients may be more willing to explore alternative modes of communication. Patients and caregivers who have lived with a neurogenic language disorder for a more extensive time period are more likely to have a realistic understanding of the nature of the patients' language impairments and the impact of these impairments on daily communication. They also may be more cognizant of the chronicity of the neurogenic language disorder, often having undergone many hours of rehabilitation yet still experiencing communication difficulties. Additionally, patients and caregivers living with chronic neurogenic language disorders may have discovered for themselves the benefits of **multimodal communication** but are in need of instruction in effective use of these strategies.

Funding Treatment after the Acute Phase of Recovery

It was once commonly believed that little could be done to help individuals with residual impairments months to years after onset of a neurogenic language disorder. Thus, third-party payers such as Medicare and private insurance traditionally have been unwilling to fund speech-language therapy once the condition was considered chronic (e.g., three to six months post onset). If necessary, clinicians may advocate for the individual's right to appropriate services, regardless of time post onset. If third-party funding cannot be secured, some individuals with neurogenic language disorders may choose to fund their own services, particularly if they perceive that treatment will significantly impact their functional communication and participation in desired activities.

Cognitive Strategies

A number of strategies are available that can be taught to patients with neurogenic language disorders to augment direct retraining of their cognitive abilities or to help them compensate for cognitive impairments that do not appear amenable to direct retraining. At least some of these strategies are similar to those already described with respect to communication. For instance, utilizing multimodality communication can benefit patients with deficits of attention, memory, or executive functioning (e.g., organization deficits). As an example, these patients might be taught to take notes during daily activities (e.g., telephone conversations, business meetings) as a strategy to help them attend throughout the activity, recall information being conveyed during the activity, or outline or organize information pertaining to the activity.

Other cognitive strategies differ from communication strategies in that they involve teaching patients to utilize their linguistic skills to guide or support their compromised cognitive abilities. In particular, verbal mediation has proven to be an effective strategy to help patients compensate for a number of cognitive impairments, including attention, memory, and executive function deficits. For example, Ylvisaker and Feeney (1998) described a case study of a patient with TBI who was taught to utilize successfully the self-cue of "Gotta check it out, man" (p. 18). This patient used this verbal cue to assist himself in making plans and decisions throughout his daily schedule and social interactions, which in turn helped him to reduce confusion and his inappropriate responses to that confusion (i.e., verbal aggression and social withdrawal). He was taught to use the self-cue by having those with whom he interacted remind him to "check it out" before he completed a task or gave a response, or alternately after he completed a task or response, ask him whether or not he had "checked it out" with his caregivers or certain peers. The patient also was provided with the opportunity to review periodically videotaped samples of him completing everyday tasks and in social interactions to determine if he was appropriately utilizing this verbal mediation strategy.

Cognitive strategies also are available for particular cognitive deficits (Sohlberg & Mateer, 2001a; Tompkins, 1995; Ylvisaker et al., 1998). For memory problems, there are several internal or covert strategies, such as mental rehearsal, covert self-instruction, imagery, and elaboration (see Chapter 9 for a discussion of these strategies); more overt memory strategies train patients to ask for information to be repeated or restated, or to repeat aloud information several times as part of the rehearsal process (note that these strategies would also benefit patients with auditory comprehension problems). Patients with fatigue or sustained attention problems might benefit from pacing strategies. These include learning to take rest breaks on a regular basis throughout the day at predetermined time intervals (e.g., every 20 minutes) or after completing a certain amount or set number of activities (e.g., after writing one paragraph; after completing morning hygiene activities). Another form of pacing involves teaching patients to identify what times of the day are most or least productive for them, and then to adjust their daily schedules accordingly. For instance, a patient with TBI returning to university might use the strategy of scheduling classes in the morning and study sessions in the late afternoon because he is most fatigued and easily distracted in the early afternoon after lunch and in the evening. Finally, a few strategies for addressing neglect include teaching patients to: (1) sit with their trunks turned to their neglected side, (2) select and place anchors on their neglected side prior to completing a task, and (3) use their neglected hand to complete tasks when possible.

Clinicians should keep in mind that extensive practice is necessary to help patients automate strategy use. Therefore, strategy training should begin as early as possible, even while patients are receiving direct and intensive cognitive retraining. That is, often strategies are targeted only after patients have plateaued in treatment activities designed to stimulate or re-establish cognitive functioning. Strategy training, however, can complement these types of treatment activities and offer patients a means by which to compensate for cognitive deficits that are still being directly retrained.

External Devices

Numerous external devices are available to help patients compensate for their linguistic and/or cognitive impairments (see Table 11-1). As with augmentative communication systems, external aids can vary from simple, low-technology sticky notes to sophisticated, high-technology pocket-sized computerized notebooks. They also can vary in that some devices are helpful in a variety of settings (e.g., computerized personal planner), whereas others provide assistance while completing only certain tasks (e.g., key finder). Given the number of device options avail-

Table 11-1. **Examples of External Devices**

DEVICES	POTENTIAL USES
Calendars/appointment books	Record important dates and appointments to aid memory, organization, and plannin
	Orient to day, week, month, and year
To-do lists	Record daily or weekly chores or schedule to aid memory, organization, and planning
	Can rank items in chronological order or in order of importance
	Place in each room of the house to aid recall of daily activities to be completed in that room (e.g., brush teeth, wash face, shave, etc. on list placed on bathroom mirror)
Photograph Albums	Include labeled pictures and labels of important people and events to aid memory and word finding
Memory or communication books/wallets/boxes	Include labeled pictures, short poems, small items, maps, books/wallets/boxes etc. to aid memory, attention, word-finding, and conversational skills
Electronic speller	Aids in correcting plausible spelling errors
"Windowed" cover sheet	Covers all other words or lines of text on a page to reduce visual distractions and thus aid reading
Daily/weekly pillbox	Aids in recall for taking medications
Visual Cues	
Labels/flags	Place on appliances to aid recall of turning appliance on/off
	Place on cupboards/drawers/closets to aid recall of what is in them
Instructions	Place list of simple instructions (laminated will last longer) on appliances or other electronic devices (e.g., DVD player) used on a regular basis to aid recall of how to use device or problem solving if device is not working
Alarms	Set alarms to remind about when tasks should be initiated
Kitchen timers	and/or completed to aid memory, initiation, and planning
Alarm clocks	
Alarm watches	
Electronic/computerized planners	
Ear plugs/headset	Aid in reducing auditory distractions and thus facilitate attention
Electronic and computerized planners	Program important dates and appointments to aid memory, initiation, organization, and planning
	Program names and addresses of family, friends, business associates, etc. to aid memory and word finding
Pagers/cell phones	Aid in recall, initiation, and completion of daily activities

able, selection of which aids are most appropriate for a given patient should be based on factors such as:

1. the patient's linguistic abilities (e.g., if a patient is unable to read, devices such as written to-do lists would be inappropriate);

2. the patient's cognitive abilities (e.g., if a patient has severely impaired learning abilities, devices that require multiple steps to use may be inappropriate);

3. the patient's motor abilities (e.g., if a patient has impaired fine motor skills, a device such as a palm-top personal computer that requires precise, complex manual manipulations would be inappropriate);

4. the patient's sensory and perceptual skills (e.g., a patient with a concomitant hearing loss may have difficulty using devices that provide only auditory cues or feedback);

5. cost, particularly if the patient must pay for the device(s) out-of-pocket;

6. strategies or devices that the patient used premorbidly, and thus may already be familiar with and already own;

7. the patient's preference, as when the patient likes the device, he or she will be more motivated to use the device;

8. caregivers' preference, as when they like the device, they will be more likely to encourage the patient to use it, and thus help with generalization and maintenance of device use; and

9. the patient's daily needs (e.g., one external memory device may be suitable for use in the patient's home, but another external memory device is needed when the patient is driving).

Additionally, it is particularly important for clinicians to determine whether patients present with anosognosia, or impaired awareness, of their deficits. External devices are typically inappropriate for patients with poor deficit awareness, as they will not recognize the need for the device and consequently will lack the motivation to use the device (Ownsworth & McFarland, 1999).

Not only are there many devices from which to choose, there also are several options in terms of how these devices can be used, and thus, how patients can be trained. For example, the goal of training may be that (1) patients will be responsible for using the device independently, (2) caregivers will assist patients with device use, or (3) caregivers will be responsible for implementing device use. Patients with severe memory and/or executive function impairments are often unable to use external devices independently because they forget to use the device, lose the device, or cannot problem solve to determine under what circumstances they will need to use the device. Consequently, for these patients, training will focus on teaching the caregivers when and how to use the device to facilitate the patients' cognitive and/or linguistic abilities. Generally, training the use of an external device will involve treatment sessions focused on teaching patients and/or caregivers how (e.g., steps necessary to program and consequently access information in a pocket-sized computerized planner) and when to use the device (e.g., in what physical and social settings will device use be necessary and appropriate), as well as sessions focused on practice with the device so as to foster independent and maintained device use (for more specific descriptions of training procedures, see Donaghy & Williams, 1998 or Sohlberg & Mateer, 2001a).

Although external devices are commonly used in clinical practice, examination of the research literature indicates that this approach to compensating for impaired linguistic and/or cognitive abilities has been the focus of relatively few empirical investigations. A notable exception is research pertaining to the Neuropage system (Evans et al., 1998; Wilson et al., 1997; 2001). Neuropage consists of both computer and paging devices: Reminders of a given patient's needs are entered into the computer, and then the computer via a modem contacts the paging company on certain days and at certain times to send those reminders to the patient's pager. The pager is equipped with an auditory or vibratory alarm to notify patients that they need to look to see what reminder has been sent. Several studies have shown that patients of varying age, etiology (i.e., TBI, stroke, progressive neurological disease), and degree of cognitive impairment may benefit from this or similar paging systems. Importantly, these benefits have included greater levels of independence while completing daily activities such as using public transportation, taking medications, and carrying out self-care and hygiene activities. Furthermore, some patients have been able to maintain their improvements even when they are no longer using the pager. This device has not proven helpful, however, for patients with poor insight who did not understand why they needed the device and thus were reluctant to utilize the system. Similar benefits also have recently been reported when patients with severe memory disorders were trained to use a Sony IC Recorder (ICD-50), a small, portable electronic device that can present approximately 300 spoken messages at preprogrammed times on a daily or weekly basis (Yasuda et al., 2002). Because the ICD-50 provides spoken cues, it is appropriate for patients who have reading or visual impairments that can interfere with their ability to read pager messages.

Another device that has been used frequently in both clinical and research settings is the memory or communication book, which also can be provided in alternate forms such as a memory or communication wallet or box. A typical memory or communication book will contain sentence and picture stimuli that represent events, people, pets, hobbies, and places that are important to the patient. Other pages to incorporate into the book include a calendar (e.g., weekly, monthly), map (e.g., city, state, and/or country), and blank pages on which patients and/or caregivers can record daily activities (see Figure 11-5). When these books are being used primarily to assist communication abilities, pages that list the alphabet and numbers also are often appropriate. All stimuli are placed into a three-ring binder with page protectors and tabs to divide the book into information categories (e.g., family, hobbies, "my past").

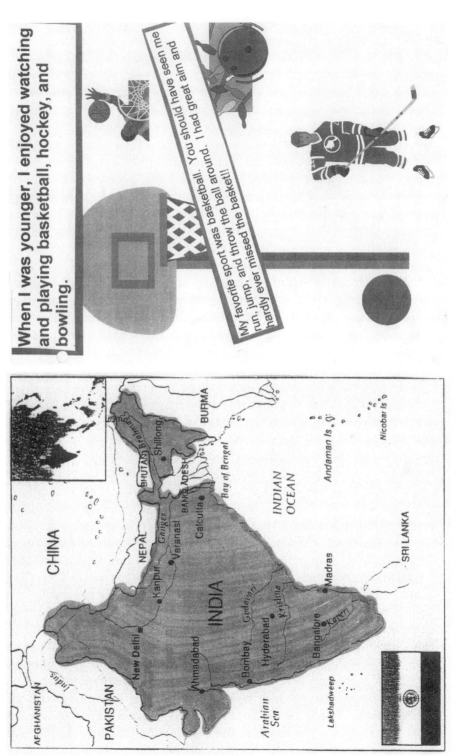

Figure 11-5. Example pages from memory books developed for patients in the middle stages of Alzheimer's disease.

Steps to creating a memory book include first interviewing patients and caregivers (i.e., family as well as other health care providers such as therapists, nursing assistants, etc.) to determine what information should be included, and how best to organize that information. Next, to make the actual book, the clinician must consider that patient's motoric, sensory, cognitive, and linguistic abilities to determine the size of the book (e.g., a small, wallet-sized book may be more appropriate for a patient who is mobile and does not want to carry around a large, cumbersome binder), the size of the pictures and written stimuli (e.g., for patients with visual impairments, large font, enlarged pictures, and/or line drawings are most appropriate), the complexity of written stimuli (e.g., for patients with aphasia and/or dementia, single words or short phrases with simple grammar are often most appropriate), and the amount of information to be included (e.g., patients with memory and/or attention impairments may be unable to learn what information is in their book and where that information is located within their book if the book contains too much information or too many information categories or pages).

The next step is to train patients and/or caregivers how and when to use the book. First, patients and caregivers should be oriented to what information has been included and where that information is located within the book. Second, patients and caregivers should be shown how to utilize the information. For example, patients with aphasia should be shown how the book can help them with their word-retrieval difficulties. Similarly, patients with TBI, right hemisphere brain damage (RHD), or mild dementia should be shown how to use the book to compensate for their short- and long-term memory problems. For patients with severe linguistic and/or cognitive deficits, training will focus more on the caregivers so that they can learn how to use the book to facilitate conversations with the patients (e.g., avoid quizzing and grilling about information in the book). When the goal of training is to facilitate the patient's independent use of the memory or communication book, clinicians must assure that sufficient practice sessions are provided, and must additionally incorporate a variety of activities and communication partners into these practice sessions so as to encourage device use in a variety of settings.

Bourgeois and colleagues (2001; 2003; Bourgeois, 1992; Hoerster, Hickey, & Bourgeois, 2001) have conducted a series of studies supporting the use of memory books, wallets, and boxes with patients who have varying types and severities of dementia. Positive outcomes include increases in the frequency and quality of dementia patients' daily social interactions, improvements in the informativeness of patients' verbal output, and decreases in patients' depression symptoms and repetitive behaviors (e.g., perseverative questions or comments). Importantly, improvements have been observed even when caregivers were provided with only nominal training. Other researchers have evaluated the effects of providing memory books to other patient populations, such as those with memory problems related to TBI or stroke (Burke, Danick, Bernis, & Dugan, 1994; Ownsworth & McFarland, 1999; Squires et al., 1996). The results of these studies indicate that when these patients were provided with adequate training and support regarding device use, gains in their daily communication, memory, attention, and executive function abilities (e.g., organization, deficit awareness), as well as their emotional well-being (e.g., decreased distress related to memory problems) were achieved. Similar positive outcomes have been reported when computerized memory "books," that is, pocket-sized personal computers, have been used with patients with TBI (Kim, Downs, Robinson-Boone, & Parks et al., 2000; Wright, Rogers, Wilson, Evans, & Emslie, 2001). Because of the general population's widespread use of pocket-sized personal computers, another benefit of these devices is that more patients may be willing to use them because of the nominal social stigma associated with them.

In summary, initial research indicates that the provision of external devices represents an effective approach for compensating for acquired linguistic and/or cognitive deficits. Further research remains necessary, however, to help determine (1) which devices might be most appropriate for which patients or symptoms, (2) long-term effects of device use (e.g., can improvements be maintained following withdrawal of the device or of training with the device), and (3) which methods are most efficient for training device use.

Practicing Compensatory Strategies

Once effective compensatory strategies are identified, clinicians should structure treatment to allow patients with neurogenic language disorders to practice using their strategies during interactions and activities that mimic typical daily situations. Such practice provides patients with an opportunity to explore which strategies are best applied under which circumstances, as well as to develop confidence and, hopefully, automaticity in using the strategies for functional communication and daily activities.

Strategy and External Device Training

Carryover and maintenance of strategy or external device use to untrained contexts is unlikely if clinicians do not properly teach patients how to use the strategy or device. Research indicates that successful strategy and external device use is most likely when training stresses the following (Singer & Bashir, 1999; Ylvisaker et al., 1998): (1) developing the patient's motivation to use the strategy or device and, relatedly, caregivers' motivation or approval of the strategy so that they will encourage the patient's strategy use in settings outside of the therapy room; (2) assuring that the patient knows how and when to use the strategy or device; and (3) providing intensive and extensive practice (e.g., as long as two years has been recommended in some cases). Clinicians should keep in mind that the following procedures should also be adhered to when training caregivers on the use of strategies (see Caregiver Training section of this chapter).

A few procedures can be implemented to assure adequate motivation to use the strategy or device (Tompkins, 1995; Ylvisaker et al., 1998). First, patients and caregivers should be allowed to participate in selecting possible strategies and devices. To help them make their choice, patients might try using a number of strategies, and then the patient, caregiver, and clinician can discuss which one or ones they felt were most helpful. Alternately, the clinician, patient, and caregiver might interview other patients already using a strategy or device regarding their perceptions of strategy or device benefits. Second, there should be some discussion about how prevalent strategy and device use is, even among people who do not have neurogenic language disorders. Such a discussion may help allay fears of social stigma or concern that strategy or device use is a sign of weakness or giving up on communicative or cognitive recovery.

The next treatment step involves teaching patients how to execute the strategy or use the external device. This can be achieved through activities such as clinician- or peer-modeling, extensive hands-on patient practice to help automate strategy or device use, and review of video- or audiotaped samples of the patient's performance when using as well as not using the strategy or device, to further the patient's understanding of the benefits of the strategy or device (Tompkins, 1995; Ylvisaker et al., 1998). Clinicians should keep in mind that because use of many strategies and devices involves several abilities or steps, a task analysis may be necessary to determine how to break down strategy or device use into smaller and distinct task components (Sohlberg & Mateer, 2001a). Treatment then proceeds by training the first subcomponents, and adding subsequent steps when the patient has mastered the initial steps. For example, the initial steps for training use of an electronic planner might include establishing where the planner will be kept (e.g., shirt pocket, purse, pants pocket), learning how to turn the device on and off, and finding the calendar display on the device. Later training steps might include programming in upcoming events and setting the alarm so that the patient can receive an auditory reminder about these events.

To assure transfer and maintenance of strategy or device use, training should include having the patient identify situations or activities in which the strategy or device would and would not be appropriate (Sohlberg & Mateer, 2001a; Tompkins, 1995); this will help foster the patient's ability to predict what task or situations will necessitate strategy or external device use. Additionally, involving caregivers (e.g., family, peers, other medical team members) in treatment sessions will provide patients with practice in variable contexts, and encourage caregivers' understanding and reinforcement of the patients' strategy or device use.

For patients with severe cognitive deficits, device or strategy use might be trained using the errorless learning, spaced retrieval, or vanishing cues techniques described in Chapter 9. Because skills acquired via these training procedures are not typically expected to generalize (i.e., they result in primarily task-specific learning), this approach is most appropriate when patients will need the strategy or device for only a small set of activities or contexts (e.g., uses a watch alarm as a reminder for taking medication only). With severely impaired patients, it also is often necessary to make caregivers responsible for prompting patients to use their strategy or device, as these patients often lack the executive skills (e.g., self-monitoring, problem solving, initiation) essential to independent strategy or device implementation.

Promoting Aphasics' Communicative Effectiveness (PACE)

Promoting Aphasics' Communicative Effectiveness (PACE; Davis & Wilcox, 1985) is a clinical protocol that provides practice for communication strategies. The goal of PACE is to structure treatment so that the communication interactions share characteristics with customary daily communication. For example, the classic PACE activity involves using cards with information printed on one side placed facedown on the table. The content of the cards is unknown to *both* the clinician and the patient. The clinician and the patient take turns selecting a card and attempting to communicate the content of the card to the other person. Similar PACE activities can be incorporated into a variety of similar task scenarios (e.g., role playing, barrier tasks), as well.

Four principles of PACE are applied during treatment interactions. The first principle is equal participation: Taking turns as sender and receiver of messages is thought to be similar to the turn-taking typical in conversational interactions. Another benefit of equal participation is that the "power" of the communicative interaction is shared more evenly between the participants (i.e., clinician and patient) than is characteristic of most therapy interactions.

The second principle is that there is an exchange of new information between the participants. In many typical therapy activities, clinicians already know what patients are trying to convey, and are thus in a position to evaluate the "correctness" of patients' communication attempts. Further, when one communication partner (usually the clinician) can predict what the other is trying to convey, the validity of the communication interaction is diminished. By practicing barrier activities (see Chapter 9) and using picture cards or other stimuli that are unknown to the clinician, the patient, or both, the information being communicated will be new or, at least, indefinite to both participants. Structuring the activity so that clinicians are truly unaware of card content can be a challenge for clinicians, as typically they have to supply the stimuli. Nonetheless, if the selection of cards is large enough and well shuffled, there is less risk that clinicians will be able to guess what is being communicated based on familiarity with the stimuli. Alternately, clinicians might elicit the assistance of caregivers in providing stimuli (e.g., family photographs) so that they are truly naïve about at least some of the treatment stimuli.

The third, and arguably most important, principle of PACE interactions is that both clinicians and patients are free to use any mode available to communicate the message. Clinicians do not direct patients to use a particular mode, even if one or two specific modes (e.g., drawing and gesturing) were previously practiced during therapy drills and determined effective. Instead, clinicians may model the use of potentially effective modes when it is their turn to send a message. This principle highlights the emphasis on effective communication, rather than skill in using a specific communicative strategy.

The final principle of PACE is that "feedback" occurs naturally as listeners indicate their understanding of the message. This feature of PACE activities is significantly different from most impairment-level treatments, during which clinicians typically provide feedback regarding specific aspects of the patients' responses (e.g., linguistic accuracy, promptness), provide cues for more "accurate" responses, or both. Once again, because in PACE, clinicians are not in the authoritative role of determining the quality of patients' communicative attempts, the power in treatment interactions is more balanced.

Although PACE activities are not perfect simulations of natural conversation, they do provide an opportunity for patients with neurogenic language disorders to apply compensatory strategies in a more typical communicative interaction. These activities also provide an opportunity for patients to explore metacommunicative and pragmatic aspects of interactions, such as recognizing communication breakdowns and using repair strategies (Davis, 2000). The principles of PACE may be incorporated into most therapeutic interactions to facilitate generalization of compensatory strategies and external devices into functional daily communication.

The effectiveness of PACE has been evaluated in several aphasia treatment studies (e.g., Li et al., 1988; Murray, 1998). The results of these investigations consistently indicate that this treatment approach positively affects the communicative abilities of patients with aphasia, particularly in terms of their communicative flexibility (i.e., they use a greater variety of communication modalities) and success (i.e., regardless of whether linguistic accuracy improved, communication partners were able to understand and respond to more of the patients' communication attempts). Whereas this approach clearly has clinical applications for other neurogenic language disorders (e.g., pragmatic difficulties of patients with TBI or RHD), treatment research involving patient populations other than those with aphasia has yet to be conducted.

GROUP TREATMENT

There is little question that patients with neurogenic language disorders benefit from one-on-one interactions with a speech-language pathologist. Individual treatment sessions provide an opportunity for clinicians and patients to focus on specific communicative or cognitive skills in a relatively risk-free context. Group treatment, however, offers several advantages that are not easily achieved by individual treatment (Graham, 1999; Parente & Stapleton, 1999; Rosenthal, 2004). For example, given increasing demands on health care funding and clinicians' time, group treatment represents a cost-effective therapy approach. Group treatment provides an opportunity for patients to communicate with and receive feedback from non-professionals in a supportive atmosphere. Not only is the clinician available for support, but so are the other group members who are experiencing similar communicative and/or cognitive challenges. Patients participating in group treatment also have the opportunity to observe their peers' use of compensatory strategies and general progress over time, which may provide an avenue for insightful assessment of their own communicative or cognitive strategies and recovery, respectively. A growing body of evidence supports the use of group treatment for a variety of patient populations, reporting, in addition to improvements in cognitive or communicative functioning, benefits such as increased socialization, decreased depression, and improved life satisfaction (Elman, 1999; Lin, Dai, & Huang, 2003; Parente & Stapleton, 1999). Accordingly, clinicians will want to be familiar with some of the unique aspects of this intervention approach.

Selecting Group Members

Several factors have been suggested as entry criteria for group membership (Marshall, 1999). Some groups might be organized according to severity of linguistic or cognitive impairment (Bernstein-Ellis & Elman, 1999) or stage of recovery (Gillis, 1999). Groups organized in this way may be particularly useful if the clinician intends to use group treatment to address specific communicative or cognitive strategies. Because group treatment relies heavily on conversation among participants, designing groups with related interests also may facilitate quality interactions. Because it may be difficult to determine the interests of patients before the groups are formed, a simple way to address this issue is to group members by age, as contemporaries often share similar historical knowledge as well as current life issues (e.g., raising a family, job concerns, retirement). Of course, practical concerns such as availability of transportation, jobs, and family responsibilities may also serve to establish group membership. It is recommended that groups be limited to five to ten members, as larger groups may not allow ample opportunity for every member to participate (Bernstein-Ellis & Elman, 1999).

Group Process

A strength of group treatment is that it can easily be adapted to meet the needs of almost any group of patients with neurogenic language disorders. For example, group sessions may be scheduled daily, weekly, or at longer intervals and may vary in duration (e.g., 60 vs. 90 minutes), depending primarily on the treatment setting and each individual participant's goals. Similarly, the group process or function will arise from the group's goals. For instance, groups to address specific communicative or cognitive strategies will likely include more structure and more direct clinician support. Such group sessions may include activities similar to what have been described for individual treatment sessions, with the modification that all group members may serve as the "speakers" and the "listeners" during the activities. Other groups focusing on realistic practice and generalization of communicative or cognitive strategies may be conversation-oriented or incorporate completion of real-world activities (e.g., a group outing to a concert; mock job interviews); given the nature of the activities in these groups, the clinician's role may differ significantly from what is typical of individual treatment sessions.

Bernstein-Ellis and Elman (1999) described group treatment strategies that may address group goals. Because group members may come to rely on the clinician to direct group interactions, it may be helpful to devise strategies that allow group members to assume leadership roles. For example, group members might take turns serving as facilitator for a given conversation or activity. Alternatively, members might take turns within a single conversation or activity, prompting participation from other members at the end of their conversation or activity turn. As the group process becomes more established, group members themselves can be responsible for monitoring participation by all members and planning group activities. For example, group members might facilitate communication in much the same way that the clinician may have during the initial stages of treatment, by encouraging multimodality communication, reminding members about trained strategies (e.g., word retrieval or memory techniques), and perhaps even cueing other group members to facilitate communication or activity completion. Group members may also provide feedback to participants who tend to dominate the conversation or activity or who are unsupportive of the group goals.

If the group chooses to explore activities other than conversation, a variety of other activities are easily incorporated into a group treatment setting (Holland & Beeson, 1999; Lin et al., 2003). For example, traditional PACE activities such as those described previously in this chapter can be implemented in a small group. Clinicians may find it useful to have a variety of PACE materials available so that the activities can be carried out in pairs or in larger groups. Because group treatment sessions provide a safe environment in which to practice communicative and cognitive strategies, clinicians may wish to incorporate role-plays and scenarios to simulate real-life situations. For patients practicing communicative strategies, group members may find it helpful to develop scripts for specific communication situations (e.g., refusing phone solicitation) and then practice those scripts in role-plays. Script development may also be useful for group members practicing executive function strategies, such as those to facilitate problem solving or organization. Group participants should be encouraged to identify relevant role-plays, scenarios, or other stimuli, and to give feedback to group members as they apply communicative and cognitive strategies during these activities.

Some real-life activities can be incorporated into group sessions without the need for simulation. For instance, card and board games are a common recreational activity for which patients with neurogenic language disorders may wish to develop or maintain communicative and cognitive strategies. It is recommended that games requiring the exchange of ideas or information (e.g., bridge, Pictionary™, charades) be selected over those that are inherently less communicative (e.g., rummy, Yahtzee™, dominoes, Old Maid) when group treatment goals are more focused on communication (Holland & Beeson, 1999). Alternately, if the goal of the group activity is to allow practice of cognitive strategies such as use of memory or problem-solving techniques, these other games may still be appropriate (Johnson & Bourgeois, 1998). Reminiscence activities also are popular in both cognitive and communicative therapy groups. These activities usually involve reviewing materials such as old photographs, songs, newspapers, or magazines to evoke group participants to share their memories of typically distant past experiences.

Considerations for Specific Patient Groups

A key feature of activity and participation-level treatments is that their application is not dependent on specific underlying impairments. However, treatment groups comprised of patients experiencing particular impairments may have unique goals or group processes, even if the activities addressing the goals are quite similar across treatment groups.

Aphasia Groups

Although patients with cognitive communicative disorders such as dementia and TBI may experience auditory comprehension difficulties, such deficits are likely more common and pronounced in patients with aphasia. Thus, the group process in aphasia groups may emphasize strategies and activities addressing comprehension as well as appropriate group interaction. In particular, patients in aphasia groups can be encouraged to develop independence in monitoring their own comprehension and initiating clarification strategies (e.g., requesting repetitions; asking communication partners to write down or draw what was being said). Language expression difficulties common to patients with aphasia are easily targeted during the general group treatment activities described in the previous sections of this chapter.

RHD and TBI Groups

Group treatment for patients with RHD and TBI often incorporates goals addressing the unique cognitive or communicative impairments (e.g., disorientation, inattention, pragmatic disruptions) or needs of these patients (e.g., because patients with TBI are often younger than other neurogenic patient populations, they often have more needs related to vocational or educational issues). The group activities addressing these issues often may, however, be the same as those incorporated into aphasia groups. The difference will be primarily with respect to which compensatory strategies each patient will need to use to participate effectively in the group interaction or activity.

Many patients with RHD and TBI will benefit from group treatment addressing orientation and attention, particularly during the early stages of recovery (Cherney & Halper, 1999; Sargeant, Webster, Salzman, White, & McGrath, 2000). These "reality orientation" groups can involve activities such as making crafts for an upcoming holiday, singing songs that pertain to the time of year, and reviewing orientation facts such as the day's date and the group's location. Daily reality orientation groups are particularly appropriate for residential care centers as orientation to time, place, and person will be common to all patients. Sharing of personal biographical information and discussion of current news events can also be incorporated into orientation groups. These group sessions are typically shorter and more frequent than groups designed for other purposes, but still provide an opportunity for patients to practice orientation strategies such as attending to environmental cues (e.g., checking outside to identify visual cues regarding time of day or season), or using external devices (e.g., checking the date on one's watch).

Group treatment also is an appropriate venue for practicing compensatory strategies addressing higher-level cognitive skills such as memory, time management, organization, goal setting, and problem solving (Dikengil, Monda, & King, 1992; Parente & Stapleton, 1999; Rath et al., 2003). The types of activities discussed previously (e.g., conversation, role-playing, PACE-like interactions, reminiscence) provide a context for targeting a variety of cognitive abilities, including recalling and sequencing information, inhibition, problem solving, planning, initiation, awareness of deficits, and self-monitoring. Because pragmatic skills are often impaired in patients with RHD or TBI, group treatment for these patients may have a greater emphasis on appropriate interaction in a variety of contexts (e.g., giving impromptu speeches, debating, role-playing service encounters), as opposed to effective transaction, which may more often be of concern for aphasia groups (Dikengil et al., 1992; Wiseman-Hakes et al., 1998).

Dementia Groups

Although group treatment for patients with dementia poses unique challenges, those with milder deficits may benefit from the opportunity to practice compensatory strategies in a group treatment setting; accordingly, for these dementia patients, group treatment goals and activities may be similar to those described previously for aphasic, RHD, and TBI patient populations (Johnson & Bourgeois, 1998; Lin et al., 2003). For example, Santo Pietro and Boczko (1998) have developed and successfully implemented a Breakfast Club treatment protocol in which a group of patients living in an extended care facility come together to prepare, serve, eat, and then clean up breakfast under the supervision of a clinician; during these breakfast-related activities, patients are encouraged through multi-modality cues to use their cognitive and communicative strategies.

For patients with more severe dementia, group treatment may provide more a context for clinician-facilitated group interaction with less emphasis on patients' ability to use compensatory strategies (Hickey & Bourgeois, 2003). Clark and Witte (1995) suggested several strategies for enhancing the effectiveness of group treatment in advanced dementia. First, perhaps more so than is necessary for other treatment groups, topics of discussion should be concrete, related to common life experiences, or both. The clinician may frequently be required to redirect the conversation to maintain topical cohesion, and to restate, rephrase, and/or simplify expressed concepts in terms of vocabulary and syntactic complexity to ensure comprehension by all group members. Stimulation techniques and scaffolding strategies (see Chapter 9) may also be incorporated to facilitate richer contributions from the group members. Reality orientation activities, similar to those described for RHD and TBI groups, are another common component of group treatment for patients in middle to later stages of dementia (Hickey & Bourgeois, 2003).

Assessing Group Outcomes

As suggested above, although group treatment can be structured to address underlying linguistic and cognitive impairments contributing to neurogenic language disorders, more often group treatment focuses on activity-level function. Thus, clinicians may find it useful to incorporate measures of functional communication as well as participation and quality of life, such as those described in Chapter 7, when evaluating the effectiveness of group treatment (Garrett, 1999; Vickers, 2004). The feedback provided by group members and their communication partners throughout the group treatment process, although not formal measures of outcome, also may help clinicians identify the most useful aspects of group treatment.

Reimbursement for Group Treatment

Most common third-party payment sources, including Medicare, Medicaid, and private insurers, usually cover group treatment services for patients with neurogenic language disorders (Busch, 1999). As is true for reimbursement of any speech-language service, the clinician must clearly demonstrate to the payer that the service was necessary, provided in a manner consistent with established practice patterns, and resulted in desired outcomes (see Chapter 12). The group treatment that is provided should be clearly related to the patient's treatment plan. In some cases, clinicians may need to provide a thorough rationale to third-party payers regarding how the group treatment addresses the functional goals of the treatment plan, as well as provide evidence that such treatment has been shown beneficial for other patients with similar communicative or cognitive impairments.

When group treatment is a part of service addressing the long-term impacts of neurogenic language disorders (e.g., Life Participation Approach to Aphasia—see below), third-party payment may be harder to secure. In such cases, patients may choose to fund their group treatment personally. Because group treatment costs are shared by all group members, clinicians may find that they can charge a lower per-person rate (e.g., $15/session, Bernstein-Ellis & Elman, 1999), making private pay affordable to many individuals. Clinicians should be careful to assure patients that although the lower fee makes group treatment a better value, it in no way means that group treatment is less valuable than individual treatment.

MODIFYING THE COMMUNICATION ENVIRONMENT

It is likely that most speech-language pathologists focus the greater part of treatment efforts on remediating underlying linguistic and cognitive impairments and training individuals with neurogenic language disorders to use compensatory strategies. However, as the ICF emphasizes, the degree to which patients are able to participate in desired activities depends also on factors external to patients. Thus, clinicians may effect positive changes in communicative and cognitive success and in overall participation and quality of life by addressing these external factors.

Training Communication Partners

As human communicators, we are all aware that effective communication depends on both the senders and receivers of messages. This applies to neurologically intact communicators as well as patients experiencing neurogenic language disorders. Communication partners unfamiliar with neurogenic language disorders may be reluctant to interact with patients experiencing these communication difficulties, in many cases due to the assumption that these patients lack the ability to communicate, intellectual competence, or both (Holland & Fridriksson, 2001; Kagan, 1995; Laroi, 2003). For elderly patients, communication interactions may be further limited by partners with misconceptions or a lack of awareness of age-related changes in communication and cognition (Armstrong & McKechnie, 2003). Additionally, given the increasing frequency with which volunteers are incorporated into treatment programs for patients with neurogenic language disorders (Hickey, Bourgeois, & Olswang, 2004; Kagan, Black, Duchan, Simmons-Mackie, & Square, 2001; Rayner & Marshall, 2003), many potential communication partners are being identified who are enthusiastic about interacting with patients but are uncertain how to ensure that these interactions are positive. Even partners who understand the nature of neurogenic language disorders or age-related communication-cognition changes may still lack skill in facilitating communication in the presence of significant language deficits (Rayner & Marshall, 2003). However, just as both participants in a typical conversation must take responsibility for effective communication, communication partners of patients with neurogenic language disorders can develop skill in "maintaining the integrity of the conversational process" (Kagan et al., 2001, p. 625).

One approach to training communication partners involves identifying communicative behaviors that disrupt communication and then working to eliminate those behaviors (Murray, 1998; Orange & Colton-Hudson, 1998; Wilkinson et al., 1998). This method has the greatest potential success when the clinician is familiar with the partners' communication patterns during interactions outside of the clinical setting so that the most disruptive behaviors can be targeted. Unfortunately, many clinicians do not have an opportunity to assess naturally occurring interactions. An alternative approach, providing structured training in the behaviors that support successful interactions, may ultimately have the same effects as the first approach, as there is evidence that "poor" speaking partners fail to demonstrate the facilitative communicative behaviors exhibited by "good" speaking partners (Simmons-Mackie & Kagan, 1999). Moreover, positive communication skill training has the advantage that trained partners will develop skills that will enable them to interact effectively in different settings, as well as with other individuals experiencing neurogenic language disorders (Hickey et al., 2004; Kagan et al., 2001; Rayner & Marshall, 2003).

In studies of conversations between patients with neurogenic language disorders and volunteers or health care workers, several communicative behaviors have been identified as facilitating effective communication (Simmons-Mackie & Kagan, 1999; Sundin, Jansson, & Norberg, 2000) (see Table 11-2). For example, conversation can be enhanced when the communication partner acknowledges the communication attempts of the patient with a neurogenic language disorder. This acknowledgment may be verbal (e.g., "I see.") or nonverbal (e.g., nodding the head) and indicates to the patient that the partner is actively engaged in the interaction. Positive communicators also provide sufficient time for patients to process conversation as well as formulate and produce their contributions to the conversation; if patients feel rushed, they are likely to feel stressed, which in turn can negatively affect their communication abilities, lead to decreased conversational participation, or both. A third facilitating behavior that serves a similar acknowledgment function is "congruent overlap." When the partner's response is simultaneous with and reinforces what the patient is expressing, it communicates a sense of unity between the conversation participants. The use of disjunct markers, or cues that what is about to be communicated is incongruent with the previous exchange, also appears to facilitate communication. These markers serve as a polite and respectful means of disagreeing with or modifying a previous contribution made by the other conversation participant. For example, in the following exchange, the marker

Table 11-2. Strategies for Facilitating Communication with Patients with Neurogenic Language Disorders (Simmons-Mackie & Kagan, 1999; Yorkson, Beukelman, Strand & Bell, 1999)

DESCRIPTION OF STRATEGY	EXAMPLE
Introduce/confirm the topic: When communication partners are aware of the topic, it is easier to predict what is being communicated.	"Are we talking about your visit to Atlanta?"
Be aware of turn-taking signals: Patients with nonfluent aphasia may be slow to initiate speech and may have difficulty getting a turn in conversation. Patients with fluent aphasia and "press of speech" may continue speaking long after they have expressed their "main point."	Indications a turn is desired • Prolonged eye contact • Leaning forward or other anticipatory posture • Deep inhalation Requesting a turn • Hold up a hand • "Excuse me."
Provide sufficient time for the patient to formulate a response. Attend to and acknowledge communication attempts: Give the speaker your attention and acknowledge communication attempts. Attend to and acknowledge all communication modes and cues.	• nodding • "I see." • "Is that so?" • verbal • intonation • gesture • context
Manage communication breakdown: Signal the individual as soon as you fail to understand, then identify specifically what you misunderstood, and utilize previously agreed-upon clarification strategies based on those practiced during treatment (the patient should be aware of and be comfortable with identified strategies—finishing the sentence, guessing, providing additional time).	Signal misunderstanding • lift a finger • raise eyebrows or use other facial expression to signal confusion Identify misunderstanding • "I didn't catch who you are talking about." • "This happened when?" • "Do you want this one or that one?"
Incorporate face-saving strategies: Minimize the interactional cost of the communication breakdown by reinforcing the competence of the patient and your relationship with him or her.	• "Whew! We really worked at that one, didn't we?" • "I see where you're going with this." • "I'm glad we figured that out."

"Well . . ." signals to the patient that the communication partner is declining the request for her to stay for dinner.

> Patient: "Gonna stay. . . dinner stay."
> Partner: "Well, I am having dinner at my sister's tonight."

Effective communication partners also demonstrate accommodation to non-standard communication modalities (Hickey et al., 2004; Simmons-Mackie & Kagan, 1999; Sundin et al., 2000). Previous sections of this chapter explored the potential benefits of multimodality communication for patients with neurogenic language disorders, but clearly these strategies can be effective only to the extent they are accepted by conversation partners. Simmons-Mackie and Kagan (1999) described a communication partner who demonstrated understanding of the patient's gestures, but still requested that the patient try to say the appropriate words. The authors pointed out that the partner was not trying to be unkind, but apparently perceived talking to be the only acceptable communication modality. With appropriate training, partners can facilitate the effectiveness of multimodal communication, perhaps as did another partner described in this study, who not only accepted alternate communication modalities but also adopted some of the alternative communicative behaviors in his own contributions to the conversation.

The final characteristic of good conversation partners described by Simmons-Mackie and Kagan (1999) is the use of "face-saving" repair strategies. These authors reported that whereas nearly all the conversation partners in their study asked clarification questions, some did so in such a way as to acknowledge the competence of the patient with the neurogenic language disorder. For example, one partner closed a long repair sequence by acknowledging the information that was successfully communicated. In contrast, another partner repeatedly asked the same clarification question even after a feasible response had been provided by the patient. The authors pointed out that this second behavior can be interpreted as a lack of confidence in the patient's response, and thus communicates a lack of appreciation for the patient's inherent competence.

The intervention program "Supportive Conversation for Adults with Aphasia" (SCA; (Kagan et al., 2001) evolved out of research into the behaviors of effective conversation partners. The philosophy of SCA is that effective conversation partners both acknowledge and reveal the competence of patients with neurogenic language disorders through appropriate communicative behaviors. Behaviors that acknowledge competence include using "natural adult talk" with tone and style appropriate for the context, and demonstrating sensitivity to the conversation partner. Sensitivity may be demonstrated by acknowledging attempts to communicate, providing encouragement, listening respectfully, avoiding rushing the patient, and bearing an appropriate amount of the communicative burden so that the patient feels neither overburdened nor patronized. SCA trains conversation partners to reveal competence in three main ways: (1) ensure that the patient understands what is being communicated, (2) ensure that the patient has a means of responding, and (3) verify that the message received was that intended by the patient. Each of these goals can be accomplished using verbal strategies (e.g., redundancy, providing fixed choice options), nonverbal approaches (e.g., using and receiving multimodal messages, providing tangible or graphic conversational aids such as maps, newspaper headlines or articles, calendars), or both. In each case, SCA encourages conversation partners to be responsive to communicative cues provided by the patient (e.g., facial expressions, inconsistent responses). For samples of positive and negative communicative behaviors for training purposes, clinicians may consult the *Increasing Communicative Access* videotape created by Kagan and colleagues (1996). Importantly, Kagan et al. (2001) found that when volunteers were provided with SCA training, the communication skills of both the trained volunteers and the patients with neurogenic language disorders improved, as evidenced by more effective interactional (i.e., interpersonal) and transactional (i.e., informational) exchanges. Similar programs developed by Hickey et al. (2004) and Rayner and Marshall (2003) also have been found to produce positive changes in not only the volunteers' communication style, but also the patients' participation levels and accuracy during conversations. It should be noted, however, that Rayner and Marshall (2003) observed some declines in positive communicative behaviors among their trained volunteers over time, suggesting that maintenance training may be necessary.

Communication partners of patients with cognitive-communicative disorders due to RHD, TBI, or dementia may benefit from instruction in different, or at least additional, strategies for facilitating effective communication than those described above for aphasia, as the communication breakdowns of these patients may involve other aspects of language (e.g., pragmatics, suprasegmental phonology), stem from different underlying impairments (e.g., attention or memory deficits), or both. For example, a variety of verbal and nonverbal communication strategies have been recommended to encourage and facilitate the activity and social participation of patients with dementia (Clark & Witte, 1995; Orange & Colton-Hudson, 1998). In addition to the communication strategies consistent with SCA, caregivers of patients with dementia should be trained to use consistent words or phrases to communicate recurrent concepts (e.g., mealtimes, leaving the home, etc.). Further, the caregivers' nonverbal communication (i.e., facial expression, intonation, gestures, and other body language) should be both calming and congruent so that all cues are communicating the same meaning, adding to communication redundancy. Additional strategies for which there is empirical support include avoiding analogies and other figurative or complex language structures, providing explicit conversational topic introductions and indications of when topic changes are occurring (e.g., "Let's talk about planning dinner . . . okay, now let's switch and talk about the phone bill."), asking questions or giving directions one at a time, eliminating distractions, and encouraging patients to circumlocute when they are experiencing word-finding difficulties (Hart & Wells, 1997; Kemper & Harden, 1999; Orange & Colton-Hudson, 1998; Small & Gutman, 2002).

Although it has often been recommended that caregivers speak slowly to enhance the comprehension of patients with dementia, recent research indicates that this strategy is ineffective, and in fact viewed as patronizing by patients with dementia (Kemper & Harden, 1999). Accordingly, this strategy should not be recommended, and clinicians should observe patient-caregiver interactions to determine if this is a negative caregiver communication behavior that needs to be addressed.

Communication partners of patients with RHD or TBI may benefit from strategies addressing the communicative behaviors common in these conditions. For both RHD and TBI, pragmatic deficits commonly contribute to communication breakdown. Because disruptive pragmatic behaviors such as interrupting or inappropriate proxemics (e.g., standing too close to communication partners) may be interpreted as rudeness (as opposed to reflecting disability), instructing communication partners about the nature of the pragmatic deficits accompanying RHD and TBI may foster greater understanding and, thus, patience with the communication behaviors of these patients (Laroi, 2003). Instruction in specific strategies for facilitating communication in the presence of pragmatic or other cognitive-communicative deficits specific to these patient populations may also be provided. Table 11-3 lists several disruptive cognitive-communicative impairments and the partner responses that may improve communication effectiveness.

Additionally, communication partners should be made aware of cognitive deficits such as visuoperceptual, attention, and memory impairments that may disrupt communicative interactions with these patients. Again, disruptive behaviors related to these cognitive impairments can be misinterpreted by family members and caregivers (Laroi, 2003). For instance, families might assume that patients' failure to complete daily chores represents resistance to authority when it is actually a product of memory difficulties. Likewise, decreased arousal and initiation may be inappropriately attributed to depression, laziness, or poor motivation. Accordingly, education about these symptoms can foster families' and caregivers' patience and acceptance of patients, which in turn will lead to increased socialization with the patients, participation in patients' treatment programs, or both. Information about specific strategies also may be provided. For example, partners may be instructed on where best to stand or present visual information to ensure perceptual awareness when interacting with patients with neglect. Maintaining eye contact, periodically saying the patient's name or touching his or her arm, and reducing or eliminating environmental distractions (visual, auditory, or both) may help maintain or redirect attention. Finally, providing periodic summaries of what has been discussed may compensate for short-term memory deficits. Whenever possible and appropriate, communication partners also may wish to provide reminders or cues to patients to use their own compensatory strategies for addressing these impairments.

Before leaving the discussion of training communication partners, it may be helpful to consider techniques clinicians may employ when instructing communication partners. Bayles and Kaszniak (1997) suggested the following steps: First, provide oral and written descriptions of the strategy followed by demonstration

Table 11-3. Example Communication Strategies Addressing Specific Cognitive-Communicative Deficits

COGNITIVE-COMMUNICATIVE DEFICIT	STRATEGY FOR COMMUNICATION PARTNER
Failure to maintain appropriate eye contact	Model appropriate contact, positioning yourself in the patient's line of sight.
Lack of conversation initiation	Introduce a broad topic, or offer choices of topic.
Inappropriate social greetings	Model appropriate greetings.
Interrupting or impaired turn-taking	Use a nonverbal signal (e.g., raising a finger or hand) to indicate your turn is not over and that the patient should wait until you have completed your turn. A similar signal may be used to indicate a turn has been inappropriately long.
Inappropriate proxemics	Reposition yourself to a more comfortable proximity, and if necessary explain why you have moved.
Failure to monitor listener responses	Use a verbal or nonverbal signal to convey a lack of understanding or a need to respond. Minimize environmental distractions.
Poor topic maintenance or perseveration	Redirect the conversation to the appropriate topic. This can be done with disjunctive markers such as "What I was saying a minute ago. . . ?" or "I think we reached closure on that issue. What did you think of. . . ?"
Inappropriate topic initiation	Redirect the conversation to an appropriate topic. Disjunctive markers such as "I'd rather talk about that later." or "We probably shouldn't talk about that now." may be used.
Difficulty interpreting prosodic cues (e.g., emphatic stress, emotional intonation)	Match your linguistic content and prosody to provide redundant cues regarding the meaning of your verbal output. Ask the patient to summarize his/her interpretation of what's been said to assure appropriate understanding.
Difficulty interpreting figurative and indirect language	Avoid using figurative and indirect linguistic devices or, if these devices are used, provide redundant cues and ask the patient to summarize his/her interpretation of what's been said to assure appropriate understanding.
Difficulty with prosody production	Encourage patient to select words that will cue you regarding what parts of the message are most important or that will explicitly tell you his/her feelings.

with the patient. The communication partner should practice the strategy with the clinician and, when skilled in using the strategy, practice with the patient. These authors further recommended that practice interactions be videotaped so that the communication partner can review and evaluate the effectiveness of the interaction. Additionally, group treatment sessions provide an opportunity for communication partners to practice communication enhancement strategies in a more natural communication setting (Clark & Witte, 1995). Practice of these skills in group treatment also serves to emphasize the interactional nature of communication and to extend the responsibility for effective communication to all communication partners. Sorin-Peters (2003) additionally advocated that when training communication partners, clinicians apply adult learning principles such as considering the partners' individual learning styles (e.g., do they learn better by doing or by observing?), encouraging partners to evaluate their own progress, and collaborating with partners to establish target communicative behaviors.

Because it is unlikely that health care workers would be able to attend individual or group therapy sessions on a regular basis, workshops may be a more appropriate means by which to educate these possible communication partners about effective cognitive and communicative strategies to enhance their interactions with patients with neurogenic language disorders. The content of these workshops may include description and examples (e.g., videotape samples) of the types of cognitive and communicative impairments that their patients may display, as well as review of the types of strategies covered in the preceding paragraphs of this chapter. Inclusion of a practical skills training component within these workshops (e.g., role playing and/or disability simulation exercises) and the provision of handouts or booklets that can be referred to after the workshop also are effective means by which to train these types of caregivers. Conveniently, there are a few commercially available workshop programs that provide guidelines for what content and activities to include (e.g., Jordan, Bell, Bryan, Maxim, & Axelrod, 2000; Ripich, 1996). Several studies have confirmed that providing these types of workshops can produce significant increases in health care workers' knowledge of neurogenic language disorders, use of positive communication strategies, and empathetic awareness of the effects of neurogenic language disorders on the lives of patients and their loved ones (Maxim et al., 2001; Pentland, Hutton, MacMillan, & Mayer, 2003; Rayner & Marshall, 2003; Shaw & May, 2001).

Modifying the Physical Environment

With the advent of the Americans with Disabilities Act and other manifestations of the disability movement, our society has a broadened awareness of how modifying the physical environment can greatly improve accessibility of products, services, and activities to individuals with physical disabilities. Curb cutouts, buildings equipped with ramps and automatic doors, Braille markings on elevator doors, auditory signals at crosswalks, closed captioning, and TTD phone lines are commonplace and expected. Unfortunately, society remains less sensitive to how the physical environment may influence the ability of individuals with more invisible disabilities, such as neurogenic language disorders, to participate in desired life activities.

Accordingly, part of treatment should be dedicated towards teaching patients and their caregivers how to alter their physical environment to maximize patients' cognitive and communicative abilities. An initial step is for the clinician to assess the physical environment to determine if modifications are necessary and, if so, which modifications will facilitate effective communication and efficient completion of daily activities. This evaluation is a part of the assessment of activity and participation (see Chapter 7) and includes considering the arrangement of the home, work, or classroom setting, mobility options, and sensoriperceptual factors such as lighting and noise levels (Gitlin, Liebman, & Winter, 2003; Lubinski, 2001).

Probably the most obvious environmental characteristic influencing communicative effectiveness and cognitive functioning is the acoustic environment. Patients with neurogenic language disorders often experience auditory comprehension deficits that are exacerbated by hearing loss related to age or noise exposure. Patients with compromised attention abilities also will be easily distracted, and thus have problems with communication and other activities in the presence of noise. Furthermore, potential communication partners also may demonstrate hearing difficulties. Accordingly, the clinician can help patients, their family members, or health care facility workers arrange the physical environment to facilitate clear transmission of auditory signals. An obvious strategy for enhancing the acoustic environment is reducing background noise such as television and stereo sounds that may compete with spoken auditory signals or cause distraction while patients are completing daily activities (Sohlberg, 2002). Other less apparent sources of noise include appliances, clocks, and traffic and other sounds that may be coming from outside of the home or work setting. It is not always necessary or even desirable to eliminate these noise sources, because they can be stimulating and provide a source of conversation (Lubinski, 1991). However, the clinician can help patients and their family members identify areas in the environment where the noise level is low or controllable. The placement of sound-absorbing materials (e.g., curtains, carpet, ceiling tiles) may further reduce noise levels (Calkins & Brush, 2003). If patients or their communication partners demonstrate hearing loss, the clinician should collaborate with an audiologist to ensure that suitable amplification devices are available and used appropriately.

Another aspect of the environment that influences communicative effectiveness and daily activity performance is lighting. Consideration of lighting is particularly important given that many patients with neurogenic language disorders have impairments (e.g., vision field cut, visuospatial neglect, glare sensitivity, decreased light accommodation, visuoperceptual limitations) that limit their visual access (Gitlin et al., 2003). Adequate lighting facilitates conversation by allowing the communication partners to observe facial expressions and other nonverbal cues and to attend to contextual cues. Other, less obvious characteristics of the visual environment may also influence the communication interactions of patients with neurogenic language disorders. For example, visual stimuli serve as a primary source of conversation topics and as an initiative to complete many daily activities. If patients do not have the same visual access to these stimuli as other individuals in the environment, they will be less able to participate in interactions or activities. The clinician can assist families and health care providers by identifying key features of the visual environment that serve as meaningful stimuli (e.g., weather, television news, photos, magazines, etc.). Visual access to these stimuli may then be enhanced by thoughtful arrangement of the communication environment. Figure 11-6 identifies potential environmental modifications that may facilitate visual access to promote effective communication and successful activity participation.

A number of additional environmental modifications may enhance orientation to person, place, and time (Gitlin et al., 2003; Lubinski, 1995). Enhancing personal orientation may be most important for patients with severe dementia, and primarily involves personalizing the environment. Placement of personal items such as photographs is a common way of facilitating orientation, and can be extended to include personal furniture, clothing, bedding, and small appliances. Allowing the patient to participate in selecting room colors or arranging items in the room can also serve to personalize the environment. Orientation to time can be heightened via natural environmental cues, such as those provided by windows (e.g., day vs. night; seasonal cues such as leaves on or off the trees), or visual access to normal daily activities (e.g., meals, regularly scheduled television programs, etc.). Clocks and calendars as well as other seasonal props (e.g., seasonal floral arrangements, holiday decorations) may also enhance temporal orientation. Finally, maintaining a consistent routine may facilitate orientation, as the patient associates specific activities (e.g., bathing, shopping) with a certain time of day or day of the week.

- Use visual contrasts (e.g., dark against light colors).
- Reduce glare by covering shiny surfaces, using indirect lighting, and/or adding window shades.
- Position important visual information at eye level, with consideration for the patient's most typical position (e.g., wheelchair vs. standing). Visual information includes clocks, calendars, photographs, sculptures, magazines, and other items in the environment that contribute to orientation or communciation.
- Provide even and adequate but not excessive lighting, allowing the patient control of lighting intensity whenever possible.
- If appropriate, position the patient so that he or she has visual accesss to the most common sources of communication topics and activities (e.g., television, window, kitchen or other common center of activity).

Figure 11-6. Environmental modifications to improve visual access. The visual environment influences oral, written, and gestural communication effectiveness.

Spatial orientation is most easily enhanced by maintaining a consistent physical environment. Placing additional cues in the environment, such as personal items or graphic signs, may also facilitate orientation. For patients with severe deficits, color-coded pathways may facilitate independence in moving from one location to another (e.g., bedroom to dining room) within a given area. These will be particularly helpful in environments where traditional spatial cues are lacking (e.g., most homes have only one hallway that leads to bedrooms and bathrooms, whereas assisted care facilities often have many hallways that may lead nearly anywhere).

Environmental modifications also may be useful in reducing the frequency and severity of certain behavioral disturbances (Chavin, 2002; Gitlin et al., 2003) For example, patients who are easily agitated may respond positively to calming background music or simulated presence audio- (e.g., audiotape of a loved one talking to the patient) or videotapes (e.g., videotape of the patient's family completing daily activities). Wandering and exiting problems may be minimized by covering doorknobs with cloth, storing keys to doors and vehicles in out-of-sight locations, installing a home alarm system, placing motion detector lights near exits, creating an area or clear pathway where patients may wander or pace safely (e.g., establishing a walking route in an assisted care facility; rearranging furniture to provide a clear path), and disguising exit doors with curtains or posters.

Patients with higher-level cognitive deficits may also benefit from environmental modifications. Parente and Herrmann (2003) identified five basic principles for organizing the environment to compensate for memory and other cognitive deficits (Figure 11-7). The first principle is consistency, which refers not only to the arrangement of the environment but also to how various items in the environment are used. For example, these authors recommended that a receptacle inside the main entrance to the house be used for keys. Likewise, a specific area could be identified where any items to be taken to work or school (e.g., lunch bag, tote, etc.) will be placed, and another area could be designated for dirty laundry. The intent of this principle is to allow habits to compensate for disruptions in memory or attention that impede a patient's ability to navigate an inconsistent environment.

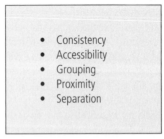

Figure 11-7. Principles for organizing the environment to compensate for memory and other cognitive deficits (Parente & Herrmann, 2003). Thoughtful organization of the physical environment can enhance patients' function and independence in the presence of memory and/or other cognitive deficits.

The second principle is accessibility. Parente and Herrmann (2003) recommended that the environment be organized so that items used frequently are located in the most physically accessible areas and less frequently used items are placed in less accessible areas. This principle is one most individuals adopt to some extent, but may need to be carefully and systematically applied in the environments of patients with visuoperceptual, attentional, memory, and/or planning or problem-solving deficits. This principle is closely related to two other principles, those of grouping and proximity. By arranging the environment so that related items are located together (i.e., grouping), with the most commonly used items most accessible within the grouping (i.e., accessibility) and maintained near the area in which they are used (i.e., proximity), patients may rely less on their own organization skills to identify needed items, or on their own visuoperceptual, attention, and memory skills to locate those items. For example, the area most accessible to the bathroom sink might include items such as soap, towels, comb, and toothbrush. Other bathroom items used less frequently and thus placed in less accessible areas might include tweezers or a hair dryer.

Separation, the final principle of organization, refers to arranging the environment so that conceptually separate items are placed in discrete locations (Parente & Herrmann, 2003). Examples include arranging clothes according to purpose (e.g., work vs. leisure clothing) or by season, or arranging the pantry so that breakfast items are on one shelf, lunch and dinner items on another shelf, and baking items on still another shelf. Parente and Herrmann pointed out that each patient may benefit from different organization strategies, and that careful observation over time may be the best method for identifying the most effective environmental organization.

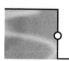

PARTICIPATION-FOCUSED TREATMENTS AND COMMUNITY RESOURCES

The last decade has seen a growing awareness of the life changes that often accompany chronic neurogenic language disorders. Because communication is so endemic to human interactions, the impact of these disorders extends beyond the ability to exchange information (Lyon, 1998). Patients coping with neurogenic language disorders may find themselves "disconnected" from their social networks, or even from their spouse or close family members. The psychosocial impacts of neurogenic language disorders are not limited to the patients experiencing the disorder, but extend to those around them as well (Laroi, 2003; Sorin-Peters, 2004). As communication and other health and social service professionals have become more aware of the chronicity of neurogenic language disorders (Lyon, 1998), systematic attempts to alleviate the life disruption of these disorders have emerged. This section will review treatments that focus primarily on improving the patients' participation in life activities, irrespective of their communicative effectiveness.

LIFE PARTICIPATION APPROACH TO APHASIA

A relatively recent movement in the delivery of services to patients with neurogenic language disorders is the Life Participation Approach to Aphasia (LPAA; Chapey et al., 2001). Although this approach was originally conceived as a service delivery model for patients with aphasia, the philosophy driving LPAA is applicable to the management of all neurogenic language disorders, and several existing treatment approaches for TBI and dementia contain elements consistent with LPAA tenets (e.g., Mahendra & Arkin, 2004; Ylvisaker & Feeney, 1998). LPAA does not prescribe specific clinical methods, but rather encompasses a set of values that guide the management of neurogenic language disorders.

One core value of LPAA is that the primary goal is the enhancement of life participation by patients experiencing neurogenic language disorders. This includes appropriate assessment of life participation and of how the presence of a neurogenic language disorder is affecting participation, as well as the identification of strategies for improving life participation. LPAA also acknowledges that the effects of neurogenic language disorders are broader than those experienced by the individual with the condition, and thus, a second core value is to provide support for family and other individuals who interact with the patients. Relatedly, LPAA recognizes that improving life participation for patients may include targeting personal and external factors as well as the underlying functional impairments contributing to participation limitations. Finally, LPAA emphasizes providing service at all stages of recovery or disease progression. Patients with neurogenic language disorders experience life changes common to many individuals, changes such as moving to a new home, changes in marital status, gaining family members through birth and marriage, employment changes such as retirement, financial changes, and health changes. Such changes may alter the degree to which a neurogenic language disorder is impacting the patient's life participation, and thus may warrant intervention. LPAA embraces the notion that the primary criteria for treatment eligibility be need and potential benefit rather than time post onset.

Side Bar

Participation Treatments Expand the Role of the Speech-Language Pathologist

In Chapter 7, we introduced Ray, who sought assistance with regaining his driver's license. Ray had received impairment-level treatment in the days and weeks following his stroke, but these services had been discontinued when he was discharged from the rehabilitation center. The severe aphasia Ray continued to experience a year after his stroke minimally impacted his participation in independent living and social interactions, but his lack of a driver's license was a significant impediment.

(continued)

The focus of Ray's treatment was preparation for the written examination that was required to regain his driver's license. Intervention activities included reviewing the DMV driving handbook, developing strategies for comprehending the questions and response choices, and identifying reliable response modes for expressing choices of the correct response. Ray participated in sixteen treatment sessions before attempting the written test. The test center offered several accommodations during the written test, including reading the questions aloud and yes/no responses to each of the choices. Additionally, a speech language pathologist assisted in administering the test to help facilitate Ray's comprehension and expression.

Consistent with LPAA, Ray received services during a period of time post onset when intervention has traditionally not been offered, even though treatment had been previously discontinued. Additionally, treatment focused on compensatory techniques and environmental modifications expressly for the purpose of improving a specific aspect of life participation, with little concern for improving underlying language ability.

To complete the story, Ray passed the written test and went on to pass the driving portion of the test as well. He was issued a restricted driver's license that allowed him to drive on non-interstate highways within fifty miles of his home. The restriction was imposed because of Ray's inability to read printed road signs. However, this restriction did not pose a significant barrier to Ray's participation in desired activities, so his goals for treatment were met.

SOCIAL MODEL

A philosophy related to LPAA is that embraced by social models of intervention: Social models emphasize how the presence of a neurogenic language disorder affects patients' communication in social contexts, as well as how social contexts facilitate or inhibit patients' participation. Simmons-Mackie (2001) identified several principles embraced by social models. First, it is often assumed that the primary purpose of communication is the exchange of information, or **transaction.** Although transaction is an important function of communication, another equally important function is reciprocal activity to establish and maintain relationships, or **interaction.** Social models recognize the importance of adequate communication for accomplishing social goals and emphasize the need to address this aspect of communication during intervention.

Second, similar to LPAA, social models emphasize the need to address communication and cognition in relevant contexts. Traditional impairment level treatments, including many of those reviewed in Chapter 9, often involve highly structured communicative or cognitive tasks targeting specific linguistic or cognitive processes, disconnecting the processing from its typically occurring or **authentic context.** For example, a common communicative context is conversation, thus treatment within a social model emphasizes practicing communication strategies in the context of conversation. To assure that the context is realistic, clinicians can involve patients and caregivers in generating conversational topics or target activities of daily living, and should encourage practice in settings outside of the therapy room (Sorin-Peters, 2004). Relatedly, social models acknowledge that communication in authentic contexts is rarely "perfect," but rather is characterized by disfluencies, interruptions, and corrections (Simmons-Mackie, 2001). Because these imperfections are accepted as normal aspects of daily communication, patients with neurogenic language disorders and their caregivers are encouraged to focus less on perfect word choices or grammar and more on successful transactions and interactions.

Social models also are consistent with LPAA in acknowledging that neurogenic language disorders affect individuals in addition to the patients who are experiencing the disorders, and that the effects extend beyond the immediate home environment to the larger social context. Thus, intervention within social models may include training communication partners and modifying the environment, such as discussed earlier in this chapter. The emphasis within the framework of social models is on enabling patients with a neurogenic language disorder as well as other individuals affected by the neurogenic language disorder to participate fully in the communicating society.

SUPPORT GROUPS AND COMMUNITY RESOURCES

Although neurogenic language disorders are relatively common, many people experiencing and affected by these impairments know very little about the nature and impact of these conditions until they themselves are experiencing them. Thus, a sense of being the only one coping with these conditions may be more common than it is for individuals with more well-known and visible disabilities (Rosenthal, 2004). Support groups consisting of patients affected by neurogenic language disorders can be very helpful in assisting other patients in adjusting to and coping with the presence of a communicative or cognitive disability. Similarly, support groups for caregivers of those with neurogenic language disorders can play an important role in helping caregivers adjust to and accept the many changes that accompany the onset of a neurogenic language disorder.

Several types of support groups exist for patients with neurogenic language disorders and their caregivers. These groups typically function to provide information about the neurogenic language disorder or disease, discuss coping and management strategies, and help patients and caregivers identify other appropriate community resources (e.g., respite care programs, home health care services, legal consultants). For example, many communities have established stroke support groups that serve patients experiencing a variety of the impairments common in stroke. Although not every member of the group is affected by neurogenic language disorders, group members may share experiences related to changes in health status, employment, navigating health care systems, and securing funding for rehabilitation costs. Groups established for specific neurogenic language disorders such as aphasia, RHD, dementia (in particular, Alzheimer's disease), and TBI, and for caregivers of patients with these disorders also are available in many communities.

In addition to local support groups, many national associations serve patients affected by neurogenic language disorders. Most of these associations have as their primary mission the direct support of patients affected by neurogenic language disorders by providing easily understood information about the condition and contact information for local support groups and association representatives. Often the organizations maintain web sites that include discussion forums and other avenues for connecting with other patients or caregivers affected by the condition (see Table 11-4). These organizations also often seek to educate the public and health care providers about the condition as well as to fund research related to

Table 11-4. Example List of Internet Resources

EXAMPLE LISTS OF INTERNET RESOURCES	
Sites for Individuals Affected by Stroke	
National Stroke Association	www.stroke.org
American Stroke Association (a division of the American Heart Association)	www.strokeassociation.org www.americanheart.org
American Stroke Foundation	www.americanstroke.org
Washington University Internet Stroke Center	www.strokecenter.org
Sites for Individuals Affected by Aphasia	
National Aphasia Association	www.aphasia.org
Aphasia Hope Foundation	www.aphasiahope.org
Sites for Individuals Affected by RHD	
ASHA Public Information about RHD	www.asha.org/public/speech/disorders/right_brain.htm
Sites for Individuals Affected by TBI	
Brain Injury Association of America	www.biausa.org
Brain Injury Society	www.bisociety.org
Sites of Individuals Affected by Dementia	
Alzheimer's Association	www.alz.org
Alzheimer's Disease International	www.alz.co.uk
Alzheimer's Disease Education & Referral Center	www.alzheimers.org
Dementia Information from the Neurology Channel	www.neurologychannel.com/dementia

the condition. Clinicians may wish to refer to the American Speech-Language-Hearing Association web site, which includes a comprehensive and up-to-date list of these organizations.

In addition to specific groups and organizations serving to support patients and caregivers affected by neurogenic language disorders, many other community resources may be useful as patients resume their participation in usual activities. Each state operates a department of vocational rehabilitation that assists patients with disabilities as they re-enter the work force. Services provided by vocational rehabilitation centers include identifying and facilitating the implementation of appropriate accommodations (including financial support for augmentative communication or external cognitive devices) so that patients can return to their previous occupations. If necessary, patients also can receive education and/or training in a new field.

Older patients with neurogenic language disorders may benefit from attending a senior center or related program that provides social programs for the elderly. Not only are these centers generally supportive of patients with disabilities, but many older adults without disabilities attend activities at the center, providing a rich social context for patients with neurogenic language disorders. These centers may be particularly useful in helping patients identify hobbies and other recreational activities that are compatible with their current physical, cognitive, and communicative abilities. Larger communities may have similar centers for young adults and professional-aged individuals.

COMPLEMENTARY AND ALTERNATIVE TREATMENTS

Complementary and alternative medicine (CAM) represents one of the most rapidly growing approaches to preventing and treating a spectrum of medical and psychological problems, including neurogenic language disorders, with approximately 60% of the U.S. adult population reporting that they have utilized at least one CAM approach in the last year, and visits to CAM providers exceeding those to primary care physicians (Barnes, Powell-Griner, McFann, & Nahin, 2004; Zollman & Vickers, 1999). According to the National Center for Complementary and Alternative Medicine (NCCAM; 2002), CAM encompasses a diverse collection of health care systems (e.g., traditional Chinese medicine, folk healing), therapies (e.g., hypnosis, natural environment therapy, massage), and products (e.g., herbal medications, homeopathic preparations) for maximizing, restoring, or maintaining physical and mental well-being that have been developed and primarily utilized outside of conventional medical institutions. Despite the heterogeneity of these approaches, all focus on providing individualized treatment of patients, and on emphasizing "holistic" treatment in terms of not only remediating medical or physical ailments, but also fostering mental and spiritual well-being (Barnes et al., 2004). Accordingly, many of these treatments aim to go beyond effecting change at only the ICF level of body function, and strive to enhance patients' recovery at ICF activity and participation levels as well. Because of increased consumer interest in CAM techniques, and because of growing empirical support for the use of at least some of these techniques, a brief description of a few CAM approaches that have been used with neurogenic patient populations is provided below.

RELAXATION THERAPY

Relaxation therapy, which includes meditation, progressive muscle relaxation, and biofeedback, is one of the most commonly practiced forms of CAM (Barnes et al., 2004; NCCAM, 2002). Very generally, these therapies involve sustaining attention to a verbal (e.g., word, phrase, prayer) or nonverbal (e.g., tone, mental image) stimulus or muscle activity while concurrently inhibiting thoughts or sensory input that may interfere with the attentional focus on the target stimulus or activity (Murray & Kim, 2004). Practice of these relaxation techniques can produce physiological changes (e.g., reduced heart and breathing rates) to counter stress, and has been found to address a variety of conditions such as chronic pain, anxiety, depression, and cardiovascular disease that commonly coexist with neurogenic language disorders (Jorm, Christensen, Griffiths, & Rodgers, 2002; Wetherall, 1998).

Initial research indicates that relaxation therapy might help ameliorate linguistic and cognitive symptoms associated with a number of neurological disorders. For example, meditation has been used in combination with other CAM or conventional (e.g., memory strategy education) procedures to enhance the word retrieval, memory, and attention abilities of patients with aphasia (Ince, 1968), mild cognitive impairment (Rapp et al., 2002), or TBI (Wilson & Robertson, 1992). **Guided imagery** (GI) also has been used with neurogenic patient populations. This relaxation technique requires patients to select a pleasant and calm location or event, and then imagine being at that location or event (Barnes et al., 2004). When combined with other CAM or conventional treatments, GI has been found to improve social interaction (Welden & Yesavage, 1982), quality of life (Bedard et al., 2003), and the informativeness of verbal output (Murray & Ray, 2001) in patients with dementia, TBI, or aphasia. More substantial positive effects have been associated with **progressive muscle relaxation** (PMR), which involves successively contracting and relaxing certain muscle groups (Barnes et al., 2004). For example, both Marshall and Watts (1976) and Suhr et al. (1999) found that PMR by itself facilitated the linguistic (i.e., naming, verbal fluency, and other spoken language abilities) and cognitive (i.e., memory) abilities of patients with aphasia or Alzheimer's disease. Another relaxation therapy that has proven effective with neurogenic patient populations is **biofeedback.** This technique involves teaching patients conscious self-regulation of physiological functions (e.g., brain wave activity, skin temperature) that are related to stress levels by connecting patients to simple electronic devices that monitor the target physiological functions (Barnes et al., 2004). Whereas most biofeedback research has focused on motoric changes in patients with neurogenic disorders (e.g., Yoo, Park, & Chung, 2001), a study by Holland and colleagues (1999) indicated that two TBI patients with severe cognitive-communicative disorders not only learned how to utilize biofeedback, but also consequently exhibited decreased anxiety, increased therapy compliance, and achieved faster therapy progress while using this CAM technique.

It is also noteworthy that relaxation therapy has been successfully used to alleviate stress and other negative symptoms in caregivers of patients with neurogenic language disorders. For example, Mizuno, Hosaka, Ogihara, Higano, and Mano, (1999) enrolled one group of caregivers of dementia patients in a five-week intervention program consisting of education (e.g., information about dementia, associations between stress and disease), group discussions on caregiving problems, and relaxation therapy, while another group of caregivers on their waiting list served as controls. Caregivers who completed the intervention program displayed significantly improved emotional and immune functioning compared to the control group. Additionally, caregivers who continued to use relaxation techniques at home were able to maintain or make additional improvements at two months post-treatment.

SENSORY STIMULATION

Of the various CAM approaches tried with neurogenic patient populations, **sensory stimulation** techniques have been utilized most frequently both clinically and in the research literature. As shown in Table 11-5, there are a variety of sensory stimulation treatments, all of which are based on exposing patients to, and allowing them to interact with, often in a non-directive manner, stimuli that will excite one or more senses. The rationale for sensory stimulation is that patients with neurogenic disorders often not only present with disease- and/or age-related declines in their sensory and perceptual abilities, but also may live in sensory-deprived environments, particularly those who reside in long-term care facilities (Kovach, 2000). These biologically- and environmentally-related sensory deficiencies can lead to a state of sensory deprivation, which in turn has been found to evoke or aggravate behavioral, social, cognitive, and psychiatric problems. Accordingly, preventing or ameliorating sensory deprivation should have beneficial effects upon patients' physical and mental well being.

Indeed, several sensory stimulation treatments, including light (e.g., Yamadera et al., 2000), toy (e.g., Murray et al., 2003), music (e.g., Nayak, Wheeler, Shiflett, & Agonstinelli, 2000), robotic pet (e.g., Libin & Cohen-Mansfield, 2004), and pet (e.g., Richeson, 2003) therapies have been successfully utilized with neurogenic patients. Most research, however, has focused on the provision of multisensory stimulation, which is also referred to as Snoezelen (Lancioni, Cuvo, & O'Reilly, 2002). In this treatment approach, patients are exposed to an environment or collection of stimuli designed to stimulate all sensory channels. For example, a long-term care facility may have a Snoezelen room that contains spot lights, mirror

Table 11-5. Sensory Stimulation Treatments

TYPE OF THERAPY	BRIEF DESCRIPTION AND EFFECTS
Multi-sensory stimulation or Snoezelen	Structured or unstructured exposure to visual (e.g., colored lights), auditory (e.g., music), tactile (e.g., fabric samples with different textures), olfactory (e.g., scented oils), proprioceptive (e.g., a swinging chair), and/or gustatory (e.g., different flavored candies) stimuli to decrease disruptive behaviors, and increase communicative output, cognitive functioning, socialization, and emotional well-being
Toy stimulation	Provision of toys, in particular plush animal toys or baby dolls, which patients care for and interact with to decrease disruptive behaviors, and increase communicative output and emotional well-being
Pet or animal-assisted therapy	Inclusion of trained pets (e.g., dog, cat, fish) in traditional behavioral treatment to enhance linguistic and/or cognitive abilities, improve emotional functioning, and decrease disruptive behaviors
Music therapy	Patients produce or listen to music to facilitate their linguistic and/or cognitive abilities, decrease disruptive behaviors, and improve emotional functioning
Light therapy or phototherapy	Structured exposure to bright light emitted from light boxes, light rooms, or light visors to improve sleep/wake cycle regularity and consequently improve general cognitive, behavioral, and emotional functioning
Robotherapy	Provision of robotic pets that patients care for and interact with to decrease disruptive behaviors and increase communicative output and emotional well-being
Natural environment therapy	Exposure to objects, colors, sounds, and so forth that are indigenous to patients' daily environments prior to being admitted to an acute or chronic care facility

balls, and/or optic fiber sprays to stimulate vision, music equipment to stimulate audition, essential oil samples to stimulate smell, vibrating chairs and/or fabric samples to stimulate touch, and food samples to stimulate taste. A key component to this approach, particularly when it is provided to patients with dementia, is that patients are given the choice to interact with whatever stimuli appeal to them. Positive outcomes reported in studies involving patients with varying forms of moderate to severe dementia (e.g., Alzheimer's disease, Huntington's disease, multi-infarct dementia) include decreases in disruptive behaviors, apathy, negative emotions (e.g., anxiety), and perseveration, and increases in socialization, memory, attention, communicative output and fluency, mobility, activities of daily living, quality of life, and caregiver morale when even brief periods of multisensory stimulation were provided (Cornell, 2004; Kovach, 2000; Leng et al., 2003). These improvements are typically temporary, but even transient positive changes have clinical significance for those caring for these patients.

Multisensory stimulation also has been provided to patients who have suffered a severe stroke or TBI in an attempt to increase the rate and extent of recovery from coma and persistent vegetative state. Treatment procedures for this patient population differ from those described above for patients with dementia in that the sensory stimuli are selected and applied by the clinician or caregiver on typically a more intensive schedule (e.g., one to two hour-long sessions per day) and in a more structured manner. Positive outcomes such as increased levels of cognitive functioning and decreased coma lengths have been frequently reported (e.g., Oh & Seo, 2003; Wilson et al., 1993). Despite the predominance of encouraging findings for patients with dementia, severe TBI, or stroke, most previous studies had weak research designs (e.g., use of unstandardized measures, biased observers, and/or small or imprecisely described subject samples). Therefore, more methodologically rigorous investigations must be completed before definitive conclusions regarding the effectiveness of multisensory stimulation can be made (Chung, Lai, Chung, & French, 2004; Lombardi, Taricco, De Tanti, Telaro, & Liberati, 2002).

ACUPUNCTURE

Acupuncture involves stimulating the skin, and consequently the nerves, at designated anatomic locations or acupoints in order to reestablish blocked or intermittent flow of body energy, referred to as "chi" or "qi" (Barnes et al., 2004; Murray & Kim, 2004). There are numerous forms of acupuncture that vary in terms of stimulation method (e.g., needling/manual or electric needle insertion, finger pressure/acupressure, heat application/moxibustion) and location and number of acupoints. Recent empirical studies have verified that stimulation of these peripheral acupoints does indeed activate higher levels of the nervous system (e.g., spinal cord, midbrain, cortical regions) as well as cause the release of neurotransmitters and neurohormones (e.g., enkephalines, serotonin) (Lo & Cui, 2003).

Whereas the use of acupuncture to treat certain medical conditions (e.g., chronic pain, nausea) has substantial empirical support (Rabinstein & Shulman, 2003), application of this CAM technique to remediate neurogenic language disorders has so far produced mixed findings (Murray & Kim, 2004). For instance, in several studies conducted by Chinese researchers to evaluate the effects of acupuncture on aphasia, it is not clear whether the positive changes reported reflected improved motor speech versus improved motor speech and spoken language, or whether the positive changes were maintained over time (Zhang, 1989; Zhang & Zhao, 1990). Likewise, research with TBI or Parkinson's disease patients has primarily evaluated changes in motor symptoms, and failed to include linguistic or cognitive outcome measures (Murray & Kim, 2004). More encouraging findings, however, have been reported when **transcutaneous electrical nerve stimulation** (TENS) has been used with neurogenic patient populations. TENS is similar to electro-acupuncture, as it involves stimulating the skin at certain frequencies and skin sites (which tend to overlap with acupoints). Improvements in memory, verbal fluency, and emotional-behavioral symptoms in patients with Alzheimer's disease (Scherder, Bouma, & Steen, 1992; 1995), and reductions in left neglect in patients with RHD (Vallar, Rusconi, & Bernardini, 1996), have been reported following TENS. Further research is needed, however, to determine optimal stimulation schedules and to examine how long these positive changes are maintained.

EXERCISE

Augmenting conventional behavioral linguistic or cognitive treatments with physical exercise has been found to benefit patients representing a range of static and progressive neurological disorders. Various forms of exercise have been incorporated into treatment, including yoga, tai chi, dancing, walking, biking, and strength/weight training. The addition of exercise to linguistic and cognitive rehabilitation programs is supported by several lines of research, including: (1) the prevalence of suboptimal levels of physical activity among the elderly, particularly those with neurological disorders (e.g., Becker, Bar-Or, Mendelson, & Najenson, 1978); (2) in animal and some human studies, exercise has been found to enhance cerebral blood flow, promote immune system functioning, and evoke structural and neurochemical changes in brain regions that are known to support linguistic and cognitive functioning, including the hippocampus and prefrontal cortex (e.g., Rogers, Schroeder, Secher, & Mitchell, 1990); and (3) exercise has been found to help healthy adults, as well as those with a variety of medical conditions (e.g., depression, anxiety, diabetes mellitus, osteoarthritis, incontinence), improve or maintain their physical, cognitive, and emotional status (e.g., Bassey, 2000).

With respect to neurogenic language disorders, most research on the effects of exercise has involved patients with TBI or dementia. In terms of TBI, a few studies have documented the benefits of exercise on the physical well-being of these patients, particularly in terms of reductions in fatigue, which in turn may positively affect cognitive and linguistic functioning (Moran, 1976; Wolman, Cornall, Flucher, & Greenwood, 1994). For example, Grealy and colleagues (1999) directly examined the effects of exercise on the cognitive abilities of patients in the acute or chronic stages of recovery from TBI. Two groups of patients with TBI were involved in this study: one group that only received traditional rehabilitation procedures and one that received both traditional rehabilitation procedures as well as a virtual reality exercise program. The four-week exercise program consisted of riding a recumbent, nonimmersive virtual reality exercise bicycle at least three times per week for up to 25 minutes per session. The virtual reality component consisted of a color monitor that displayed graphics pertaining to a bicycle ride on an island, in a town and countryside, or on a snowy mountain; patients were also provided kinesthetic (e.g., bike seat would tilt when they did a turn), tactile (e.g., a fan would blow on them to simulate air flow), and auditory (e.g., they heard sounds relating to the pictured scenes) stimulation. A comparison of the treatment and control group's pre- and post-treatment test performances indicated that the treatment group displayed superior improvements on tests of verbal and visual learning that were attributed to improved working memory abilities, as well as significantly faster reaction times.

The results of several investigations have established that exercise can enhance cognitive functioning in patients with mild to severe forms of dementia (Bonner & Cousins, 1996; Lindenmuth & Lindenmuth, 1994; Palleschi, Vetta, & deGennaro, 1996). For example, Arkin (Arkin, 2003; Arkin & Mahendra, 2001; Mahendra & Arkin, 2004) has published a series of studies on the positive effects of her Elder Rehab program on the linguistic, cognitive, physical, and emotional functioning of community-dwelling patients in the early to middle stages of Alzheimer's disease. Arkin's treatment program consists of: (1) two to three weekly exercise sessions consisting of aerobic exercise (i.e., walking, stationary biking), strength training, and flexibility and balance exercises; (2) one weekly volunteer work session at which patients help out at community agencies; (3) one weekly recreational activity such as going to a museum or concert; and (4) language (e.g., providing opinions and advice concerning controversial topics, generating the pros and cons of situations and issues, object description tasks) and memory exercises (i.e., listening to tape-recorded narratives about their life and family and answering questions pertaining to these tapes) completed either during or prior to exercise sessions. For all components of the program, either student volunteers or caregivers accompany the patients. Comparisons of pre- and post-intervention assessment results have indicated that patients with dementia show significant improvements in their physical fitness and depression levels, and have higher or maintained general cognitive abilities, and spoken language production (e.g., informativeness levels) and comprehension (i.e., proverb interpretation) skills.

The above findings are encouraging with respect to the positive effects of exercise on the linguistic and cognitive abilities of patients with TBI or dementia. Although it seems likely that these positive outcomes could also be achieved in patients with aphasia or cognitive-communicative disorders related to RHD, no research to support this contention has yet been conducted. Likewise with respect to dementia, most research has involved patients with Alzheimer's disease; thus, how patients with other dementing illnesses respond to exercise needs to be examined.

In summary, despite growing empirical support for using CAM to supplement more traditional behavioral linguistic or cognitive treatments for neurogenic language disorders, further research is required to resolve a number of issues. First, it is not yet known whether certain CAM approaches might prove more suitable for certain neurogenic patient populations or certain linguistic or cognitive symptoms. Second, investigation of the long-term effects of CAM is needed (e.g., Are positive effects maintained following termination of the CAM technique? How much CAM intervention is needed to foster maintenance of positive treatment effects?). Third, many previous studies had weak designs (e.g., failed to control for placebo or practice effects; relied on subjective measures), and thus investigations with strong, controlled designs are still needed. Finally, future research should focus on extending our understanding of the effects of CAM to a broader range of neurogenic disorders and linguistic and cognitive abilities.

COUNSELING AND EDUCATION

It is somewhat misleading to introduce the topic of counseling and education in Chapter 11, as this aspect of service to patients and caregivers affected by neurogenic language disorders is crucial from the moment speech-language pathologists meet patients and their families. Although neurogenic language disorders are relatively common, many individuals know very little about these conditions and may experience considerable anxiety related to the "unknown." Moreover, physicians and other members of the care team may be more concerned or familiar with immediate physical health concerns, and thus fail to address issues related to communication and cognition. Thus, it is important that clinicians be prepared to provide information to patients and their caregivers or families immediately upon meeting them as well as throughout the recovery process, or, in the case of progressive disorders (e.g., Alzheimer's disease, Huntington's disease), throughout disease evolution.

The amount and type of information individuals need varies according to a variety of factors, so clinicians will need to be sensitive to relevant cues (e.g., signs of confusion, fatigue, and/or impatience) when providing information. During the days early post onset or immediately following diagnosis with a progressive disease, most families will benefit from basic information about the neurogenic language disorder, explanation of professional jargon, and description and demonstration of simple strategies for facilitating communicative interactions with their loved ones. It is likely that this information will need to be provided more than once, as the stress associated with medical crisis affects the ability of individuals to understand and retain the vast amount of information that will be presented to them by a variety of different medical professionals (Hinckley, 2000). Providing written material in addition to verbal explanations is highly recommended, as it may help individuals comprehend the information being presented and will allow them to reread and refer back to the information as often as they need (Sorin-Peters, 2004); additionally, they will be able to share this written material with family members and other significant others who are unable to speak directly with the health care team.

When the immediate health crisis has passed, family members will likely request information about when communication or cognition will return to normal (Holland & Fridriksson, 2001). In the case of progressive disorders, patients and families will want to know how quickly abilities will deteriorate. Often clinicians will be unable to provide a prognosis so early in recovery or the disease process, but it may be possible to discuss the factors that influence the rate and degree of recovery or disease progression (see Chapters 5 and 6 for a description of linguistic and cognitive prognostic indicators, respectively) and begin to explore treatment options with patients and their families. Because status changes are common in the early days of recovery from static disorders (e.g., stroke, TBI), clinicians also should be prepared to explain variability so that patients, their caregivers, or both do not become discouraged or overly optimistic when communication or cognitive abilities change temporarily.

As patients continue through the recovery process, they may benefit from more detailed information about treatment options. Similarly, family members may request information about the treatments their loved ones are receiving; in particular, the purpose of many treatment activities or compensatory strategies may not be obvious to non-speech-language pathologists. For patients experiencing degenerative conditions, counseling and education should include information to help the patient and family members prepare for the inevitable decline in cognitive and communicative abilities and, accordingly, for continual changes in therapy goals (which, it should be emphasized, focus on maintaining rather than necessarily improving current functioning) and procedures. When discussing treatment procedures and progress, clinicians should always assure that they not only identify linguistic and cognitive areas in need of remediation, but also emphasize areas of strength by describing how patients' abilities have progressed or been maintained over the course of treatment (Holland & Fridriksson, 2001).

At every stage in the clinical process, the clinician should provide referrals to appropriate resources, including support groups, which are discussed in greater detail in an earlier section of this chapter. Clinicians also may wish to provide a printed list of key Internet resources, with the understanding that additional resources may be identified through an Internet search. Table 11-4 includes a sample list of sites clinicians might include. Given the relative speed with which Internet resources appear and disappear, it is recommended that these lists be updated at least annually. A variety of print resources also are available. For example, a very useful resource developed specifically for patients affected by neurogenic language disorders is *Coping with Aphasia* (Lyon, 1998). In language appropriate for non-communication professionals, this book addresses a plethora of concerns experienced throughout the various stages of recovery. Although this book focuses on aphasia, much of the information is applicable to any condition of sudden onset. Also available are a number of personal accounts written by individuals affected by neurogenic language disorders (see Table 11-6).

Finally, clinicians should be cautioned that because the speech-language pathologist may be the health care professional with whom individuals have the greatest contact, patients and their families may request information and/or counseling outside the scope of practice of the speech-language pathologist. It is not

Table 11-6. **Examples of Published Personal Accounts of Individuals with Neurogenic Language Disorders**

TITLE	AUTHOR	PUBLISHER
Stroke, Aphasia		
Pathways: Moving beyond stroke and aphasia	Ewing, S.A. and Pfalzgraf, B. (1991)	Wayne State University Press
The invaluable guide to LIFE after stroke: An owner's manual	Josephs, A. (1992)	Amadeus Press
Return to Ithaca	Newborn, B. (1997)	Penguin
Stroke: From crisis to victory	Lavin, J. (1985)	Scholastic Library
My stroke of luck	Douglas, K (2003)	Perennial
RHD		
Right hemisphere stroke: A victim reflects on rehabilitative medicine	Johnson, F. K. (1990)	Wayne State University Press
TBI		
Over my head	Osborn, C. (2000)	Andrews McMeel
In search of wings: A journey back from traumatic brain injury	Bryant, B. (1992)	Wings
I'll carry the fork!: Recovering a life after brain injury	Swanson, K. L. (1999)	Rising Star
Surviving black ice: A survivor's insight to life after head injury	Fierce, D. W. (2002)	Writer's Block Press
Dementia		
My journey in Alzheimer's disease	Davis, R. (1989)	Tyndale House
Living in the labyrinth: A personal journey through the maze of Alzheimer's	McGowin, D. F. (1994)	Delta
Living with Alzheimer's: Ruth's story	Danforth, A. (1986)	Howarth Press

uncommon to receive questions related to insurance, medication, other symptoms (e.g., sexual dysfunction, psychiatric disorders, or family adjustment issues), other therapies, or even laboratory test results. In these cases the clinician should be prepared to refer patients and their families to the appropriate professional. More specifically, clinicians should develop a list of health care professionals who are experienced not only in their own area (e.g., family therapy, counseling, social work, psychiatry), but also in issues specific to neurogenic language disorders (e.g., how aphasia may affect a marriage; how TBI can impact a patient's ability to fulfill her parental role; how to assess depression in the presence of severe language impairment), including previous familiarity with adapting their services to meet patients' communicative strengths and weaknesses (e.g., the professional is experienced in using multimodality communication strategies).

SUMMARY

In this chapter, a number of strategies for assisting patients with neurogenic language disorders in communicating effectively and participating fully in desired activities, even in the presence of significant impairments, have been reviewed. It should be clear to the reader that managing neurogenic language disorders extends not only beyond remediation of the impairments exhibited by the patient, but also beyond even the patient: Clinicians may effect significant changes in a patient's activity and participation by directing efforts toward the communication context, including communication partners and the larger social environment. A beginning literature supports the benefits of activity and participation level treatments, and as the ICF framework becomes more widely applied in American health care, it is likely that reimbursement for these treatments will be more commonplace. In the meantime, clinicians must continue to advocate on a case-by-case basis for the most appropriate intervention plans.

Chapter 12

Modern Health Care and the Future of Neurogenic Language Disorders

LEARNING OBJECTIVES

After reading this chapter you should be able to:

- Describe the difference between fee for service and managed care.

- Define prospective payment and capitated payment.

- Discuss the impact of managed care on speech-language pathology services.

- List the components of the continuum of care.

- Describe the variations in speech-language pathology services across the continuum of care.

KEY TERMS

acute care
adaptive
cap
capitated payment
continuum of care
diagnosis-related group (DRG)
evidence-based practice

fee-for-service
functional measures
home health
long-term care
managed care
minimum data set
outpatient

prospective payment
rehabilitation
resource utilization group (RUG)
restorative
skilled nursing facility

INTRODUCTION

The past two decades have seen significant changes to the American health care system, the most noteworthy of which is the advent of managed care. There is little question that these changes have impacted speech-language pathology services provided to individuals with neurogenic language disorders, regardless of their stage of recovery, in the case of static disorders (e.g., stroke, traumatic brain injury) or disease progression in the case of progressive conditions (e.g., Alzheimer's disease, frontotemporal dementia). This chapter provides an overview of the key concepts in managed care, discusses its impact on the management of neurogenic language disorders, and offers strategies for maximizing the effectiveness of speech-language pathology services in the realm of managed care.

CONCEPTS IN MANAGED CARE

To best understand managed care, it is helpful to review the health care financing paradigm that was predominant prior to the advent of managed care. Before 1990, most health care services were financed in a **fee-for-service** model. In this framework, third-party payers reimbursed health care providers retrospectively (i.e., after the fact) for services based on per-visit or per-procedure rates. Services were typically authorized, provided that the patient continued to benefit from the services, with only very high **caps or limits** (e.g., $100,000) placed on the total amount of funding available for care. Under this system, clinicians could demonstrate that patients were continuing to benefit from services in a variety of ways. For example, treatment resulting in client improvement on a standardized test like the *Boston Diagnostic Aphasia Examination* would be eligible for reimbursement, as would treatments resulting in decreased word retrieval latencies during informal confrontation naming tasks. Additionally, the service provider and/or patient had considerable flexibility in determining which treatments to utilize, as long as improvement was shown. A key feature of the fee-for-service model is that providers can increase revenue by increasing services (e.g., increasing the frequency or total duration of treatment), again, as long as they can demonstrate that the patient is continuing to benefit from the services provided. Thus, it is not surprising that under this system, in the case of aphasia treatment, therapy services ranged in duration from two weeks to two years (Sands, Sarno, & Sankweiler, 1969) and could be expected to include at least 20 and as many as 60 treatment sessions over the course of recovery (Sarno, Silverman, & Sands, 1970; Vignolo, 1964).

Nominal limits on treatment duration and full reimbursement of treatment services by third-party payers generally benefited both providers and patients. This fee-for-service model, however, resulted in skyrocketing health care costs and prompted a call for health care reform. A primary alternative to fee-for-service is **managed care,** which differs from fee-for-service in several key ways. First, providers are not reimbursed on a per-visit basis. Instead, managed care utilizes **prospective** and/or **capitated** reimbursement. Under prospective payment systems, providers are paid a preset fee that is determined either by the diagnosis of the patient, as in **diagnosis-related groups** (DRGs), or by the **rehabilitation**/skilled care needs of the patient, or **resource utilization group** (RUG), such as under Medicare's prospective payment system (PPS) (see Table 12-1). A prospective payment is not itemized, but rather is a lump-sum payment intended to cover the costs for all services that a patient will utilize, given his or her DRG or RUG. Thus, the financial risk lies with the provider. This is illustrated by the following example.

Imagine two individuals who present to the emergency room with a left hemisphere stroke. The managed care agency will pay the acute care hospital to which they are admitted a set amount (e.g., $10,000) for each patient's care. It is important to remember that the fee is the same, regardless of the number of services the patient actually utilizes. Thus, if Patient A has a typical hospital course, undergoing

Table 12-1. **Common Acronyms Associated With Health Care Financing Under Managed Care**

ACRONYM	REFERENCE	DEFINITION
DRG	Diagnosis-Related Group	Designates the reimbursement rate for patients receiving Medicare Part A coverage in acute care settings, based on the diagnosis or diagnoses of individual patients
HCFA	Health Care Financing Agency	Agency of the federal government responsible for administering Medicare and Medicaid
PPS	Prospective Payment System	Providers are paid a predetermined rate based on the diagnosis or rehabilitation needs of the patient
RUG	Resource Utilization Group	Designates the reimbursement rate for patients receiving Medicare Part A coverage for acute rehabilitation centers or skilled nursing facilities, based on the skilled nursing and rehabilitation needs of individual patients

the standard number of diagnostic tests and treatment protocols, she will likely be discharged after 48 hours and incur $6,800 (for example) of actual costs. For Patient A, the hospital would earn a profit of $3,200, because the cost of caring for her is less than what is paid by the insurance company.

Patient B, however, may have a nonstandard hospital course, perhaps related to a particularly severe or unfortunately located lesion resulting in dense hemiparesis, global aphasia, and significant dysphagia. This patient will undergo numerous diagnostic tests, including additional x-rays and a neurosurgical consult. His severe dysphagia may result in aspiration pneumonia and subsequent placement of a feeding tube. Therefore, his stay in acute care may extend to six days or more before being discharged to the skilled nursing facility. For the sake of illustration, assume the total cost for Patient B's care is $23,000. Fortunately for the patient, he is not responsible for paying the $13,000 that the managed care company will not cover. Unfortunately, the hospital would incur a loss of $13,000, as the cost of this patient's care exceeded the fee paid by the managed care company.

Side Bar

DRGs and RUGs: What's the Difference?

DRGs and RUGs are both related prospective payments systems utilized by both federally funded health care agencies (i.e., Medicare and Medicaid) and some private insurance companies, but each is based on a unique classification system. DRGs are utilized primarily for acute care hospital stays and are based on specific diagnostic codes (e.g., International Classification

(continued)

of Disease–ICD–10, World Health Organization, 2003) (See Figure 12-1). For example, a patient with a stroke might be classified according to the DRG for "Intracerebral Hemorrhage in Hemisphere, Cortical" or "Cerebral Infarction due to Thrombosis of Cerebral Arteries."

In contrast, RUGs are determined not only based on specific diagnoses (e.g., hemiplegia, pneumonia) but also with respect to unique symptoms (e.g., wandering, fever) and services required (e.g., dressing changes, oxygen therapy), including type and intensity of rehabilitation needs (e.g., speech therapy four times per week). Subacute care centers such as nursing homes and home health agencies are the most likely to encounter RUG reimbursement systems.

Because of the variety of factors considered in the assignment of RUG, the risk of the reimbursement rate differing substantially from the actual cost of care is relatively low. Unfortunately, the process for identifying the appropriate RUG assignment involves completion of a complex assessment process (i.e., **minimum data set**) and can be quite lengthy. Assignment of DRGs, while relatively straightforward, involves a greater risk of mismatch between reimbursement rate and actual cost of care.

A similar financial risk is associated with capitated payment systems. Capitated payment is similar to prospective payment in that the managed care company pays the provider prospectively (i.e., "up front") for services provided. Under capitated contracts, a provider agrees to serve a specific population for a preset fee. Capitated contracts are typically large-scale agreements, but might be best understood using a small-scale analogy. In the past, large companies (e.g., steel manufacturers) would often hire a physician to provide care for all the company employees. The doctor was paid a salary, and that salary was the same regardless of whether he saw four or four hundred patients in one month. This same principle applies to capitated contracts, but now the "doctor for hire" is usually an entire health care system or HMO, and the "company" may be a single large employer or a group of employers who have joined

Alzheimers Disease	Encephalitis
Brain Hemorrhage	Open Brain Injury
Brain Injury	Pick's Diseasse
Cerebral Cortex Contusion	Specific Cerebrovascular Accidents
Concussion	Transien Ischemic Attack
Degenerative Nervous System Disorders	Traumatic Brain Hemorrhage

Figure 12-1. Examples of Diagnosis-Related Groups (DRG). Each patient's DRG determines the payment to the health care agency by the third-party payer, regardless of the actual cost of the patient's care.

together to increase their bargaining power. As with prospective payment, the providers have the potential to make a profit if the cost of providing care to the designated population is less than the capitated payment. On the other hand, if more services are used than the providers bargained for, they stand to lose money as well.

It is evident from these descriptions that under the fee-for-service system, it was in the best interest of the providers to increase their services, whereas the opposite is true under managed care. This issue has significant implications for the delivery of speech-language pathology services in today's health care environment, an issue that will be discussed in greater detail in a later section of this chapter.

Whereas reimbursement strategies are an important aspect of managed care (and often receive the most attention), several other characteristics of managed care warrant mentioning. A focus on **functional measures** of treatment outcomes is a hallmark of managed care. Functional measures, as discussed in Chapter 7, are those that address the ICF levels of activity and participation. Previously, under fee-for-service models, providers could document progress by measuring performance solely on impairment-level measures such as tests of word finding or measures of tongue strength. Whereas it is often anticipated that improvements at the impairment level impact the patient's functional abilities, as indicated in several discussions throughout this book, it is not possible to predict perfectly activity and participation from impairment (e.g., Ross & Wertz, 1999). The insistence on functional outcome measures is an acknowledgment of this imperfect relationship.

At present, particularly within the field of speech-language pathology, many outcome measures are reported retrospectively. That is, speech-language pathologists assess function, provide treatment, and then demonstrate how treatment has impacted function. In the future, however, speech-language pathologists will be reimbursed for providing only those treatments that have *already* been shown to be beneficial. This is known as **evidence-based practice** (described in detail in Chapter 8), and it is already in place within many aspects of health care. Evidence-based practice eventually will dictate that providers consider not only treatment efficacy and effectiveness, but also efficiency.

A final feature of managed care is the strategic use of the **continuum of care** (Figure 12-2). The continuum of care is the range of care settings in which health care is delivered. A typical continuum of care, at least for static conditions such as stroke or traumatic brain injury, begins with admission to the emergency room and continues on to the intensive care unit. The patient might then be transferred to the medical wing and from there to a rehabilitation floor. Discharge from rehabilitation might be to skilled nursing, long-term care, home health, or outpatient services. Each level of care along the continuum is characterized by the provision of particular levels of skilled care, and thus is more or less expensive. As might be anticipated, care in the intensive care unit is more expensive than care provided as an outpatient. Because managed care has a primary goal of reducing health care costs, providing care in the least expensive but most medically appropriate environment is a priority.

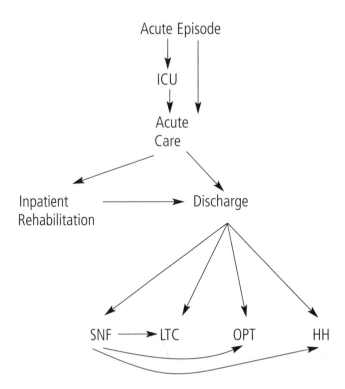

Figure 12-2. Continuum of care. ICU = Intensive Care Unit, SNF = Skilled Nursing Facility, LTC = Long-Term Care Facility, OPT = Outpatient, HH = Home Health.

IMPACT OF MANAGED CARE ON SERVICES FOR NEUROGENIC LANGUAGE DISORDERS

Managed care has impacted the delivery of rehabilitation services, including speech-language pathology, in a variety of ways. First, managed care has led to reductions in both lengths of stay in health care facilities and overall durations of treatment (Leibovitz et al., 2001). This main effect has several ramifications for different aspects of service, each of which is discussed below.

Reduced lengths of stay in acute care suggest that individuals experiencing stroke or other acute neurological insult might be hospitalized only two or three days before being transferred along the continuum of care. During this short time period, speech-language pathologists will focus their efforts on careful assessment, and it is unlikely that a formal treatment plan will be developed or initiated (Holland & Fridriksson, 2001). In other settings, such as rehabilitation and skilled nursing, shorter lengths of stay have the potential to have the opposite effect: that is, a *de-*

emphasis on assessment. In these settings, clinicians recognize that great functional gains must be demonstrated in a short amount of time, so they may initiate treatment as quickly as possible to capitalize on the time available. Another factor driving clinicians in these settings to forego detailed assessment is that the prospective payment system authorized by Medicare bases reimbursement rates on treatment minutes only. Thus, despite the inappropriateness of selecting treatment procedures without appropriate assessment results to guide that selection, the facility will not be paid for any time the clinician spends assessing the patient, and will thus be reluctant to pay clinicians for assessment services. Another result of the pressure to reduce length of stay is that priority is given to any treatment that will impact the patient's need for skilled medical treatment (moving them down the continuum of care) or that prevents additional medical complications (saving on diagnostic and treatment costs). With respect to speech-language pathology services, the result is that referrals for dysphagia assessment and treatment may take priority over communication services. In essence, patients who are unable to *eat* are both more expensive to care for (e.g., increased nursing needs, special dietary requirements, placement and maintenance of feeding tubes) and stay in the hospital longer than patients who are unable to *speak* or *understand*. Thus, dysphagia management may be perceived (and in many cases misperceived) as more valuable than communication management, particularly in acute care settings (Hallowell & Clark, 2002).

Related to shorter lengths of stay is the trend for reduced overall durations of treatment throughout the continuum of care. Because prospective payment and capitated payment systems reimburse providers at a flat rate, accomplishing goals in fewer sessions may mean the difference between profit and loss, which ultimately may mean the difference between employment and unemployment for the clinician. Clinicians will likely feel strong pressure from their employers to determine treatment durations based on reimbursement schedules versus patients' needs (Henri & Hallowell, 1999), but must reconcile that pressure with clinical ethics to provide the most appropriate treatment.

Lastly, another impact of managed care on speech-language pathology services is the requirement of documented functional outcomes. Managed care has essentially revolutionized the way speech-language pathologists as well as other rehabilitation professionals document the effectiveness of their services. Specifically, clinicians can no longer write goals or report progress in terms that make sense only to other clinicians (e.g., "Mr. Smith will produce embedded clauses with third person reflexive pronouns during idiom descriptions with 95% accuracy."). Rather, goals and progress reports must indicate how patients' functional abilities are changing as a result of intervention (e.g., "Mr. Smith will obtain billing information from three local businesses utilizing the strategies practiced during treatment sessions: scripts, alphabet cueing, and drawing.") (see Table 12-2). In essence, clinicians must highlight the effects of services on the patient's daily activities and participation, rather than on underlying impairments. Impairments may improve subsequent to treatment, but clinicians must show that is not the *only* positive effect of treatment.

Table 12-2. Clinical Goals under Managed Care

GOALS/OUTCOMES CONSISTENT WITH AIMS OF MANAGED CARE	GOALS/OUTCOMES INCONSISTENT WITH AIMS OF MANAGED CARE
Ms. Jones will independently use target strategies to complete written tasks involving both left and right hemispace.	Ms. Jones will reduce hemispatial neglect.
Mr. Smith will participate in a ten-minute discussion of work-related topics, using target strategies to maintain topics and repair communication breakdowns.	Mr. Smith will respond appropriately to yes/no questions.
Ms. Harris will successfully use a public transportation system to attend a cultural event.	Ms. Harris will improve reasoning skills.

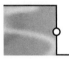

STRATEGIES FOR OPTIMIZING SERVICES FOR NEUROGENIC LANGUAGE DISORDERS

In order for the management of neurogenic language disorders to maintain feasibility and credibility in today's healthcare environment, speech-language clinicians will need to structure their services to align with the goals of managed care. Several key strategies will help in this endeavor.

First, managed care dictates that speech-language pathologists target and show evidence of functional changes in their patients' lives. More specifically, as indicated above, clinicians must document specifically how treatments are impacting patients at the ICF levels of activity and participation. At least for the present, this type of documentation will be justification for our services.

In the future, however, evidence-based practice policies will additionally dictate that clinicians be able to demonstrate *a priori* that a treatment they plan to use has documented efficacy for the types of communicative and/or cognitive problems for which it will be prescribed. This movement has several implications for the field of speech-language pathology. First, it suggests that clinicians need to be familiar with the efficacy literature (see Chapter 8). Because this literature is expanding daily, clinicians will need to stay current, setting aside time to review and understand the literature, and to attend conferences where state-of-the-art therapies are critically discussed. It also means that clinicians need to *become* researchers. Clinicians should take advantage of opportunities for single-subject experiments to assess the benefit of one or more treatment strategies in a sound design that can be reported and replicated. These contributions are critical to the livelihood of our profession, particularly in the area of neurogenic language disorders.

Related to the issues discussed above is the need for clinicians to market actively the services provided to individuals with communication and/or cognitive difficulties. Clinicians must ensure that physicians, nurses, social workers, other health care providers (e.g., occupational therapists, neuropsychologists), case managers, and, perhaps most importantly, patients and their caregivers understand how neurogenic language disorders impact activity and participation and how our services positively influence the lives of the patients we serve. Marketing may be particularly important in relation to specific services. For example, physicians and other health care providers may be unfamiliar with speech-language pathology services to individuals with dementia or other cognitive-communicative disorders, or of the role of speech-language pathologists in the management of the progressive disorders. This can be accomplished in a variety of ways. The following suggestions are not meant to be exhaustive, but instead provide a place to start and will perhaps inspire even more creative ideas.

Side Bar

More Than a Swallow-ologist

The need for marketing is illustrated quite clearly by the following two situations. First, early in my clinical career, after I had evaluated the swallowing function of an individual who had experienced a stroke, I spoke to the physician about addressing the patient's communication. The physician asked for more information, and when I explained how the patient was having difficulty understanding and expressing himself and how I could help the patient with these difficulties, the physician replied, "Huh, I didn't know you guys did anything except swallowing."

More recently, I was conducting a study comparing the language abilities of patients with Parkinson's disease to those of patients with Huntington's disease. Although the types of language problems associated with Parkinson's or Huntington's diseases are not yet well described, significant empirical and clinical evidence indicates that these diseases can cause significant motor speech and swallowing problems and dementia. However, only two out of more than 30 patient participants had received speech-language pathology services (both for swallowing vs. cognitive-communicative issues) prior to their participation in the study, even though many demonstrated significant dysarthria and cognitive problems.

The first example shows how, because our services in the area of dysphagia are in such high demand, our expertise in the areas of communication and cognition is becoming de-emphasized, and perhaps overlooked completely. The second example indicates that we need not only to increase health care professionals' understanding of the breadth of services provided by speech-language pathologists, but also improve the general public's awareness of the field of speech-language pathology so that they can request our services.

Perhaps the most effective way of marketing services is to speak directly to potential referral sources, preferably face to face. When professional colleagues know the speech-language pathologist and the services he or she provides, just seeing the clinician in the hallways might spark a referral. Professional relationships will only be strengthened as colleagues become aware of the professional and effective care speech-language pathologists provide, as well as the impact of services for communicative and cognitive disorders on the patient's overall health and wellness.

Other opportunities to highlight services are available during national "awareness" times, such as Stroke Awareness Month (May), Aphasia Awareness Month (June), and Better Speech and Hearing Month (May). These are convenient occasions to display posters and distribute marketing materials, to offer educational programs and in-services, and to remind administrators, other care providers, patients, and their families about neurogenic language disorders and the types of services that speech-language pathologists can provide to manage these disorders.

Patient and professional advocacy is another activity that is becoming increasingly important in the advent of managed care. Advocacy is particularly important with respect to patients with neurogenic language disorders, given that these patients are often less able than other patient groups to self-advocate for appropriate services and financial coverage. Many marketing and education activities may also serve the purpose of advocacy as referral sources become more aware of the value of speech-language services. Clinicians may find it necessary to advocate for specific patient needs (e.g., comprehensive assessment, continued treatment, augmentative communication systems), which may involve speaking directly with primary care physicians, administrators, and/or third-party payment providers. A useful resource for clinicians practicing patient advocacy is the Advocacy Committee of the American Speech-Language-Hearing Association's (ASHA) Special Interest Division 2: Neurophysiology and Neurogenic Speech and Language Disorders. Although some of the resources provided by the Advocacy Committee are available through the ASHA web site, most are available only through the Division newsletter, which is a benefit of Division membership. Clinicians can learn more about Division 2 through the ASHA web site.

In addition to marketing and advocacy, reducing treatment costs through innovative methods is also a professional priority. One of the best ways to reduce treatment costs is through prevention and wellness promotion activities. It may seem counterintuitive to devise ways for people to *not* need speech-language pathology services, but because additional revenue is not necessarily gained for additional treatment services, it is in our best interest, and certainly in the best interest of our patients and the general public, to do everything possible to maintain their cognitive and communicative health.

Side Bar

The Benefit of Prevention

Imagine a dentist who has agreed to provide all of the fillings and/or other treatments to a group of people. For this service she is paid, up front, $10,000. Further imagine that it costs the dentist $10 to perform regular cleaning and prophylaxis, but $95 to place a

(continued)

filling, and $450 to administer a root canal. It is very much in the dentist's best interest to practice prevention to reduce overall costs, while helping the patients' dental health along the way. Under managed care, the speech-language pathologist's situation is exactly as it is for this dentist.

Opportunities to practice "preventative speech-language pathology" may not be immediately obvious. Expanding the vision of speech-language pathology services, however, may reveal several ways to promote cognitive and communicative wellness. First, clinicians can increase the public's awareness of the types of medical conditions and diseases that impact communication and cognition. Any wellness or prevention programs that address these conditions and diseases will also address communication and cognition. Therefore, communication and cognitive wellness can be targeted during Brain Awareness Week, Parkinson's Day, High Blood Pressure Month, and Wear Your Helmet Year, just as examples. Wellness activities should target individuals across the lifespan, in recognition that it is not just adults who experience acquired neurogenic language problems (Clark, 1999). Increasing public awareness through wellness promotion may also have a positive impact on future referrals—patients or caregivers who know about speech-language pathologists are more apt in the future to request speech-language pathology services if the situation warrants.

Clinicians also may promote wellness through educational programs designed to teach individuals how to cope with existing cognitive and/or communicative impairments. These programs might target individuals with the impairments, their families, friends, co-workers, and employers (see Chapter 11). These programs may have as great an impact on patients' participation as any direct treatment provided.

It would be inappropriate to leave a discussion of innovative and cost-reducing programs without mentioning speech-language pathology assistants (SLPAs). Although the roles and responsibilities of SLPAs have been described by ASHA (1996, 2000), many health care providers have not yet incorporated the services of these individuals, possibly due to the ambivalence with which the field of speech-language pathology, at least in the United States, has received the concept of SLPAs. Whereas it is not our intention to advocate one way or another on this issue, it is important to point out that the utilization of SLPAs has the potential to reduce treatment costs. It is clear that a paraprofessional working at a rate of $15 per hour can provide more treatment hours for $100 compared to the professional working at a rate of $35 per hour. However, the cost savings is maintained only if quality treatment is administered and the patient demonstrates functional gains as a result. When SLPAs provide treatment, it is the responsibility of the speech-language pathologist to ensure quality care by carefully assessing the patient, developing an appropriate treatment plan, and providing appropriate supervision (ASHA, 1996, 2000). Ideally, the use of SLPAs will improve the efficiency of services, and help maintain the livelihood of the profession in the current health care environment.

One caution regarding the use of SLPAs in medical settings is noteworthy. ASHA, as well as some states, has legislated that SLPAs may not provide services in the area of dysphagia (ASHA, 2000; North Carolina Board of Examiners, 1999). Stated another way, *only* speech-language pathologists can provide dysphagia services, whereas screening and treatment of other disorder areas (including neurogenic language disorders) *can* be carried out by SLPAs. A likely, although probably unintended, result of this mandate is that the most highly skilled professional services will be provided to individuals with dysphagia, whereas support personnel will carry out services to individuals with other impairments. This scenario certainly has the potential to even further devalue the services speech-language pathologists provide in the areas of neurogenic speech and language disorders, while continuing to emphasize dyphagia services. Research is currently underway examining the feasibility of SLPAs providing limited services to individuals with dysphagia, the results of which may alter future policies. Until then, however, speech-language pathologists need to be cognizant of the implications for the restricted use of SLPAs.

MANAGEMENT STRATEGIES ACROSS THE CONTINUUM OF CARE

The final section of this chapter describes how the nature of services to individuals with neurogenic language disorders varies across the continuum of care. It will become clear that factors such as the medical status of the patient, length of stay, reimbursement formulae, and availability of support (health care providers and family) all impact how care is delivered in different settings. The care settings described in this section are those included in traditional health care models, but readers are reminded that services also may be provided in nontraditional settings (e.g., life participation approaches, see Chapter 11).

INTENSIVE CARE

In the **intensive care unit** (ICU), the patient is generally medically unstable, and consequently, the primary health-care goal is life preservation. Depending on the nature of patients' medical conditions, they may undergo a variety of diagnostic tests or experience a multitude of treatments. For example, a stroke patient will likely undergo several imaging studies during the first few hours to days following admission to determine the nature and extent of the stroke. A patient with head trauma may require orthopedic or neurosurgery, and may have additional complications such as the presence of a tracheostomy and mechanical ventilation. Length of stay in the ICU depends on the nature and severity of the illness or trauma, but a stay of one to two days would not be uncommon following an ischemic stroke, and head trauma may warrant ICU stays of five to seven days.

Referrals to speech-language pathology for patients in the ICU are not uncommon, and the clinician's role in this setting is rather unique. Perhaps in this setting more than any other, communication with the referring physician is critical, so that the speech-language pathologist clearly understands what is being requested. Some physicians will request that clinicians address swallowing in the ICU but defer communication services until the patient is transferred to the medical floor, whereas other physicians will request communication assessment immediately. Frequently physicians are seeking additional information that will help them with differential diagnosis, and other times the request is to begin rehabilitation. The speech-language pathologist should be certain what is requested before proceeding.

If the request is to provide information to assist in differential diagnosis, then careful assessment of all modalities at the impairment level is warranted. Keep in mind that the clinician, as the communication expert, may have the best understanding about the potential relationships between observed behaviors and neurogenic pathology. Whereas it is inappropriate to make a medical diagnosis, it is quite appropriate to suggest possible pathologies, such as "The patient exhibits anosognosia concurrent with a gross left neglect. She demonstrates a flat affect and responds inappropriately to indirect requests. . . These characteristics are consistent with damage to the nondominant hemisphere."

An important aspect of care during this critical time is ongoing assessment. When a patient's medical status is poor and rapidly changing, the most telling signs of improvement or decline may be changes in communication, swallowing, or cognitive function. The astute clinician must constantly assess the patient for evolution of symptoms that might indicate a change in medical status, the need for additional medical intervention, or both. The clinician should feel comfortable alerting the physician or attending nurse to changes in status, and must be able to describe specifically the nature of these changes and the cause for concern. It has been our experience that as other health care providers see the relevance of the observations speech-language pathologists make, a greater respect for our services develops.

For some patients it will be appropriate to begin rehabilitation in the ICU, especially if the patient appears aware of his or her surroundings but is unable to communicate. In this case, establishing a communication system as soon as possible will have an immeasurable impact on the patient's well-being, the anxiety of the family, and will even impact the care the patient receives, as the physicians and other care providers have a means of communicating with the patient. Often the first communication system developed will be nonverbal, perhaps using eye-gaze or pointing. Equally important is educating family and health care providers on the reliability of patients' yes/no responses and comprehension accuracy. The reader is encouraged to review Chapter 11 and explore additional sources on augmentative and alternative communication systems (e.g., Beukelman, Yorkston & Reichle, 2000) for more information on this aspect of care.

Side Bar

The Risks of *Mis*communication

Patients with aphasia are often excellent at hiding or minimizing the severity of their communication impairments. Consequently, families as well as health care professionals who are naïve about aphasic symptoms may easily misperceive the extent of patients' communication difficulties. For example, a spouse of one of the patients in our aphasia support group recently related an incident that occurred while her husband was in the hospital immediately following his stroke. One day she entered his hospital room while a nurse was collecting medical information from her husband. The nurse appeared to know that he had aphasia, as she was relying on primarily yes/no questions to complete his case history (i.e., avoiding the need for him to provide extensive verbal responses); however, the nurse was not aware that he had an unreliable yes/no response and significant auditory comprehension problems that compromised his understanding even at the single word level. If his wife had not entered his hospital room when she did, this patient could have received inappropriate medical treatment as the nurse was asking about whether or not he had any allergies—he responded no, when indeed he did have allergies, including some with respect to certain medications. Accordingly, educating all potential communication partners about patients' cognitive and communicative strengths and weaknesses is an essential component of treatment for any neurogenic language disorder.

ACUTE CARE

Acute care refers to the services provided on a typical hospital ward. Most patients in acute care are no longer considered to be in a life-threatening condition, although they may still be quite ill or injured. A typical stay in acute care following stroke is three to seven days, and the medical goals at this time are differential diagnosis and stabilization of the patient's medical status so that he or she can be discharged.

Speech-language pathology referrals at this time are typically for the purpose of differential diagnosis of the cognitive and/or communicative impairments and to provide recommendation for discharge plans. It is not likely that the patient will remain in acute care long enough for the development and/or execution of a formal treatment plan; thus, the role of speech-language pathologists in this setting can be considered "consultative" (Johnson, Valachovic, & George, 1998). Likewise, in the case of patients with TBI who might still be demonstrating post-traumatic amnesia (see Chapter 2), formal assessment is inappropriate at this stage of recovery because of patients' significant confusion and low frustration tolerance. Relatedly, during this time, even though patients may be medically stable or, in the case of

TBI, out of the post-traumatic amnesia phase, patients with neurogenic language disorders may have decreased alertness and reduced stamina, which means that sessions with patients are often only 10 to 20 minutes in length. This is not an extensive period of time in which to conduct an assessment, so clinicians must learn to be creative in their assessment strategies. One way to work effectively within these time restrictions is to schedule short but frequent visits throughout the day. This has an advantage of increasing contact time and also allows the clinician to observe variations in performance related to time of day, fatigue, medication schedule, the presence of family members, and other factors.

Another way to maximize time with acute care patients is to modify assessment tools to meet the time restrictions inherent to this setting. Recall from Chapters 5 and 6 that most assessment batteries and other standardized tools for assessing communication and cognition may take up to 60 minutes to administer to patients who can maintain alertness and attentional focus. Therefore, in the acute care setting it is usually better to select instruments that are less time-consuming, such as those listed in Figure 12-3 (see also Tables 5-1 and 6-1). Another strategy experienced clinicians may adopt is to develop informal protocols that provide the desired information in a reduced amount of time. Informal protocols must be systematic and comprehensive enough to be reasonably valid and reliable, and yet assess communication as efficiently as possible. Figure 12-4 is an example of an informal protocol that addresses the communication behaviors of interest in an aphasia assessment (e.g., comprehension, naming, speech fluency, repetition, reading/writing). Similar informal protocols may be developed to address the cognitive and communicative behaviors more likely to be affected by right hemisphere brain damage, TBI, or dementia. The effectiveness of informal protocols depends largely on the observation skill of the clinician. An astute clinician can make a number of judgments about a patient's communication and cognitive abilities during the period of time when the clinician enters the room, turns on the lights, and positions the patient. The development of these informal assessment skills is key to effective practice in acute care.

In addition to differential diagnosis, another important goal of assessment in acute care is to develop discharge recommendations. Under managed care, it is the goal to restore the greatest amount of function for the least cost, or in the least

---

Bedside Evaluation Screening Test of Aphasia–2 (West, Sands, & Ross-Swain, 1998)

Brief Test of Head Injury (Helm-Estabrooks & Hotz, 1991)

Burns Brief Inventory of Communication and Cognition (Burns, 1997)

Mini Inventory of Right Brain Injury–2 (Pimental & Knight, 2000)

Figure 12-3. Examples of brief assessment tools for neurogenic language disorders.

Aphasia Evaluation Protocol

Client: _____ Date: _____ Examiner: _____

Fluency

Conversational Speech/Events:
- ☐ telegraphic
- ☐ effortful
- ☐ paraphasia
- ☐ perseveration
- ☐ circumlocution

Naming (name & function)

Common/Uncommon Objects:

☐ Watch		☐
☐ Shirt		☐
☐ Table		☐
☐ Chair		☐
☐ _____		☐

(function)

Repetition

Repeating Words:
- ☐ cap
- ☐ boat
- ☐ laughing
- ☐ piano
- ☐ forty-two

Notes/Observations:

Comprehension

Yes/No Questions:
- ☐ Are you sitting in a chair?
- ☐ Are we in Paris, France?
- ☐ Is it nighttime?
- ☐ Are you wearing a swimsuit?
- ☐ Do cars fly?
- ☐ Is your hair purple?

Common/Uncommon Pics:

☐ key		☐
☐ fork		☐
☐ pencil		☐
☐ phone		☐
☐ cup		☐

(function)

Repeating Phrases:
- ☐ time to go
- ☐ Personal computer

Sentences:
- ☐ Put it in the microwave.
- ☐ She is not very happy.

Wh- Questions:
- ☐ Why do you store ice in the freezer
- ☐ What would you do if you lost a friend's phone number?
- ☐ What do you use to hit a nail?

Body Parts:
- ☐ nose
- ☐ eye
- ☐ chin
- ☐ foot
- ☐ elbow

Reading (read word, find pic)
- ☐ Bed
- ☐ Clock
- ☐ Window
- ☐ Pillow
- ☐ Door

Following Directions:
- ☐ Touch your nose
- ☐ Look at the door
- ☐ Touch your head, then your mouth
- ☐ Touch your chair, then clap twice
- ☐ Look at the door, look at me, then close your eyes

Writing
- ☐ Name (wrote, dictated, copied)
- ☐ Address
- ☐ Shapes (if can't do name)

Sentences:
- ☐ Touch your nose.
- ☐ Point to the door.

☐ Melissa Lindsey, 2004

Figure 12-4. Informal assessment protocol. This protocol targets communication behaviors most often disrupted in aphasia.

expensive setting along the continuum of care. The speech-language assessment should lead to recommendations regarding the need for cognitive and/or communication treatment, the environment in which the treatment would be best provided, and the prognosis for functional improvement. The prognostic factors discussed in Chapters 4, 5, and 6 should be among those considered by the clinician when making discharge recommendations.

As was discussed for ICU, rehabilitation in acute care should begin as soon as it is appropriate, especially if the patient requires an augmentative communication system. Clinicians should further provide family members and care staff with instruction in the use of any developed systems. The importance of patient and family education at this point cannot be understated (Holland & Fridriksson, 2001). Often in ICU, family members are so concerned about whether the patient will survive that the impact of any cognitive or communicative impairments is not considered. Thus, it is often in acute care when the patient and family begin to realize that communication or cognition have not returned to normal and may not do so for some time, if ever. The clinician should provide as much information as possible about the nature of the patient's impairments, highlighting strengths and needs, and provide a reasonable prognosis, if possible, based on the information available. It is often hard to make a good prognosis in acute care, especially if the patient is very early post onset, and occasionally the clinician will have to say, "It's too early to tell." At such times, clinicians can share with families the factors that will impact the prognosis, and provide information about the services that will be provided during the patient's stay.

Finally, the importance of ongoing assessment during the acute care phase is similar to that discussed for ICU. Patients with neurogenic disorders often move back and forth between ICU and the medical floor as their conditions destabilize, and it is the speech-language pathologist's responsibility to continue to assess communication and certain cognitive abilities, and to provide recommendations as indicated throughout this process.

INPATIENT REHABILITATION UNIT

Many patients who experience neurologic insult will benefit from intensive rehabilitation services, typically provided in an inpatient rehabilitation unit. Patients are transferred to a rehabilitation or "rehab" unit when they are considered medically stable and can participate in two to four hours of treatment per day. Inpatient rehabilitation stays for patients with acute neurologic disease are often 10 to 28 days in length (Indredavik, Fjaertoft, Ekeberg, Loge, & Morch, 2000; Roth & Lovell, 2003), during which the goal is to regain function.

Speech-language pathology services in rehab often begin with assessment. If appropriate, information may be provided from the acute care facility, in which case it may be possible to begin treatment immediately, with ongoing assessment incorporated into the treatment sessions. Treatment in rehab settings is intense, often twice daily for up to 60 minutes each session, and this is for each discipline involved (e.g., occupational therapy (OT), physical therapy (PT), and speech-language pathology).

Rehabilitation for individuals with neurologic insult is a team effort. Treatment goals are often jointly developed, and progress toward these goals is discussed regularly during multidisciplinary rounds. In some cases it may be advantageous to implement joint treatment sessions with other disciplines, for example when goals are vocationally focused (e.g., "The patient will use his augmentative communication device to access the computer network at his place of employment.").

Treatment in rehab settings is often both **restorative** (i.e., targeting the impairment) and **adaptive** (i.e., targeting activity and participation), although the goals in both cases are to improve overall functioning. Treatment may be individual, group, or both. Patients will typically make large gains while in rehab, as the benefits of spontaneous recovery and intensive treatment are exploited.

Patients are discharged from the rehabilitation unit when it is judged that their rehabilitation needs have been met, or when additional treatments can be provided more efficiently in a less expensive setting. As was true in acute care, the speech-language pathologist will provide input regarding the most appropriate disposition from rehab, including recommendations for additional treatment.

SKILLED NURSING FACILITIES

Patients who are medically stable enough to be discharged from acute care but still not well enough to participate in the intensive treatment regimen characteristic of inpatient rehabilitation units may be admitted to a **skilled nursing facility** (SNF). Patients in an SNF require skilled nursing care and may receive rehabilitation services, although typically not as intensely as what is provided in rehab. Stays in SNFs may be 10 to 28 days, during which time the goals are to continue to improve the patient's medical status as well as functional abilities.

For patients who are recovering from acute neurological illness, communication and cognitive services in SNFs are very similar to those provided in rehab units, although likely with less intensity. Because Medicare reimburses SNF facilities based on the amount of rehabilitation services the patient receives, however, clinicians may be encouraged by administrators to provide as much treatment as the patient can tolerate and benefit from.

Some patients are admitted to SNFs because of decline in function due to degenerative disease (e.g., Alzheimer's disease or Parkinson's disease). For these patients, the focus of services may be maintenance rather than improvement of function. When such is the case, the clinician will need not only to address current function, but plan for future declines in function. For patients with degenerative disease, treatment in SNFs is nearly always adaptive rather than restorative. As was true with acute care and rehab, it will be necessary for clinicians in SNF settings to participate in discharge planning and to provide education to the family and care givers in how to best facilitate communication with the patient.

LONG-TERM CARE FACILITIES

When individuals can no longer live independently or be cared for in the home, they may be admitted to a **long-term care** (LTC) facility. Unlike SNFs, where patients receive skilled nursing care, LTC facilities typically provide limited nursing and rehabilitation services. The goal in LTC is to maintain medical stability and facilitate quality of life. Many patients admitted to LTC facilities will remain there until death, which can be months or even years after admission. Most patients in LTC are not expected to make substantial gains in function, so speech-language pathology services typically focus on maintaining functional cognitive and communicative abilities for as long as possible. Treatments are almost always adaptive in nature.

Because many patients in LTC often suffer from degenerative disease, it will be necessary for the speech-language pathologist to provide ongoing assessment of communication, swallowing, and possibly cognition in order to recommend changes in care as needed. Often this ongoing assessment takes the form of systematic screening of all residents, with special consideration given to those with relevant admitting diagnoses. Periodically, patients in LTCs will experience an acute neurologic insult, such as a stroke or TBI. In that event, the speech-language pathologist will be responsible for assessing and treating the patient, always keeping in mind baseline function when developing a prognosis and treatment plan.

Treatment in LTCs often takes the form of environmental manipulation and staff education, as opposed to direct intervention with individual patients. Many patients in LTC cannot benefit from direct intervention, even adaptive strategies, because of severe cognitive deficits. In such cases, the clinician may still impact their functional abilities by modifying their surroundings and instructing their families and caregivers in how to best facilitate communication and cognitive functioning. Group treatment is another possible treatment option, at least for some patients, particularly given the social benefits associated with group participation (see Chapter 11).

HOME HEALTH

Some patients will benefit from nursing and rehabilitation services provided in the home (i.e., **home health** services). Typically, home health rehabilitation services are offered to individuals who have been discharged from acute care, rehab, or skilled nursing. Patients who might benefit from additional treatment but are unable to leave their homes to receive the services may be eligible for home health. Additionally, individuals with degenerative disease who continue to live at home may also benefit from home health services. The goal of home health care is to maintain or improve medical status while maintaining or improving functional abilities. For most individuals, home health rehabilitation services may last 14 to 30 days, although some people retain skilled home nursing care for longer durations.

Services in home health settings will range from daily intensive restorative treatment (e.g., for individuals recovering from acute illness) to weekly or monthly adaptive treatment focusing on environmental modification and caregiver training (e.g., for individuals at the end stages of degenerative disease). Home health services offer the advantage of being provided in the environment that is typically most conducive to the patient's function, and will often involve the caregiver more directly than is generally possible in other settings. However, these same factors can be disadvantages if the home environment and/or the caregiver do not facilitate communication or cognitive functioning. In such cases, the clinician would likely target these factors as well as those directed at modifying the patient's cognitive or communicative behaviors.

Coordination of services with other disciplines is particularly important in the home health setting. Because many different therapists and caregivers may be going in and out of the home throughout the week, it is often difficult for the patient or the family to keep track of goals, treatment schedules, or both. Treatment in home health will be most successful if the various care providers are aware of all the services the patient is receiving (e.g., to avoid duplicating or omitting assessment and/or treatment of certain symptoms), and if all of these services are coordinated and targeted toward common functional goals.

OUTPATIENT SERVICES

The final setting to be discussed in this chapter is the **outpatient** setting. Patients who live at home and have transportation to a treatment facility may receive outpatient services. Most patients receiving outpatient services are considered medically stable, but primarily need to regain function. Outpatient rehabilitation services may last four to 12 weeks, or potentially longer if the patient continues to show functional gains and has the financial resources to pay for continued services.

Outpatient services may be recommended for individuals discharged from other facilities following acute episodes or for individuals in the early stages of degenerative disease. In both cases, it is likely that a thorough evaluation of communication and cognitive function is warranted before the initiation of treatment. In the first case, information will be gained regarding current status and amount of recovery since the onset. In the second case, a baseline will be established from which it will be possible to compare future rate and amount of decline in function.

Treatment of cognitive and communicative problems in outpatient settings is usually both restorative and adaptive in nature. Outpatient services can be very beneficial because at this point in their recovery, most patients and caregivers are in a position to take strategies utilized in treatment, try them out at home or at work, and then report back during future sessions. Outpatient treatment sessions may involve family members and can be specifically targeted for vocational goals. Outpatient services also have the advantage of being the least expensive of all care settings (particularly when services are provided at a university clinic), so many patients can afford more treatment than could be obtained in other settings.

LOOKING AHEAD

The goal of this chapter was to provide a picture of the "real-world" clinical environments in which clinicians often provide care to patients with neurogenic language disorders. In many ways, the current health care environment is not conducive to what might be considered ideal to the management of neurogenic language disorders. Certainly many speech-language pathologists, patients, and their families may feel that the mandates of managed care impose inappropriate limits on the amount and nature of the speech-language services that will be funded by third-party payers. One might argue that the medical environment, regardless of the reimbursement situation, is not ideal for the management of cognitive or communication disorders.

Nonetheless, there are a number of reasons to be optimistic about the future. As indicated in Chapter 8, the research base documenting the benefits of treatment for neurogenic language disorders continues to expand, providing speech-language pathologists with the information necessary to appropriately select, implement, and obtain reimbursement for management strategies. As highlighted in this chapter, there also are several approaches that clinicians can adopt to increase public awareness of not only neurogenic language disorders, but also the services that our profession can provide to help prevent, assess, and treat those disorders. Better understanding and appreciation of our field should lead to greater demand for speech-language pathology services and, consequently, increased pressure on funding agencies to support speech-language pathology services. Additionally, developing technologies, including functional imaging and genetic mapping, continue to enhance our understanding of the nature and causes of neurogenic language disorders, as well as the physiologic mechanisms supporting recovery. Finally, as described in Chapters 9, 10, and 11, the variety of management strategies continues to expand. We look forward to a future in which seemingly divergent treatments (e.g., pharmacotherapy, behavioral intervention, life-participation approaches, alternative medicine) will be integrated to optimize patient outcomes, even for those battling progressive diseases. As the benefits of such integrated management become evident, concurrent reimbursement strategies should follow.

Glossary

acetylcholine A neurotransmitter that is found throughout the brain, spinal cord, and autonomic nervous system.

activities and participation ICF construct that describes an individual's ability to engage in personal, social, vocational, and recreational activities.

activity ICF construct relating to a patient's ability to complete specific tasks such as speaking or writing.

acupuncture A technique involving stimulating the skin, and consequently the nerves, at designated anatomic locations referred to as acupoints.

acute care Stage in the continuum of care in which most patients' conditions are not currently life-threatening but are in need of daily physician and continual nursing care.

adaptive Treatment strategies that compensate for impairments but do not induce permanent improvements in underlying structure or function.

ageism The systematic stereotyping and discrimination of people on the basis of their age.

agonists Drugs designed to increase the amount or efficiency of neurotransmitters.

agoraphobia An unexplained fear of open spaces.

agrammatism The production of short utterances that consist primarily of content words such as nouns and verbs, contain relatively few function words, such as articles and conjunctions, have either simplified or incomplete grammatical structure, and represent a restricted range of sentence types or forms.

agraphia Impaired written expression. Also called acquired dysgraphia.

alexia Disruption in written language comprehension. Also known as acquired dyslexia.

allesthesia The misattribution of sensory information from one side of the body (i.e., the unattended or neglected side of the body) to stimulation of the other side of the body.

Alzheimer's disease (AD) The most common cause of irreversible dementia and dementia in general. Its etiology remains unknown, although genetic and other physiological causes are still being investigated. Confirmation of an AD diagnosis can only be made upon autopsy.

amphetamine A drug that increases levels of dopamine and norepinephrine within the brain.

aneurysm A weak or thin spot on a blood vessel that causes the vessel to dilate or balloon.

angular gyrus Area of the brain within the parietal lobe that, with the supramarginal gyrus, contributes to written language comprehension.

angular gyrus syndrome A collection of symptoms (i.e., disorientation, anomia, and acalculia) caused by multiple lesions to posterior and inferior parietal regions of the left hemisphere.

anomia Difficulty recalling the names of people, objects, locations, concepts, and actions.

anomic aphasia Aphasia characterized by a relatively isolated impairment of naming, with fluent language output and relatively good comprehension of spoken and written language.

anosognosia An impaired awareness or denial of one's own deficits.

antagonists Drugs that reduce the amount or efficiency of neurotransmitters.

anterograde amnesia A memory problem that relates to difficulties storing and retrieving long-term memories or, more generally, new information, subsequent to the onset of brain damage or disease.

anterograde memories Long-term memories that are stored after brain damage has occurred, or after the onset of the neurological disease process.

anticoagulants Medications such as heparin or warfarin that prevent thrombus formation and release of emboli.

antiplatelet medications Drugs such as aspirin or clopidogrel that help reduce the buildup of plaque on existing thrombotic areas.

apathy The lack of feeling or emotion; indifference.

aphasia A disruption in using and understanding language following neurological injury or disease that is not related to general intellectual decline or sensorimotor deficits.

apraxia of speech A difficulty with volitionally positioning muscles as well as planning and sequencing muscle movements for the production of phonemes and phoneme sequences.

arcuate fasciculus Fibrous tract that connects Wernicke's and Broca's areas.

arteriogram The radiological procedure used to visualize the arteries.

arteriovenous malformation (AVM) A congenital defect in the communication links between arteries and veins that results in weakened arterial walls, and may lead to hemorrhagic stroke.

association areas Cortical areas surrounding Broca's and Wernicke's areas and involved in language processing.

ataxia Disturbance in movement accuracy, force, and timing due to lesions of the cerebellum.

attention switching The process of moving attentional focus from one task, stimulus, or stimulus property to another.

auditory agnosia Difficulty recognizing and applying meaning to auditory information despite normal hearing sensitivity and accurate recognition of the same stimuli in other sensory modalities.

augmentative communication A communication system whereby written words or pictured symbols are selected to facilitate language expression or comprehension.

authentic assessment An assessment based on ethnographic and conversational analysis research methods.

authentic context The typically occurring context of linguistic or cognitive processes.

barrier games Activities used for addressing a variety of pragmatic and discourse goals in which a solid barrier is placed between the patient and the clinician to create a communicative need and that, in the absence of nonverbal cues, require utilization of specific and efficient language output.

basal ganglia Subcortical structure with contributions to linguistic and cognitive processing and motor skills. They include structures such as the caudate nucleus, putamen, globus pallidus, subthalamic nucleus, and substantia nigra.

basement or floor effect Test performance profile in which patients predominantly receive scores of zero.

benign Term for tumors that are noncancerous and do not spread or metastasize to other parts of the body.

biofeedback A relaxation technique used to teach patients conscious self-regulation of physiological functions that are related to stress levels by connecting patients to simple, electronic devices that monitor the target physiological functions.

body function A construct of the ICF that describes the functional integrity of tissues and organs.

body structure A construct of the ICF that describes the integrity of tissues and organs.

bradykinesia Slowed movement associated with Huntington's disease, Parkinson's disease, and other neurological diseases.

brain attacks New term for a stroke, introduced to encourage patients experiencing symptoms of stroke to get immediate medical help.

Broca's aphasia Aphasia characterized by nonfluent language output and relatively spared language comprehension compared to output fluency difficulties.

Broca's area Area of the brain in the inferior lateral frontal lobe and generally proposed to play a primary role in language expression.

bromocriptine A drug that increases levels of dopamine within the brain.

canonical A sentence using the active voice.

capitated payment Health care financing system in which providers agree to serve a given population for a preset fee.

caps or limits Designates a maximum amount of third-party funding available for medical or rehabilitative services.

carotid arterial system Arterial system that begins as the left and right common carotid arteries and supplies most of the cerebral hemispheres.

catastrophic reaction Difficulty maintaining biologic homeostasis and a form of massive denial. Symptoms include sudden and violent switching into a state of intense negativity.

catecholamine system Consists of a certain group of neurotransmitters and the neurons that release those neurotransmitters. These neurotransmitters are related because they are all made from a common chemical pathway. Dopamine, norepinephrine, and epinephrine are the most common catecholamine neurotransmitters.

ceiling Refers to 100% accuracy on test performance.

choline acetyltransferase A chemical responsible for making acetylcholine, an excitatory neurotransmitter known to be important for learning and memory.

cholinergic system Consists of the neurotransmitter acetylcholine and the neurons that release acetycholine.

chorea A motoric disturbance associated with Huntington's disease and other neurological disorders that is characterized by rapid, involuntary, purposeless movements of the extremities, head, neck, or trunk. These movements are irregular and asymmetrical.

Circle of Willis A ring of arteries located at the base of brain, which connects the carotid and vertebrobasilar artery systems. Provides the brain with collateral circulation that can help compensate for a blockage in one of the major cerebral arteries.

circumlocutions The use of descriptions, definitions, or sound effects for target words.

clinical trial Research examining the benefit of intervention generally involving large sample sizes, randomized subject assignment, and other experimental controls.

closed head injury A traumatic brain injury in which the skull is not pierced by the external force and thus stays intact.

cognition The process by which sensory information is transformed, condensed, elaborated, stored, retrieved, and exploited, thus allowing understanding and interaction with the environment.

cognitive flexibility A type of executive function that allows for changing or adapting behavior in the event of failure.

cognitive neuropsychological treatments Aphasia treatments in which models of normal and/or disordered language are used to motivate selection of treatment targets and procedures.

cohesion Refers to the linguistic means by which words and sentences are meaningfully linked to each other within a text or spoken discourse sample.

coma A condition characterized by the lack of or minimally organized or purposeful response to external stimuli within one's environment.

communication A fundamental human behavior involving the exchange of ideas.

complementary and alternative medicine (CAM) A diverse collection of health care systems, therapies, and products developed outside of conventional medical institutions that are used to prevent and treat a spectrum of medical and psychological problems using a holistic approach.

computerized tomography An imaging technique that allows scientists to identify brain lesions in live patients. Also known as CT scans.

conduction aphasia Aphasia characterized by disproportionately severe deficits during repetition, but with relatively good comprehension, fluent spontaneous speech, and mild to moderate naming deficits.

construct validity Psychometric property that indicates how well a test relates to other measures of the same construct.

content validity Psychometric property that indicates how well a test measures all of the behaviors that it purports to measure.

continuum of care Description of the settings available for the provision of medical and rehabilitation services, varying in cost and intensity of care.

contra coup effect or injury The term used when cerebral contusions occur both at the site of impact (i.e., "coup") and at the opposite side of the brain (i.e., "contra").

contusions Bruises that form around the site of impact of a traumatic brain injury due to laceration of blood vessels.

cortical dementia The dementia associated with Alzheimer's disease, Pick's disease, and other neurological disorders that cause brain damage at primarily cortical levels.

cortical stimulation A method of inferring brain function accomplished by applying electrical stimulation to the brain in order to disrupt typical functioning.

criterion-related validity Also called predictive validity, this psychometric property refers to how well a test predicts whether a patient has a deficit.

critical appraisal Thoughtful analysis of the relevance, validity, and accuracy of the research evidence.

crossed aphasia A rare aphasia with varied impairments resulting from lesions to the nondominant, and thus typically right hemisphere.

cueing hierarchy A technique used to stimulate word retrieval skills in which cues that facilitate word retrieval are arranged in a hierarchy according to the level of external support they provide.

declarative memory A form of long-term memory that holds information that can be stored and accessed explicitly or consciously.

dementia A chronic, progressive deterioration of memory and at least one other area such as personality, communication ability, or executive control functioning.

dementia of the frontal lobe type (DFT) or fronto-temporal dementia A dementia associated with behavioral symptoms such as socially inappropriate behavior and disinhibition in the absence of neuropathological markers of Pick's or Alzheimer's diseases.

depression Mood disorder characterized by feelings of sadness and worthlessness, sleep disturbances, changes in eating habits, and fatigue.

derivational affix Morpheme that when added to a word, transforms that word into different word forms (e.g., a noun becomes an adjective).

diagnosis-related group (DRG) Designates the reimbursement rate for patients receiving Medicare Part A coverage in acute care settings, based on the diagnosis or diagnoses of individual patients.

diffuse axonal shearing or injury Microscopic damage associated with traumatic brain injury that includes the shearing of axons from their myelin sheath or tearing of the axons themselves, and that frequently affects brain tissue at gray-white matter junctions (e.g., inferior frontal lobe, cerebellar peduncles).

diplopia Double vision, typically associated with brain stem damage.

disability A concept introduced by the International Classification of Impairment, Disability, and Handicap (ICIDH, 1980) that is roughly synonymous with the newer ICF term of activity limitation.

divided attention A complex attentional skill of attending to and completing concurrently more than one task, or simultaneously attending to and processing multiple stimuli.

donepezil A drug that prevents the breakdown of acetylcholine, and thus increases levels of this neurotransmitter.

dopamine A neurotransmitter that is found in particularly high concentrations within frontal regions of the cortex and numerous subcortical areas. It is part of the catecholamine system.

dose The intensity and duration of an intervention.

dysarthria A motor speech disorder caused by impairments of speech musculature tone (i.e., reduced or excessive tone) and/or control (i.e., incoordination, imprecise movements).

dysphagia Swallowing problems found in patients with neurological diseases such as stroke, Huntington's disease, Parkinson's disease, traumatic brain injury (TBI), and amyotrophic lateral sclerosis (ALS). Without treatment, dysphagia may lead to malnutrition, pneumonia, and other medical complications.

ecological validity Psychometric property that refers to how well patients' test performances predict their behavior in daily, real-world settings.

edema Swelling that is the product of increased intra- or extracellular fluid in the brain or other bodily tissues.

effectiveness Evidence that an intervention is beneficial when applied under typical clinical conditions.

efficacy Evidence that an intervention is beneficial when applied under ideal conditions.

efficiency Characteristic of an intervention that encompasses the size of benefit as well as the effort expended.

electroencephalography (EEG) A method by which gross electrical activity in the brain is measured.

embolus A clot that forms or a piece of fatty plaque that breaks off from elsewhere in the circulatory system, and then travels to block off a smaller artery that supplies blood to the brain.

empty speech Term used to describe fluent speech lacking in information content.

encoding The process of maintaining information in working memory and then transferring that information into long-term memory stores.

endarterectomy A surgical procedure that removes plaque buildup within the carotid artery system.

environmental factors A construct of the ICF that describes contributions such as assistive mobility devices, physical geography, lighting, support systems, attitudes, and policies as they relate to the individual's ability to participate fully in desired activities.

episodic memory A subdivision of declarative memory that contains context-dependent or autobiographical memories.

errorless learning An approach based upon implicit learning mechanisms in which patients are prevented from making errors via the use of cues that are gradually withdrawn.

evidence-based practice The systematic review and appraisal of research evidence as a component of clinical decision making.

executive functioning The set of high-level, inter-related cognitive abilities responsible for generating, selecting, planning, and monitoring goal-directed and adaptive responses that in turn sustain completion of independent, purposeful, and/or novel behavior.

expressive aphasia Used to describe the language characteristics of significantly impaired language output capabilities.

fee-for-service Health care financing strategy in which providers are reimbursed for individual instances of service provision.

fluency Refers to phrase length in the speech production of patients with aphasia as well as characteristics of melodic line, articulatory agility, speech rate, and grammatical form.

fluent aphasia Aphasia characterized by ease of speech production with adequate melodic line, rhythm, rate, flow, and phrase length.

focused attention The ability to concentrate on and prioritize certain features of the external or internal environment in the presence of competing features or stimuli. Also called selective attention.

functional magnetic resonance imaging (fMRI) Provides images of changes in blood oxygenation within the brain that are used to identify brain areas that are active during specific cognitive and linguistic tasks.

functional measures Measures of performance obtained during activities typical of daily life, including activities related to personal, social, professional, or recreational pursuits.

genres Refers to types of discourse, such as traditional narrative, procedural, expository, service encounters, expert interviews, and gossiping.

glioblastomas Malignant (i.e., cancerous) brain tumors that are treated with chemotherapy, radiation, and/or surgery.

global aphasia Aphasia type marked by significant impairments in all language modalities and functions.

guided imagery (GI) A relaxation technique requiring patients to select a pleasant and calm location or event, and then imagine being at that location or event.

handicap A concept introduced by the International Classification of Impairment, Disability, and Handicap (ICIDH, 1980) that is roughly synonymous with the newer ICF term of participation restriction.

hematoma The buildup of blood that escapes from an artery and then surrounds brain tissue.

hemiakinesia Characterized by underuse or, in some cases, complete lack of use of one side of the body, even in the absence of hemiparesis. Also referred to as hemihypokinesia or motor extinction, impersistence, or neglect.

hemianesthesia Somatosensory problems (e.g., reduced sense of temperature and pain) on only one side of the body.

hemiballismus Sudden, centrifugally spreading, throwing movements of extremities on one side. It is caused by lesions to the contralateral subthalamic nucleus.

hemi-inattention A common symptom of neglect syndrome that includes problems such as poor response to or report of stimuli presented contralateral to the side of brain damage. It results in poor performance of tasks or activities in the contralateral hemispace that cannot be attributed to motor or sensory impairments.

hemiparesis A muscular weakness on one side of the body.

hemiplegia Paralysis of one side of the body.

hemorrhagic stroke A stroke due to a cerebral artery bursting and causing blood to escape and flood surrounding brain tissue.

home health A stage in the continuum of care in which medical and rehabilitative services are provided in the patient's home.

homonymous hemianopia A visual field cut in which the patient cannot see one half (left or right) of the visual field in each eye.

human immunodeficiency virus (HIV) The virus that causes acquired immune deficiency syndrome (AIDS) and that may invade the brain and cause widespread damage (particularly to white matter and subcortical brain structures) and, consequently, dementia (sometimes referred to as HIV encephalopathy).

Huntington's disease (HD) A progressive neurological disease that causes gradual deterioration of the caudate nuclei, and eventually cortical cell loss as well. Frequent symptoms include chorea, dysarthria, gait and posture problems, dysphagia, bradykinesia, and social disinhibition.

hypoxia Decreased oxygen in brain tissue.

impairment A construct of the ICF that describes the impact of disease or injury on the body and its functions.

indefinite substitutions The use of nonspecific words or descriptions for target words.

infarct The area of dead brain tissue that results from ischemia or cerebral blood flow disruption.

inflectional affix Morpheme that provides syntactic information (e.g., verb tense) when added to a word.

Informativeness The accuracy and appropriateness of the lexical-semantic content in spoken or written language samples.

inhibition An executive function requiring the ability to regulate and repress automatic, routine, or extraneous processing or behaviors.

intensive care unit (ICU) The specialized center in a hospital where medically unstable patients receive care and whose primary health care goal is life preservation.

interaction The establishment and maintenance of relationships as a function of communicative exchanges.

internal capsule Subcortical structure consisting of axons from cortical neurons.

International Classification of Function (ICF) A model created by the World Health Organization (WHO) for describing the impact of disease or injury on the body and its functions, as well as patients' ability to complete tasks or activities relevant to their personal, social, education, and/or vocational pursuits.

intracerebral hemorrhage A hemorrhage in which blood invades tissue within the brain.

irreversible dementia Dementia in which cognitive symptoms are persistent. Most causes of irreversible dementia are progressive neurologic diseases. Sometimes referred to as "primary degenerative dementia."

ischemic brain damage Cell death or infarction due to inadequate blood supply to the brain.

ischemic stroke A stroke caused by a deficiency in blood flow to the brain due to blockage of a cerebral artery.

jargon Production of entire sentences in which all content words, and in some cases functor words as well, are replaced with neologisms.

Korsakoff's disease A disease caused by chronic alcohol abuse that results in damage to diencephalic structures (e.g., hypothalamus, mammillary bodies) and widespread cortical atrophy. It is associated with irreversible and progressive dementia.

lability A difficulty controlling one's emotion that often occurs following brain damage. May result in unprovoked laughing or crying.

lacunar stroke Blockage of small penetrating arteries that supply blood to structures deep within the brain. Associated with lesions that are two to 15 mm^2.

language The primary communication tool that utilizes socially shared, rule-based symbols to represent concepts.

language competence Implies possession of underlying language skills, processes, or representations.

language performance The ability to exhibit access to or execution of intact language rules and contents.

lesion method A technique for studying localization of brain function, by which changes in behavior following brain injury and/or disease are noted and the control of those behaviors is deductively attributed to the injured neural area.

limb apraxia A motoric problem characterized by difficulty executing acquired and volitional movements of the fingers, wrists, elbows, and/or shoulders. It is most frequently observed in patients with left hemisphere brain damage.

long term care A state in the continuum of care in which basic custodial care is provided in a residential setting.

macular degeneration A progressive breakdown or damage to the macula, a portion of the retina. Symptoms include blurring of vision, dim colors, and difficulty reading.

magnetic resonance imaging (MRI) A non-invasive imaging technique that allows scientists to identify brain lesions in live patients.

magnetoencephalography (MEG) The measurement of the magnetic fields generated by electrical activity of the brain.

malignant Term for brain tumors that are cancerous and often recur despite treatment efforts. They may invade other parts of the body, or themselves be the product of a cancer elsewhere in the body that has infiltrated the brain.

managed care A general term used to describe the current American health care system; implies external management of health care practices and financing.

mania A psychiatric disorder characterized by mental and physical hyperactivity, disorganization of behavior, and elevation of mood.

mapping therapy A theoretically motivated approach to treating deficits of grammatical production and/or comprehension in which patients with aphasia are taught to improve their ability to map the relationship between words' thematic roles and their location within a sentence.

Melodic Intonation Therapy (MIT) Stimulation treatment developed to improve word retrieval and speech prosody of patients with severe nonfluent aphasia.

memory Cognitive function responsible for storing, retaining, and retrieving processed information.

meningioma A brain tumor that arises from the arachnoid tissue that sheaths the brain.

meningitis An infection that causes inflammation of the pia and arachnoid tissues that cover the brain.

methylphenidate A drug more commonly known as Ritalin. It increases levels of dopamine and norepinephrine within the brain.

micrographia A mechanical disruption of writing that results in extreme reductions in letter size. It is a frequent symptom of Parkinson's disease.

minimum data set Framework for guiding the assessment process for the purpose of assigning an appropriate resource utilization group.

mnemonic strategies Techniques to enhance memory encoding (or storing) and retrieval skills.

multi-infarct dementia (MID) An irreversible dementia caused by multiple strokes at both cortical and subcortical levels.

multimodal communication Strategies that can be taught to patients with neurogenic language disorders to augment direct retraining of their cognitive abilities or to help them compensate for attention, memory, or executive functioning impairments.

Multiple Oral Rereading (MOR) Treatment designed to increase use of whole-word reading that utilizes repeated oral reading of a pre-selected text to increase reading rate.

neglect dygraphia Writing difficulty related to neglecting the left side of words or the left side of the page.

neglect dyslexia Reading difficulty related to not attending to the left side of words or the left side of the page.

neglect syndrome Refers to a set of attention problems associated with predominantly right hemisphere damage (although it can also occur following left hemisphere damage) in which patients are slow or inaccurate at reporting, reacting to, orienting to, or seeking out stimuli that are presented contralateral to the side of their brain damage.

neologisms Substitution of nonwords.

neurofibrillary tangles Unusual triangular and looped fibers in the cytoplasm of neurons that are a pathological marker of Alzheimer's disease.

neuroprotective agents Drugs such as nimodipine (i.e., a calcium blocker) and citicoline (i.e., an acetylcholine precursor) that are designed to protect brain tissue directly adjacent to the infarct (i.e., penumbra) from the fatal chemi-

cal changes that occur when its blood flow is reduced.

neuropsychologists Professionals who assess cognitive abilities including perception, attention, memory, executive functions, and sometimes language.

neurotransmitters Chemical substances that are released by neurons to facilitate message transmission among neurons. They may also facilitate communication between neurons and muscles or neurons and glands.

no responses A type of error associated with word retrieval problems.

noncanonical A sentence using the passive voice.

nondeclarative memories A form of long-term memory that can be evoked and, in some cases, stored unconsciously.

nonfluent aphasia Aphasia characterized by speech produced haltingly and with great effort.

norepinephrine/noradrenalin A neurotransmitter that is found throughout the cortex, cerebellum, spinal cord, and autonomic nervous system. It is part of the catecholamine system.

nystagmus An involuntary, rapid, and rhythmic movement of the eyeball, which may be horizontal, vertical, rotatory, or mixed.

occupational therapists Professionals who assess fine motor and sensorimotor abilities, skills involved in completing activities of daily living, and sometimes the cognitive abilities of perception, attention, and problem solving.

open head injury A traumatic brain injury in which the skull is fractured or penetrated by an external force and the contents of the skull are exposed.

organization The executive process by which one structures or categorizes incoming information, as well as a response to that information.

orientation A type of cognitive function in which a person demonstrates the ability to orient himself or herself to time, people, and places.

outcomes The end results of program efforts; specifically, changes in patients' communicative and cognitive functioning.

outcomes measurement The process of assessing the end result of an intervention

outpatient A stage in the continuum of care in which patient care is provided at a centralized non-residential setting (e.g., clinic).

pantomime A form of gestural communication that involves a series of relatively transparent movements that are associated with a given activity or situation.

paragrammatism Speech characterized by substitution of inappropriate syntactic elements.

paraphasia Errors in naming.

Parkinson's disease (PD) A progressive, neurological disease associated with deterioration of subcortical structures such as the substantia nigra, and decreased levels of the neurotransmitter dopamine. Common symptoms include dysarthria, bradykinesia, resting tremor, rigidity, gait and posture disturbances, micrographia, and depression.

participation ICF construct addressing the impact of impairments and activity limitations on a patient's ability to participate in desired life activities.

participation measures Assess the degree to which individuals participate in the activities characteristic of their daily lives.

pharmacotherapy A treatment approach in which medications are used to resolve physiological problems such as decreased levels of certain chemicals in the brain that are proposed to underlie behavioral symptoms associated with brain damage or disease.

phonemic paraphasia Sound errors involving substitutions, additions, omissions, and/or rearrangements of target word phonemes. Also known as literal paraphasia.

Pick's disease A relatively rare disease that typically occurs between the ages of 40 to 60 years and more frequently affects women than men. Causes progressive deterioration of primarily frontal regions of the brain and produces an irreversible dementia.

planning A type of executive function that allows for devising strategies and sequencing the steps of those strategies to achieve intended goals.

positron emission tomography (PET) An invasive imaging technology utilizing injected radioactive isotopes to track blood flow in the brain.

post-traumatic amnesia (PTA) Refers to an acute and commonly temporary phase of recovery from traumatic brain injury in which patients who have typically just emerged from coma are extremely confused, distractible, and disoriented.

premorbid abilities Patient's skill level (e.g., motoric, sensory, cognitive abilities) prior to the onset of brain damage or disease.

presbycusis Progressive deterioration of hearing sensitivity, especially in the high frequencies, due to aging.

presbyopia A deficit of vision due to aging. Specific symptoms include increased sensitivity to glare, and difficulty with accommodation and recession of the near point of vision, so that objects very near the eyes cannot be seen distinctly without the use of convex glasses.

primary progressive aphasia (PPA) A degenerative condition generally associated with left hemisphere pathology and characterized by progressive impairment of comprehension, naming, speech fluency, and reading and writing skills, but relative sparing in other areas of cognition.

problem solving Executive function processes that include problem identification, and generation, selection, and implementation of solutions.

procedural memory A form of nondeclarative, long-term memory that holds memory for motor and cognitive skills that are habitual and that require little effort to recall.

process measures Measures designed to assess the degree to which a given policy or procedure is being carried out according to specification.

progressive muscle relaxation (PMR) A type of relaxation therapy which involves sustaining attention to the activity of successively contracting and relaxing certain muscle groups while concurrently inhibiting thoughts or sensory input that may interfere with the attentional focus on the target.

prospective memory A memory function that allows recalling and carrying out future intentions.

prospective payment A health care financing system in which the reimbursement rate is determined according to an estimate of cost of care.

pseudodementia Overt cognitive problems such as impaired memory and reasoning that are found in some depressed elderly patients, and that may be reversed if patients receive proper and prompt medical treatment for their depression.

pure agraphia Isolated impairments of writing in the absence of any other language impairment.

pure alexia Isolated reading difficulties in the absence of any other language impairment. Also called word blindness.

pure aphasia Isolated impairments of specific language functions.

pure word deafness Profound auditory comprehension deficits without evidence of impairment in other language functions or hearing sensitivity.

qualitative information Information regarding *how* a patient performs a given task and thus concerning the identification of influential task parameters and patient strategies.

quality of life measures A description of an individual's overall satisfaction and ability to enjoy life.

random paraphasias Substitutions of words that lack apparent semantic relations to the target words.

reauditorization A treatment technique designed to improve auditory comprehension abilities by having patients first read aloud target items, and then repeat these items aloud when provided with a spoken model and a picture stimulus.

receptive aphasia Aphasia characterized by significant impairments in auditory and written comprehension.

rehabilitation A stage in the continuum of care in which patients receive intense rehabilitation services in a residential setting.

relational or closed class words Refers to the relatively small set of words such as prepositions, pronouns, determiners, and conjunctions that convey primarily morphosyntactic information.

reliability Psychometric property that indicates how similar test results are across repeated administrations of the test under comparable testing conditions.

repetition The ability to repeat words or phrases without processing for meaning.

resource utilization group (RUG) Designates the reimbursement rate for patients receiving Medicare Part A coverage in acute care settings, based on the rehabilitation/skilled care needs of the patient.

Response Elaboration Training (RET) Program designed to improve utterance length and information content, primarily in patients with nonfluent aphasia, that utilizes incidental learning, reinforcement of patient-initiated output, and emphasis on utterance content.

restorative Treatment strategies intended to effect long-lasting improvements in underlying body structure and function.

retrieval The process by which long-term memories are transferred to consciousness.

retrograde amnesia Characterized by continuous or interrupted deficits of long-term memories that were stored prior to the onset of brain injury or disease.

retrograde memories Those memories acquired prior to brain damage or neurological disease onset.

reversible dementia Dementia that can be improved or, in some cases, completely resolved with appropriate medical treatment.

RHD Acronym for right hemisphere damage. Denotes the linguistic and cognitive impairments typical of patients with right hemisphere brain damage.

segmental Sound elements of words or syllables.

selective attention The ability to concentrate on and prioritize certain features of the external or internal environment in the presence of competing features or stimuli. Also called focused attention.

selective serotonin reuptake inhibitors A class of drugs that prevent the reuptake of serotonin, a neurotransmitter found throughout the brain and spinal cord. By preventing reuptake, these drugs function to increase the level or potency of serotonin. They are commonly used to treat depression and have relatively few side effects.

self-monitoring The executive ability to appraise and adjust one's performance and behavior on the basis of environmental feedback, knowledge of task difficulty, and awareness of one's own strengths and weaknesses.

Semantic Feature Analysis (SFA) Program designed to encourage word generation in patients with aphasia or TBI by activating the semantic network (via elicitation of semantic features).

semantic memory A subdivision of declarative memory that holds context-independent, factual memories.

semantic paraphasia Word choice error that is semantically related to the target word.

senile plaques Aggregations of degenerating neurons and the remains of degenerating nerve fibers that are a pathological marker of Alzheimer's disease.

sensory stimulation A complementary and alternative medicine approach that exposes patients to and allows them to interact with, often in a non-directive manner, stimuli that will excite one or more senses, such as light or music therapy.

short-term memory The transient store of information for a short time span of a few minutes.

single photon emission computed tomography (SPECT) An invasive imaging technology utilizing injected radioactive isotopes to track blood flow in the brain.

skilled nursing facility A stage in the continuum of care in which continual nursing care is provided in a residential setting.

skull fracture A break or crack in a bone of the skull that can occur following a traumatic brain injury.

spaced retrieval A memory treatment that involves patients practicing with the aid of cues to recall information or to use a strategy over progressively longer time intervals.

speech acts Theoretical units of communication that encompass the various message meanings (intended and actually perceived) by the message sender and message receiver and what the rules governing the linguistic utterance are.

standardization Property in which a test has been given to a large sample of individuals who represent the cross-section of the population with whom the test will be used in clinical practice.

stimulation treatments Aphasia treatments that emphasize the role of stimulus factors in a patient's current linguistic abilities. Exposure to stimulus and task hierarchies is the means by which compromised language functions and modalities are rehabilitated.

stroke Any disruption in blood flow to the brain. Also called a cerebrovascular accident or brain attack.

subarachnoid hemorrhage A hemorrhage in which blood spills into the pia-arachnoid space surrounding the brain.

subcortical aphasia Aphasia resulting from damage to noncortical sites such as the thalamus or basal ganglia and characterized by various language impairments.

subcortical dementia The dementia associated with Parkinson's disease, Huntington's disease, multiple sclerosis, and other diseases that cause brain damage at primarily subcortical levels.

substantive or open class The set of words including verbs, nouns, adjectives, and adverbs that primarily convey lexical-semantic information.

superior longitudinal fasciculus Fibers that allow intrahemisphere communication by connecting the frontal cortex with the parietal, temporal, and occipital cortices.

supramarginal gyrus Area of the brain within the parietal lobe that, with the angular gyrus, contributes to written language comprehension.

suprasegmental Intonation, stress, and pauses in speech production.

sustained attention The ability to maintain attention and, thus, consistent performance over long periods of time.

team approach Treatment approach designed to establish and maintain collaboration among professionals from a variety of health care disciplines, including speech-language pathology, psychology, audiology, occupational therapy, and physical therapy.

thalamus Subcortical structure that has been proposed to play a crucial role in a number of cognitive functions, including attention and verbal memory.

thrombolytic drugs Medicines such as rtPA (recombinant tissue plasminigen activator) that break up blood clots by speeding up the body's natural clot dissolving process.

thrombosis An arterial blockage due to a buildup of atherosclerotic or fatty plaque on an artery that provides blood flow to the brain.

tics A term referring to involuntary compulsive movements of small muscle groups of the face.

transaction The communicative exchange of information.

transcortical mixed aphasia Aphasia characterized by severe impairments in comprehension, fluency, and naming, but with repetition ability better than what the other language deficits would suggest. Also known as isolation aphasia.

transcortical motor aphasia Nonfluent aphasia similar to Broca's aphasia and characterized by better verbal output for repeated phrases and sentences than for spontaneous verbal output.

transcortical sensory aphasia Fluent aphasia similar to Wernicke's aphasia and characterized by poor comprehension with better repetition abilities than spontaneous speech abilities.

transcranial magnetic stimulation A method of inferring brain function by altering the function of cortical neurons using magnetic fields.

transcutaneous electrical nerve stimulation (TENS) A technique similar to electro-acupuncture that involves stimulating the skin at certain frequencies and skin sites to affect brain functioning.

transient ischemic attack (TIA) A small and temporary disruption of blood flow to the brain that does not cause permanent brain damage.

traumatic brain injury (TBI) An insult to the brain produced by external forces that may cause a variety of temporary or permanent physical, cognitive, emotional, and behavioral impairments.

Treatment of Underlying Forms (TUFF) A theoretically motivated approach to treating deficits of grammatical production and/or comprehension. Its goal is to remediate patients' ability to process phrase movement by increasing their awareness and understanding of verbs, verb argument structure, and how certain sentence constituents move to form noncanonical sentence types.

tumors or neoplasms Tissue masses that arise from an abnormally fast rate of cell reproduction.

validity The truthfulness or soundness of a finding or measure.

vegetative state Term used to describe patients who appear to waken from coma but who demonstrate no willful interaction with their external or internal environments and no communication ability.

vertebrobasilar arterial system Arterial system that arises from the left and right subclavian arteries. Provides blood supply to the occipital lobes as well as medial and inferior portions of temporal lobes and subcortical structures such as the thalamus.

visual agnosia A disturbance in recognizing or associating meaning with visual stimuli even though visual sensitivity is adequate to see the stimuli.

Voluntary Control of Involuntary Utterances (VCIU) Treatment program designed to stimulate propositional (i.e., voluntary) verbal output in patients whose current spoken language abilities are restricted to involuntary production of a small set of real words.

watershed areas Lateral areas of the hemispheres that are located where distributions of major cerebral arteries overlap, and thus have a backup blood supply.

Wernicke's aphasia Fluent aphasia characterized by marked comprehension, naming, and repetition impairments.

Wernicke's area Area of the brain located in the posterior aspects of the superior temporal lobe and linked to language comprehension.

working memory The process by which information is temporarily stored while it is concurrently being processed or manipulated.

References

Aarsland, D., Hutchinson, M., & Larsen, J. P. (2003). Cognitive, psychiatric and motor response to galantamine in Parkinson's disease with dementia. *International Journal of Geriatric Psychiatry, 18,* 937–941.

Abel, S., Schultz, A., Radermacher, I., Willmes, K., & Huber, W. (2003). Increasing versus vanishing cues in naming therapy. *Brain and Language, 87,* 143–144.

Abou-Khalil, R., & Abou-Khalil, B. (2003). Cortical stimulation mapping and speech production. *Perspectives on Neurophysiology and Neurogenic Speech and Language Disorders, 13,* 10–15.

Adamovich, B. (1990, June). Paper presented at the Clinical Aphasiology Conference. Santa Fe, NM.

Adamovich, B. B., & Henderson, J. (1992). *Scales of cognitive ability for traumatic brain injury.* Chicago, IL: Riverside Publishing.

Adams, C., Lloyd, J., Aldred, C., & Baxendale, J. (2003). *Evaluating intervention for children with pragmatic language impairment.* Poster presented at National Convention of the American Speech-Language-Hearing Association, Chicago, IL.

Adams, W., & Sheslow, D. (2003). *Wide Range Assessment of Memory and Learning–2.* Lutz, FL: Psychological Assessment Resources.

Aftonomos, L. B., Appelbaum, J. S., & Steele, R. D. (1999). Improving outcomes for persons with aphasia in advanced community-based treatment programs. *Stroke, 30,* 1370–1379.

Aftonomos, L. B., Steele, R., Appelbaum, J., & Harris, V. (2001). Relationships between impairment-level assessments and functional-level assessments in aphasia: Findings from LCC treatment programmes. *Aphasiology, 15,* 951–964.

Agency for Healthcare Policy and Research (1990). *Medical treatment effectiveness research [Agency for Health Care Policy and Research Program note]*. Rockville, MD: Department of Health and Human Services, Public Health Service.

Agency for Healthcare Research and Quality (2002). *Systems to rate the strength of scientific evidence: Summary*. [Online] Retrieved 08/27/04: http://www.ahrq.gov/clinic/tp/strengthtp.htm

Aine, C. (1995). A conceptual overview and critique of functional neuroimaging techniques in humans: MRI/fMRI and PET. *Critical Reviews in Neurobiology, 9,* 229–309.

Albers, G. W., & Tijssen, J. G. (1999). Antiplatelet therapy: New foundations for optimal treatment decisions. *Neurology, 53,* S25–S31.

Albert, M. L., Bachman, D. L., Morgan, A., & Helm-Estabrooks, N. (1988). Pharmacotherapy for aphasia. *Neurology, 38,* 877–879.

Albert, M. L., Sparks, R., & Helm, N. (1988). Melodic intonation therapy for aphasia. *Archives of Neurology, 29,* 130–131.

Albin, R. L., Young, A. B., & Penney, J. B. (1995). The functional anatomy of disorders of the basal ganglia. *Trends in Neuroscience, 18,* 63–64.

Alderman, N. (1996). Central executive deficit and response to operant conditioning methods. *Neuropsychological Rehabilitation, 6,* 161–186.

Alderman, N., Fry, R. K., & Youngson, H. A. (1995). Improvement of self-monitoring skills, reduction of behavior disturbance and the dysexecutive syndrome: Comparison of response cost and a new programme of self-monitoring training. *Neuropsychological Rehabilitation, 5,* 193–221.

Alexander, M. P., Hiltbrunner, B., & Fischer, R. S. (1989). Distributed anatomy of transcortical sensory aphasia. *Archives of Neurology, 46,* 885–892.

Alexander, M. P., Naeser, M. A., & Palumbo, C. L. (1987). Correlations of subcortical CT lesion sites and aphasia profiles. *Brain, 110,* 961–991.

Alexander, M. P., Naeser, M. A., & Palumbo, C. (1990). Broca's area aphasias: Aphasia after lesions including the frontal operculum. *Neurology, 40,* 353–362.

Alexopolous, G. S., Abrams, R. C., Young, R. C., & Shamoian, C. A. (1988). Cornell scale for depression in dementia. *Biological Psychiatry, 23,* 271–284.

Al-Khawaja, I., Wade, D. T., & Collin, C. F. (1996). Bedside screening for aphasia: A comparison of two methods. *Journal of Neurology, 243,* 201–204.

Amann, B., Sterr, A., Thoma, H., Messer, T., Kapfhammer, H. P., & Grunze, H. (2000). Psychopathological changes preceding motor symptoms in Huntington's disease: A report of four cases. *World Journal of Biological Psychiatry, 1,* 55–58.

American Academy of Neurology Therapeutics and Technology Assessment Subcommittee (1994). Assessment: Melodic intonation therapy. *Neurology, 44,* 566–568.

American Psychiatric Association (1994). *Diagnostic and Statistical Manual of Mental Disorders* (4th ed.). Washington, DC: Author.

American Speech-Language-Hearing Association (1996). Guidelines for the training, credentialing, use, and supervision of speech-language pathology assistants. *ASHA, 38,* 21–34.

American Speech-Language-Hearing Association (2000). *Council on Professional Standards in Speech-Language Pathology and Audiology: Background information and criteria for registration of speech-language pathology assistants*. Rockville, MD: Author.

American Speech-Language Hearing Association (2001). *Scope of practice in speech-language pathology*. Rockville, MD: Author.

American Speech-Language Hearing Association (2004). *Evidence-based practice in communication disorders: An introduction (Technical Report)*. [Online] Retrieved 09/15/04: http://www.asha.org/members/deskref-journals/deskref/default

Anderson, J. M., Gilmore, R., Roper, S., Crosson, B., Bauer, R. M., Nadeau, S., et al. (1999). Conduction aphasia and the arcuate fasciculus: A reexamination of the Wernicke-Geschwind model. *Brain and Language, 70*, 1–12.

Andersson, S., & Fridlund, B. (2002). The aphasic person's view of the encounter with other people: A grounded theory analysis. *Journal of Psychiatric Mental Health Nursing, 9*, 285–292.

Annoni, J. M., Khateb, A., Gramigna, S., Staub, F., Carota, A., Maeder, P., et al. (2003). Chronic cognitive impairment following laterothalamic infarcts: A study of 9 cases. *Archives of Neurology, 60*, 1439–1443.

Apel, K., & Trisha Self, T. (2003). Evidence-based practice: The marriage of research and clinical service. *ASHA Leader, 8*, 6.

Aphasia Tutor [Computer software]. (2004). Blacksburg, VA: Bungalow Software.

Appelros, P., Karlsson, G. M., Seiger, A., & Nydevik, I. (2002). Neglect and anosognosia after first-ever stroke: Incidence and relationship to disability. *Journal of Rehabilitation Medicine, 34*, 215–220.

Ardila, A., & Rosselli, M. (1993). Spatial agraphia. *Brain and Cognition, 22*, 137–147.

Ardila, A., Rosselli, M., & Strumwasser, S. (1991). Neuropsychological deficits in chronic cocaine abusers. *International Journal of Neuroscience, 57*, 73–79.

Arkin, S. (1991) Memory training in early Alzheimer's disease: An optimistic look at the field. *American Journal of Alzheimer's and Related Disorders Care and Research, 6*, 17–25.

Arkin, S. (1998). Alzheimer memory training: Positive results replicated. *American Journal of Alzheimer's Disease, 13*, 102–104.

Arkin, S. (2003). Student-led exercise sessions yield significant fitness gains for Alzheimer's patients. *American Journal of Alzheimer's Disease and Other Dementias, 18*, 159–170.

Arkin, S., & Mahendra, N. (2001). Discourse analysis of Alzheimer's patients before and after intervention: Methodology and outcomes. *Aphasiology, 15*, 533–569.

Armstrong, L. (1996). *Armstrong Naming Test*. London: Whurr Publishers.

Armstrong, L., & McKechnie, K. (2003). Intergenerational communication: Fundamental but under-exploited theory for speech and language therapy with older people. *International Journal of Language and Communication Disorders, 38*, 13–29.

Arnett, P. A., Rao, S. M., Hussain, M., Swanson, S. J., & Hammeke, T. A. (1996). Conduction aphasia in multiple sclerosis: A case report with MRI findings. *Neurology, 47*, 576–578.

Arnold, L. (1999). *The source for aphasia therapy*. East Moline, IL: Linguisystems.

Arrindell, W. A., Meeuwesen, L., & Huyse, F. J. (1991). The Satisfaction With Life Scale (SWLS): Psychometric properties in a non-psychiatric medical outpatients sample. *Personality and Individual Differences, 12*, 117–123.

Avery, J., & Kennedy, M. R. (2002). Intervention for memory disorders after TBI. *Special Interest Division 2: Neurophysiology and Neurogenic Speech and Language Disorders Newsletter, 12*, 9–14.

Axelrod, B. N., Jiron, C. C., & Henry, R. R. (1993). Performance of adults ages 20 to 90 on the abbreviated Wisconsin Card Sorting Test. *The Clinical Neuropsychologist, 7*, 205–209.

Azouvi, P. Couillet, J., Leclereq, M., Martin, Y., Asloun, S., & Rousseaux, M. (2004). Divided attention and mental effort after severe traumatic brain injury. *Neuropsychologia, 42*, 1260–1268.

Azouvi, P., Samuel, C., Louis-Dreyfus, A., Bernati, T., Bartolomeo, P., Beis, J., et al. (2002). Sensitivity of clinical and behavioral tests of spatial neglect after right hemisphere stroke. *Journal of Neurology, Neurosurgery, and Psychiatry, 73,* 160–166.

Baddeley, A. (1990). *Human memory: Theory and practice.* Hove, UK: Lawrence Erlbaum Associates.

Baddeley, A. (2003). Working memory and language: An overview. *Journal of Communication Disorders, 36,* 189–208.

Baddeley, A., Emslie, H., & Nimmo-Smith, I. (1994). *Doors and People.* Bury St. Edmunds, Suffolk, England: Thames Valley Test Company.

Baddeley, A., Emslie, H., Kolodny, J., & Duncan, J. (1998). Random generation and the executive control of working memory. *The Quarterly Journal of Experimental Psychology, 51A,* 819–852.

Baines, K. A., Martin, A. W., & Heeringa, H. M. (1999). *Assessment of Language-Related Functional Activities.* Austin, TX: Pro-Ed.

Baker, F. A. (2000). Modifying the Melodic Intonation Therapy program for adults with severe non-fluent aphasia. *Music Therapy Perspectives, 18,* 110–114.

Bakheit, A. M. O., Barrett, L., & Wood, J. (2004). The relationship between the severity of post-stroke aphasia and state self-esteem. *Aphasiology, 18,* 759–764.

Ballard, C. G. (2004). Definition and diagnosis of dementia with Lewy bodies. *Dementia and Geriatric Cognitive Disorders, 17,* 15–24.

Ballard, K. J., & Thompson, C. K. (1999). Treatment and generalization of complex sentence production in agrammatism. *Journal of Speech, Language, and Hearing Research, 42,* 690–707.

Bardo, J. V., Delis, D., & Kaplan, E. (2002*). Role of executive functions in language: Evidence from a new verbal reasoning test.* Poster presentation at the annual International Neuropsychology Society conference, Toronto, Canada.

Barker-Collo, S. L. (2001). The 60-item Boston Naming Test: Cultural bias and possible adaptations for New Zealand. *Aphasiology, 15,* 85–92.

Barnes, P. M., Powell-Griner, E., McFann, K., & Nahin, R. L. (2004). Complimentary and alternative medicine use among adults: United States, 2002. *Advance data from vital and health statistics, No. 343.* Hyattsville, MD: National Center for Health Statistics.

Barona, A., Reynolds, C., & Chastain, R. (1984). A demographically based index of premorbid intelligence for the WAIS-R. *Journal of Clinical and Consulting Psychology, 52,* 885–887.

Barrett, A. M. (2000). Treatment of unilateral neglect in patients with right hemisphere brain damage. *Special Interest Division 2: Neurophysiology and Neurogenic Speech and Language Disorders Newsletter, 10,* 18–26.

Barrett, A. M., Crucian, G. P., Beversdorf, D. Q., & Heilman, K. M. (2001). Monocular patching may worsen sensory-attentional neglect: A case report. *Archives of Physical Medicine and Rehabilitation, 82,* 516–518.

Barrie, M. A. (2002). Objective screening tools to assess cognitive impairment and depression. *Topics in Geriatric Rehabilitation, 18,* 28–46.

Barriere, I., & Lorch, M. (2003). Considerations on agraphia in light of a new observation of pure motor agraphia. *Brain and Language, 85,* 262–270.

Bartha, L., & Benke, T. (2003). Acute conduction aphasia: An analysis of 20 cases. *Brain and Language, 85,* 93–108.

Bartolomeo, P., Chokron, S., & Gainotti, G. (2001). Laterally directed arm movements and right unilateral neglect after left hemisphere damage. *Neuropsychologia, 39,* 1013–1021.

Bassey, E. J. (2000). The benefits of exercise for the health of older people. *Reviews in Clinical Gerontology, 10,* 17–31.

Basso, A. (1992). Prognostic factors in aphasia. *Aphasiology, 6,* 337–348.

Basso, A., Capitani, E., Laiacona, M., & Luzzatti, C. (1980). Factors influencing type and severity of aphasia. *Cortex, 16,* 631–636.

Basso, A., Capitani, E., & Moraschini, S. (1982). Sex differences in recovery from aphasia. *Cortex, 18,* 469–475.

Basso, A., & Caporali, A. (2001). Aphasia therapy or the importance of being earnest. *Aphasiology, 15,* 307–332.

Basso, A., Della Sala, S., & Farabola, M. (1987). Aphasia arising from purely deep lesions. *Cortex, 23,* 29–44.

Bastiaanse, R., & Edwards, S. (2001). Word order and finiteness in Dutch and English Broca's and Wernicke's aphasia. *Brain and Language, 79,* 72–74.

Bastiaanse, R., Edwards, S., & Rispens, J. (2002). *Verb and Sentence Test.* Bury St. Edmunds, Suffolk, England: Thames Valley Test Company.

Bate, A. J., Mathias, J. L., & Crawford, J. R. (2001). Performance on the Test of Everyday Attention and standard tests of attention following severe traumatic brain injury. *The Clinical Neuropsychologist, 15,* 405–422.

Bates, E. (1976). *Language in context.* New York: Academic Press.

Bauer, R. M., Zawacki, T. (1997). Auditory agnosia and amusia. In T. E. Feinburg & M. J. Farah (eds.), *Behavioral neurology and neuropsychology* (pp. 267–276), New York: McGraw-Hill.

Bayles, K. A. (2003). Effects of working memory deficits on the communicative functioning of Alzheimer's dementia patients. *Journal of Communication Disorders, 36,* 209–219.

Bayles, K., Azuma, T., Cruz, R., Tomoeda, C., Wood, J., & Montgomery, E. (1999). Gender differences in language of Alzheimer's disease patients revisited. *Alzheimer's Disease and Associated Disorders, 13,* 138–146.

Bayles, K., & Tomoeda, C. (1993). *Arizona Battery for Communication Disorders of Dementia.* Tucson, AZ: Canyonlands Publishing.

Bayles, K., & Tomoeda, C. (1994). *Functional Linguistic Communication Inventory.* Tucson, AZ: Canyonlands Publishing.

Bayles, K. A., & Kaszniak, A. W. (1987). *Communication and cognition in normal aging and dementia.* Boston: College-Hill.

Bayles, K. A., & Kim, E. S. (2003). Improving the functioning of individuals with Alzheimer's disease: Emergence of behavioral interventions. *Journal of Communication Disorders, 36,* 327–343.

Baylor, C. R. (2003). Structural CT and MRI: The basics. *Special Interest Division 2: Neurophysiology and Neurogenic Speech and Language Disorders Newsletter, 13,* 18–24.

Beats, B. C., Sahakian, B. J., & Levy, R. (1996). Cognitive performance in tests sensitive to frontal lobe dysfunction in the elderly depressed. *Psychological Medicine, 26,* 591–604.

Beaumont, J. G., Marjoribanks, J., Flury, S., & Lintern, T. (1999). A screening test of auditory comprehension for individuals with severe physical disability. *British Journal of Clinical Psychology, 38,* 1–4.

Beaumont, J. G., Marjoribanks, J., Flury, S., & Lintern, T. (2002). *Putney Auditory Comprehension Screening Test.* Bury St. Edmunds, Suffolk, England: Thames Valley Test Company.

Beck, A. T., Steer, R. A., & Brown, G. K. (1996). *Beck Depression Inventory–II Manual*. San Antonio, TX: The Psychological Corporation.

Becker, E., Bar-Or, O., Mendelson, L., & Najenson, T. (1978). Pulmonary function and responses to exercise of patients following craniocerebral injury. *Scandinavian Journal of Rehabilitation Medicine, 10,* 47–50.

Bedard, M., Felteau, M., Mazmanian, D., Fedyk, K., Klein, R., Richardson, J., et al. (2002). Pilot evaluation of a mindfulness-based intervention to improve quality of life among individuals who sustained brain injuries. *Disability and Rehabilitation, 25,* 722–731.

Beeson, P. (1998). Treatment for letter-by-letter reading: A case study. In N. Helm-Estabrooks & A. L. Holland (Eds.), *Clinical decision making in aphasia treatment* (pp. 153–177). Clifton Park, NY: Singular Thomson Delmar Learning.

Beeson, P. M. (1999). Treating acquired writing impairment: Strengthening graphemic representations. *Aphasiology, 9–11,* 767–786.

Beeson, P., & Insalaco, D. (1998). Acquired alexia: Lessons from successful treatment. *Journal of the International Neuropsychological Society, 4,* 621–635.

Beeson, P., & Rapcsak, S. Z. (2002). Clinical diagnosis and treatment of spelling disorders. In A. E. Hillis (Ed.), *The handbook of adult language disorders: Integrating cognitive neuropsychology, neurology, and rehabilitation* (pp. 101–120). New York: Psychology Press.

Beeson, P., Rising, K., & Volk, J. (2003). Writing treatment for severe aphasia: Who benefits? *Journal of Speech, Language, and Hearing Research, 46,* 1038–1060.

Beeson, P. M., Bayles, K. A., Rubens, A. B., & Kaszniak, A. (1993). Memory impairments and executive control in individuals with stroke-induced aphasia. *Brain and Language, 45,* 253–275.

Beeson, P. M., & Hillis, A. E. (2001). Comprehension and production of written words. In R. Chapey (Ed.), *Language intervention strategies in aphasia and related neurogenic communication disorders* (pp. 572–595). Philadelphia: Lippincott, Williams, & Wilkins.

Behrmann, M., & Lieberthal, T. (1989). Category-specific treatment of a lexical-semantic deficit: A single case study of global aphasia. *British Journal of Disorders of Communication, 24,* 281–299.

Beis, J. M., Andre, J. M., Baumgarten, A., & Challier, B. (1999). Eye patching in unilateral spatial neglect: Efficacy of two methods. *Archives of Physical Medicine and Rehabilitation, 80,* 71–76.

Bell, B. D. (1994). Pantomime recognition impairment in aphasia: An analysis of error types. *Brain and Language, 47,* 269–278.

Benedict, R. H. B. (1997). *Brief Visuospatial Memory Test–Revised*. Lutz, FL: Psychological Assessment Resources.

Benson, D. F., Cummings, J. L., & Tsai, S. Y. (1982). Angular gyrus syndrome simulating Alzheimer's disease. *Archives of Neurology, 38,* 616–620.

Benton, A. L., Hamsher, K., Rey, G. J., & Sivan, A. B. (1994). *Multilingual Aphasia Examination* (3rd ed.), San Antonio, TX: The Psychological Corporation.

Benton, A. L., Hamsher, K., & Sivan, A. B. (2001). *Multilingual Aphasia Examination* (4th ed.). Lutz, FL: Psychological Assessment Resources.

Benton, A. L., Hamsher, K. deS., Varney, N. R., & Spreen, O. (1983). *Contributions to neuropsychological assessment*. New York: Oxford University Press.

Benton, A. L., Smith, K., & Lang, M. (1972). Stimulus characteristics and object naming in aphasic patients. *Journal of Communication Disorders, 5,* 19–24.

Benton, E., & Bryan, K. (1996). Right cerebral hemisphere damage: Incidence of language problems. *International Journal of Rehabilitation Research, 19,* 47–54.

Ben-Yishay, Y., & Daniels-Zide, E. (2000). Examined lives: Outcomes after holistic rehabilitation. *Rehabilitation Psychology, 45,* 112–129.

Berardelli, A., Noth, J., Thompson, P. D., Bollen, E. L. E. M., Curra, A., Deuschl, G., et al. (1999). Pathophysiology of chorea and bradykinesia in Huntington's disease. *Movement Disorders, 14,* 398–403.

Berg, I. J., Koning-Haanstra, M., & Deelmman, B. G. (1991). Long-term effects of memory rehabilitation: A controlled study. *Neuropsychological rehabilitation, 1,* 97–111.

Bergner, M., Bobbitt, R. A., Carter, W. B., & Gibson, B. S. (1981). The Sickness Impact Profile: Development and final revision of a health status measure. *Medicare Care, 19,* 787–805.

Bernicot, J., & Dardier, V. (2001). Communication deficits: Assessment of subjects with frontal lobe damage in an interview setting. *International Journal of Language and Communication Disorders, 36,* 245–263.

Bernstein-Ellis, E., & Elman, R. J. (1999). Aphasia group communication treatment: The aphasia center of California approach. In R. J. Elman (Ed.), *Group treatment of neurogenic communication disorders: The expert clinician's approach* (pp. 47–55). Boston: Butterworth-Heinemann.

Beschin, N., & Robertson, I. H. (1997). Personal versus extrapersonal neglect: A group study of their dissociation using a reliable clinical test. *Cortex, 33,* 379–384.

Beukelman, D. R., Yorkston, K. M., & Reichle, J. (Eds.) (2000). *Augmentative and alternative communication for adults with acquired neurologic disorders.* Baltimore: Paul H. Brookes Publishing.

Beuthien-Baumann, B., Handrick, W., Schmidt, T., Burchert, W., Oehme, L., Kropp, J., et al. (2003). Persistent vegetative state: Evaluation of brain metabolism and brain perfusion with PET and SPECT. *Nuclear Medicine Communications, 24,* 643–649.

Biddle, A. K., Watson, L. R., Hooper, C. R., Lohr, K. N., & Sutton, S. F. (2002). *Criteria for determining disability in speech-language disorders: Evidence report/technology assessment no. 52.* Rockville, MD: Agency for Healthcare Quality and Research.

Binder, J. R., Frost, J. A., Hammeke, T. A., Cox, R. W., Rao, S. M., & Prieto, T. (1997). Human brain language areas identified by functional magnetic resonance imaging. *Journal of Neuroscience, 17,* 353–362.

Bird, T., Knopman, D., VanSwieten, J., Rosso, S., Feldman, H., Tanabe, H., et al. (2003). Epidemiology and genetics of frontotemporal dementia/Pick's disease. *Annals of Neurology, 54,* S29–S31.

Bishop, D. S., & Pet, R. (1995). Psychobehavioral problems other than depression in stroke. *Topics in Stroke Rehabilitation, 2,* 56–68.

Black, S. E., Behrmann, M., Bass, K., & Hacker, P. (1989). Selective writing impairment: Beyond the allographic code. *Aphasiology, 3,* 265–277.

Blessed, G., Tomlinson, B. E., & Roth, M. (1968). The association between quantitative measures of dementia and of senile change in the cerebral grey matter of elderly subjects. *British Journal of Psychiatry, 114,* 797–811.

Blomert, L. (1998). Recovery from language disorders: Interactions between brain and rehabilitation. In B. Stemmer & H. A. Whitaker (Eds.), *Handbook of neurolinguistics* (pp. 547–557). New York: Academic Press.

Blomert, L., Kean, M-L., Koster, C., Schokker, J. (1994). Amsterdam-Nijmegen Everyday Language Test: Construction, reliability, and validity. *Aphasiology, 8,* 381–407.

Blomert, L., Koster, C., van Mier, J., & Kean, M-L. (1987). Verbal communication abilities of aphasic speakers: The everyday language test. *Aphasiology, 1,* 463–474.

Blonder, L. X., Bowers, D., & Heilman, K. M. (1991). The role of the right hemisphere in emotional communication. *Brain, 114,* 1115–1127.

Blumstein, S. E. (1998). Phonological aspects of aphasia. In M. T. Sarno (Ed.), *Acquired aphasia* (3rd ed., pp. 157–185). New York: Academic Press.

Blumstein, S. E., Katz, B., Goodglass, H., Shrier, R., & Dworetsky, B. (1985). The effects of slowed speech on auditory comprehension in aphasia. *Brain and Language, 24,* 246–265.

Bogod, N. M., Mateer, C. A., & MacDonald, S. W. S. (2003). Self-awareness after traumatic brain injury: A comparison of measures and their relationship to executive functions. *Journal of the International Neuropsychological Society, 9,* 450–458.

Boller, F., Becker, J. T., Holland, A. L., Forbes, M. M., Hood, P. C., & McGonigle-Gibson, K. L. (1991). Predictors of decline in Alzheimer's disease. *Cortex, 27,* 9–17.

Bombardier, C. H., & Thurber, C. A. (1998). Blood alcohol level and early cognitive status after traumatic brain injury. *Brain Injury, 12,* 32–48.

Bonakdarpour, B., Eftekharzadeh, A., & Ashayeri, H. (2003). Melodic intonation therapy in Persian aphasia patients. *Aphasiology, 17,* 75–95.

Bonner, A. P., & Cousins, S. O. (1996). Exercise and Alzheimer's disease: Benefits and barriers. *Activities and Adaptation in Aging, 20,* 21–32.

Bourgeois, M. (1992). Evaluating memory wallets in conversations with persons with dementia. *Journal of Speech and Hearing Research, 35,* 1344–1357.

Bourgeois, M., Camp, C., Rose, M., White, B., Malone, M., Carr, J., et al. (2003). A comparison of training strategies to enhance use of external aids by persons with dementia. *Journal of Communication Disorders, 36,* 361–378.

Bourgeois, M., Dijkstra, K., Burgio, L., & Allen-Burge, R. (2001). Memory aids as an augmentative and alternative communication strategy for nursing home residents with dementia. *AAC: Augmentative and Alternative Communication, 17,* 196–210.

Bourgeois, M., & Melton, A. (2004). *Training compensatory memory strategies via the telephone for persons with TBI.* Presentation at the Clinical Aphasiology Conference, Park City, UT.

Bowen, A., McKenna, K., & Tallis, R. C. (1999). Reasons for the variability in the reported rate of occurrence of unilateral neglect after stroke. *Stroke, 30,* 1196–1202.

Bowers, L., Barrett, M., Huisingh, R., Orman, J., & LoGiudice, C. (1991). *TOPS—Adolescent: Test of Problem Solving.* East Moline, IL: Linguisystems.

Bowers, L., Huisingh, R., LoGiudice, C., & Orman, J. (2005). *The WORD Test 2: Adolescent.* East Moline, IL: LinguiSystems.

Boyd, T. M., & Sautter, S. W. (1994). Route-finding: A measure of everyday executive functioning in the head-injured adult. *Applied Cognitive Psychology, 72,* 171–181.

Boyle, M. (2001). Semantic feature analysis: The evidence for treating lexical impairments in aphasia. *Neurophysiology and Neurogenic Speech and Language Disorders, 11,* 23–28.

Bracy, C. B., & Drummond, S. S. (1993). Word retrieval in fluent and nonfluent dysphasia: Utilization of pictogram. *Journal of Communication Disorders, 26,* 113–128.

Bracy, O. (1983). Computer based cognitive rehabilitation. *Cognitive Rehabilitation, 1,* 7–8.

Bracy, O. (1994). *PSSCogRehab.* Indianapolis, IN: Psychological Software Services.

Bradburn, N. M. (1969). *The structure of psychological well-being.* Chicago: Aldine Publishing Company.

Bragoni, M., Altieri, M., DiPiero, V., Padovani, A., Mostardini, C., & Lenzi, G. L. (2000). Bromocriptine and speech therapy in nonfluent chronic aphasia after stroke. *Neurological Sciences, 21,* 19–22.

Brandt, J., & Benedict, R. H. B. (2001). *Hopkins Verbal Learning Test–Revised.* Lutz, FL: Psychological Assessment Resources.

Brandt, J., Spencer, M., & Folstein, M. (1988). The Telephone Interview for Cognitive Status. *Neuropsychiatry and Neuropsychology, 1,* 111–117.

Braswell, D., Hartry, A., Hoornbeek, S., Johansen, A., Johnson, L., Schultz, J., et al. (1992). *The Profile of Executive Control System.* Gaylord, MI: Northern Rehabilitation Services.

Braunling-McMorrow, D., Lloyd, K., & Fralish, K. (1986). Teaching social skills to head-injured adults. *Journal of Rehabilitation, 52,* 39–44.

Brickenkamp, R., & Zillmer, E. (1998). *d2 Test of Attention.* Lutz, FL: Psychological Assessment Resources.

Broadbent, D. B., Cooper, P. F., FitzGerald, P., & Parkes, K. R. (1982). The Cognitive Failures Questionnaire and its correlates. *British Journal of Clinical Psychology, 21,* 1–16.

Brooks, J., Fos, L. A., Greve, K. W., & Hammond, J. S. (1999). Assessment of executive function in patients with mild traumatic brain injury. *The Journal of Trauma: Injury, Infection, and Critical Care, 46,* 159–163.

Brookshire, R. H. (1997). *Introduction to neurogenic communication disorders* (5th ed.). St. Louis: Mosby.

Brookshire, R. H. (2003). *Introduction to neurogenic communication disorders* (6th ed.). St. Louis: Mosby.

Brookshire, R. H., & Nicholas, L. E. (1994). Speech sample size and test-retest stability of connected speech measures for adults with aphasia. *Journal of Speech and Hearing Research, 37,* 399–407.

Brookshire, R. H., & Nicholas, L. E. (1995). Performance deviations in the connected speech of adults with no brain damage and adults with aphasia. *American Journal of Speech-Language Pathology, 4,* 118–123.

Brookshire, R. H., & Nicholas, L. E. (1997). *The Discourse Comprehension Test* (rev. ed.). Minneapolis, MN: BRK Publishers.

Brown, J. W., Leader, B. J., & Blum, C. S. (1983). Hemiplegic writing in severe aphasia. *Brain and Language, 19,* 204–215.

Brown, L., Sherbenou, R. J., & Johnsen, S. K. (1997). *Test of Nonverbal Intelligence* (3rd ed.). Austin, TX: Pro-Ed.

Brown, T. E. (1996). *Brown Attention-Deficit Disorder Scales.* San Antonio, TX: The Psychological Corporation.

Brown, V. L., Hammill, D. D., & Wiederholt, J. L. (1995). *Test of Reading Comprehension* (3rd ed.). Austin, TX: Pro-Ed.

Brumfitt, S., & Sheeran, P. (1999). The development and validation of the visual analogue self-esteem scale (VASES). *British Journal of Clinical Psychology, 38,* 387–400.

Brush, J. A., & Camp, C. J. (1998a). Spaced-retrieval training during dysphagia therapy: A case study. *Clinical Gerontologist, 19,* 96–99.

Brush, J. A., & Camp, C. J. (1998b). Using spaced-retrieval as an intervention during speech-language therapy. *Clinical Gerontologist, 19,* 51–64.

Brush, J. A., & Camp, C. J. (1999). Effective interventions for persons with dementia: Using spaced retrieval and Montessori techniques. *Special Interest Division 2: Neurophysiology and Neurogenic Speech and Language Disorders Newsletter, 9,* 27–32.

Bryan, K. L. (1995). *The Right Hemisphere Language Battery* (2nd ed.). London: Whurr Publishers.

Bryan, K. L., & Hale, J. B. (2001). Differential effects of left and right cerebral vascular accidents on language competency. *Journal of the International Neuropsychological Society, 7,* 655–664.

Bryant, B. R., Wiederholt, J. L., & Bryant, D. P. (2004). *Gray Diagnostic Reading Tests–2.* Austin, TX: Pro-Ed.

Buchman, A. S., Garron, D. C., Trost-Cardamone, J. E., Wichter, M. D., & Schwartz, M. (1986). Word deafness: One hundred years later. *Journal of Neurology, Neurosurgery, and Psychiatry, 49,* 489–499.

Bucks, R. S., Willison, J. R., & Byrne, L. M. T. (2000). *Location Learning Test.* Bury St. Edmunds, Suffolk, England: Thames Valley Test Company.

Buklina, S. B. (2003). Impairments in premorbid knowledge recall in patients with hemispheric and intraventricular brain damage. *Neuroscience and Behavioral Physiology, 33,* 933–938.

Burgess, P., & Shallice, T. (1997). *The Hayling and Brixton Tests.* Bury St. Edmunds, Suffolk, England: Thames Valley Test Company.

Burgess, P., Alderman, N., Evans, J., Emslie, H., & Wilson, B. (1998). The ecological validity of tests of executive function. *Journal of the International Neuropsychological Society, 4,* 547–558.

Burgio, F., & Basso, A. (1997). Memory and aphasia. *Neuropsychologia, 35,* 759–766.

Burke, J. M., Danick, J. A., Bernis, B., & Durgin, C. J. (1994). A process approach to memory book training for neurological patients. *Brain Injury, 8,* 71–81.

Burn, D. J., & McKeith, I. G. (2003). Current treatment of dementia with Lewy bodies and dementia associated with Parkinson's disease. *Movement Disorders, 18 (Suppl. 6),* S72–S79.

Burns, M. S. (1997). *Burns Brief Inventory of Communication and Cognition.* San Antonio, TX: The Psychological Corporation.

Burrell, K. L., Linebaugh, C. W., & Cozens-Hoffman, C. (1996). The effects of auditory distractors on the auditory and reading comprehension of adults with unilateral right hemisphere damage. *Clinical Aphasiology, 24,* 255–270.

Burvill, P. W., Johnson, G. A., Jamrozik, K. D., Anderson, C. S., Stewart-Wynne, E. G., & Chakera, T. M. H. (1995). Anxiety disorders after stroke: Results from the Perth Community Stroke Study. *The British Journal of Psychiatry, 166,* 328–332.

Busch, C. (1999). Group treatment reimbursement issues. In R. J. Elman (Ed.), *Group treatment of neurogenic communication disorders: The expert clinician's approach* (pp. 31–35). Boston: Butterworth-Heinemann.

Busch, C. R., Brookshire, R. H., & Nicholas, L. E. (1988). Referential communication abilities of aphasic speakers. *Journal of Speech and Hearing Disorders, 53,* 475–482.

Buschke, H. (1973). Selective reminding for analysis of memory and learning. *Journal of Verbal Learning and Verbal Behavior, 12,* 543–550.

Bush, B. A., Novack, T. A., Malec, J. F., Stringer, A. Y., Millis, S. R., & Madan, A. (2003). Validation of a model for evaluating outcome after traumatic brain injury. *Archives of Physical Medicine and Rehabilitation, 84,* 1803–1807.

Butcher, J. N., Dahlstrom, W. G., & Graham, J. R. (1989). *Minnesota Multiphasic Personality Inventory-2 (MMPI-2): Manual for administration and scoring.* Minneapolis, MN: University of Minnesota Press.

Butler, J. A. (2002). How comparable are tests of apraxia? *Clinical Rehabilitation, 16,* 389–398.

Butler, O. T., Anderson, L., Furst, C. J., & Namerow, N. S. (1989). Behavioral assessment in neuropsychological rehabilitation: A method for measuring vocational related skills. *Clinical Neuropsychologist, 3,* 235–243.

Butler, R. W., & Copeland, D. R. (2002). Attentional processes and their remediation in children treated for cancer: A literature review and the development of a therapeutic approach. *Journal of the International Neuropsychology Society, 8,* 115–124.

Butters, N., Delis, D. C., & Lucas, J. A. (1995). Clinical assessment of memory disorders in amnesia and dementia. *Annual Reviews in Psychology, 46,* 493–523.

Butters, N., Lopez, O. L., & Becker, J. T. (1996). Focal temporal lobe dysfunction in probable Alzheimer's disease predicts a slow rate of cognitive decline. *Neurology, 46,* 687–692.

Butters, N., Samuels, I., Goodglass, H., & Brody, B. (1970). Short-term visual and auditory memory disorders after parietal and frontal lobe damage. *Cortex, 6,* 44–459.

Byng, S. (1988). Sentence processing deficits: Theory and therapy. *Cognitive Neuropsychology, 5,* 629–676.

Byng, S., Kay, J., Edmundson, A., & Scott, C. (1990). Aphasia tests reconsidered. *Aphasiology, 4,* 67–91.

Byrne, G. J. (2000). Drug treatment in dementia. *Current Opinion in Psychiatry, 13,* 415–421.

Calabresi, P., Cupini, L. M., Centonze, D., Pisani, F., & Bernardi, G. (2003). Antiepileptic drugs as a possible neuroprotective strategy in brain ischemia. *Annals of Neurology, 53,* 693–702.

Calkins, M. P., & Brush, J. A. (2003). Designing for dining. *Alzheimer's Care Quarterly, 4,* 73–76.

Campbell, C. R., & Jackson, S. T. (1995). Transparency of one-handed Amer-Ind hand signals to nonfamiliar viewers. *Journal of Speech and Hearing Research, 38,* 1284–1289.

Campbell, V. A., Crews, J. E., Moriarty, D. G., Zack, M. M., & Blackman, D. K. (1999). Surveillance for sensory impairment, activity limitation, and health-related quality of life among older adults-United States, 1993–1997. *MMWR Surveillance Summaries, 48,* 131–156.

Canadian Study of Health and Aging Working Group. (1994). Canadian study of health and aging: Study methods and prevalence of dementia. *Canadian Medical Association Journal, 150,* 899–913.

Cannata, A. P., Alberoni, M., Franceschi, M., & Mariani, C. (2002). Frontal impairment in subcortical ischemic vascular dementia in comparison to Alzheimer's disease. *Dementia and Geriatric Cognitive Disorders, 13,* 101–111.

Caplan, B. (1987). Assessment of unilateral neglect: A new reading test. *Journal of Clinical and Experimental Neuropsychology, 9,* 359–364.

Caplan, D. (1981). On the cerebral localization of linguistic functions: Logical and empirical issues surrounding deficit analysis and functional localization. *Brain and Language, 14,* 120–137.

Caplan, D. (1993). Toward a psycholinguistic approach to acquired neurogenic language disorders. *American Journal of Speech-Language Pathology, 2,* 59–83.

Caplan, D., & Bub, D. (1990). *Psycholinguistic assessment of aphasia.* Mini-seminar presented at the annual convention of the American Speech-Language-Hearing Association, Seattle, WA.

Caplan, D., & Hanna, J. E. (1998). Sentence production by aphasic patients in a constrained task. *Brain and Language, 63,* 184–218.

Caplan, D., & Utman, J. A. (1992). Selective acoustic phonetic impairment and lexical access in an aphasic patient. *Journal of the Acoustic Society of America, 95,* 512–517.

Caplan, D., Waters, G. S., & Hildebrandt, N. (1997). Determinants of sentence comprehension in aphasic patients in sentence-picture matching tasks. *Journal of Speech, Language, and Hearing Research, 40,* 542–555.

Captain's Log [Computer software]. (1985). Richmond, VA: BrainTrain.

Caramazza, A., & Berndt, R. S. (1985). A multicomponent deficit view of agrammatic Broca's aphasia. In M. L. Kean (Ed.), *Agrammatism* (pp. 27–63). Orlando: Academic Press.

Caramazza, A., Berndt, R. S., & Basili, A. G. (1983). The selective impairment of phonological processing: A case study. *Brain and Language, 18,* 128–174.

Caramazza, A., & Hillis, A. E. (1991). Lexical organization of nouns and verbs in the brain. *Nature, 349,* 788–790.

Caramazza, A., & Miceli, G. (1991). Selective impairment of thematic role assignment in sentence processing. *Brain and Language, 41,* 402–436.

Caramazza, A., Papagno, C., & Ruml, W. (2000). The selective impairment of phonological processing in speech production. *Brain and Language, 75,* 428–450.

Cardenas, D. D. (1987). Antipsychotics and their use after traumatic brain injury. *Journal of Head Trauma Rehabilitation, 2,* 43–49.

Carlesimo, G. A., Sabbadini, M., Bombardi, P., Di Porto, E., Loasses, A., & Caltagirone, C. (1998). Retrograde memory deficits in severe closed-head injury patients. *Cortex, 34,* 1–23.

Carlomagno, S., Iavarone, A., & Colombo, A. (1994). Cognitive approaches to writing rehabilitation: From single case to group studies. In M. Riddoch & G. W. Humphreys (Eds.), *Cognitive neuropsychology and cognitive rehabilitation* (pp. 485–502). Hillsdale, NJ: Erlbaum.

Carmines, E. G., & Zeller, R. A. (1979). *Reliability and validity assessment.* Newbury Park, CA: Sage Publications.

Carrow-Woolfolk, E. (1995). *OWLS: Listening Comprehension Scale and Oral Expression Scale.* Circle Pines, MN: American Guidance Service.

Carrow-Woolfolk, E. (1996). *OWLS: Written Expression Scale.* Circle Pines, MN: American Guidance Service.

Cary, L. M. (1995). Somatosensory loss after stroke. *Critical Review of Physical and Rehabilitative Medicine, 7,* 51–91.

Caselli, R. J. (2000). Visual syndromes as the presenting feature of degenerative brain disease. *Seminars in Neurology, 20,* 139–144.

Caspari, I., Parkinson, S. R., LaPointe, L. L., & Katz, R. C. (1998). Working memory and aphasia. *Brain and Cognition, 37,* 205–223.

Cassidy, T. P., Lewis, S., & Gray, C. S. (1998). Recovery from visuospatial neglect in stroke patients. *Journal of Neurology, Neurosurgery, and Psychiatry, 64,* 555–557.

Centers for Disease Control and Prevention. (2003). *Traumatic brain injury.* Available: http://www.cdc.gov/ncipc/factsheets/tbi.htm.

Central Brain Tumor Registry for the United States (2005). *Fact sheet.* Available: http://www.cbtrus.org/factsheet/factsheet.html.

Chan, A. S., Salmon, D. P., Butters, N., & Johnson, S. A. (1995). Semantic network abnormality predicts rate of cognitive decline in patients with probable Alzheimer's disease. *Journal of the International Neuropsychological Society, 1,* 297–303.

Chan, R. C. K, & Manly, T. (2002). The application of "dysexecutive syndrome" measures across cultures: Performance and checklist assessment in neurologically healthy and traumatically brain-injured Hong Kong Chinese volunteers. *Journal of the International Neuropsychological Society, 8,* 771–780.

Chapey, R. (1986). An introduction to language intervention strategies in adult aphasia. In R. Chapey (Ed.), *Language intervention strategies in adult aphasia* (2nd ed., pp. 2–11). Baltimore: Williams & Wilkins.

Chapey, R., Duchan, J. F., Elman, R. J., Garcia, L. J., Kagan, A., Lyon, J. G., et al. (2001). Life participation approach to aphasia: A statement of values for the future. In R. Chapey (Ed.), *Language intervention strategies in aphasia and related neurogenic communication disorders* (4th ed., pp. 235–245). Philadelphia: Lippincott, Williams & Wilkins.

Chapey, R., & Hallowell, B. (2001). Introduction to language intervention strategies in adult aphasia. In R. Chapey (Ed.), *Language intervention strategies in aphasia and related neurogenic communication disorders* (pp. 3–17). Philadelphia: Lippincott, Williams & Wilkins.

Chapman, S. B., Culhane, K. A., Levin, H. S., Harward, H., Mendelsohn, D., Weing-Cobbs, L., et al. (1992). Narrative discourse after closed head injury in children and adolescents. *Brain and Language, 43,* 42–65.

Chapman, S. B., Wanek, A., & Sharpe, S. (1994). *Narrative discourse in pediatric head injury: What a story!* Paper presented at the annual Colorado Speech and Hearing Association convention, Denver, CO.

Chapman, S. B., Weiner, M., Rackley, A., Hynan, L., & Zientz, J. (2004). Effects of cognitive-communication stimulation for Alzheimer's disease patients treated with donepezil. *Journal of Speech, Language, and Hearing Research, 47,* 1149–1163.

Chavin, M. (2002). Music as communication. *Alzheimer's Care Quarterly, 3,* 145–156.

Chen, S. H., Thomas, J. D., Glueckauf, R. L., & Bracy, O. L. (1997). The effectiveness of computer-assisted cognitive rehabilitation for persons with traumatic brain injury. *Brain Injury, 11,* 197–209.

Chen, S. T., Sultzer, D. L., Hinkin, C. H., Mahler, M. E., & Cummings, J. L. (1998). Executive dysfunction in Alzheimer's disease: Association with neuropsychiatric symptoms and functional impairment. *The Journal of Neuropsychiatry and Clinical Neurosciences, 10,* 426–432.

Chenery, H. J., Copland, D. A., & Murdoch, B. E. (2002). Complex language functions and subcortical mechanisms: Evidence from Huntington's disease and patients with non-thalamic subcortical lesions. *International Journal of Language and Communication Disorders, 37,* 459–474.

Cherney, L. R. (1998). Pragmatics and discourse: An introduction. In L. R. Cherney, B. Shadden, & C.A. Coelho (Eds.). *Analyzing discourse in communicatively impaired adults.* Gaithersburg, MD: Aspen.

Cherney, L. R. (2002). Unilateral neglect: A disorder of attention. *Seminars in Speech and Language, 23,* 117–128.

Cherney, L. R., & Halper, A. S. (1999). Group treatment for individuals with right hemisphere damage. In R. J. Elman (Ed.), *Group treatment of neurogenic communication disorders: The expert clinician's approach* (pp. 121–137). Boston: Butterworth-Heinemann.

Cherney, L. R., & Halper, A. S. (2000). Assessment and treatment of functional communication following right hemisphere damage. In L. E. Worrall & C. M. Frattali (Eds.), *Neurogenic communication disorders: A functional approach* (pp. 276–292). New York: Thieme.

Cherney, L. R., & Halper, A. S. (2001). Unilateral visual neglect in right hemisphere stroke: A longitudinal study. *Brain Injury, 15,* 585–592.

Cherney, L. R., Halper, A. S., Kwasnika, C. M., Harvey, R. L., & Zhang, M. (2001). Recovery of functional status after right hemisphere stroke: Relationship with unilateral neglect. *Archives of Physical Medicine and Rehabilitation, 82,* 322–328.

Cherney, L. R., Shadden, B., & Coelho, C. A. (Eds.). (1998). *Analyzing discourse in communicatively impaired adults.* Gaithersburg, MD: Aspen.

Cheung, R. W., Cheung, M. C., & Chan, A. S. (2004). Confrontation naming in Chinese patients with left, right or bilateral brain damage. *Journal of the International Neuropsychological Society, 10,* 46–53.

Chittum, W. R., Johnson, K., Chittum, J. M., Guercio, J. M., & McMorrow, M. J. (1996). Road to Awareness: An individualized training package for increasing knowledge and comprehension of personal deficits in persons with acquired brain injury. *Brain Injury, 10,* 763–776.

Chiu, Y. C., Algase, D., Whall, A., Liang, J., Liu, H. C., Lin, K. N., et al. (2004). Getting lost: Directed attention and executive functions in early Alzheimer's disease patients. *Dementia and Geriatric Cognitive Disorders, 17,* 174–180.

Christensen, H., Griffiths, K., MacKinnon, A., & Jacomb, P. (1997). A quantitative review of cognitive deficits in depression and Alzheimer-type dementia. *Journal of the International Neuropsychological Society, 3,* 631–651.

Christensen, H., Hofer, S. M., MacKinnon, A. J., Korten, A. E., Jorm, A. F., & Henderson, A. S. (2001). Age is no kinder to the better educated: Absence of an association investigated using latent growth techniques in a community sample. *Psychological Medicine, 31,* 15–28.

Christopoulou, C., & Bonvillian, J. D. (1985). Sign language, pantomime, and gestural processing in aphasic persons: A review. *Journal of Communication Disorders, 18,* 1–20.

Chung, J. C. C., Lai, C., Chung, P. M., & French, H. P. (2004). Snoezelen for dementia. *The Cochrane Database of Systematic Reviews.*

Cicerone, K. D. (2002). Remediation of "working attention" in mild traumatic brain injury. *Brain Injury, 16,* 185–195.

Cicerone, K. D., Dahlberg, C., Kamar, K., Langenbahn, D. M., Malec, J. F., Bergquist, T. F. et al. (2000). Evidence-based cognitive rehabilitation: Recommendations for clinical practice. *Archives of Physical Medicine and Rehabilitation, 81,* 316–321.

Cicerone, K. D., & Giacino, J. T. (1992). Remediation of executive function deficits after traumatic brain injury. *Neuropsychological Rehabilitation, 2,* 12–22.

Cifu, D. X., Kreutzer, J. S., Marwitz, J. H., Rosenthal, M., Englander, J., & High, W. (1996). Functional outcomes of older adults with traumatic brain injury: A prospective, multicenter analysis. *Archives of Physical Medicine and Rehabilitation, 77,* 883–888.

Cifu, D. X., & Steward, D. G. (1999). Factors affecting functional outcome after stroke: A critical review of rehabilitation interventions. *Archives of Physical Medicine and Rehabilitation, 80 (Suppl. 1),* S35–S39.

Clare, L., Wilson, B. A., Carter, G., Breen, K., Gosses, A., & Hodges, J. R. (2000). Intervening with everyday memory problems in dementia of Alzheimer type: An errorless learning approach. *Journal of Clinical & Experimental Neuropsychology, 22,* 132–147.

Clark, H. M. (1999). *Brain Awareness Week: Health promotion project for students.* Poster presented at the annual convention of the American Speech-Language-Hearing Association, San Francisco, CA.

Clark, L. W., & Witte, K. (1995). Nature and efficacy of communication management in Alzheimer's Disease. In R. Lubinski (Ed.), *Dementia and communication* (pp. 238–256). Clifton Park, NY: Singular Thomson Delmar Learning.

Clark, M. S., & Smith, D. S. (1999). Psychological correlates of outcome following rehabilitation from stroke. *Clinical Rehabilitation, 13,* 129–140.

Clark, W. M., & Lutsep, H. L (1999). Medical treatment strategies: Intravenous thrombolysis, neuronal protection, and anti-reperfusion injury agents. *Neuroimaging Clinics of North America, 9,* 465–437.

Clifford, D. B. (2000). Humanimmunodeficiency virus-associated dementia. *Archives of Neurology, 57,* 321–324.

Cocchini, G., Beschin, N., & Della Sala, S. (2002). Chronic anosognosia: A case report and theoretical account. *Neuropsychologia, 40,* 2030–2038.

Cochran, J. W. (2001). Effect of modafinil on fatigue associated with neurological illnesses. *Journal of Chronic Fatigue Syndrome, 8,* 65–70.

Code, C., Muller, D. J., & Herrmann, M. (1999). Perceptions of psychosocial adjustment of aphasia: Application of the Code-Muller Protocols. *Seminars in Speech and Language, 20,* 51–63.

Coelho, C. (2002). Story narratives of adults with closed head injury and non-brain-injured adults: Influence of socioeconomic status, elicitation task, and executive functioning. *Journal of Speech, Language and Hearing Research, 45,* 1232–1248.

Coelho, C. A., & Duffy, R. J. (1987). The relationship of the acquisition of manual signs to severity of aphasia: A training study. *Brain and Language, 31,* 328–345.

Coelho, C. A., Liles, B. Z., Duffy, R. J., Clarkson, J. V., & Elia, D. (1994). Longitudinal assessment of narrative discourse in a mildly aphasic adult. *Clinical Aphasiology, 22,* 145–155.

Coelho, C. A., McHugh, R. E., & Boyle, M. (2000). Semantic feature analysis as a treatment for aphasic dysnomia: A replication. *Aphasiology, 14,* 233–242.

Cognitive Package [Computer software]. (2004). Blacksburg, VA: Bungalow Software.

Cohn, E. S. (1999). Hearing loss with aging. *Clinics in Geriatric Medicine, 15,* 145–161.

Cole-Virtue, J., & Nickels, L. (2004). Spoken word to picture matching from PALPA: A critique and some new matched sets. *Aphasiology, 18,* 77–102.

Conley, A., & Coelho, C. A. (2003). Treatment of word retrieval impairment in chronic Broca's aphasia. *Aphasiology, 17,* 203–212.

Conlon, C. P., & McNeil, M. R. (1991). The efficacy of treatment for two globally aphasic adults using visual action therapy. *Clinical Aphasiology, 19,* 185–195.

Connor, L., Olber, L. K., Tocco, M., Fitzpatrick, P. M., & Albert, M. L. (2001). Effect of socioeconomic status on aphasia severity and recovery. *Brain and Language, 78,* 254–257.

Connor, L. T., Helm-Estabrooks, N., & Palumbo, C. L. (2001). Severe auditory comprehension impairment with no lesion of Wernicke's area. *Brain and Language, 79,* 48–50.

Conway, T. W., Heilman, P., Rothi, L. J. G., Alexander, A. W., Adair, J., Crosson, B. A., et al. (1998). Treatment of a case of phonological alexia with agraphia using the Auditory Discrimination in Depth Program. *Journal of the International Neuropsychological Society, 4,* 608–620.

Cooke, A., DeVita, C., Gee, J., Alsop, D., Detre, J., Chen, W., et al. (2003). Neural basis for sentence comprehension deficits in frontotemporal dementia. *Brain and Language, 85*, 211–221.

Coppens, P., Hungerford, S., Yamaguchi, S., & Yamadori, A. (2002). Crossed aphasia: An analysis of the symptoms, their frequency, and a comparison with left-hemisphere aphasia symptomatology. *Brain and Language, 83*, 425–463.

Cornell, A. (2004). Evaluating the effects of Snoezelen on women who have a dementing illness. *International Journal of Psychiatric Nursing Research, 9*, 1045–1062.

Corwin, J., & Blysma, F. W. (1993). Translations of excerpts from Andre Rey's *Psychological examination of traumatic encephalopathy* and P. A. Osterrieth's *The Complex Figure Copy Test. The Clinical Neuropsychologist, 7*, 3–15.

Coull, J. T. (1998). Neural correlates of attention and arousal: Insights from electrophysiology, functional neuroimaging and psychopharmacology. *Progress in Neurobiology, 55*, 343–361.

Cramon, D. Y. Von, & Matthes-von Cramon, G. (1992). Reflections on the treatment of brain-injured patients suffering from problem-solving disorders. *Neuropsychological Rehabilitation, 2*, 207–230.

Crary, M. A., Haak, N. J., & Malinsky, A. E. (1989). Preliminary psychometric evaluation of an acute aphasia screening protocol. *Aphasiology, 3*, 611–618.

Crepeau, F., Scherzer, B., Belleville, S., & Desmarais, G. (1997). A qualitative analysis of central executive disorders in a real-life work situation. *Neuropsychological Rehabilitation, 7*, 147–165.

Crerar, M. A., Ellis, A. W., & Dean, E. C. (1996). Remediation of sentence processing deficits in aphasia using a computer-based microworld. *Brain and Language, 52*, 229–275.

Crockford, C., & Lesser, R. P. (1994). Assessing functional communication in aphasia: Clinical utility and time demands of three methods. *European Journal of Disorders of Communication, 29*, 165–182.

Cronbach, L. J. (1990). *Essentials of psychological testing* (4th ed.). New York: Harper and Row.

Crook, T., Ferris, S., McCarthy, M., & Rae, D. (1980). Utility of digit recall tasks for assessing memory in the aged. *Journal of Consulting and Clinical Psychology, 48*, 228–233.

Croot, K. (2002). Diagnosis of AOS: Definition and criteria. *Seminars in Speech and Language, 23*, 267–280.

Crosson, B. (1985). Subcortical functions in language: A working model. *Brain and Language, 25*, 257–292.

Crosson, B. (2000). Systems that support language processes: Verbal working memory. In S. Nadeau, L. Rothi, & B. Crosson (Eds.). *Aphasia and language: Theory to practice* (pp. 399–418). New York: Guilford Press.

Crowley, J. A., & Miles, M. A. (1991). Cognitive remediation in pediatric head injury: A case study. *Journal of Pediatric Psychology, 16*, 611–627.

Crucian, G. P., & Okun, M. S. (2003). Visual-spatial ability in Parkinson's disease. *Frontiers in Bioscience, 8*, 992–997.

Crum, R. M., Anthony, J. C., Bassett, S. S., & Folstein, M. F. (1993). Population-based norms for the Mini-Mental State Examination by age and educational level. *Journal of the American Medical Association, 269*, 2386–2391.

Cuenod, C. A., Bookheimer, S. Y., Hertz-Pannier, L., Zeffiro, T. A., Theodore, W. H., & Le Bihan, D. (1995). Functional MRI during word generation, using conventional equipment: A potential tool for language localization in the clinical environment. *Neurology, 45,* 1821–1827.

Culbertson, W., Tanner, D. C., Peck, A. K., & Hopper, A. T. (1998). Orientation testing and responses of brain-injured subjects. *Journal of Medical Speech-Language Pathology, 6,* 93–103

Cullbertson, W. C., & Zillmer, E. A. (1999). *Tower of LondonDX: Research Version.* North Tonawanda, NY: Multi-Health Systems.

Cummings, J. L. (1997). Neuropsychiatric manifestations of right hemisphere lesions. *Brain and Language, 57,* 22–37.

Cummings, J. L. (1988). Intellectual impairment in Parkinson's disease: Clinical, pathologic and biochemical correlates. *Journal of Geriatric Psychiatry and Neurology, 1,* 24–36.

Cummings, J. L. (2000). Cognitive and behavioral heterogeneity in Alzheimer's disease: Seeking the neurobiological basis. *Neurobiology of Aging, 21,* 845–861.

Cummings, J. L., & Burns, M. S. (1996). Neurological syndromes associated with right hemisphere damage. In A. S. Halper, L. R. Cherney, & M. S. Burns (Eds.), *Clinical management of right hemisphere dysfunction* (pp. 9–20). Gaithersburg, MD: Aspen.

Cummings, J. L., Mega, M., Gray, K., Rosenberg-Thompson, S., Carusi, D. A., & Gornbein, J. (1994). The Neuropsychiatric Inventory: Comprehensive assessment of psychopathology in dementia. *Neurology, 44,* 2308–2314.

Cunningham, R., Farrow, V., Davies, C., & Lincoln, N. (1995). Reliability of the assessment of communicative effectiveness in severe aphasia. *European Journal of Disorders of Communication, 30,* 1–16.

Dabul, B. (2000). *Apraxia Battery for Adults–2.* Austin, TX: Pro-Ed.

Daker-White, G., Beattie, A. M., Gilliard, J., & Means, R. (2002). Minority ethnic groups in dementia care: A review of service needs, service provision and models of good practice. *Aging and Mental Health, 6,* 101–108.

Daley, M. P., & Fouche, J. H. (1999). *Critical thinking for activities of daily living and communication.* Austin, TX: Pro-Ed.

Damasio, A. R. (1981). The nature of aphasia: Signs and syndromes. In M. T. Sarno (Ed.), *Acquired aphasia* (pp. 51–65). Austin, TX: Pro-Ed.

Damasio, A. R. (1995). *Descartes' Error: Emotion, reason, and the human brain.* New York: Quill.

Daniloff, J. K., Fritelli, G., Buckingham, H. W., Hoffman, P. R., & Daniloff, R. G. (1986). Amer-Ind versus ASL: Recognition and imitation in aphasic subjects. *Brain and Language, 28,* 95–113.

Daniloff, J. K., Noll, J. D., Fristoe, M., & Lloyd, L. L. (1982). Gesture recognition in patients with aphasia. *Journal of Speech and Hearing Disorders, 47,* 43–49.

Darley, F. (1982). *Aphasia.* Philadelphia: W. B. Saunders.

Darley, F. A., Aronson, A. E., & Brown, J. R. (1975). *Motor speech disorders.* Philadelphia: W.B. Saunders.

Darley, F. L., Keith, R. L., & Sasanuma, S. (1977). The effect of alerting and tranquilizing drugs upon the performance of aphasic patients. *Clinical Aphasiology, 7,* 91–96.

Davis, G. A. (2000). *Aphasiology: Disorders and clinical practice.* Boston: Allyn & Bacon.

Davis, G. A., & Coelho, C. A. (2004). Referential cohesion and logical coherence of narration after closed head injury. *Brain and Language, 89,* 508–523.

Davis, G. A., & Wilcox, M. J. (1985). *Adult aphasia rehabilitation: Applied pragmatics.* Clifton Park, NY: Singular Thomson Delmar Learning.

Dearden, N. M. (1998). Mechanisms and prevention of secondary brain damage during intensive care. *Clinical Neuropathology, 17,* 221–228.

DeDe, G., Parris, D., & Waters, G. (2003). Teaching self-cues: A treatment approach for verbal naming. *Aphasiology, 17,* 465–480.

De Deyn, P., De Reuck, J., Orgogozo, J. M., Vlietinck, R., & Deberdt, W. (1997). Treatment of acute ischemic stroke with piracetam. *Stroke, 28,* 2347–2352.

Deelman, B. G. (2001). Prospective memory training in older adults. *Educational Gerontology, 27,* 455–478.

DeFilippis, N. A., & McCampbell, E. (1997). *Booklet Category Test* (2nd ed.). Lutz, FL: Psychological Assessment Resources.

D'Elia, L. F., Satz, P., Uchiyama, C. L., & White, T. (1996). *Color Trails Test.* Lutz, FL: Psychological Assessment Resources.

Delis, D. C., Kaplan, E., & Kramer, J. H. (2001). *Delis-Kaplan Executive Function System- Examiner's Manual.* San Antonio, TX: The Psychological Corporation.

Delis, D. C., Kramer, J. H., Kaplan, E., & Ober, B. A. (2000). *California Verbal Learning Test* (2nd ed.). San Antonio, TX: The Psychological Corporation.

Delis, D. C., Squire, L. R., Bihrle, A., & Massman, P. (1992). Componential analysis of problem-solving ability: Performance of patients with frontal lobe damage and amnesic patients on a new sorting test. *Neuropsychologia, 30,* 683–697.

Della Barba, G., Frasson, E., Mantovan, M. C., Gallo, A., & Denes, G. (1996). Semantic and episodic memory in aphasia. *Neuropsychologia, 34,* 361–367.

Della Sala, S., Gray, C., Baddeley, A., & Wilson, L. (1997). *Visual Patterns Test.* Bury St. Edmunds, Suffolk, England: Thames Valley Test Company.

Deloche, G., Dordain, M., & Kremin, H. (1993). Rehabilitation of confrontation naming in aphasia: Relations between oral and written modalities. *Aphasiology, 7,* 201–216.

Deloche, G., Hannequin, D., Dordain, M., Perrier, D., Pichard, B., Quint, S., et al. (1996). Picture confrontation oral naming: Performance differences between aphasics and normals. *Brain and Language, 53,* 105–120.

de Partz, M. P. (1986). Re-education of a deep dyslexic patient: Rationale of the method and results. *Cognitive Neuropsychology, 3,* 149–177.

de Partz, M. P., Seron, X., & van der Linden, M. (1992). Re-education of a surface dysgraphia with a visual imagery strategy. *Cognitive Neuropsychology, 9,* 369–401.

DeRenzi, E. (1997a). Prosopagnosia. In T. E. Feinberg & M. J. Farah (Eds.), *Behavioral neurology and neuropsychology* (pp. 245–255). New York: McGraw-Hill.

DeRenzi, E. (1997b). Visuospatial and constructional disorders. In T. E. Feinberg & M. J. Farah (Eds.), *Behavioral neurology and neuropsychology* (pp. 297–307). New York: McGraw-Hill.

de Riesthal, M., & Wertz, R. T. (2004). Prognosis for aphasia: Relationship between selected biographical and behavioral variables and outcome and improvement. *Aphasiology, 18* 899–915.

Derogatis, L. R. (1975). *Brief Symptom Inventory.* Baltimore: Clinical Psychometric Research.

Diamond, P. T., Holroyd, S., Macciochi, S. N., & Felsenthal, G. (1995). Prevalence of depression and outcome on the geriatric rehabilitation unit. *American Journal of Physical Medicine and Rehabilitation, 74,* 214–217.

Dick, J. P., Builoff, R. J., Stewart, A., Blackstock, J., Bielawaska, C., Paul, E., et al. (1984). Mini-Mental State Examination in neurological patients. *Journal of Neurology, Neurosurgery, and Psychiatry, 47,* 496–499.

Dickson, D. W. (2001). Neuropathology of Pick's disease. *Neurology, 56 (Suppl. 4)*, S16–S20.

Diener, E., Emmons, R. A., Larsen, R. J., & Griffin, S. (1985). The Satisfaction with Life Scale. *Journal of Personality Assessment, 49*, 71–75.

Dikengil, A., Monda, D., & King, C. (1992). Communication functional skills group: An integrated group therapy approach to injury rehabilitation. *The Journal of Cognitive Rehabilitation, 10*, 28–31.

Dikmen, S., & Machamer, J. E. (1995). Neurobehavioral outcomes and their determinants. *Journal of Head Trauma Rehabilitation, 10*, 74–84.

Dikmen, S., Machamer, J. E., Winn, H. R., & Temkin, N. R. (1995). Neuropsychological outcome at one year post head injury. *Neuropsychology, 9*, 80–90.

DiSimoni, F. G. (1989). *Comprehensive Apraxia Test*. Dalton, PA: Praxis House.

Doesborgh, S. J., Mieke, van de Sandt-Koenderman, M., Dippel, D. W., van Harskamp, F., Koudstaal, P. J., & Visch-Brink, E. G. (2004). Effects of semantic treatment on verbal communication and linguistic processing in aphasia after stroke: A randomized controlled trial. *Stroke, 35*, 141–146.

Dogil, G., Frese, I., Haider, H., Rohm, D., & Wokurek, W. (2004). Where and how does grammatically geared processing take place—and why is Broca's area often involved. A coordinated fMRI/ERBP study of language processing. *Brain and Language, 89*, 337–345.

Dollaghan, C. A. (2004). Evidence-based practice in communication disorders: What do we know, and when do we know it? *Journal of Communication Disorders, 37*, 391–400.

Donaghy, S., & Williams, W. (1998). A new protocol for training severely impaired patients in the usage of memory journals. *Brain Injury, 12*, 1061–1070.

Donkervoort, M., Dekker, J., van den Ende, E., Stehmann-Saris, J. C., & Deelman, B. G. (2000). Prevalence of apraxia among patients with a first left hemisphere stroke in rehabilitation centers and nursing homes. *Clinical Rehabilitation, 14*, 130–136.

Dore, J. (1974). A pragmatic description of early language development. *Journal of Psycholinguistic Research, 3*, 343–350.

Douglas, J., O'Flaherty, C., & Snow, P. (2000). Measuring perception of communicative ability: The development and evaluation of the La Trobe communication questionnaire. *Aphasiology, 14*, 251–268.

Dowden, P. A., Marshall, R. C., & Tompkins, C. A. (1981) Amer-Ind sign as a communicative facilitator for aphasic and apraxic patients. *Clinical Aphasiology, 11*, 133–140.

Doyle, P. J., Goda, A. J., & Spencer, K. A. (1995). The communicative informativeness and efficiency of connected discourse by adults with aphasia under structured and conversational sampling conditions. *American Journal of Speech-Language Pathology, 4*, 130–134.

Doyle, P. J., Goldstein, H., & Bourgeois, M. (1987). Experimental analysis of syntax training in Broca's aphasia: A generalization and social validation study. *Journal of Speech and Hearing Disorders, 52*, 143–155.

Doyle, P. J., McNeil, M. R., Mikolic, J. M., Prieto, L., Hula, W. D., Lustig, A. P., et al. (2004). The Burden of Stroke Scale (BOSS) provides valid and reliable score estimates of functioning and well-being in stroke survivors with and without communication disorders. *Journal of Clinical Epidemiology, 57*, 997–1007.

Doyle, P. J., Tsironas, D., Goda, A. J., & Kalinyak, M. (1996). The relationship between objective measures and listeners' judgments of the communicative informativeness of the connected discourse of adults with aphasia. *American Journal of Speech-Language Pathology, 5*, 53–60.

Dragon NaturallySpeaking Preferred, version 4.01. (1999). United Kingdom: Lernout and Hauspie Speech Products and Dragon Systems.

Dreher, J. C., & Grafman, J. (2003). Dissociating the roles of the rostral anterior cingulated and the lateral prefrontal cortices in performing two tasks simultaneously or successively. *Cerebral Cortex, 13,* 329–339.

Drew, R. L, & Thompson, C. K. (1999). Model-based semantic treatment for naming deficits in aphasia. *Journal of Speech, Language, and Hearing Research, 42,* 972–989.

Dronkers, N. N. (1996). A new brain region for coordinating speech articulation. *Nature, 384,* 159–161.

Drummond, S. S. (1993). *Dysarthria Examination Battery.* San Antonio, TX: The Psychological Corporation.

Ducharme, J. M. (1999). A conceptual model for treatment of externalizing behaviour in acquired brain injury. *Brain Injury, 13,* 645–668.

Duff, K., Patton, D., Schoenberg, M. R., Mold, J., Scott, J. G., & Adams, R. L. (2003). Age- and education-corrected independent normative data for the RBANS in a community dwelling elderly sample. *The Clinical Neuropsychologist, 17,* 351–366.

Duff, M., Proctor, A., & Haley, K. (2002). Mild traumatic brain injury: Assessment and treatment procedures used by speech-language pathologists. *Brain Injury, 16,* 773–787.

Duffy, J. R., & Peterson, R. C. (1992). Primary progressive aphasia. *Aphasiology, 6,* 1–16.

Duffy, J. R., & Coelho, C. A. (2001). Schuell's stimulation approach to rehabilitation. In R. Chapey (Ed.), *Language intervention strategies in aphasia and related neurogenic communication disorders* (4th ed., pp. 341–382). Philadelphia: Lippincott, Williams & Wilkins.

Duffy, J. R., & Watkins, L. B. (1984). The effect of response choice relatedness on pantomime and verbal recognition ability in aphasic patients. *Brain and Language, 21,* 291–306.

Duffy, R. J., & Duffy, J. R. (1984). *Assessment of Nonverbal Communication.* Austin, TX: Pro-Ed.

Dugbartey, A. T., Rosenbaum, J. G., Sanchez, P. N., & Townes, B. D. (1999). Neuropsychological assessment of executive functions. *Seminars in Clinical Neuropsychiatry, 4,* 5–12.

Dunn, L. M., & Dunn, E. S. (1997). *Peabody Picture Vocabulary Test III.* Circle Pines, MN: American Guidance Service.

Dunst, C. J., Trivette, C. M., & Cutspec, P. A. (2002). Toward an operational definition of evidence-based practices. *Centerscope, 1,* 1–10.

Edgeworth, J., Robertson, I. H., & MacMillan, T. (1998). *The Balloons Test.* Bury St. Edmunds, Suffolk, England: Thames Valley Test Company.

Edwards, S. (1995). Profiling fluent aphasic spontaneous speech: A comparison of two methodologies. *European Journal of Disorders of Communication, 30,* 333–345.

Ehmann, T. S., Beninger, R. J., Gawel, M. J., & Riopelle, R. J. (1990). Coping, social support and depressive symptoms in Parkinson's disease. *Journal of Geriatric Psychiatry and Neurology, 3,* 85–90.

Eisenson, J. (1994). *Examining for Aphasia* (3rd ed.). Austin, TX: Pro-Ed.

Elderkin-Thompson, V., Boone, K. B., Hwang, S., & Kumar, A. (2004). Neurocognitive profiles in elderly patients with frontotemporal degeneration or major depressive disorder. *Journal of the International Neuropsychological Society, 10,* 753–771.

Ellis, H. C., & Hunt, R. R. (1993). *Fundamentals of human memory and cognition.* Dubuque, IA: William C. Brown.

Elman, R. J. (Ed.). (1999). *Group treatment of neurogenic communication disorders: The expert clinician's approach.* Boston: Butterworth-Heinemann.

Enderby, P. (1983). *Frenchay Dysarthria Assessment.* San Diego, CA: College Hill Press.

Enderby, P., Broeckx, J., Hospers, W., Schildermans, F., & Deberdt, W. (1994). Effect of piracetam on recovery and rehabilitation after stroke: A double-blind, placebo-controlled study. *Clinical Neuropharmacology, 17,* 320–331.

Enderby, P., & Crow, E. (1996). Frenchay Aphasia Screening Test: Validity and comparability. *Disability and Rehabilitation, 18,* 238–240.

Enderby, P., Wood, V., Wade, D., Langton Hewer, R. (1997). *The Frenchay Aphasia Screening Test.* Philadelphia: Taylor & Francis.

Engle, R. W. (2002). Working memory capacity as executive attention. *Current Directions in Psychological Science, 11,* 19–23.

Ennis, M. R. (2001). Comprehension approaches for word retrieval training in aphasia. *Neurophysiology and Neurogenic Speech and Language Disorders, 11,* 18–23.

Ericksen, J., Cifu, D. X., & Burnett, D. (2001). The role of neuropharmacologic agents in return to work after traumatic brain injury. *Brain Injury Source, 5,* 32–34.

Erkulwater, S., & Pillai, R. (1989). Amantadine and the end stage dementia of Alzheimer's type. *Southern Medical Journal, 82,* 550–554.

Escobar, J. I., Burnam, A., Karno, M., Forsythe, A., Landsverk, J., & Golding, J. M. (1986). Use of the Mini-Mental State Examination in a community population of mixed ethnicity. *Journal of Nervous and Mental Disease, 174,* 607–614.

Evanofski, M. (1997). *Attention workbook volume 1* (2nd ed.). Dedham, MA: AliMed.

Evans, J., Wilson, B. A., Needham, P., & Brentnall, S. (2003). Who makes good use of memory aids? Results of a survey of people with acquired brain injury. *Journal of the International Neuropsychological Society, 9,* 925–935.

Evans, J. J., Emslie, H. C., & Wilson, B. A. (1998). External cueing systems in the rehabilitation of executive impairments of action. *Journal of the International Neuropsychology Society, 4,* 399–408.

Evans, J. J., Wilson, B. A., Schuri, Y., Andrade, J., Baddeley, A. D., Bruna, O., et al. (2000). A comparison of "errorless" and "trial-and-error" learning methods for teaching individuals with acquired memory deficits. *Neuropsychological Rehabilitation, 10,* 67–101.

Evans, R., Bishop, D., & Haselkorn, J. (1991). Factors predicting satisfactory home care after stroke. *Archives of Physical Medicine and Rehabilitation, 72,* 144–147.

Farah, M. J., & Feinberg, T. E. (1997). Visual object agnosia. In T. E. Feinberg & M. J. Farah (Eds.), *Behavioral neurology and neuropsychology* (pp. 239–244). New York: McGraw-Hill.

Farlow, M., Gracon, S. I., Hershey, L. A., Lewis, K. W., Sadowsky, C. H., & Dolan-Reno, J. (1992). A controlled trial of tacrine in Alzheimer's disease. *Journal of the American Medical Association, 268,* 2523–2529.

Fasotti, L., Kovacs, F., Eling, P., & Brouwer, W. H. (2000). Time pressure management as a compensatory strategy training after closed head injury. *Neuropsychological Rehabilitation, 10,* 47–65.

Fassbinder, W., & Tompkins, C. A. (2001). Slowed lexical-semantic activation in individuals with right hemisphere brain damage? *Aphasiology, 15,* 1079–1090.

Feher, E. P., Mahurin, R. K., Doody, R. S., Cooke, N., Sims, J., & Pirozzolo, F. J. (1992). Establishing the limits of the Mini-Mental State: Examination of 'subtests.' *Archives of Neurology, 49,* 87–92.

Feinberg, T., & Goodman, B. (1984). Affective illness, dementia, and pseudodementia. *Journal of Clinical Psychiatry, 45,* 99–103.

Ferro, J. M., Mariano, G., & Madureira, S. (1999). Recovery from aphasia and neglect. *Cerebrovascular Disease, 9 (Suppl. 5),* 6–22.

Filley, C. M. (2000). Clinical neurology and executive dysfunction. *Seminars in Speech and Language, 21,* 95–108.

Filley, C. M. (2002). The neuroanatomy of attention. *Seminars in Speech and Language, 23,* 89–98.

Fillingham, J. K., Hodgson, C., Sage, K., & Lambon Ralph, M. A. (2003). The application of errorless learning to aphasic disorders: A review of theory and practice. *Neuropsychological Rehabilitation, 13,* 337–363.

Fink, R. B., Brecher, A., Schwartz, M. F., & Robey, R. R. (2002). A computer-implemented protocol for treatment of naming disorders: Evaluation of clinician-guided and partially self-guided instruction. *Aphasiology, 16,* 1061–1086.

Fink, R. B., Schwartz, M. F., & Myers, J. L. (1998). Investigations of the sentence-query approach to mapping therapy. *Brain and Language, 65,* 203–207.

Fink, R. B., Schwartz, M. F., Rochon, E., Myers, J. L., Socolof, G. S., & Bluestone, R. (1995). Syntax stimulation revisited: An analysis of generalization treatment effects. *American Journal of Speech-Language Pathology, 4,* 99–104.

Fischer, R. S., & LaFleche, G. C. (1998). Executive functioning and rehabilitation outcome. *Journal of the International Neuropsychological Society, 4,* 68.

Fischer, S., Trexler, L. E., & Gauggel, S. (2004). Awareness of activity limitations and prediction of performance in patients with brain injuries and orthopedic disorders. *Journal of the International Neuropsychological Society, 10,* 190–199.

Fisher, M. (2003). Recommendations for advancing development of acute stroke therapies: Stroke therapy academic industry roundtable 3. *Stroke, 34,* 1539–1546.

Fleming, J. M., Strong, J., & Ashton, R. (1996). Self-awareness of deficits in adults with traumatic brain injury: How best to measure? *Brain Injury, 10,* 1–15.

Floel, A., Poeppel, D., Buffalo, E. A., Braun, A., Wu, C. W., Seo, H. J., et al. (2004). Prefrontal cortex asymmetry for memory encoding of words and abstract shapes. *Cerebral Cortex, 14,* 404–409.

Florance, C. (1981). Methods of communication analysis used in family interaction therapy. *Clinical Aphasiology, 11,* 204–211.

Foldi, N. S., LoBosco, J. J., & Schaefer, L. A. (2002). The effect of attentional dysfunction in Alzheimer's disease: Theoretical and practical implications. *Seminars in Speech and Language, 23,* 139–150.

Folstein, M. F., Folstein, S. E., & McHugh, P. R. (1975). "Mini-Mental State:" A practical method for grading the cognitive state of patients for the clinician. *Journal of Psychiatric Research, 12,* 189–198.

Folstein, M. F., Folstein, S. E., & McHugh, P. R. (2001). *Mini-Mental State Examination.* Lutz, FL: Psychological Assessment Resources.

Formisano, R., Carlesimo, G. A., Sabbadini, M., Loasses, A., Penta, F., Vinicola, V., et al. (2004). Clinical predictors and neuropsychological outcome in severe traumatic brain injury patients. *Acta Neurochirurgica, 146,* 457–462.

Forrester, G., & Geffen, G. (1995). *Julia Farr Services Post-Traumatic Amnesia Scale.* Unley, Australia: Julia Farr Foundation.

Francis, D. R., Clark, N., & Humphreys, G. W. (2003). The treatment of an auditory working memory deficit and the implications for sentence comprehension abilities in mild receptive aphasia. *Aphasiology, 17,* 723–750.

Frank, E. M., & Barrineau, S. (1996). Current speech-language protocols for adults with traumatic brain injury. *Journal of Medical Speech-Language Pathology, 4,* 81–101.

Franklin, S. (1989). Dissociations in auditory word comprehension: Evidence from nine fluent aphasic patients. *Aphasiology, 3,* 189–207.

Fraser, S., Glass, J. N., & Leathem, J. M. (1999). Everyday memory in an elderly New Zealand population: Performance on the Rivermead Behavioral Memory Test. *New Zealand Journal of Psychology, 28,* 118–123.

Frassinetti, F., Angeli, V., Menghello, F., Avanzi, S., & Ladavas, E. (2002). Long-lasting amelioration of visuospatial neglect by prism adaptation. *Brain, 125,* 608–623.

Fratiglioni, L., & Rocca, W. A. (2001). Epidemiology of dementia. In F. Bolla & S. F. Cappa (Eds.), *Handbook of neuropsychology* (Vol. 6, pp. 193–215). New York: Elsevier Science.

Frattali, C. M. (1994). Functional assessment. In R. Lubinski and C. Frattali (Eds.). *Professional issues in speech-language pathology and audiology* (pp. 306–320). Clifton Park, NY: Singular Thomson Delmar Learning.

Frattali, C. M., (1998a). Measuring modality-specific behaviors, functional abilities, and quality of life. In C. M. Frattali (Ed.), *Measuring outcomes in speech-language pathology* (pp. 55–88). New York: Thieme.

Frattali, C. M. (Ed.). (1998b). *Measuring outcomes in speech-language pathology.* New York: Thieme New York.

Frattali, C. M., Thompson, C., Holland, A., Wohl, A., & Ferketic, M. (1995) *American Speech-Language-Hearing Association Functional Assessment of Communication Skills for Adults.* Rockville, MD: ASHA.

Frattali, C. M., & Worral, L. E. (2001). Evidence-based practice: Applying science to the art of clinical care. *Journal of Medical Speech Language Pathology, 9,* ix–xiv.

Freed, D. (2004). Two case studies of family influence on treatment outcome after stroke. *Special Interest Division 2: Neurophysiology and Neurogenic Speech and Language Disorders Newsletter, 14,* 16–19.

Freed, D., Celery, K., & Marshall, R. C. (2004). Effectiveness of personalized and phonological cueing on long-term naming performance by aphasic subjects: A clinical investigation. *Aphasiology, 18,* 743–757.

Freed, D. B., Marshall, R. C., & Chuhlantseff, E. A. (1996). Picture naming variability: A methodological consideration of inconsistent naming responses in fluent and nonfluent aphasia. *Clinical Aphasiology, 24,* 193–205.

Freedman, M., Alexander, M. P., & Naeser, M. A. (1984). Anatomic basis of transcortical motor aphasia. *Neurology, 34,* 409–417.

Freedman, M., Leach, L., Kaplan, E., Winocur, G., Shulman, K. I., & Delis, D. C. (1994). *Clock drawing: A neuropsychological analysis.* New York: Oxford University Press.

Friederici, A., & Frazier, L. (1992). Thematic analysis in agrammatic comprehension: Syntactic structure and task demands. *Brain and Language, 42,* 1–29.

Friedman, R. B., & Lott, S. N. (2000). Rapid word identification in pure alexia is lexical but not semantic. *Brain and Language, 72,* 219–237.

Friedman, R. B., Ween, J. E., & Albert, M. L. (1993). Alexia. In K. Heilman & E. Valenstein (Eds.), *Clinical neuropsychology* (pp. 37–62). New York: Oxford University Press.

Fromm, D., & Holland, A. (1989). Functional communication in Alzheimer's disease. *Journal of Speech and Hearing Disorders, 54,* 535–540.

Fujioka, M., Okuchi, K., Hiramatsu, K. L., Sakaki, T., Sakaguchi, S., & Ishii, Y. (1997). Specific changes in human brain after hypoglycemic injury. *Stroke, 28,* 584–587.

Funnell, E., & Hodges, J. R. (1996). Deficits of semantic memory and executive control: Evidence for differing effects upon naming in dementia. *Aphasiology, 10,* 687–709.

Gaddie, A., Kearns, K. P., & Yedor, K. (1991). A qualitative analysis of response elaboration training effects. *Clinical Aphasiology, 19,* 171–183.

Gainotti, G., Azzoni, A., Razzano, C., Lanzillotta, M., Marra, C., & Gasparini, F. (1997). The post-stroke depression rating scale: A test specifically devised to investigate affective disorders of stroke patients. *Journal of Clinical and Experimental Neuropsychology, 19,* 340–356.

Gainotti, G., D'Erme, P., Villa, G., & Carlo, C. (1986). Focal brain lesions and intelligence: A study with a new version of Raven's Colored Matrices. *Journal of Clinical and Experimental Neuropsychology, 8,* 37–50.

Gallo, J. J., Rabins, P. V., & Anthony, J. C. (1999). Sadness in older persons: 13-year follow-up of a community sample in Baltimore, Maryland. *Psychological Medicine, 29,* 341–350.

Garrett, K. L. (1999). Measuring outcomes of group therapy. In R. J. Elman (Ed.), *Group treatment of neurogenic communication disorders: The expert clinician's approach* (pp. 17–29). Boston: Butterworth-Heinemann.

Garrett, M. F. (1988). Processes in language production. In F. J. Newmeyer (Ed.), *Linguistics: The Cambridge survey: III. Language: Psychological and biological aspects* (pp. 69–96). Cambridge: Cambridge University Press.

Gates, A., & Bradshaw, J. L. (1977). The role of the cerebral hemispheres in music. *Brain and Language, 4,* 403–431.

German, D. J. (1990). *The Test of Adolescent and Adult Word-Finding.* Austin, TX: Pro-Ed.

Gernsbacher, M. A., & Kaschak, M. P. (2003). Neuroimaging studies of language production and comprehension. *Annual Review of Psychology, 54,* 91–114.

Gerritsen, M. J. J., Berg, I. J., Deelman, B. G., Visser-Keizer, A. C., & Meyboom-de Jong, B. (2003). Speed of information processing after unilateral stroke. *Journal of Clinical and Experimental Neuropsychology, 25,* 1–13.

Ghika-Schmid, F., van Melle, G., Guex, P., & Bogousslavsky, J. (1999). Subjective experience and behavior in acute stroke: The Lausanne Emotion in acute stroke study. *Neurology, 52,* 22–28.

Giacino, J. T., & Cicerone, K. D. (1998). Varieties of deficit unawareness after brain injury. *Journal of Head Trauma Rehabilitation, 13,* 1–15.

Gierut, J. A. (2001). Complexity in phonological treatment: Clinical factors. *Language, Speech, and Hearing Services in Schools, 32,* 229–241.

Gil, M., Cohen, M., Korn, C., & Groswasser, Z. (1996). Vocational outcome of aphasic patients following severe traumatic brain injury. *Brain Injury, 10,* 39–45.

Gilleard, C. J. (1997). Education and Alzheimer's disease: A review of recent international epidemiological studies. *Aging and Mental Health, 1,* 33–46.

Gillis, R. J. (1999). Traumatic brain injury: Cognitive-communicative needs and early intervention. In R. J. Elman (Ed.), *Group treatment of neurogenic communication disorders: The expert clinician's approach* (pp. 141–151). Boston: Butterworth-Heinemann.

Gioia, G., Isquith, P. K., Guy, S. C., Kenworthy, L. (2001). *Behavior Rating Inventory of Executive Function.* Melbourne, Australia: PsychPress.

Gitlin, L. N., Liebman, J., & Winter, L. (2003). Are environmental interventions effective in the management of Alzheimer's disease and related disorders? A synthesis of evidence. *Alzheimer's Care Quarterly, 4,* 85–107.

Gladsjo, J. A., Miller, S. W., & Heaton, R. K. (1999). *Norms for letter and category fluency: Demographic corrections for age, education, and ethnicity.* Lutz, FL: Psychological Assessment Resources.

Gladstone, D. J., Danells, C. J., Armesto, A., McIlroy, W. E., Staines, R., & Graham, S. J. (2004). Physiotherapy couples with dextroamphetamine for motor rehabilitation after hemiparetic stroke: A randomized controlled trial. *Stroke, 35,* 239.

Gleason, J. B., Goodglass, H., Green, E., Ackerman, N., & Hyde, M. R. (1975). The retrieval of syntax in Broca's aphasia. *Brain and Language, 2,* 451–471.

Glisky, E. L. (1992). Computer-assisted instruction for patients with traumatic brain injury: Teaching of domain-specific knowledge. *Journal of Head Trauma Rehabilitation, 7,* 1–12.

Glisky, E. L., & Schacter, D. L. (1989). Extending the limits of complex learning in organic amnesia: Computer training in a vocational domain. *Neuropsychologia, 27,* 107–120.

Glisky, E. L., Schacter, D. L., & Tulving, E. (1986). Learning and retention of computer-related vocabulary in amnesic patients: Method of vanishing cues. *Journal of Clinical and Experimental Neuropsychology, 8,* 292–312.

Glosser, G., Baker, K. M., de Vries, J. J., Alavi, A., Grossman, M., & Clark, C. M. (2002). Disturbed visual processing contributes to impaired reading in Alzheimer's disease. *Neuropsychologia, 40,* 902–909.

Glosser, G., & Deser, T. (1990). Patterns of discourse production among neurological patients with fluent language disorders. *Brain and Language, 40,* 67–88.

Glosser, G., & Goodglass, H. (1990). Disorders in executive control functions among aphasic and other brain-damaged patients. *Journal of Clinical and Experimental Neuropsychology, 12,* 485–501.

Glosser, G., Wiener, M., & Kaplan, E. (1988). Variations in aphasic language behaviors. *Journal of Speech and Hearing Research, 53,* 115–124.

Glosser, G., Wolfe, N., Albert, M. L., Lavine, L., Steele, J. C., Calne, D. B., et al. (1993). Cross-cultural cognitive examination: Validation of a dementia screening instrument for neuroepidemiological research. *Journal of the American Geriatrics Society, 41,* 931–939.

Gold, M., VanDam, D., & Silliman, E. R. (2000). An open-label trial of bromocriptine in nonfluent aphasia: A qualitative analysis of word storage and retrieval. *Brain and Language, 74,* 141–156.

Goldberg, E., Podell, K., Bilder, R., & Jaeger, J. (2000). *Executive Control Battery.* Lutz, FL: Psychological Assessment Resources.

Golden, C. (2002). *Stroop Color and Word Test.* Lutz, FL: Psychological Assessment Resources.

Goldenberg, G., Dettmers, H., Grothe, C., & Spatt, J. (1994). Influence of linguistic and non-linguistic capacities on spontaneous recovery of aphasia and on success of language therapy. *Aphasiology, 8,* 443–456.

Goldenberg, G., & Spatt, J. (1994). Influence of size and site of cerebral lesions on spontaneous recovery of aphasia and on success of language therapy. *Brain and Language, 47,* 684–698.

Goldfarb, R., & Bader, E. (1979). Espousing melodic intonation therapy in aphasia rehabilitation: A case study. *International Journal of Rehabilitation Research, 2,* 333–342.

Golding, E. (1989). *Middlesex Elderly Assessment of Mental State.* Bury St. Edmunds, Suffolk, England: Thames Valley Test Company.

Goldman, W. P., Baty, J., Buckles, V. D., Sahrmann, S., & Morris, J. C. (1998). Cognitive and motor functioning in Parkinson disease: Subjects with and without questionable dementia. *Archives of Neurology, 55,* 674–680.

Goldstein, K., & Scheerer, M. (1948). Abstract and concrete behavior in experimental study with special tests. *Psychological Monograph, 53,* 1–151.

Goldstein, K. H., & Scheerer, M. (1953). Tests of abstract and concrete behavior. In A. Weider (Ed.), *Contributions toward medical psychology: Theory and psychodiagnostic methods* (pp. 702–730). New York: Ronald Press.

Goldstein, L. B., & Gradison, M. (1999). Stroke-related knowledge among patients with access to medical care in the Stroke Belt. *Journal of Stroke Cerebrovascular Disorders, 8,* 349–352.

Golisz, K. M. (1998). Dynamic assessment and multicontext treatment of unilateral neglect. *Topics in Stroke Rehabilitation, 5,* 11–28.

Golper, L. C. (1996). Language assessment. In G. L. Wallace (Ed.), *Adult aphasia rehabilitation* (pp. 57–86). Boston: Butterworth-Heinemann.

Golper, L. C. (2001). Teams and partnerships in aphasia intervention. In R. Chapey (Ed.), *Language intervention strategies in adult aphasia* (4th ed., pp. 194–207). New York: Lippincott, Williams & Wilkins.

Golper, L. C., Rau, M. T., Erskins, B., Langhans, J. J., & Houlihan, J. (1987). Aphasic patients' performance on a Mental Status Examination. *Clinical Aphasiology, 16,* 124–135.

Golper, L. C., Wertz, R. T., Frattali, C. M., Yorkston, K. M., Myers, P., Katz, R., et al. (2001). Evidence-based practice guidelines for the management of communication disorders in neurologically impaired individuals: Project introduction. Academy of Neurologic Communication Disorders and Sciences.

Goodglass, H. (1981). The syndromes of aphasia: Similarities and differences in neurolinguistic features. *Topics in Language Disorders, 1,* 1–14.

Goodglass, H. (1993). *Understanding aphasia.* New York: Academic Press.

Goodglass, H. (1998). Stages of lexical retrieval. *Aphasiology, 4–5,* 287–298.

Goodglass, H., & Berko, J. (1960). Agrammatism and inflectional morphology in English. *Journal of Speech and Hearing Research, 3,* 257–267.

Goodglass, H., & Kaplan, E. (1983). *Boston Diagnostic Examination for Aphasia.* Philadelphia: Lea & Febiger.

Goodglass, H., & Kaplan, E. (1983). *The assessment of aphasia and related disorders* (2nd ed.). Philadelphia: Lea & Febiger.

Goodglass, H., Kaplan, E., & Barresi, B. (2001). *Boston Diagnostic Aphasia Examination* (3rd ed.). Philadelphia: Lippincott, Williams & Wilkins.

Goodman, H., & Englander, J. (1992). Traumatic brain injury in elderly individuals. *Physical Medicine and Rehabilitation Clinics of North America, 3,* 441–453.

Goodman, R. A., & Caramazza, A. (1986a). *The Johns Hopkins University Dysgraphia Battery.* Baltimore: The Johns Hopkins University.

Goodman, R. A., & Caramazza, A. (1986b). *The Johns Hopkins University Dyslexia Battery.* Baltimore: The Johns Hopkins University.

Gordon, J. K. (1998). The fluency dimension in aphasia. *Aphasiology, 12,* 673–688.

Gordon, W. A., Hibbard, M. R., Egelko, S., Diller, L., Shaver, M. S, Lieberman, A., et al. (1985). Perceptual remediation in patients with right brain damage: A comprehensive program. *Archives of Physical Medicine and Rehabilitation, 66,* 353–359.

Gordon, W. P. (1983). Memory disorders in aphasia: I. Auditory immediate recall. *Neuropsychologia, 21,* 325–339.

Gorelick, P. B., Born, G.V. R., D'Agostino, R. B., Hanley, D. F., Moye, L., & Pepine, C. J. (1999). Therapeutic benefit: Aspirin revisited in light of the introduction of clopidogrel. *Stroke, 30,* 1716–1721.

Grabowski, J., & Damasio, A. (1997). Definition, clinical features and neuroanatomical basis of dementia. In M. Esiri & J. Morris (Eds.), *The neuropathology of dementia* (pp. 1–20). Cambridge, MA: University Press.

Grace, J., & Malloy, P. (1992). *Frontal Lobe Personality Scale (FLOPS).* Providence, RI: Brown University.

Graham, D. I. (1999). Pathophysiological aspects of injury and mechanisms of recovery. In M. Rosenthal, J. S. Kreutzer, E. R. Griffith, & Pentland, B. (Eds.), *Rehabilitation of the adult and child with traumatic brain injury* (3rd ed., pp. 19–41). Philadelphia: F. A. Davis.

Graham, D., I., Adams, J. H., Nicoll, J. A. R., Maxwell, W. L., & Gennarelli, T. A. (1995). The nature, distribution, and causes of traumatic brain injury. *Brain Pathology, 4,* 397–406.

Graham, M. A. (1999). Aphasia group therapy in a subacute setting: Using the American Speech-Language-Hearing Association Functional Assessment of Communication Skills. In R. J. Elman (Ed.), *Group treatment of neurogenic communication disorders: The expert clinician's approach* (pp. 37–45). Boston: Butterworth-Heinemann.

Granadier, R. J. (2000). Ophthalmology update for primary practitioners. Part1. Update on optic neuritis. *Disease-A-Month, 46,* 508–532.

Grant, D. A., & Berg, E. A. (1993). *Wisconsin Card Sorting Test.* Tampa, FL: Psychological Assessment Resources.

Grayson, E., Hilton, R., & Franklin, S. (1997). Early intervention in a case of jargon aphasia: Efficacy of language comprehension therapy. *European Journal of Disorders of Communication, 32,* 257–276.

Grealy, M. A., Johnson, D. A., & Rushton, S. K. (1999). Improving cognitive function after brain injury: The use of exercise and virtual reality. *Archives of Physical Medicine and Rehabilitation, 80,* 661–667.

Greenwald, M. L., & Gonzalez-Rothi, L. J. (1998). Lexical access via letter naming in a profoundly alexic and anomic patient: A treatment study. *Journal of the International Neuropsychological Society, 4,* 595–607.

Grice, H. P. (1975). Logic and conversation. In P. Cole & J. Morgan (Eds.), *Studies in syntax and Semantics: Vol. 3. Speech acts* (pp. 41–58). New York: Academic Press.

Griffin, S. L., van Reekum, R., & Masanic, C. (2003). A review of cholinergic agents in the treatment of neurobehavioral deficits following traumatic brain injury. *Journal of Neuropsychiatry and Clinical Neuroscience, 15,* 17–26.

Grigsby, J., Kaye, K., & Robbins, L. J. (1992). Reliabilities, norms and factor structure of the Behavioral Dyscontrol Scale. *Perceptual and Motor Skills, 74,* 883–892.

Grodzinsky, Y. (1984). The syntactic characterization of agrammatism. *Cognition, 16,* 99–120.

Guilford, J. (1967). *The nature of human intelligence.* New York: McGraw-Hill.

Gronwall, D. (1977). Paced Auditory Serial Addition Test: A measure of recovery from concussion. *Perceptual and Motor Skills, 44,* 367–373.

Groot, Y. C., Wilson, B. A., Evans, J., & Watson, P. (2002). Prospective memory functioning in people with and without brain injury. *Journal of the International Neuropsychological Society, 8,* 645–654.

Grossman, M. (2002). Frontotemporal dementia: A review. *Journal of the International Neuropsychological Society, 8,* 566–583.

Groves-Wright, K., Neils-Strunjas, J., Burnett, R., & O'Neill, M. J. (2004). A comparison of verbal and written language in Alzheimer's disease. *Journal of Communication Disorders, 37,* 109–130.

Guilford, J. (1967). *The nature of human intelligence.* New York: McGraw-Hill.

Guilford, J. P., & Hoepfner, R. (1971). *The analysis of intelligence.* New York: McGraw-Hill.

Guitton, D., Buchtel, H. A., & Douglas, R. M. (1985). Frontal lobe lesions in man cause difficulties in suppressing reflexive glances and in generating goal-directed saccades. *Experimental Brain Research, 58,* 455–472.

Gupta, S. R., & Mlcoch, A. G. (1992). Bromocriptine treatment of nonfluent aphasia. *Archives of Physical Medicine and Rehabilitation, 73,* 373–376.

Gupta, S. R., Mlcoch, A. G., Scolaro, C., & Moritz, T. (1995). Bromocriptine treatment of nonfluent aphasia. *Neurology, 45,* 2170–2173.

Gurland, G. B., Chwat, S. E., & Wollner, S. G. (1982). Establishing a communication profile in adult aphasia: Analysis of communicative acts and conversation consequences. *Clinical Aphasiology, 12,* 97–112.

Guyatt, G. H., Haynes, R. B., Jaeschke, R. Z., Cook, D. J., Green, L., Naylor, C. D., et al. (2000). Users' guides to the medical literature: XXV. Evidence-based medicine: Principles for applying the Users' Guides to patient care. Evidence-Based Medicine Working Group. *JAMA, 284,* 1290–1296.

Guyatt, G. H., Sinclair, J., Cook, D. J., & Glasziou, P. (1999). Users' guides to the medical literature: XVI. How to use a treatment recommendation. Evidence-Based Medicine Working Group and the Cochrane Applicability Methods Working Group. *JAMA, 281,* 1836–1843.

Haaland, K. Y., Vranes, L. F., Goodwin, J. S., & Garry, P. J. (1987). Wisconsin card sort test in a healthy elderly population. *Journal of Gerontology, 42,* 345–346.

Hacke, W., Ringleb, P., & Stingele, R. (1999). Update in thrombolytic therapy. *Revue Neurologique, 155,* 662–665.

Hagen, C. (1981). Language disorders secondary to closed head injury. *Topics in Language Disorders, 1,* 73–87.

Hajek, V. E., Kates, M. H., Donnelly, R., & McGree, S. (1993). The effect of visuospatial training in patients with right hemisphere stroke. *Canadian Journal of Rehabilitation, 6,* 175–186.

Hall, K. S, Ogunniyi, A. O, Hendrie, H. C., & Brittain, H. M. (1996). A cross cultural community based study of dementias: Methods and performance of the survey instrument Indianapolis, U.S.A., and Ibadan, Nigeria. *International Journal of Methods in Psychiatric Research, 6,* 1–14.

Halliday, M. A. K. (1994). *An introduction to functional grammar* (2nd ed.). London: Edward Arnold.

Hallowell, B., & Clark, H. M. (2002). *Dysphagia is taking over: Lowered priorities for aphasia services under managed care*. Paper presented at the 2002 Clinical Aphasiology Conference, Ridgedale, MO.

Halper, A. S., Cherney, L. R., Burns, M. S., & Mogil, S. I. (1996). *Clinical management of right hemisphere dysfunction* (2nd ed.). Rockville, MD: Aspen.

Halper, A. S., Cherney, L. R., Drimmer, D. P., & Chang, O. (1996). Right hemisphere stroke: Performance trends on word list recall and recognition. *Archives of Physical Medicine and Rehabilitation, 77,* 837.

Hamberger, M. J., & Seidel, W. T. (2003). Auditory and visual naming tests: Normative and patient data for accuracy, response time, and tip-of-the-tongue. *Journal of the International Neuropsychological Society, 9,* 479–489.

Hamilton, M. (1959). The assessment of anxiety states by rating. *British Journal of Medical Psychology, 32,* 50–55.

Hamilton, M. (1960). A rating scale for depression. *Journal of Neurology, Neurosurgery, and Psychiatry, 23,* 56–62.

Hammill, D. D., Brown, V. L., Larsen, S. C., & Wiederholt, J. L. (1994). *Test of Adolescent and Adult Language* (3rd ed.). Austin, TX: Pro-Ed.

Hammill, D. D., & Larsen, S. C. (1996). *Test of Written Language* (3rd ed.). Austin, TX: Pro-Ed.

Hammill, D. D., Pearson, N. A., & Widerholt, J. L. (1997). *Comprehensive Test of Nonverbal Intelligence*. Austin, TX: Pro-Ed.

Hanlon, R. E., Brown, J. W., & Gerstman, L. J. (1990). Enhancement of naming in nonfluent aphasia through gesture. *Brain and Language, 38,* 298–314.

Hanna, G., Schell, L. M., & Schreiner, R. (1977). *The Nelson Reading Skills Test*. Chicago, IL: Riverside Publishing.

Hardin, K., & Ramsberger, G. (2004). *Attentional training in aphasia: A case study*. Presentation at the Clinical Aphasiology Conference, Park City, UT.

Harrison, F. C., Zafonte, R., Mann, N., Dijkers, M., Englander, J., & Kreutzer, J. (1998). Brain injury as a result of violence: Preliminary findings from the traumatic brain injury model systems. *Archives of Physical Medicine and Rehabilitation, 79,* 730–737.

Hart, B., & Wells, D. L. (1997). The effects of language used by caregivers on agitation in residents with dementia. *Clinical Nurse Specialist, 11,* 20–23.

Hart, J., & Gordon, B. (1990). Delineation of single-word semantic comprehension deficits in aphasia with anatomical correlation. *Annals of Neurology, 27,* 226–231.

Hart, T., Whyte, J., Polansky, M., Millis, S., Hammond, F. M., Sherer, M., et al. (2003). Concordance of patient and family report of neurobehavioral symptoms at one year after traumatic brain injury. *Archives of Physical Medicine and Rehabilitation, 84,* 204–213.

Hartley, L. L. (1995). *Cognitive-communicative abilities following brain injury*. Clifton Park, NY: Singular Thomson Delmar Learning.

Hartley, L. L., & Jensen, P. J. (1991). Narrative and procedural discourse after closed head injury. *Brain Injury, 5,* 267–285.

Hartman-Maeir, A., Soroker, N., Ring, H., & Katz, N. (2002). Awareness of deficits in stroke rehabilitation. *Journal of Rehabilitation Medicine, 34,* 158–164.

Hartmann, A., Hupp, T., Koch, H. C., Dollinger, P., Stapf, C, Schmidt, R., Hofmeister, C., Thompson, J. L., Marx, P., & Mast, H. (1999). Prospective study on the complication rate of carotid surgery. *Cerebrovascular Diseases, 9,* 152–156.

Hawkins, K. A., & Bender, S. (2002). Norms and the relationship of Boston Naming Test performance to vocabulary and education: A review. *Aphasiology, 16,* 1143–1153.

Heaton, R. K., Grant, I, Butters, N., White, D. A., Kirson, D., Atkinson, J. H., McCutchan, J. A., Taylor, M. J., Kelly, M. D., Ellis, R. J., et al. (1995). The HNRC 500: Neuropsychology of HIV infection at different disease stages. *Journal of the International Neuropsychological Society, 1,* 231–251.

Heaton, R. K., Miller, W., Taylor, M. J., & Grant, I. (2004). *Revised comprehensive norms for an Expanded Halstead-Reitan Battery: Demographically adjusted neuropsychological norms for African American and Caucasian adults.* Lutz, FL: Psychological Assessment Resources.

Heeschen, C., & Kolk, H. (1988). Agrammatism and paragrammatism. *Aphasiology, 2,* 299–302.

Heilman, K. M., Rothi, L., Campanella, D., & Wolfson, S. (1979). Wernicke's and global aphasia without alexia. *Archives of Neurology, 36,* 129–133.

Heilman, K. M., Watson, R. T., & Rothi, L. G. (1997). Disorders of skilled movements: Limb apraxia. In T. E. Feinberg & M. J. Farah (Eds.), *Behavioral neurology and neuropsychology* (pp. 227–235). New York: McGraw-Hill.

Heilman, K. M., Watson, R. T., & Valenstein, E. (1985). Neglect and related disorders. In K. M. Heilman & E. Valenstein (Eds.), *Clinical neuropsychology* (pp. 279–336). New York: Oxford University Press.

Helm, N. A., & Barresi, B. (1980). Voluntary Control of Involuntary Utterances: A treatment approach for severe aphasia. *Clinical Aphasiology, 10,* 308–315.

Helm-Estabrooks, N. (1981). *Helm elicited language program for syntax stimulation.* Austin, TX: Pro-Ed.

Helm-Estabrooks, N. (1991). *Test of Oral and Limb Apraxia.* Austin, TX: Pro-Ed.

Helm-Estabrooks, N. (1992). *Aphasia Diagnostic Profiles.* Austin, TX: Pro-Ed.

Helm-Estabrooks, N. (1995). *Cognitive linguistic task book.* Sandwich, MA: Cape Cod Institute for Communication Disorders.

Helm-Estabrooks, N. (1998). A "cognitive" approach to treatment of an aphasic patient. In N. Helm-Estabrooks & A. L. Holland (Eds.), *Approaches to the treatment of aphasia* (pp. 69–89). Clifton Park, NY: Singular Thomson Delmar Learning.

Helm-Estabrooks, N. (2001). *Cognitive Linguistic Quick Test.* San Antonio, TX: The Psychological Corporation.

Helm-Estabrooks, N., & Albert, M. L. (1991). *Manual of aphasia therapy.* Austin, TX: Pro-Ed.

Helm-Estabrooks, N., & Albert, M. L. (2004). *Manual of aphasia and aphasia therapy* (2nd ed.). Austin, TX: Pro-Ed.

Helm-Estabrooks, N., Connor, L. T., & Albert, M. L. (2000). Treating attention to improve auditory comprehension in aphasia. *Brain and Language, 74,* 469–472.

Helm-Estabrooks, N., Emery, P., & Albert, M. L. (1987). Treatment of Aphasic Perseveration (TAP) program: A new approach to aphasia therapy. *Archives of Neurology, 44,* 1253–1255.

Helm-Estabrooks, N., Fitzpatrick, R., & Barresi, B. (1982). Visual Action Therapy for global aphasia. *Journal of Speech and Hearing Disorders, 44,* 385–389.

Helm-Estabrooks, N., Fitzpatrick, P. M., & Barresi, B. (1981). Response of an agrammatic patient to a syntax stimulation program for aphasia. *Journal of Speech and Hearing Disorders, 46,* 422–427.

Helm-Estabrooks, N., & Holtz, G. (1991). *Brief Test of Head Injury.* Austin, TX: Pro-Ed.

Helm-Estabrooks, N., & Nicholas, M. (2000). *Sentence Production Program for Aphasia.* Austin, TX: Pro-Ed.

Helm-Estabrooks, N., Nicholas, M., & Morgan, A. (1989). *Melodic Intonation Therapy program*. Austin, TX: Pro-Ed.

Helm-Estabrooks, N., & Ramsberger, G. (1986a). Aphasia treatment delivered by telephone. *Archives of Physical Medicine and Rehabilitation, 67*, 51–53.

Helm-Estabrooks, N., & Ramsberger, G. (1986b). Treatment of agrammatism in long-term Broca's aphasia. *British Journal of Disorders of Communication, 21*, 39–45.

Helm-Estabrooks, N., Ramsberger, G., Morgan, A. R., & Nicholas, M. (1989). *Boston Assessment of Severe Aphasia*. Austin, TX: Pro-Ed.

Henderson, L. W., Frank, E. M., Pigatt, T., Abramson, R. K., & Houston, M. (1998). Race, gender, and educational level effects on Boston Naming Test scores. *Aphasiology, 12*, 901–911.

Henri, B. P., & Hallowell, B. (1999). Mastering managed care: problems and possibilities. In B. S. Cornett (Ed.), *Clinical practice management for speech-language pathologists* (pp. 3–28). Gaithersburg, MD: Aspen.

Herbert, R., Best, W., Hickin, J., Howard, D., & Osborne, F. (2003). Combining lexical and interactional approaches to therapy for word finding deficits in aphasia. *Aphasiology, 17*, 1163–1186.

Herrmann, M., Britz, A., Bartels, C., & Wallesch, C. W. (1995). The impact of aphasia on the patient and family in the first year post-stroke. *Topics in Stroke Rehabilitation, 2*, 5–19.

Herrmann, M., Johannsen-Horback, H., & Wallesch, C. (1993). The psychosocial aspects of aphasia. In D. Lafond, R. DeGiovani, Y. Joannette, J. Ponzio, & M. Sarno (Eds.), *Living with aphasia: Psychosocial issues* (pp. 17–36). Clifton Park, NY: Singular Thomson Delmar Learning.

Hertanu, J., & Moldover, J. (1996). Rehabilitation of patients with cardiovascular problems. *Archives of Physical Medicine Rehabilitation, 77*, S38–S43.

Hickey, E. M., & Bourgeois, M. S. (2003). Beyond swallowing: Communication intervention in nursing homes. *Special Interest Division 2: Neurophysiology and Neurogenic Speech and Language Disorders Newsletter, 13*, 5–9.

Hickey, E. M., Bourgeois, M. S., & Olswang, L. B. (2004). Effects of training volunteers to converse with nursing home residents with aphasia. *Aphasiology, 5–7*, 625–637.

Hickin, J., Best, W., Herbert, R., Howard, D., & Osborne, F. (2002). Phonological therapy for word-finding difficulties: A re-evaluation. *Aphasiology, 16*, 981–999.

Hier, D. B., Mondlock, J., & Caplan, L. R. (1983). Recovery of behavioural abnormalities after right hemisphere stroke. *Neurology, 33*, 345–350.

Hilari, K., Byng, S., Lamping, D. L., & Smith, S. C. (2003). Stroke and Aphasia Quality of Life Scale-39 (SAQLS-39) Evaluation of acceptability, reliability, and validity. *Stroke, 34*, 1944–1950.

Hill, R. D., Wahlin, A., Winblad, B., & Backman, L. (1995). The role of demographic and lifestyle variables in utilizing cognitive support for episodic remembering among very old adults. *Journal of Gerontology: Psychological Sciences, 50*, 219–227.

Hillis, A. E. (1989). Efficacy and generalization of treatment for aphasic naming errors. *Archives of Physical Medicine Rehabilitation, 70*, 632–636.

Hillis, A. E. (1991). Effects of separate treatments for distinct impairments within the naming process. *Clinical Aphasiology, 19*, 255–265.

Hillis, A. E. (1993). The role of models of language processing in rehabilitation of language impairments. *Aphasiology, 7*, 5–26.

Hillis, A. E., Barker, P. B., Wityk, R. J., Aldrich, E. M., Restrepo, L., Breese, E. L., et al. (2004). Variability in subcortical aphasia is due to variable sites of cortical hypoperfusion. *Brain and Language, 89,* 524–530.

Hillis, A. E., & Caramazza, A. (1994). Theories of lexical processing and rehabilitation of lexical deficits. In M. Riddoch & G. W. Humphreys (Eds.), *Cognitive neuropsychology and cognitive rehabilitation* (pp. 449–484). Hillsdale, NJ: Erlbaum.

Hillis, A. E., & Caramazza, A. (1995). A framework for interpreting distinct patterns of hemispatial neglect. *Neurocase, 1,* 189–207.

Hillis, A. E., Rapp, B., Romani, C., & Caramazza, A. (1990). Selective impairment of semantics in lexical processing. *Cognitive Neuropsychology, 7,* 191–243.

Hillis Trupe, A. E. (1986). Effectiveness of retraining phoneme to grapheme conversion. *Clinical Aphasiology, 16,* 163–171.

Hinckley, J. J. (1998). Investigating the predictors of lifestyle satisfaction among younger adults with chronic aphasia. *Aphasiology, 12,* 509–518.

Hinckley, J. J. (2000). Effective tools for family education. *Advance for Speech-Language Pathologists & Audiologists, 16.*

Hinke, R. M., Hu, X., Stillman, A. E., Kim, S. G., Merkle, H., Salmi, R., et al. (1993). Functional magnetic resonance imaging of Broca's area during internal speech. *Neuroreport, 4,* 675–678.

Hirsch, F. M., & Holland, A. L. (1999). *How can we assess the quality of life of aphasic individuals? A study of five available measures.* Poster presented at the 1999 Clinical Aphasiology Conference, Key West, FL.

Hirsch, F. M., & Holland, A. L. (2000). Beyond activity: Measuring participation in society and quality of life. In L. E. Worrall & C. M. Frattali (Eds.). *Neurogenic communication disorders: A functional approach* (pp. 35–54). New York: Thieme.

Hjaltason, H., Tegner, R., Tham, K., Levander, M., & Ericson, K. (1996). Sustained attention and awareness of disability in chronic neglect. *Neuropsychologia, 34,* 1229–1233.

Ho, L. W., Carmichael, J., Swartz, J., Wyttenbach, A., Rankin, J., & Rubinsztein, D. C. (2001). The molecular biology of Huntington's disease. *Psychological Medicine, 31,* 3–14.

Hodges, J. (2004). *Addenbrooke's Cognitive Examination.* Bury St. Edmunds, Suffolk, England: Thames Valley Test Company.

Hodges, J. R. (2001). Frontotemporal dementia (Pick's disease): Clinical features and assessment. *Neurology, 56,* S6–S10.

Hoen, B., Thelander, M., & Worsley, J. (1997). Improvement in the psychological well-being of people with aphasia and their families: Evaluation of a community-based programme. *Aphasiology, 11,* 681–691.

Hoerster, L., Hickey, E., & Bourgeois, M. (2001). Effects of memory aids on conversations between nursing home residents with dementia and nursing assistants. *Neuropsychological Rehabilitation, 11,* 399–427.

Holland, A. L. (1980) *Communicative Abilities in Daily Living.* Austin, TX: Pro-Ed.

Holland, A. L. (1991). *Assessing pragmatic skills in aphasia.* Presentation at the annual convention of the Canadian Association of Speech-Language Pathologists and Audiologist, Montreal, Canada.

Holland, A. L. (1996). Pragmatic assessment and treatment for aphasia. In G. L. Wallace (Ed.), *Adult aphasia rehabilitation* (pp. 161–173). Boston: Butterworth-Heinemann.

Holland, A. L., & Beeson, P. M. (1999). Aphasia groups: The Arizona experience. In R. J. Elman (Ed.), *Group treatment of neurogenic communication disorders: The expert clinician's approach* (pp. 77–83). Boston: Butterworth-Heinemann.

Holland, A. L., Fratalli, C. M., & Fromm, D. (1999). *Communication Activities of Daily Living* (2nd ed.). Austin, TX: Pro-Ed.

Holland, A. L., & Fridriksson, J. (2001). Aphasia management during the early phases of recovery following stroke. *American Journal of Speech-Language Pathology, 10,* 19–28.

Holland, A. L., Fromm, D., DeRuyter, F., & Stein, M. (1996). Treatment efficacy: Aphasia. *Journal of Speech and Hearing Research, 39,* S27–S36.

Holland, A. L., Greenhouse, J., Fromm, D., & Swindell, C. S. (1989). Predictors of language restitution following stroke: A multivariate analysis. *Journal of Speech and Hearing Research, 32,* 232–238.

Holland, A. L., & Hinckley, J. J. (2002). Assessment and treatment of pragmatic aspects of communication in aphasia. In A. E. Hillis (Ed.), *The handbook of adult language disorders: Integrating cognitive neuropsychology, neurology, and rehabilitation* (pp. 413–427). New York: Psychology Press.

Holland, D., Witty, T., Lawler, J., & Lanzisera, D. (1999). Biofeedback-assisted relaxation training with brain injured patients in acute stages of recovery. *Brain Injury, 13,* 53–57.

Holtzapple, P., Pohlman, K., LaPointe, L. L., & Graham, L. F. (1989). Does SPICA mean PICA? *Clinical Aphasiology, 18,* 131–144.

Holtzer, R., Burright, R. G., & Donovick, P. J. (2004). The sensitivity of dual-task performance to cognitive status in aging. *Journal of the International Neuropsychology Society, 10,* 230–238.

Hoofien, D., Gilboa, A., Vakil, E., & Barak, O. (2004). Unawareness of cognitive deficits and daily functioning among persons with traumatic brain injuries. *Journal of Clinical and Experimental Neuropsychology, 26,* 278–290.

Hooker, K., Bowman, S. R., Coehlo, D. P., Lim, S. R., Kaye, J., Guariglia, R., et al. (2002). Behavioral change in persons with dementia: Relationships with mental and physical health of caregivers. *Journals of Gerontology Series B: Psychological Sciences and Social Sciences, 57,* P453–P460.

Hooper, H. E. (1983). *Hooper Visual Organization Test.* Los Angeles: Western Psychological Services.

Hopper, T. (2004). *Learning by individuals with dementia: The effects of spaced-retrieval training.* Presentation at the Clinical Aphasiology Conference, Park City, UT.

Hopper, T., Bayles, K. A., Harris, F., & Holland, A. (2001). The relationship between Minimum Data Set ratings and scores on measures of communication and hearing among nursing home residents with dementia. *American Journal of Speech-Language Pathology, 10,* 370–381.

Hopper, T., & Holland, A. (1998). Situation-specific treatment for aphasia. *Aphasiology, 12,* 933–944.

Hosking, S. G., Marsh, N. V., & Friedman, P. J. (2000). Depression at 3 months poststroke in the elderly: Predictors and indicators of prevalence. *Aging, Neuropsychology, and Cognition, 7,* 205–216.

Hough, M. S. (1993). Treatment of Wernicke's aphasia with jargon: A case study. *Journal of Communication Disorders, 26,* 101–111.

Hough, M. S., DeMarco, S., & Schmitzer, A. B. (1997). *Episodes of word retrieval failures after right hemisphere brain-damage.* Paper presented at the annual conference of the American Speech-Language-Hearing Association, Boston, MA.

Houghton, P. M., Pettit, J. M., & Towey, M. P. (1982). Measuring communicative competence in global aphasia. *Clinical Aphasiology, 12,* 28–39.

Howard, D., & Patterson, K. E. (1992). *Pyramids and Palm Trees.* Bury St. Edmunds, Suffolk, England: Thames Valley Test Company.

Hua, M., Chang, S., & Chen, S. (1997). Factor structure and age effects with an aphasia test battery in normal Taiwanese adults. *Neuropsychology, 11,* 156–162.

Huber, W. Poeck, K., Weniger, D., & Willmes, K. (1983). *Der Aachener Aphasie Test.* Gottingen: Hogrefe.

Huber, W., Poeck, K., & Willmes, K. (1984). The Aachen Aphasia Test. In F. C. Rose (Ed.), *Progress in aphasiology.* New York: Raven Press.

Huber, W., Willmes, K., Poeck, K., Van Vleymen, B., & Deberdt, W. (1997). Piracetam in aphasia: A double-blind study. *Archives of Physical Medicine and Rehabilitation, 72,* 245–250.

Hughes, J. D., Jacobs, D. H., & Heilman, K. M. (2000). Neuropharmacology and linguistic neuroplasticity. *Brain and Language, 71,* 96–101.

Hunkin, N. M., Squires, E. J., Aldrich, F. K., & Parkin, A. J. (1998). Errorless learning and the acquisition of word processing skills. *Neuropsychological Rehabilitation, 8,* 433–449.

Hurford, P., Stringer, A. Y., & Jann, B. (1998). Neuropharmacologic treatment of hemineglect: A case report comparing bromocriptine and methylphenidate. *Archives of Physical Medicine and Rehabilitation, 79,* 346–349.

Ince, L. P. (1968). Desensitization with an aphasic patient. *Behavioral Research and Therapy, 6,* 235–237.

Indredavik, B., Fjaertoft, H., Ekeberg, G., Loge, A. D., & Morch, B. (2000). Benefit of an extended stroke unit service with early supported discharge: A randomized, controlled trial. *Stroke, 31,* 2989–2994.

Irwin, W., Wertz, R., & Avent, J. (2002). Relationships among language impairment, functional communication, and pragmatic performance in aphasia. *Aphasiology, 16,* 823–835.

Isaacson, J. E., & Rubin, A. M. (1999). Otolaryngologic management of dizziness in the older patient. *Clinics in Geriatric Medicine, 15,* 179–191.

Ishiai, S., Koyama, Y., Seki, K., Orimo, S., Sodeyama, N., Ozawa, E., et al. (2000). Unilateral spatial neglect in AD: Significance of line bisection performance. *Neurology, 55,* 364–370.

Ivnik, R. J., Malec, J. F., Smith, G. E., Tangalos, E. G., & Petersen, R. C. (1996). Neuropsychological tests norms above age 55: COWAT, BNT, MAE Token, WRAT-R Reading, AMNART, STROOP, TMT, and JLO. *The Clinical Neuropsychologist, 10,* 262–278.

Jackson, H. H. (1878). On affectations of speech from disease of the brain. *Brain, 1,* 304–330.

Jacobs, B. J. (2001). Social validity of changes in informativeness and efficiency of aphasic discourse following Linguistic Specific Treatment (LST). *Brain and Language, 78,* 115–127.

Jacobs, B. J., & Thompson, C. K. (1992, November). *Effects of semantically based training on lexical processing in severe aphasia.* Poster presentation at the annual ASHA Convention, San Antonio, TX.

Jacobs, B. J., & Thompson, C. K. (2000). Cross-modal generalization effects of training noncanonical sentence comprehension and production in agrammatic aphasia. *Journal of Speech, Language, and Hearing Research, 43,* 5–20.

Jacobs, D. H., Adair, J. C., Gold, M., Shuren, J., Williamson, D. J., Gonzalez-Rothi, L., et al. (1994). Physostigmine improves confrontation naming in two patients with anomic aphasia in an open-label, dose-escalating study. *Brain and Language, 47,* 532–535.

Jagger, J., Levine, J. I., Jane, J. A., & Rimel, R. W. (1984). Epidemiologic features of head injury in a predominantly rural population. *Journal of Trauma-Injury Infection & Critical Care, 24,* 40–44.

Janvin, C., Aarsland, D., Larsen, J. P., & Hugdahl, K. (2003). Neuropsychological profile of patients with Parkinson's disease without dementia. *Dementia & Geriatric Cognitive Disorders, 15,* 126–131.

Jehkonen, M., Ahonen, J. P., Dastidar, P., Koivisto, A. M., Laippala, P., Vilkki, J., et al. (2000). Visual neglect as a predictor of functional outcome one year after stroke. *Acta Neurologica Scandinavica, 101,* 195–201.

Jehkonen, M., Ahonen, J. P., Dastidar, P., Koivisto, A. M., Laippala, P., Vilkki, J., et al. (2001). Predictors of discharge to home during the first year after right hemisphere stroke. *Acta Neurologica Scandinavica, 104,* 136–141.

Jehkonen, M., Ahonen, J. P., Dastidar, P., Laippala, P., & Vilkki, J. (2000a). Unawareness of deficits after right hemisphere stroke: Double-dissociations of anosognosias. *Acta Neurologica Scandinavica, 102,* 378–384

Joanette, Y., & Brownell, H. H. (1990). *Discourse ability and brain damage: Theoretical and empirical perspectives.* New York: Springer-Verlag.

Joanette, Y., Goulet, P., & Hannequin, D. (1990). *Right hemisphere and verbal communication.* New York: Springer-Verlag.

Jodzio, K., Gasecki, D., Drumm, D. A., Lass, P., & Nyka, W. (2003). Neuroanatomical correlates of the post-stroke aphasias studied with cerebral blood flow SPECT scanning. *Medical Science Monitor, 9,* MT32-MT41.

Johns, J. S., Cifu, D. X., Keyser-Marcus, L., Jolles, P. R., & Fratkin, M. J. (1999). Impact of clinically significant heterotopic ossification on functional outcome after traumatic brain injury. *Journal of Head Trauma Rehabilitation, 14,* 269–276.

Johnson, A. F., Valachovic, A. M., & George, K. P. (1998). Speech-language pathology practice in the acute care setting: A consultative approach. In A. F. Johnson & B. H. Jacobson (Eds.) *Medical speech-language pathology: A practitioner's guide* (pp. 96–130) New York: Thieme.

Johnson, K., & Bourgeois, M. (1998). Language intervention for patients with dementia attending a respite program. *Special Interest Division 2: Neurophysiology and Neurogenic Speech and Language Disorders Newsletter, 8,* 11–16.

Johnson, M. L., Simpson, J. D., & O' Connell, H. S. (2003). *Structured therapy for pragmatic behavior: Working towards generalization.* Poster presented at the Annual Convention of the American Speech-Language-Hearing Association, Chicago, IL.

Johnstone, B., Childers, M. K., & Hoerner, J. (1998). The effects of normal aging on neuropsychological functioning following traumatic brain injury. *Brain Injury, 12,* 569–576.

Jordan, L., Bell, L., Bryan, K., Maxim, J., & Axelrod, L. (2000). *Communicate: Evaluation of a training package for carers of older people with communication impairments.* Middlesex: University College London/Middlesex University.

Jorgensen, H.S., Nakayama, H., Raaschou, H. O., Vive-Larsen, J., Stoier, M., & Olsen, T. S. (1995). Outcome and time course of recovery in stroke. Part 1: Outcome. The Copenhagen stroke study. *Archives of Physical Medicine and Rehabilitation, 76,* 399–405.

Jorm, A. F., Christensen, J., Griffiths, K. M., & Rodgers, B. (2002). Effectiveness of complementary and self-help treatments for depression. *Medical Journal of Australia, 176,* S84–S96.

Jost, B. C., & Grossberg, G. T. (1996). The evolution of psychiatric symptoms in Alzheimer's disease: A naturalistic study. *Journal of the American Geriatrics Society, 44,* 1078–1085.

Kabasawa, H., Matsubara, M., Kamimoto, K., Hibino, H., Banno, T., & Nagia, H. (1994). Effects of bifemelane hydrochloride on cerebral circulation and metabolism in patients with aphasia. *Clinical Therapeutics, 16,* 471–482.

Kafer, K. L., & Hunter, M. (1997). On testing the face validity of planning/problem-solving tasks in a normal population. *Journal of the International Neuropsychology Society, 3,* 108–119.

Kajs-Wyllie, M. (2002). Ritalin revisited: Does it really help in neurological injury? *Journal of Neuroscience Nursing, 34,* 303–313.

Kaga, K., Nakamura, M., Takayama, Y., & Momose, H. (2004). A case of cortical deafness and anarthria. *Acta Oto-Laryngologica, 124,* 202–205.

Kagan, A. (1995). Revealing the competence of aphasic adults through conversation: A challenge to health professionals. *Topics in Stroke Rehabilitation, 2,* 15–28.

Kagan, A., Black, S. E., Duchan, J. F., Simmons-Mackie, N., & Square, P. (2001). Training volunteers as conversation partners using "Supported Conversation for Adults with Aphasia" (SCA): A controlled trial. *Journal of Speech, Language, and Hearing Research, 44,* 624–638.

Kagan, A., Winckel, J., & Shumway, E. (1996). *Supported conversation for aphasic adults: Increasing communicative access* [video]. Toronto, Canada: North York Aphasia Center.

Kahneman, D. (1973). *Attention and effort.* Englewood Cliffs, NJ: Prentice-Hall.

Kalla, T., Downes, J. J., & van den Broek, M. (2001). The pre-exposure technique: Enhancing the effects of errorless learning in the acquisition of face-name associations. *Neuropsychological Rehabilitation, 11,* 1–16.

Kalra, L., Perez, I., Gupta, S., & Wittink, M. (1997). The influence of visual neglect on stroke rehabilitation. *Stroke, 28,* 1386–1391.

Kane, M. J., Bleckley, M. K., Conway, A. R. A., & Engle, R. W. (2001). A controlled-attention view of working-memory capacity. *Journal of Experimental Psychology: General, 130,* 169–183.

Kaplan, E., Goodglass, H., & Weintraub, S. (1983). *Boston Naming Test.* Philadelphia: Lea & Febiger.

Kaplan, E., Goodglass, H., & Weintraub, S. (2001). *Boston Naming Test* (2nd ed.). Philadelphia: Lippincott, Williams & Wilkins.

Kaplan, E., Leach, L., Rewilak, D., Richards, B., & Proulx, G. (2000). *Kaplan Baycrest Neurocognitive Assessment.* San Antonio, TX: The Psychological Corporation.

Karbe, H., Kessler, J., Herholz, K., Fink, G. R., & Heiss, W. D. (1995). Long-term prognosis of poststroke aphasia studied with positron emission tomography. *Archives of Neurology, 52,* 186–190.

Karnath, H. O. (1994). Subjective body orientation in neglect and the interactive contribution of neck muscle proprioception and vestibular stimulation. *Brain, 117,* 1001–1012.

Kaschel, R., Della Sala, S., Cantagallo, A., Fahlbock, A., Laaksonen, R., & Kazen, M. (2002). Imagery mnemonics for the rehabilitation of memory: A randomized group controlled trial. *Neuropsychological Rehabilitation, 12,* 127–153.

Katz, M. M., & Lyerly, S. B. (1963). Methods for measuring adjustment and social behaviour in the community. I. Rationale, description, discriminate validity and scale development. *Psychological Report, 13,* 503–535.

Katz, R. C. (2000). The role of computers in the treatment of people with aphasia: Reflections on the past 20 years. *Special Interest Division 2: Neurophysiology and Neurogenic Speech and Language Disorders Newsletter, 10,* 6–10.

Katz, R. C., Hallowell, B., Code, C., Armstrong, E., Roberts, P., Pound, C., et al. (2000). A multinational comparison of aphasia management practices. *International Journal of Language and Communication Disorders, 35,* 303–314.

Katz, R. C., & Wertz, R. T. (1997). The efficacy of computer-provided reading treatment for chronic aphasic adults. *Journal of Speech, Language, and Hearing Research, 40,* 493–507.

Katzan, I. L., Furlan, A. J., Lloyd, L. E., Frank, J. I., Harper, D. L., Hinchey, J. A., et al. (2000). Use of tissue-type plasminogen activator for acute ischemic stroke: The Cleveland area experience. *JAMA, 283,* 1151–1158.

Kauhanen, M. L., Korpelainen, J. T., Hiltunen, P., Maatta, R., Mononen, H., Brusin, E., et al. (2000). Aphasia, depression, and non-verbal cognitive impairment in ischaemic stroke. *Cerebrovascular Disease, 10,* 455–461.

Kay, J., Byng, S., Edmundson, A., & Scott, C. (1990). Missing the wood and the trees: A reply to David, Kertesz, Goodglass and Weniger. *Aphasiology, 4,* 115–122.

Kay, J., Lesser, R., & Coltheart, M. (1996). Psycholinguistic Assessments of Language Processing in Aphasia (PALPA): An introduction. *Aphasiology, 10,* 159–215.

Kay, J., Lesser, R., & Coltheart, M. (1997). *Psycholinguistic Assessments of Language Processing in Aphasia.* Hove, East Sussex: Psychology Press.

Kayser-Jones, J., Schell, E., Porter, C., Barbaccia, J., & Shaw, H. (1999). Factors contributing to dehydration in nursing homes: Inadequate staffing and lack of professional supervision. *Journal of the American Geriatrics Society, 47,* 1187–1194.

Kearns, K. P. (1985). Response elaboration training for patient initiated utterances. *Clinical Aphasiology, 14,* 196–204.

Kearns, K. P., & Scher, G. P. (1989). The generalization of response elaboration training effects. *Clinical Aphasiology, 18,* 223–245.

Kearns, K. P., Simmons, N. N., & Sisterhen, C. (1982). Gestural sign (Amer-Ind) as a facilitator of verbalization in patients with aphasia. *Clinical Aphasiology, 11,* 183–191.

Keenan, J. S., & Brassell, E. G. (1974). A study of factors related to prognosis for individual aphasic patients. *Journal of Speech and Hearing Disorders, 39,* 257–269.

Keenan, J. S., & Brassell, E. G. (1975). *Aphasia Language Performance Scales.* Murfreesboro, TN: Pinnacle Press.

Keil, K., & Kaszniak, A. W. (2002). Examining executive function in individuals with brain injury: A review. *Aphasiology, 16,* 305–335.

Kellogg, C. E., & Morton, N. W. (1999). *Beta III.* San Antonio, TX: The Psychological Corporation.

Kemper, S., & Harden, T. (1999). Experimentally disentangling what's beneficial about elderspeak from what's not. *Psychological Aging, 14,* 656–670.

Kennedy, M. R. T. (2000). Topic scenes in conversations with adults with right-hemisphere brain damage. *American Journal of Speech-Language Pathology, 9,* 72–86.

Kennepohl, S., Shore, D., Nabors, N., & Hanks, R. (2004). African American acculturation and neuropsychological test performance following traumatic brain injury. *Journal of the International Neuropsychological Society, 10,* 566–577.

Kent, R., Weismer, B., Kent, J., & Rosenbek, J. (1989). Toward phonetic intelligibility testing in dysarthria. *Journal of Speech and Hearing Disorders, 54,* 482–499.

Kent, R. D., Kent, J. F., Duffy, J., & Weismer, G. (1998). The dysarthrias: Speech-voice profiles, related dysfunctions, and neuropathology. *Journal of Medical Speech-Language Pathology, 4,* 165–211.

Keponen, S., Taiminen, T., Portin, R., Himanen, L., Isoniemi, H., Heinonen, H., et al. (2003). Axis I and II psychiatric disorders after traumatic brain injury: A 30-year follow-up study. *American Journal of Psychiatry, 159,* 1315–1321.

Kerkhoff, G. (2000). Multiple perceptual distortions and their modulation in patients with left visual neglect. *Neuropsychologia, 38,* 1073–1086.

Kerkhoff, G. (2001). Spatial hemineglect in humans. *Progress in Neurobiology, 63,* 1–27.

Kertesz, A. (1979). *Aphasia and associated disorders: Taxonomy, localization, and recovery.* New York: Grune and Stratton.

Kertesz, A. (1982). *Western Aphasia Battery.* New York: Grune and Stratton.

Kertesz, A. (1993). *Western Aphasia Battery Scoring Assistant.* San Antonio, TX: The Psychological Corporation.

Kertesz, A., Davidson, W., & Fox, H. (1997). Frontal behavioral inventory: Diagnostic criteria for frontal lobe dementia. *Canadian Journal of Neurological Sciences, 24,* 29–36.

Kertesz, A., Hillis, A., & Munoz, D. G. (2003). Frontotemporal degeneration, Pick's disease, Pick complex, and Ravel. *Annals of Neurology, 54,* S1–S2.

Kertesz, A., & McCabe, P. (1975). Intelligence and aphasia: Performance of aphasics on Raven's Coloured Progressive Matrices (RCPM). *Brain and Language, 2,* 387–395.

Kertesz, A., Sheppard, A., & MacKenzie, R. (1982). Localization in transcortical sensory aphasia. *Archives of Neurology, 39,* 475–478.

Kessler, J., Thiel, A., Karbe, H., & Heiss, W. D. (2000). Piracetam improves activated blood flow and facilitates rehabilitation of poststroke aphasic patients. *Stroke, 31,* 2112–2116.

Kiernan, R. J., Mueller, J., & Langston, J. W. (1995). *Cognistat (Neurobehavioral Cognitive Status Examination).* Lutz, FL: Psychological Assessment Resources.

Kilpatrick, K. (1977). *Therapy guide for language and speech disorders: Reading comprehension materials.* Akron, OH: Visiting Nurse Service.

Kim, H. J., Burke, D. T., Downs, M. M., Robinson-Boone, K., & Parks, G. J. (2000). Electronic memory aids for outpatient brain injury: Follow-up findings. *Brain Injury, 14,* 187–196.

Kim, M., & Thompson, C. K. (2004). Verb deficits in Alzheimer's disease and agrammatism: Implications for lexical organization. *Brain and Language, 88,* 1–20.

King, J. M., & Hux, K. (1996). Attention allocation in adults with and without aphasia: Performance on linguistic and nonlinguistic tasks. *Journal of Medical Speech-Language Pathology, 4,* 245–256.

King, K. A., Hough, M. S., Walker, M., Rastatter, M., & Holbert, D. (2004). *Mild traumatic brain injury: Effects on naming in word retrieval and discourse.* Poster presentation at the annual Clinical Aphasiology Conference, Park City, UT.

King, R. B. (1996). Quality of life after stroke. *Stroke, 27,* 1467–1472.

Kinsella, G. J. (1998). Assessment of attention following traumatic brain injury: A review. *Neuropsychological Rehabilitation, 8,* 351–375.

Kiran, S., & Thompson, C. K. (2003). The role of semantic complexity in treatment of naming deficits: Training semantic categories in fluent aphasia by controlling exemplar typicality. *Journal of Speech, Language, and Hearing Research, 46,* 608–622.

Kirkwood, S. C., Siemers, E., Stout, J., Hodes, M. E., Conneally, P. M., Christian, J. C., et al. (1999). Longitudinal cognitive and motor changes among presymptomatic Huntington disease gene carriers. *Archives of Neurology, 56*, 563–568.

Knauss, D. S. (1998). *Left visual inattention workbook*. San Antonio, TX: Communication Skill Builders.

Knopman, D. S., Knudson, D., Yoes, M. E., & Weiss, D. J. (2000). Development and standardization of a new telephonic cognitive screening test: The Minnesota Cognitive Acuity Screen (MCAS). *Neuropsychiatry, Neuropsychology, and Behavioral Neurology, 13*, 286–296.

Knopman, D. S., & Rubens, A. B. (1986). The validity of computed tomograhic scan findings for the localization of cerebral functions. *Archives of Neurology, 43*, 328–332.

Knott, R., Patterson, K., & Hodges, J. R. (2000). The role of speech production in auditory-verbal short-term memory: Evidence from progressive fluent aphasia. *Neuropsychologia, 38*, 125–142.

Kohler, S., Paus, T., Buckner, R. L., & Milner, B. (2004). Effects of left inferior prefrontal stimulation on episodic memory formation: A two-stage fMRI-rTMS study. *Journal of Cognitive Neuroscience, 16*, 178–188.

Koike, K. J. M., & Asp, C. W. (1981). Tennessee Test of Rhythm and Intonation Patterns. *Journal of Speech and Hearing Disorders, 46*, 81–87.

Kopelman, M. D. (1995). The Korsakoff syndrome. *The British Journal of Psychiatry, 166*, 154–173.

Korda, R. J., & Douglas, J. M. (1997). Attention deficits in stroke patients with aphasia. *Journal of Clinical and Experimental Neuropsychology, 19*, 525–542.

Kovach, C. R. (2000). Sensoristasis and imbalance in persons with dementia. *Journal of Nursing Scholarship, 32*, 379–384.

Kramer, A. M., & Coleman, E. A. (1999). Stroke rehabilitation in nursing homes: How do we measure quality? *Clinics in Geriatric Medicine, 15*, 869–884.

Krasuski, J., Horwitz, B., & Rumsey, J. M. (1996). A survey of functional and anatomical neuroimaging techniques. In G. R. Lyon & J. M. Rumsey (Eds.), *Neuroimaging: A window to the neurological foundations of learning and behavior and children* (pp. 25–52). Baltimore: Paul H. Brookes.

Kraus, J. F., & McArthur, D. L. (1996). Epidemiologic aspects of brain injury. *Neurologic Clinics, 14*, 435–450.

Kraus, J. F., & McArthur, D. L. (1999). Incidence and prevalence of, and cost associated with, traumatic brain injury. In M. Rosenthal, J. S. Kreutzer, E. R. Griffith, & Pentland, B. (Eds.), *Rehabilitation of the adult and child with traumatic brain injury* (3rd ed., pp. 3–18). Philadelphia: F. A. Davis Company.

Krauss, J. K., & Jankovic, J. (2002). Head injury and post-traumatic movement disorders. *Neurosurgery, 50*, 927–948.

Kremin, H., Perrier, D., De Wilde, M., Dordain, M., Le Bayon, A., Gatignol, P., et al. (2001). Factors predicting success in picture naming in Alzheimer's disease and primary progressive aphasia. *Brain and Cognition, 46*, 180–183.

Kreutzer, J. S., Seel, R. T., & Marwitz, J. H. (1999). *Neurobehavioral Functioning Inventory*. San Antonio, TX: The Psychological Corporation.

Kubat-Silman, A. K., Dagenbach, D., & Absher, J. R. (2002). Patterns of impaired verbal, spatial and object working memory after thalamic lesions. *Brain and Cognition, 50*, 178–193.

Laiacona, M., Luzzatti, C., Zonca, G., Guarnaschelli, C., & Capitani, E. (2001). Lexical and semantic factors influencing picture naming in aphasia. *Brain and Cognition, 46,* 184–187.

Lancioni, G. E., Cuvo, A. J., & O'Reilly, M. F. (2002). Snoezelen: An overview of research with people with developmental disabilities and dementia. *Disability and Rehabilitation, 24,* 175–184.

Landesman, S., & Cooper, P. R. (1982). Infectious complications of head injury. In P. R. Cooper (Ed.), *Head injury* (pp. 343–362). Baltimore: Williams & Wilkins.

Lange, G., Waked, W., Kirshblum, S., & DeLuca, J. (2000). Organizational strategy influence on visual memory performance after stroke: Cortical/subcortical and left/right hemisphere contrasts. *Archives of Physical Medicine and Rehabilitation, 81,* 89–94.

Langhorne, P., & Duncan, P. (2001). Does the organization of postacute stroke care really matter? *Stroke, 32,* 268–274.

Laroi, F. (2003). The family systems approach to treating families of persons with brain injury: A potential collaboration between family therapist and brain injury professional. *Brain Injury, 17,* 175–187.

Lawson, M. J., & Rice, D. N. (1989). Effects of training in use of executive strategies on a verbal memory problem resulting from closed head injury. *Journal of Clinical and Experimental Neuropsychology, 11,* 842–854.

Lecours, A. R., Mehler, J., Parente, M. A., & Beltrami, M. C. (1988). Illiteracy and brain damage: III. A contribution to the study of speech and language disorders in illiterates with unilateral brain damage. *Neuropsychologia, 26,* 575–589.

Le Dorze, G., Boulay, N., Gaudreau, J., & Brassard, C. (1994). The contrasting effects of a semantic versus a formal-semantic technique for the facilitation of naming in a case of anomia. *Aphasiology, 8,* 127–141.

Le Dorze, G., & Brassard, C. (1995). A description of the consequences of aphasia on aphasic persons and their relatives and friends, based on the WHO model of chronic diseases. *Aphasiology, 9,* 239–255.

Lee, A. C., Harris, J. P., Atkinson, E. A., & Fowler, M. S. (2001). Evidence from a line bisection task for visuospatial neglect in left hemiparkinson's disease. *Vision Research, 41,* 2677–2686.

Lees, K. R. (1998). Does neuroprotection improve stroke outcome? *The Lancet, 351,* 1447–1448.

Lehman, M. T., & Tompkins, C. A. (1998). Reliability and validity of an auditory working memory measure: Data from elderly and right-hemisphere damaged adults. *Aphasiology, 12,* 771–785.

Lehman Blake, M. (2003). Affective language and humor appreciation after right hemisphere brain damage. *Seminars in Speech and Language, 24,* 107–119.

Lehman Blake, M., Duffy, J. R., Myers, P. S., & Tompkins, C. A. (2002). Prevalence and patterns of right hemisphere cognitive/communicative deficits: Retrospective data from an inpatient rehabilitation unit. *Aphasiology, 16,* 537–547.

Leibovitz, A., Lubart, E., Rabinovich, H., Baumohl, L., Platinovich, N., & Habot, B. (2001). A 10-year perspective on the patients referred to a geriatric rehabilitation complex: The influence of managed care. *Journal of the American Medical Directors Association, 2,* 1–3.

Leischner, A. (1996). Word class effects upon the intrahemispheric graphic disconnection syndrome. *Aphasiology, 10,* 443–451.

Leng, T. R., Woodward, M. J., Stokes, M. J., Swan, A. V., Wareing, L., & Baker, R. (2003). Effects of multisensory stimulation in people with Huntington's disease: A randomized controlled pilot study. *Clinical Rehabilitation, 17,* 30–41.

Leplow, B., Dierks, C., Lehnung, M., Kenkel, S., Behrens, C., Frank, G., et al. (1997). Remote memory in patients with acute brain injuries. *Neuropsychologia, 35,* 881–892.

Lesser, R. (1990). Superior oral to written spelling: Evidence for separate buffers? *Cognitive Neuropsychology, 7,* 347–366.

Levin, B. E., & Katzen, H. L. (1995). Early cognitive changes and nondementing behavioral abnormalities in Parkinson's disease. In W. J. Weiner & A. E. Lang (Eds.), *Advances in neurology: Behavioral neurology of movement disorders* (Vol. 65, pp. 85–95). New York: Raven Press.

Levin, H. S., O'Donnell, V. M., & Grossman, R. G. (1979). The Galveston Orientation and Amnesia Test: A practical scale to assess cognition after head injury. *Journal of Nervous and Mental Disease, 167,* 675–684.

Levine, B., Robertson, I. H., Clare, L., Carter, G., Hong, J., Wilson, B. A., et al. (2000). Rehabilitation of executive functioning: An experimental-clinical validation of Goal Management Training. *Journal of the International Neuropsychological Society, 6,* 299–312.

Lewis-Jack, O. O., Campbell, A. L., Ridley, S., & Ocampo, C. (1997). Unilateral brain lesions and performance on Russell's version of the Wechsler Memory Scale in an African American population. *International Journal of Neuroscience, 9,* 229–240.

Lezak, M. (1995). *Neuropsychological assessment* (3rd ed.). New York: Oxford University Press.

Li, E. C., Kitselman, K., Dusatko, D., & Spinelli, C. (1988). The efficacy of PACE in remediation of naming deficits. *Journal of Communication Disorders, 21,* 491–503.

Li, E. C., Ritterman, S., Della Volpe, A., & Williams, S. E. (1996). Variation in grammatic complexity across three types of discourse. *Journal of Speech-Language Pathology and Audiology, 20,* 180–186.

Li, Y., Meyer, J., Haque, M., Chowdhury, M. H., Hinh, P., & Quach, M. (2002). Feasibility of vascular dementia treatment with cholinesterase inhibitors. *International Journal of Geriatric Psychiatry, 17,* 193–196.

Libin, A., & Cohen-Mansfield, J. (2004). Therapeutic robocat for nursing home residents with dementia: Preliminary inquiry. *American Journal of Alzheimer's Disease and Other Dementias, 19,* 111–116.

Lichtheim, L. (1885). On aphasia. *Brain, 7,* 433–484.

Liddell, M. B., Lovestone, S., & Owen, M. J. (2001). Genetic risk of Alzheimer's disease: Advising relatives. *The British Journal of Psychiatry, 178,* 7–11.

Lieberman, J. D., Pasquale, M., Garcia, R., Cipolle, M., Li, M., & Wasser, T. (2003). Use of admission Glasgow Coma score, pupil size, and pupil reactivity to determine outcome for traumatic patients. *The Journal of Trauma Injury, Infection and Critical Care, 55,* 437–443.

Lin, Y. C., Dai, Y. T., & Huang, S. L. (2003). The effect of reminiscence on the elderly population: A systematic review. *Public Health Nursing, 20,* 297–306.

Lindamood, C. H., & Lindamood, P. C. (1975). *Auditory discrimination in depth.* Austin, TX: Pro-Ed.

Lindenmuth, G., & Lindenmuth, E. (1994). Effects of a three-year exercise therapy program on cognitive functioning of elderly personal care home residents. *American Journal of Alzheimer's Care and Related Disorders, 9,* 20–24.

Little, A., & Doherty, B. (1996). Going beyond cognitive assessment: Assessment of adjustment, behavior, and the environment. In R. T. Woods (Ed.), *Handbook of the clinical psychology of aging* (pp. 475–506). New York: John Wiley and Sons.

Liu, C. J., McDowd, J., & Lin, K. C. (2004). Visuospatial inattention and daily life performance in people with Alzheimer's disease. *American Journal of Occupational Therapy, 58,* 202–210.

Llinas Regla, J., Lozano Gallego, M., Lopez, O. L., Gudayol Portabella, M., Lopez-Pousa, S., Vilalta Franch, J., et al. (1995). [Validation of the Spanish version of the Severe Impairment Battery]. *Neurologia, 10,* 14–18.

Lloyd, L., & Cuvo, A. (1994). Maintenance and generalization of behaviors after treatment of persons with traumatic brain injury. *Brain Injury, 8,* 529–540.

Lo, Y. L., & Cui, S. L. (2003). Acupuncture and the modulation of cortical excitability. *Neuroreport, 14,* 1229–1231.

Lomas, J., Pickard, L., Bester, S., Elbard, H., Finlayson, A., & Zoghaib, C. (1989). The Communicative Effectiveness Index: Development and psychometric evaluation of functional communication measure for adult aphasia. *Journal of Speech and Hearing Disorders, 54,* 113–124.

Lombardi, F., Taricco, M., De Tanti, A., Telaro, E., & Liberati, A. (2002). Sensory stimulation of brain-injured individuals in coma or vegetative state: Results of a Cochrane systematic review. *Clinical Rehabilitation, 16,* 464–472.

Lott, S. N., & Friedman, R. B. (1999). Can treatment for pure alexia improve letter-by-letter reading speed without sacrificing accuracy? *Brain and Language, 67,* 188–201.

Lowell, S., Beeson, P. M., & Holland, A. L. (1995). The efficacy of a semantic cueing procedure on naming performance of adults with aphasia. *American Journal of Speech-Language Pathology, 4,* 109–114.

Lubinski, R. (1991). Dysarthria: A breakdown in interpersonal communication. In D. Vogel & M. P. Cannito (Eds.), *Treating disordered speech motor control: For clinicians by clinicians* (pp. 153–181). Austin, TX: Pro-Ed.

Lubinski, R. (1994). Environmental systems approach to adult aphasia. In R. Chapey (Ed.), *Language intervention strategies in adult aphasia* (3rd ed., pp. 269–291). Baltimore: Williams & Wilkins.

Lubinski, R. (2001). Environmental systems approach to adult aphasia. In R. Chapey (Ed.), *Language intervention strategies in aphasia and related neurogenic communication disorders* (4th ed., pp. 269–296). Philadelphia: Lippincott, Williams & Wilkins.

Lucas, E. (1980). *Semantic and pragmatic language disorders: Assessment and remediation.* Rockville, MD: Aspen.

Ludwig, B. (1993). Post-traumatic seizures. *Physical Medicine and Rehabilitation: State of the Art Reviews, 7,* 461–467.

Lukovits, T., Mazzone, T., & Gorelick, P. (1999). Diabetes mellitus and cerebrovascular disease. *Neuroepidemiology, 18,* 1–14.

Luterman, D. M. (2001). *Counseling persons with communication disorders and their families.* Austin, TX: Pro-Ed.

Luukinen, H., Viramo, P., Koski, K., Laippala, P., & Kivela, S. L. (1999). Head injuries and cognitive decline among older adults: A population-based study. *Neurology, 52,* 557–562.

Luzzi, S., & Piccirilli, M. (2003). Slowly progressive pure dysgraphia with late apraxia of speech: A further variant of the focal cerebral degeneration. *Brain and Language, 87,* 355–360.

Lyketsos, C. G., Chen, L., & Anthony, J. C. (1999). Cognitive decline in adulthood: An 11.5-year follow-up of the Baltimore epidemiologic catchment area study. *The American Journal of Psychiatry, 156*, 58–65.

Lyon, J. G. (1998). *Coping with aphasia*. Clifton Park, NY: Singular Thomson Delmar Learning.

Lyon, J. G., Cariski, D., Keisler, L., Rosenbek, J., Levine, R., Kumpula, J., et al. (1997). Communication partners: Enhancing participation in life and communication for adults with aphasia in natural settings. *Aphasiology, 11*, 693–708.

Lyon, J. G., & Helm-Estabrooks, N. (1987). Drawing: Its communicative significance for expressively restricted aphasic adults. *Topics in Language Disorders, 8*, 61–71.

Machamer, J., Temkin, N., & Dikmen, S. (2002). Significant other burden and factors related to it in traumatic brain injury. *Journal of Clinical and Experimental Neuropsychology, 24*, 420–433.

Mackay, L. E., Chapman, P. E., & Morgan, A. S. (1997). *Maximizing brain injury recovery*. Gaithersburg, MD: Aspen.

MacKenzie, C. (2000). The relevance of education and age in the assessment of discourse comprehension. *Clinical Linguistics and Phonetics, 14*, 151–161.

Mackenzie, C., Begg, T., Lees, K., & Brady, M. (1999). The communication effects of right brain damage on the very old and the not so old. *Journal of Neurolinguistics, 12*, 79–93.

MacLennan, D. L., Nicholas, L. E., Morley, G. K., & Brookshire, R. H. (1991). The effects of bromocriptine on speech and language function in a man with transcortical motor aphasia. *Clinical Aphasiology, 21*, 145–155.

Maddicks, R., Marzillier, S. L., & Parker, G. (2003). Rehabilitation of unilateral neglect in the acute recovery stage: The efficacy of limb activation therapy. *Neuropsychological Rehabilitation, 13*, 391–408.

Maeshima, S., Toshiro, H., Sekiguchi, E., Okita, R., Yamaga, H., Ozaki, F., et al. (2002). Transcortical mixed aphasia due to cerebral infarction in left inferior frontal lobe and temporo-parietal lobe. *Neuroradiology, 44*, 133–137.

Mahendra, N., & Arkin, S. (2003). Effects of four years of exercise, language, and social interventions on Alzheimer discourse. *Journal of Communication Disorders, 36*, 395–422.

Mahendra, N., & Arkin, S. (2004). Exercise and volunteer work: Contexts for AD language and memory interventions. *Seminars in Speech and Language, 25*, 151–165.

Maher, L. M., Clayton, M. C., Barrett, A. M., Schober-Peterson, D., & Rothi, L. J. G. (1998). Rehabilitation of a case of pure alexia: Exploiting residual abilities. *Journal of the International Neuropsychological Society, 4*, 636–647.

Malia, K. B., Bewick, K. C., Raymond, M. J., & Bennet, T. L. (1997). *Brainwave-Revised*. Austin, TX: Pro-Ed.

Man, D. W., & Li, R. (2001). Assessing Chinese adults' memory abilities: Validation of the Chinese version of the Rivermead Behavioral Memory Test. *Clinical Gerontologist, 24*, 27–36.

Mangino, M., Middlemiss, C. (1997). Alzheimer's disease: Preventing and recognizing a misdiagnosis. *The Nurse Practitioner, 22*, 58–75.

Manly, T. (2002). Cognitive rehabilitation for unilateral neglect: Review. *Neuropsychological Rehabilitation, 12*, 289–310.

Manly, T., Hawkins, K., Evans, J., Woldt, K., & Robertson, I. H. (2002). Rehabilitation of executive function: Facilitation of effective goal management on complex tasks using periodic auditory alerts. *Neuropsychologia, 40*, 271–281.

Manly, T., Joost, H., Davison, B., Gaynord, B., Greenfield, E., Parr, A., et al. (2004). An electronic knot in the handkerchief: "Content free cueing" and the maintenance of attentive control. *Neuropsychological Rehabilitation, 14,* 89–117.

Manochiopinig, S., Reed, V. A., Sheard, C., & Choo, P. (1997). Significant others' perceptions of speech pathology services for Thai aphasic speakers. *Aphasiology, 11,* 210–217.

Mapou, R. L., Kramer, J. H., & Blusewicz, M. J. (1989). Performance on the California Discourse Memory Test following closed head injury. *Journal of Clinical and Experimental Neuropsychology, 11,* 58.

Marin, D., Sewell, M., & Schlechter, A. (2002). Alzheimer's disease: Accurate and early diagnosis in the primary care setting. *Geriatrics, 57,* 427–s433.

Markowitsch, H. (1998). Cognitive neuroscience of memory. *Neurocase, 4,* 429–435.

Markwardt, F. C. (1997). *Peabody Individual Achievement Test-Revised.* Circle Pines, MN: American Guidance Service.

Marsh, N. V., Kersel, D. A., Havill, J. H., & Sleigh, J. W. (1998). Caregiver burden at one year following severe traumatic brain injury. *Brain Injury, 12,* 1045–1059.

Marsh, N. V., Kersel, D. A., Havill, J. H., & Sleigh, J. W. (2002). Caregiver burden during the year following severe traumatic brain injury. *Journal of Clinical and Experimental Neuropsychology, 24,* 434–447.

Marshall, J. C., & Halligan, P. W. (1988). Blindsight and insight in visuo-spatial neglect. *Nature, 336,* 766–767.

Marshall, R. C. (1997). Aphasia treatment in the early postonset period: Managing our resources effectively. *American Journal of Speech-Language Pathology, 6,* 5–11.

Marshall, R. C. (1999). A problem-focused group treatment program for clients with mild aphasia. In R. J. Elman (Ed.), *Group treatment of neurogenic communication disorders: The expert clinician's approach* (pp. 57–65). Boston: Butterworth-Heinemann.

Marshall, R. C. (2001). Management of Wernicke's aphasia: Context-based approach. In R. Chapey (Ed.), *Language intervention strategies in aphasia and related neurogenic communication disorders* (4th ed., pp. 435–456). Philadelphia: Lippincott, Williams & Wilkins.

Marshall, R. C., Karow, C. M., Freed, D., & Babcock, P. (2002). Effects of personalized cue form on the learning of subordinate category names by aphasic and non-brain-damaged subjects. *Aphasiology, 16,* 763–771.

Marshall, R. C., Karow, C. M., Morelli, C. A., Iden, K. K., & Dixon, J. (2003). A clinical measure for the assessment of problem solving in brain-injured adults. *American Journal of Speech-Language Pathology, 12,* 333–348.

Marshall, R. C., & Neuburger, S. (1984). Extended comprehension training reconsidered. *Clinical Aphasiology, 14,* 181–187.

Marshall, R. C., & Watts, M. T. (1976). Relaxation training: Effects of communicative ability of aphasic adults. *Archives of Physical Medicine and Rehabilitation, 57,* 464–467.

Martelli, M. (1999, December). Protocol for increasing initiation, decreasing adynamia. *HeadsUp: RSS Newsletter,* 2 & 9.

Martin, I., & McDonald, S. (2003). Weak coherence, no theory of mind, or executive dysfunction? Solving the puzzle of pragmatic language disorders. *Brain and Language, 85,* 451–466.

Masanic, C. A., Bayley, M. T., & van Reekum, R. (2001). Open-label study of donepezil in traumatic brain injury. *Archives of Physical Medicine and Rehabilitation, 82,* 896–901.

Massaro, M. E., & Tompkins, C. A. (1992). Feature analysis for treatment of communication disorders in traumatically brain injured patients: An efficacy study. *Clinical Aphasiology, 22,* 245–256.

Mateer, C. A. (1999). Executive function disorders: Rehabilitation challenges and strategies. *Seminars in Clinical Neuropsychiatry, 4,* 50–59.

Mateer, C. A., Kerns, K. A., & Eso, K. L. (1999). Management of attention and memory disorders following traumatic brain injury. *Journal of learning Disabilities, 29,* 618–632.

Mateer, C. A., Polen, S. B., Ojemann, G. A., & Wyler, A. R. (1982). Cortical localization of finger spelling and oral language: A case study. *Brain and Language, 17,* 46–57.

Mateer, C. A., Rapport, R. L., & Kettrick, C. (1984). Cerebral organization of oral and signed language responses: Case study evidence from amytal and cortical stimulation studies. *Brain and Language, 21,* 123–135.

Mathias, J. L., Beall, J., & Bigler, E. D. (2004). Neuropsychological and information processing deficits following mild traumatic brain injury. *Journal of the International Neuropsychological Society, 10,* 286–297.

Matser, J. T., Kessels, A.G., Jordan, B. D., Lezak, M. D., & Troost, J. (1998). Chronic traumatic brain injury in professional soccer players. *Neurology, 51,* 791–796.

Matthews, C. G., Harley, J. P., & Malec, J. F. (1992). Guidelines for computer-assisted neuropsychological rehabilitation and cognitive remediation. In K. M. Adams & B. P. Rouke (Eds.), *The TCN guide to professional practice in clinical neuropsychology* (pp. 120–136). Amsterdam: Swets & Zeitlinger.

Mattis, S. (2001). *Dementia Rating Scale-2.* Lutz, FL: Psychological Assessment Resources.

Maxim, J., Bryan, K., Axelrod, L., Jordan, L., & Bell, L. (2001). Speech and language therapists as trainers: Enabling care staff working with older people. *International Journal of Language and Communication, 33,* 194–199.

Maxwell, W. L., Watt, C., Graham, D. I., & Gennarelli, T. A. (1993). Ultrastructural evidence of axonal shearing as a result of lateral acceleration of the head in non-human primates. *Acta Neuropathologica, 86,* 136–144.

Mayberg, H. S., & Solomon, D. H. (1995). Depression in Parkinson's disease: A biochemical and organic viewpoint. In W. J. Weiner & A. E. Lang (Eds.), *Advances in neurology: Behavioral neurology of movement disorders* (Vol. 65, pp. 49–60). New York: Raven Press.

Mayer, J. F., & Murray, L. L. (2002). Approaches to the treatment of alexia in chronic aphasia. *Aphasiology, 16,* 727–744.

Mayer, J. F., & Murray, L. L. (2003). Functional measures of naming in aphasia: Word-retrieval in confrontation naming versus connected speech. *Aphasiology, 17,* 481–498.

Mayer, J. F., Murray, L. L., & Karcher, L. A. (2004). *Treatment of anomia in severe aphasia.* Clinical Aphasiology Conference, Park City, UT.

Mayer, N. H., Keenan, M. E., & Esquenzi, A. (1999). Limbs with restricted or excessive motion after traumatic brain injury. In M. Rosenthal, E. R. Griffith, J. S. Kreutzer, & B. Pentland (Eds.), *Rehabilitation of the adult and child with traumatic brain injury* (3rd ed., pp. 503–535). Philadelphia: F. A. Davis.

Mayeux, R., Stern, Y., Rosenstein, R., Marder K., Hauser A., Cote, L., et al. (1988). An estimate of the prevalence of dementia in idiopathic Parkinson's disease. *Archives of Neurology, 45,* 260–262.

Maynard, C. K. (2003). Differentiate depression from dementia. *The Nurse Practitioner, 28,* 18–27.

Mazaux, J. M., & Orgozo, J. M. (1981). *Boston Diagnostic Aphasia Examination: Échelle française.* Paris: Éditions scientifiques et psychologiques.

Mazzocchi, F., & Vignolo, L. A. (1979). Localization of lesions in aphasia: Clinical-CT scan correlations in stroke patients. *Cortex, 15,* 627–653.

McAllister, T. W., Flashman, L. A., Sparling M. B., & Sayking, A. J. (2004). Working memory deficits after traumatic brain injury: Catecholaminergic mechanisms and prospects for treatment: A review. *Brain Injury, 18,* 331–350.

McCooey, R., Toffolo, D., & Code, C. (2000). A socioenvironmental approach to functional communication in hospital in-patients. In L. Worrall & C. M. Frattali (Eds.), *Neurogenic communication disorders: A functional approach* (pp. 295–311). New York: Thieme.

McDonald, B. C., Flashman, L. A., & Saykin, A. J. (2002). Executive dysfunction following traumatic brain injury: Neural substrates and treatment strategies. *Neurorehabilitation, 17,* 333–344.

McDonald, S. (1992). Communication disorders following closed head injury: New approaches to assessment and rehabilitation. *Brain Injury, 6,* 283–292.

McDonald, S. (1993). Pragmatic skills after closed head injury: Ability to meet the informational needs of the listener. *Brain and Language, 44,* 28–46.

McDonald, S. (2000). Exploring the cognitive basis of right-hemisphere pragmatic language disorders. *Brain and Language, 75,* 82–107.

McDonald, S., Flanagan, S., & Rollins, J. (2002). *The Awareness of Social Inference Test.* Bury St. Edmunds, Suffolk, England: Thames Valley Test Company.

McDonald, S., & Pearce, S. (1998). Requests that overcome listener reluctance: Impairment associated with executive dysfunction in brain injury. *Brain and Language, 61,* 88–104.

McDonald, S., Togher, L., & Code, C. (Eds.). (1999). *Communication disorders following traumatic brain injury.* East Sussex, UK: Psychology Press.

McDowell, I., Kristjansson, B., Hill, G. B., & Hebert, R. (1997). Community screening for dementia: The Mini-Mental State Exam and Modified Mini-Mental State Exam compared. *Journal of Clinical Epidemiology, 50,* 377–383.

McGann, W., & Werven, G. (1999). *Social communication skills for children: A workbook for principle-centered communication.* Austin, TX: Pro-Ed.

McGuire, L.M., Burright, R. G., Williams, R., & Donovick, P. J.(1998). Prevalence of traumatic brain injury in psychiatric and non-psychiatric subjects. *Brain Injury, 12,* 207–214.

McKhann, G., Drachman, D., Folstein, M., Katzman, R., Price, D., & Stadlan, E. M. (1984). Clinical diagnosis of Alzheimer's disease: Report of the NINCDS-ADRDA Work Group under the auspices of Department of Health and Human Services Task Force on Alzheimer's Disease. *Neurology, 34,* 939–44.

McKitrick, L. A., & Camp, C. J. (1993). Relearning the names of things: The spaced-retrieval intervention implemented by caregivers. *Clinical Gerontologist, 14,* 60–62.

McLaughlin, S. A., Rogers, M. A., & Shibata, D. K. (2003). A primer on functional magnetic resonance imaging (fMRI). *Perspectives on Neurophysiology and Neurogenic Speech and Language Disorders, 13,* 25–33.

McNair, D. M., Lorr, M., & Droppleman, L. F. (1981). *Profile of Mood States.* San Diego, CA: Educational and Industrial Testing Service.

McNeil, M. R. (1982). The nature of aphasia in adults. In N. J. Lass (Ed.), *Speech, language, and hearing* (Vol. 2, pp. 692–740). W. B. Saunders.

McNeil, M. R., Odell, K., & Tseng, C. (1991). Toward the integration of resource allocation into and general theory of aphasia. *Clinical Aphasiology, 20,* 21–36.

McNeil, M. R., & Prescott, T. E. (1978). *Revised Token Test*. Baltimore: University Park Press.

McNeil, M. R., Small, S. L., Masterson, R. J., & Fossett, T. R. (1995). Behavioral and pharmacological treatment of lexical-semantic deficits in a single patient with primary progressive aphasia. *American Journal of Speech-Language Pathology, 4*, 76–87.

McReynolds, L. V., & Kearns, K. P. (1983). *Single subject experimental designs in communicative disorders*. Austin, TX: Pro-Ed.

Melamed, L. E. (2000). *Kent Visual Perceptual Test*. Odessa, FL: Psychological Assessment Resources.

Melamed, S., Grosswasser, Z., & Stern, M. J. (1992). Acceptance of disability, work involvement, and subjective rehabilitation status of traumatic brain-injured patients. *Brain Injury, 6*, 233–243.

Menn, L., Ramsberger, G., Helm-Estabrooks, N. (1994). A linguistic communication measure for aphasic narratives. *Aphasiology, 8*, 343–359.

Mentis, M., & Prutting, C. (1991). Analysis of topic as illustrated in a head-injured and normal adult. *Journal of Speech and Hearing Research, 34*, 583–595.

Merrick, E. E., Donders, J., & Wiersum, M. (2003). Validity of the WCST-64 after traumatic brain injury. *The Clinical Neuropsychologist, 17*, 153–158.

Messenger, B., & Ziarnek, N. (2004). *Functional rehabilitation activity manuals*. Wake Forest, NC: Lash & Associates.

Mesulam, M. M. (1981). A cortical network for directed attention and unilateral neglect. *Annals of Neurology, 10*, 309–325.

Metter, E. J., Kempler, D., Jackson, C., Hanson, W. R., Mazziotta, J. C., & Phelps, M. E. (1989). Cerebral glucose metabolism in Wernicke's, Broca's, and conduction aphasia. *Archives Neurology, 46*, 27–34.

Metter, E. J., Riege, W. H., Hanson, W. R., Kuhl, D. E., Phelps, M. E., Squire, L. R., et al. (1983). Comparison of metabolic rates, language, and memory in subcortical aphasias. *Brain and Language, 19*, 33–47.

Meyers, J. E., & Meyers, K. R. (1995). *Rey Complex Figure Test and Recognition Trial*. Odessa, FL: Psychological Assessment Resources.

Meythaler, J. M., Depalma, L., Devivo, M. J., Guin-Renfroe, S., & Novack, T. A. (2001). Sertraline to improve arousal and alertness in severe traumatic brain injury secondary to motor vehicle crashes. *Brain Injury, 15*, 321–331.

Miller, E. (1992). Psychological approaches to the management of memory impairments. *British Journal of Psychiatry, 160*, 1–6.

Miller, N. (2002). The neurological bases of apraxia of speech. *Seminars in Speech and Language, 23*, 223–230.

Mitchum, C. C., & Berndt, R. S. (1991). Diagnosis and treatment of the non-lexical route in acquired dyslexia: An illustration of the cognitive neuropsychological approach. *Journal of Neurolinguistics, 6*, 103–137.

Mitchum, C. C., & Berndt, R. S. (1995). The cognitive neuropsychological approach to treatment of language disorders. *Neuropsychological Rehabilitation, 5*, 1–16.

Miyake, A., Emerson, M. J., & Friedman, N. P. (2000). Assessment of executive functions in clinical settings: Problems and recommendations. *Seminars in Speech and Language, 21*, 169–183.

Mizuno, E., Hosaka, T., Ogihara, R., Higano, H., & Mano, Y. (1999). Effectiveness of a stress management program for family caregivers of the elderly at home. *Journal of Medical and Dental Sciences, 46*, 145–153.

Mlcoch, A. G., & Metter, E. J. (2001). Medical aspects of stroke rehabilitation. In R. Chapey (Ed.), *Language intervention strategies in adult aphasia* (4th ed., pp. 37–54). Baltimore: Lippincott, Williams & Wilkins.

Mohr, J. P. (1976). Broca's area and Broca's aphasia. In H. Whitaker & H. Whitaker (Eds.), *Studies in neurolinguistics* (Vol. 1, pp. 201–235). New York: Academic Press.

Molrine, C. J., & Pierce, R. S. (2002). Black and white adults' expressive language performance on three tests of aphasia. *American Journal of Speech-Language Pathology, 11,* 139–150.

Moran, A. J. (1976). Six cases of severe head injury treated by exercise in addition to other therapies. *Medical Journal of Australia, 1,* 396–397.

Moran, C., & Gillon, G. (2004). Language and memory profiles of adolescents with traumatic brain injury. *Brain Injury, 18,* 273–288.

Morgan, A. L. R., & Helm-Estabrooks, N. (1987). Back to the drawing board: A treatment program for nonverbal aphasic patients. *Clinical Aphasiology, 19,* 64–72.

Morley, J. E. (1999). An overview of diabetes mellitus in older persons. *Clinics in Geriatric Medicine, 15,* 211–224.

Morris, J., Franklin, S., Ellis, A. W., Turner, J. E., & Bailey, P. J. (1996). Remediating a speech perception deficit in an aphasic patient. *Aphasiology, 10,* 137–158.

Mortley, J., Enderby, P., & Petheram, B. (2001). Using a computer to improve functional writing in a patient with severe dysgraphia. *Aphasiology, 15,* 443–461.

Mullen, R. (2004). Evidence for whom? ASHA's National Outcomes Measurement System. *Journal of Communication Disorders, 37,* 413–417.

Murray, L. L. (1998). Longitudinal treatment of primary progressive aphasia: A case study. *Aphasiology, 12,* 651–672.

Murray, L. L. (1999). Attention and aphasia: Theory, research and clinical implications. *Aphasiology, 13,* 91–112.

Murray, L. L. (2000). The effects of varying attentional demands on the word-retrieval skills of adults with aphasia, right hemisphere brain damage or no brain damage. *Brain and Language, 72,* 40–72.

Murray, L. L. (2000). Spoken language production in Huntington's and Parkinson's diseases. *Journal of Speech, Language and Hearing Research, 43,* 1350–1366.

Murray, L. L. (2002). Attention deficits in aphasia: Presence, nature, assessment and treatment. *Seminars in Speech and Language, 23,* 107–116.

Murray, L. L. (2002). Cognitive distinctions between depression and early Alzheimer's disease in the elderly. *Aphasiology, 16,* 573–586.

Murray, L. L. (2004a). Cognitive treatments for aphasia: Should we and can we help attention and working memory problems? *Medical Journal of Speech-Language Pathology, 12,* xxi–xxxviii.

Murray, L. L. (2004b). *Semantic processing in aphasia and right hemisphere brain damage: The effects of increased attention demands.* Clinical Aphasiology Conference, Park City, UT.

Murray, L. L., Ballard, K., & Karcher, L. (2004). Linguistic Specific Treatment: Just for Broca's aphasia? *Aphasiology, 18,* 785–809.

Murray, L. L., & Chapey, R. (2001). Assessment of language disorders in adults. In R. Chapey (Ed.), *Language intervention strategies in adult aphasia* (4th ed., pp. 55–126). New York: Lippincott, Williams & Wilkins.

Murray, L. L., Dickerson, S., Lichtenberger, B., & Cox, C. (2003). Effects of toy stimulation on the cognitive, communicative, and emotional functioning of adults in the middle stages of Alzheimer's disease. *Journal of Communication Disorders, 36,* 101–127.

Murray, L. L., Holland, A. L., & Beeson, P. M. (1998). Spoken language of individuals with mild fluent aphasia under focused and divided attention conditions. *Journal of Speech, Language, and Hearing Research, 41,* 213–227.

Murray, L. L., & Karcher, L. (2000). Treating written verb retrieval and sentence construction skills: A case study. *Aphasiology, 14,* 585–602.

Murray, L. L., & Kean, J. (2004). Resource theory and aphasia: Time to abandon or time to revise? *Aphasiology, 18,* 830–835.

Murray, L. L., Keeton, R. J., & Karcher, L. (in press). Treating attention in mild aphasia: Evaluation of Attention Process Training–II. *Journal of Communication Disorders.*

Murray, L. L., & Kim, H. Y. (2004). A review of select alternative treatment approaches for acquired neurogenic disorders: Relaxation therapy and acupuncture. *Seminars in Speech and Language, 25,* 133–149.

Murray, L. L., & Kim, H. Y. (2005). Phonological naming treatment for a Korean-speaking patient with severe fluent aphasia. *Asia Pacific Journal of Speech, Language and Hearing, 9,* 143–168.

Murray, L. L., & Ramage, A. E. (2000). Assessing the executive function abilities of adults with neurogenic communication disorders. *Seminars in Speech and Language, 21,* 153–168.

Murray, L. L., Ramage, A. E., & Hopper, T. (2001). Memory impairments in adults with neurogenic communication disorders. *Seminars in Speech and Language, 22,* 127–136.

Murray, L. L., & Ray, A. H. (2001). A comparison of relaxation training and syntax stimulation for chronic nonfluent aphasia. *Journal of Communication Disorders, 34,* 87–113.

Murray, L. L., & Stout, J. C. (1999). Discourse comprehension in Huntington's and Parkinson's diseases. *American Journal of Speech-Language Pathology, 8,* 137–148.

Myers, P. (1999). *Right hemisphere damage: Disorders of communication and cognition.* Clifton Park, NY: Singular Thomson Delmar Learning.

Myers, P. S., & Brookshire, R. H. (1994). The effects of visual and inferential complexity on the picture descriptions of non-brain-damaged and right-hemisphere-damaged adults. *Clinical Aphasiology, 22,* 25–34.

Mykhalovskiy, E., & Weir, L. (2004). The problem of evidence-based medicine: Directions for social science. *Social Science and Medicine, 59,* 1059–1069.

Naeser, M., & Helm-Estabrooks, N. (1985). CT scan lesion localization and response to Melodic Intonation Therapy with nonfluent aphasia cases. *Cortex, 21,* 203–223.

Naeser, M. A., Alexander, M. P., Helm-Estabrooks, N., Levine, H. L., Laughlin, S. A., & Geschwind, N. (1982). Aphasia with predominantly subcortical lesion sites: description of three capsular/putaminal aphasia syndromes. *Archives of Neurology, 39,* 2–14.

Naeser, M. A., Baker, E. H., Palumbo, C. L., Nicholas, M., Alexander, M. P., Samaraweera, R., et al. (1998). Lesion site patterns in severe, nonverbal aphasia to predict outcome with a computer-assisted treatment program. *Archives of Neurology, 55,* 1438–1448.

Naeser, M. A., & Palumbo, C. L. (1994). Neuroimaging and language recovery in stroke. *Journal of Clinical Neurophysiology, 11,* 150–174.

Naeser, M. A., Palumbo, C. L., Helm-Estabrooks, N., Stiassny-Eder, D., & Albert, M. L. (1989). Severe nonfluency in aphasia. Role of the medial subcallosal fasciculus and other white matter pathways in recovery of spontaneous speech. *Brain, 112* (Pt 1), *1–38.*

Nagaratnam, N., & Lewis-Jones, M. (1998). Predictive properties of referral communications for mental illness and dementia in a community. *Dementia and Geriatric Cognitive Disorders, 9,* 117–120.

Nagaratnam, N., Phan, T. A., Barnett, C., & Ibrahim, N. (2002). Angular gyrus syndrome mimicking depressive pseudodementia. *Journal of Psychiatry and Neuroscience, 27,* 364–368.

Nagaratnam, N., Plew, J., & Cooper, S. (1998). Pure agraphia following periendarterectomy stroke. *Internationl Journal of Clinical Practice, 52,* 203–204.

Nakase-Thompson, R., Sherer, M., Yablon, S. A., Manning, E., Vickery, C., & Eng, W. (2003). *Assessment of language among neurorehabilitation admissions: Convergent and divergent validity of the Mississippi Aphasia Screening Test.* Poster presentation at the annual International Neuropsychology Society conference, Waikiki, HI.

National Center for Complementary and Alternative Medicine. (2002). *What is Complementary and Alternative Medicine? Publication No. D156.* Bethesda, MD: Author.

National Head Injury Foundation Task Force (NHIF) on Special Education. (1989). *An educator's manual: What educators need to know about students with traumatic brain injury.* Southborough, MA: NHIF.

National Institute of Aging. (2003). *Alzheimer's disease progress report 2001–2001* (NIH Publication No. 03-5333). Washington, DC: U.S. Department of Health and Human Services.

National Institute of Neurological Disorders and Stroke. (2001). *Huntington's disease: Hope through research.* Available: http://www.ninds.nih.gov/health_and_medical/pubs/huntington_disease-htr.htm.

National Institute of Neurological Disorders and Stroke. (2002). *Traumatic brain injury: Hope through research* (NIH Publication No. 02-158). Bethesda, MD: Author.

National Institute of Neurological Disorders and Stroke. (2003). *Parkinson's disease: Hope through research.* Available: http://www.ninds.nih.gov/health_and_medical/pubs/parkinson_disease_htr.htm.

National Institutes of Health Consensus Development Panel on Rehabilitation of Persons with Traumatic Brain Injury. (1999). Rehabilitation of persons with traumatic brain injury. *JAMA, 282,* 974–983.

National Stroke Association. (2002). *All about stroke.* Available: http://www.stroke.org.

Nayak, S., Wheeler, B. L., Shiflett, S., & Agostinelli, S. (2000). Effect of music therapy on mood and social interaction among individuals with acute traumatic brain injury and stroke. *Rehabilitation Psychology, 45,* 274–283.

Nehemkis, A. M., & Lewinsohn, P. M. (1972). Effects of left and right cerebral lesions on the memory process. *Perceptual Motor Skills, 35,* 787–798.

Neils, J., Baris, J. M., Carter, C., Dellaira, A. L., Nordloh, S., Weiler, E., et al. (1995). Effects of age, education, and living environment on Boston Naming Test performance. *Journal of Speech and Hearing Research, 38,* 1143–1149.

Neils-Strunjas, J. (1998). Clinical assessment strategies: Evaluation of language comprehension and production by formal test batteries. In B. Stemmer & H. A. Whitaker (Eds.), *Handbook of neurolinguistics* (pp. 71–82). New York: Academic Press.

Neisser, U. (1967). *Cognitive psychology.* New York: Appleton-Century-Crofts.

Nelson, A., Fogel, B. S., & Faust, D. (1986). Bedside cognitive screening instruments: A critical assessment. *Journal of Nervous and Mental Disorders, 174,* 73–83.

Nelson, E. C., Wasson, J., Kirk, J., Keller, A., Clark, D., Dietrich, A., et al. (1987). Assessment of function in routine clinical practice: Description of the COOP Chart method and preliminary findings. *Journal of Chronic Diseases, 40,* 55S-69S.

Nelson, H. E. (1976). A modified Wisconsin Card Sorting Test sensitive to frontal lobe defects. *Cortex, 12,* 313–324.

Nelson, L. D., Mitrushina, M., Satz, P., Sowa, M., & Cohen, S. (1993). Cross-validation of the Neuropsychology Behavior and Affect Profile in stroke patients. *Psychological Assessment, 5,* 374–376.

Nelson, L. D., Satz, P., Mitrushina, M., Van Gorp, W., Cicchetti, D., Lewis, R., et al. (1989). Development and validation of the Neuropsychology Behavior and Affect Profile. *Psychological Assessment, 1,* 266–272.

Newcombe, F., Oldfield, R. C., Ratcliff, G. G., & Wingfield, A. (1971). Recognition and naming of object-drawing by men with focal brain wounds. *Journal of Neurosurgery and Psychiatry, 34,* 329–340.

Ni, W., Constable, R. T., Mencl, W. E., Pugh, K. R., Fulbright, R. K., Shaywitz, S. E., et al. (2000). An event-related neuroimaging study distinguishing form and content in sentence processing. *Journal of Cognitive Neuroscience, 12,* 120–133.

Nicholas, L. E., & Brookshire, R. H. (1993). A system for quantifying the informativeness and efficiency of the connected speech of adults with aphasia. *Journal of Speech and Hearing Research, 36,* 338–350.

Nicholas, L. E., & Brookshire, R. H. (1995a). Comprehension of spoken narrative discourse by adults with aphasia, right-hemisphere brain damage, or traumatic brain injury. *American Journal of Speech-Language Pathology, 4,* 69–81.

Nicholas, L. E., & Brookshire, R. H. (1995b). Presence, completeness, and accuracy of main concepts in the connected speech of non-brain-damaged adults and adults with aphasia. *Journal of Speech and Hearing Research, 38,* 145–156.

Nicholas, L. E., MacLennan, D. L., & Brookshire, R. H. (1986). Validity of multiple-sentence reading comprehension tests for aphasic adults. *Journal of Speech and Hearing Disorders, 51,* 82–87.

Nicholas, M., & Elliott, S. (1999). *C-Speak Aphasia: A communication system for adults with aphasia.* Solana Beach, CA: Mayer-Johnson.

Nicholas, M. L., Helm-Estabrooks, N., Ward-Lonergan, J., & Morgan, A. R. (1993). Evolution of severe aphasia in the first two years post onset. *Archives of Physical Medicine and Rehabilitation, 74,* 830–836.

Nicholson, K. G., Baum, S., Kilgour, A., Koh, C. K., Munhall, K. G., & Cuddy, L. L. (2003). Impaired processing of prosodic and musical patterns after right hemisphere damage. *Brain and Cognition, 52,* 382–389.

Nickels, L. A. (1995). Getting it right? Using aphasic naming errors to evaluate theoretical models of spoken word production. *Language and Cognitive Processes, 10,* 13–45.

Nickels, L. A., & Best, W. (1996). Therapy for naming disorders (Part I): Principles, puzzles, and progress. *Aphasiology, 10,* 21–47.

Nickels, L. A., & Cole-Virtue, J. (2004). Reading tasks from PALPA: How do controls perform on visual lexical decision, homophony, rhyme, and synonym judgements? *Aphasiology, 18,* 103–126.

Nickels, L. A., & Howard, D. (1995). Aphasic naming: What matters? *Neuropsychologia, 33,* 1281–1303.

Niemann, H., Ruff, R. M., & Baser, C. A. (1990). Computer-assisted attention retraining in head-injured individuals: A controlled efficacy study of an outpatient program. *Journal of Consulting and Clinical Psychology, 58,* 811–817.

Niemeier, J. P. (1998). The Lighthouse Strategy: Use of a visual imagery technique to treat visual inattention in stroke patients. *Brain Injury, 12,* 399–406.

Noe, E., Marder, K., Bell, K. L., Jacobs, D. M., Manly, J., & Stern, Y. (2004). Comparison of dementia with Lewy bodies to Alzheimer's disease and Parkinson's disease with dementia. *Movement Disorders, 19,* 60–67.

Norman, D. A., & Shallice, T. (1986). Attention to action: Willed and automatic control of behavior. In R. J. Davidson, G. E. Schwartz, & D. Shapiro (Eds.), *Consciousness and self-regulation* (pp. 1–18). New York: Plenum Press.

North Carolina Board of Examiners (1999). Speech-language pathology assistants. *North Carolina Board of Examiners Directory* (1999 ed.). Greensboro, N.C.: North Carolina Board of Examiners.

Nussbaum, P. D. (1994). Pseudodementia: A slow death. *Neuropsychology Review, 4,* 71–90.

Nussbaum, P. D. (1998). Neuropsychological assessment of the elderly. In G. Goldstein, P. D., Nussbaum, & S. R. Beers (Eds.), *Neuropsychology* (pp. 83–105). New York: Plenum Press.

Nyberg, L., Forkstam, C., Petersson, K. M., Cabeza, R., & Ingvar, M. (2002). Brain imaging of human memory systems: Between-systems similarities and within-system differences. *Cognitive Brain Research, 13,* 281–292.

Nybo, T., & Koskiniemi, M. (1999). Cognitive indicators of vocational outcome after severe traumatic brain injury (TBI) in childhood. *Brain Injury, 13,* 759–66.

Oberg, L. W., & Turkstra, L. S. (1998). The use of elaborative encoding to facilitate vocabulary learning after adolescent traumatic brain injury: Two case illustrations. *Journal of Head Trauma Rehabilitation, 3,* 44–62.

Obler, L. K., & Albert, M. L. (1979). *The Action Naming Test.* Boston, MA: VA Medical Center.

O'Brien, J. T., Erkinjuntti, T., Reisberg, B., Roman, G., Sawada, T., Pantoni, L., et al. (2003). Vascular cognitive impairment. *The Lancet: Neurology, 2,* 89–98.

O'Connor, R. E., McGraw, P., & Edelsohn, L. (1999). Thrombolytic therapy for acute ischemic stroke: Why the majority of patients remain ineligible for treatment. *Annals of Emergency Medicine, 33,* 9–14.

Odell, K. H., & Flynn, M. (1998). Treatment outcomes in individuals with right hemisphere brain damage. Presented at the annual conference of the American Speech-Language-Hearing Association, San Antonio, TX.

Oelschlaeger, M. L., & Thorne, J. C. (1999). Application of the correct information unit analysis to the naturally occurring conversation of a person with aphasia. *Journal of Speech, Language and Hearing Research, 42,* 636–648.

Ogrezeanu, V., Voinescu, I., Mihailescu, L., & Jipescu, I. (1994). "Spontaneous" recovery in aphasics after single ischaemic stroke. *Romanian Journal of Neurology and Psychiatry, 32,* 77–90.

Oh, H., & Seo, W. (2003). Sensory stimulation programme to improve recovery in comatose patients. *Journal of Clinical Nursing, 12,* 394–404.

Ojemann, G. A., & Mateer, C. (1979). Human language cortex: localization of memory, syntax, and sequential motor-phoneme identification systems. *Science, 205,* 1401–1403.

Ojemann, G. A., & Whitaker, H. A. (1978). Language localization and variability. *Brain and Language, 6,* 239–260.

Oliveira, R. M., Gurd, J. M., Nixon, P., Marshall, J. C., & Passingham, R. E. (1997). Micrographia in Parkinson's disease: The effect of providing external cues. *Journal of Neurology, Neurosurgery, and Psychiatry, 63,* 429–433.

Orange, J. B., & Colton-Hudson, A. (1998). A case study of a spousal communication education and training program for Alzheimer's disease. *Special Interest Division 2: Neurophysiology and Neurogenic Speech and Language Disorders Newsletter, 8,* 22–29.

Ostrosky-Solis, F., Ardila, A., & Rosselli, M. (1997). *Evaluación Neuropsicológica Breve en Español.* San Antonio, TX: The Psychological Corporation.

O'Sullivan, T., & Fagan, S. C. (1998). Drug-induced communication and swallowing disorders. In A. F. Johnson & B. H. Jacobson (Eds.), *Medical speech-language pathology: A practitioner's guide* (pp. 176–191). New York: Thieme.

Owens, R. E. (1984). *Language development: An introduction.* Toronto: Charles E. Merrill.

Owens, R. E., Metz, D. E., & Haas, A. (2003). *Introduction to communication disorders: A life span perspective.* Boston: Allyn & Bacon.

Ownsworth, T. L., & McFarland, K. (1999). Memory remediation in long-term acquired brain injury: Two approaches in diary training. *Brain Injury, 13,* 605–626.

Ozeren, A., Sarica, Y., Mavi, Y., & Demirkiran, M. (1995). Bromocriptine is ineffective in the treatment of chronic nonfluent aphasia. *Acta Neurologica Belgium, 95,* 235–238.

Paghera, B., Marien, P., & Vignolo, L. A. (2003). Crossed aphasia with left spatial neglect and visual imperception: a case report. *Neurological Science, 23,* 317–322.

Palleschi, L., Vetta, F., & deGennaro, E. (1996). Effects of aerobic training on the cognitive performance of elderly patients with senile dementia of the Alzheimer's type. *Archives of Gerontology and Geriatrics, Suppl. 5,* 47–50.

Palmese, C. A., & Raskin, S. A. (2000). The rehabilitation of attention in individuals with mild traumatic brain injury using the APT-II programme. *Brain Injury, 14,* 535–548.

Pang, D. (1985). Pathophysiologic correlates of neurobehavioral syndromes following closed head injury. In M. Ylvisaker (Ed.), *Head injury rehabilitation: Children and adolescents* (pp. 3–70). San Diego: College-Hill Press.

Paolucci, S., Antonucci, G., Guariglia, C., Magnotti, L., Pizzamiglio, L., & Zoccolotti, P. (1996). Facilitory effect of neglect rehabilitation on the recovery of left hemiplegic stroke patients: A cross-over study. *Journal of Neurology, 243,* 308–314.

Paolucci, S., Antonucci, G., Pratesi, L., Traballesi, M., Lubich, S., & Grasso, M. G. (1998). Functional outcome in stroke inpatient rehabilitation: Predicting no, low, and high response patients. *Cerebrovascular Diseases, 8,* 228–234.

Paradis, M., & Libben, G. (1987). *The assessment of bilingual aphasia.* Hillsdale, NJ: Erlbaum.

Paradis, M., & Libben, G. (1993). *Evaluacion de la afasia en los bilingues.* Barcelona, Spain: Masson.

Parenté, R., & Anderson-Parenté, J. K. (1991). *Retraining memory: Techniques and applications.* Houston, TX: CSY.

Parente, R., Anderson-Parente, J., & Stapleton, M. (2001). The use of rhymes and mnemonics for teaching cognitive skills to persons with acquired brain injury. *Brain Injury Source, 5,* 16–19.

Parente, R., & Herrmann, D. (2003). *Retraining cognition: Techniques and applications* (2nd ed.). Austin, TX: Pro-Ed.

Parente, R., & Stapleton, M. (1999). Development of a cognitive strategies group for vocational training after traumatic brain injury. *Neurorehabilitation, 13,* 13–20.

Park, N. W., & Ingles, J. L. (2001). Effectiveness of attention rehabilitation after an acquired brain injury: A meta-analysis. *Neuropsychology, 15,* 199–210.

Park, N. W., Moscovitch, M., & Robertson, I. H. (1999). Divided attention impairments after traumatic brain injury. *Neuropsychologia, 37,* 1119–1133.

Park, N. W., Proulx, G. B., & Towers, W. M. (1999). Evaluation of the Attention Process Training programme. *Neuropsychological Rehabilitation, 9,* 135–154.

Parrot Software [computer software]. (1982–2003). West Bloomfield, MI: Author.

Pashek, G. V., & Bachman, D. L. (2003). Cognitive, linguistic, and motor speech effects of donepezil hydrocholoride in a patient with stroke-related aphasia and apraxia of speech. *Brain and Language, 87,* 179–180.

Pashler, H. (1994a). Dual-task interference in simple tasks: Data and theory. *Psychological Bulletin, 116,* 220–244.

Pashler, H. (1994b). Graded capacity-sharing in dual-task interference? *Journal of Experimental Psychology: Human Perception and Performance, 20,* 330–342.

Pasquier, F., Fukui, T., Sarazin, M., Pijnenburg, Y., Diehl, J., Grundman, M., et al. (2003). Laboratory investigations and treatment in frontotemporal dementia. *Annals of Neurology, 54,* S32–S35.

Patel, M., Coshall, C., Rudd, A. G., & Wolfe, C. D. A. (2003). Natural history of cognitive impairment after stroke and factors associated with its recovery. *Clinical Rehabilitation, 17,* 158–166.

Patrick, P. D., Buck, M. L., Conaway, M. R., & Blackman, J. A. (2003). The use of dopamine enhancing medications with children in low response states following brain injury. *Brain Injury, 17,* 497–506.

Patterson, R., & Wells, A. (1995). Involving the family in planning for life with aphasia. *Topics in Stroke Rehabilitation, 2,* 39–46.

Paul-Brown, D., Frattali, C. M., Holland, A. L., Thompson, C. K., Caperton, C. J., & Slater, S. C. (2004). *Quality of communication life scale.* Rockville, MD: American Speech-Language-Hearing Association.

Paulsen, J. S., Ready, R. E., Hamilton, J. M., Mega, M. S., & Cummings, J. L. (2001). Neuropsychiatric aspects of Huntington's disease. *Journal of Neurology, Neurosurgery, and Psychiatry, 71,* 310–314.

Paulsen, J. S., Ready, R. E., Stout, J. C., Salmon, D. P., Thal, L. J., Grant, I., et al. (2000). Neurobehaviors and psychotic symptoms in Alzheimer's disease. *Journal of the International Neuropsychological Society, 6,* 815–820.

Payne, J. C. (1994). *Communication profile: A functional skills survey.* San Antonio, TX: Communication Skill Builders.

Payne, J. C. (1997). *Adult neurogenic language disorders: Assessment and treatment. A comprehensive ethnobiological approach.* Clifton Park, NY: Singular Thomson Delmar Learning.

Peach, R. K. (2001). Further thoughts regarding management of acute aphasia following stroke. *American Journal of Speech-Language Pathology, 10,* 29–36.

Peach, R. K., & Wong, P. C. M. (2004). Integrating the message level into treatment for agrammatism using story retelling. *Aphasiology, 18,* 429–441.

Pease, D. M., & Goodglass, H. (1978). The effects of cueing on picture naming in aphasia. *Cortex, 14,* 178–189.

Peavy, G. M. (1998). *Severe Cognitive Impairment Profile.* Lutz, FL: Psychological Assessment Resources.

Pedersen, P. M., Jorgensen, H. S., Nakayama, H., Raaschou, H. O., & Olsen, T. S. (1995). Aphasia in acute stroke: Incidence, determinants, and recovery. *Annals of Neurology, 38,* 659–666.

Pedersen, P. M., Jorgensen, H. S., Nakayama, H., Raaschou, H. O., & Olsen, T. (1996). Frequency, determinants, and consequences of anosognosia in acute stroke. *Journal of Neurological Rehabilitation, 10,* 243–250.

Pedersen, P. M., Jorgensen, H. S., Nakayama, H., Raaschou, H. O., & Olsen, T. S. (1997). Hemineglect in acute stroke: Incidence and prognostic implications. *American Journal of Physical Medicine and Rehabilitation, 76,* 122–127.

Pedersen, P. M., Vinter, K., & Olsen, T. S. (2004). Aphasia after stroke: Type, severity and prognosis. The Copenhagen aphasia study. *Cerebrovascular Disorders, 17,* 35–43.

Pedersen, P. M., Wandel, A., Jorgensen, H. S., Nakayama, H., Raaschou, H. O., & Olsen, T. S. (1996). Ipsilateral pushing in stroke: Incidence, relation to neuropsychological symptoms, and impact on rehabilitation. *Archives of Physical Medicine and Rehabilitation, 77,* 25–28.

Penfield, W., & Roberts, L. (1959). *Speech and brain mechanisms.* Princeton, NJ: Princeton University Press.

Penn, C. (1988). The profiling of syntax and pragmatics in aphasia. *Clinical Linguistics and Phonetics, 2,* 179–207.

Penn, C., Jones, D., & Joffe, V. (1997). Hierarchial discourse therapy: A method for the mild patient. *Aphasiology, 11,* 601–632.

Penner, I., Rausch, M., Kappos, L., Opwis, K., & Radu, E. W. (2003). Analysis of impairment related functional architecture in MS patients during performance of different attention tasks. *Journal of Neurology, 250,* 461–472.

Pennings, J. L., Bachulis, B. L., Simons, C. T., & Slazinski, T. (1993). Survival after severe brain injury in the aged. *Archives of Surgery, 128,* 787–793.

Pentland, B., Hutton, L., MacMillan, A., & Mayer, V. (2003). Training in brain injury rehabilitation. *Disability and Rehabilitation, 25,* 544–548.

Pentland, B., & Whittle, I. R. (1999). Acute management of brain injury. In M. Rosenthal, J. S. Kreutzer, E. R. Griffith, & Pentland, B. (Eds.), *Rehabilitation of the adult and child with traumatic brain injury* (3rd ed., pp. 42–52). Philadelphia: F. A. Davis.

Peper, M., & Irle, E. (1997). Categorical and dimensional coding of emotional intonations in patients with focal brain lesions. *Brain and Language, 58,* 233–264.

Perbal, S., Couillet, J., Azouvi, P., & Pouthas, V. (2003). Relationships between time estimation, memory, attention and processing speed in patients with severe traumatic brain injury. *Neuropsychologia, 41,* 1599–1610.

Perkins, L., Whitworth, A., & Lesser, R. (1997). *Conversation Analysis Profile for People with Cognitive Impairment.* Philadelphia: Taylor & Francis.

Pfeiffer, E. (1975). A short portable mental status questionnaire for the assessment of organic brain deficit in elderly patients. *Journal of the American Geriatrics Society, 23,* 433–441.

Pictionary, I. (1993, 1999). Pictionary.

Pimental, P. A., & Kingsbury, N. A. (1989). *Mini Inventory of Right Brain Injury.* Austin, TX: Pro-Ed.

Pimental, P. A., & Kingsbury, N. A. (2000). *Mini Inventory of Right Brain Injury-II.* Austin, TX: Pro-Ed.

Pizzamiglio, I., Mammucari, A., & Razzano, C. (1985). Evidence for sex differences in brain organization in recovery in aphasia. *Brain and Language, 25*, 213–223.

Plante, E. (2004). Evidence-based practice in communication sciences and disorders. *Journal of Communication Disorders, 37*, 389–390.

Plenger, P. M., Dixon, C. E., Castillo, R. M., Frankowski, R. F., Yablon, S. A., & Levin, H. S. (1996). Subacute methylphenidate treatment for moderate to moderately severe traumatic brain injury: A preliminary double-blind placebo-controlled study. *Archives of Physical Medicine and Rehabilitation, 77*, 536–540.

Polster, M. R., & Rose, S. B. (1998). Disorders of auditory processing: Evidence for modularity in audition. *Cortex, 34*, 47–65.

Ponsford, J., & Kinsella, G. (1991). The use of a rating scale of attentional behavior. *Neuropsychological Rehabilitation, 1*, 241–257.

Ponsford, J. L., Olver, J. H., & Curran, C. (1995). A profile of outcome: Two years after traumatic brain injury. *Brain Injury, 9*, 1–10.

Popovici, M., Mihailescu, L., & Voinescu, I. (1992). Melodic Intonation Therapy in the rehabilitation of Romanian aphasics with buccolingual apraxia. *Review of Romanian Neurology and Psychiatry, 30*, 99–113.

Porch, B. E. (1981). *Porch Index of Communicative Ability: Vol. 2. Administration, scoring, and interpretation* (3rd ed.). Palo Alto, CA: Consulting Psychologists Press.

Porteus, S. D. (1965). *Porteus Maze Test. Fifty years application.* Palo Alto, CA: Pacific.

Potter, J., Deighton, T., Patel, M., Fairhurst, M., Guest, R., & Donnelly, N. (2000). Computer recording of standard tests of visual neglect in stroke patients. *Clinical Rehabilitation, 14*, 441–446.

Pound, C. (1996). Writing remediation using preserved oral spelling: A case for separate output buffers. *Aphasiology, 10*, 283–296.

Pouratian, N., Cannestra, A. F., Bookheimer, S. Y., Martin, N. A., & Toga, A. W. (2004). Variability of intraoperative electrocortical stimulation mapping parameters across and within individuals. *Journal of Neurosurgery, 101*, 458–466.

Powell, G. E., Bailey, S., & Clark, E. (1980). A very short form of the Minnesota Aphasia Test. *British Journal of Social and Clinical Psychology, 19*, 189–194.

Powell, T., & Malia, K. (2003). *The brain injury workbook.* Oxen, UK: SpeechMark.

Prigatano, G. P. (1991). Disturbances in self-awareness of deficit after traumatic brain injury. In G. P. Prigatano & D. L. Schacter (Eds.), *Awareness of deficit after brain injury* (pp. 111–126). New York: Oxford University Press.

Prins, R., & Bastiaanse, R. (2004). Analysing the spontaneous speech of aphasic speakers. *Aphasiology, 18*, 1075–1091.

Prutting, C. (1979). The action of moving forward progressively from one point to another on the way to completion. *Journal of Speech and Hearing Research, 14*, 776–792.

Prutting, C. A., & Kirchner, D. M. (1987). A clinical appraisal of the pragmatic aspects of language. *Journal of Speech and Hearing Disorders, 52*, 105–119.

Purdy, M. (2002). Executive function ability in persons with aphasia. *Aphasiology, 16*, 549–557.

Puskaric, N. J., & Pierce, R. S. (1997). Effects of constraint and expectation on reading comprehension in aphasia. *Aphasiology, 11*, 249–261.

Putnam, S. H., & Fichtenberg, N. L. (1999). Neuropsychological examination of the patient with traumatic brain injury. In M. Rosenthal, E. R. Griffith, J. S. Kreutzer, & B. Pentland (Eds.), *Rehabilitation of the adult and child with traumatic brain injury* (3rd ed., pp. 147–166). Philadelphia: F. A. Davis.

Rabins, P. V. (1983). Reversible dementia and the misdiagnosis of dementia: A review. *Hospital Community Psychiatry, 9,* 830–835.

Rabinstein, A. A., & Shulman, L. (2003). Acupuncture in clinical neurology. *Neurology, 9,* 137–148.

Radanovic, M., & Scaff, M. (2003). Speech and language disturbances due to subcortical lesions. *Brain and Language, 84,* 337–352.

Radloff, L. W., & Teri, L. (1986). Assessing depression in older adults: The CES-D scale. *Clinical Gerontologist, 5,* 119–137.

Ramage, A., Beeson, P., & Rapcsak, S. Z. (1998). *Dissociation between oral and written spelling: Clinical characteristics and possible mechanisms.* Presentation at the Clinical Aphasiology Conference, Asheville, NC.

Ramasubbu, R., & Patten, S. B. (2003). Effect of depression on stroke morbidity and mortality. *Canadian Journal of Psychiatry, 48,* 250–257.

Ramsberger, G. (1994). Functional perspective for assessment and rehabilitation of persons with severe aphasia. *Seminars in Speech and Language, 15,* 1–16.

Ramsberger, G., & Helm-Estabrooks, N. (1989). Visual Action Therapy for bucco-facial apraxia. *Clinical Aphasiology, 00,* 395–400.

Ramsing, S., Blomstrand, C., & Sullivan, M. (1991). Prognostic factors for return to work in stroke patients with aphasia. *Aphasiology, 5,* 583–588.

Randolph, C. (1998). *Repeatable Battery for the Assessment of Neuropsychological Status.* San Antonio, TX: The Psychological Corporation.

Rao, P. R. (1995). Drawing and gesture as communication options in a person with severe aphasia. *Topics in Stroke Rehabilitation, 2,* 49–56.

Rapp, S., Brenes, G., & Marsh, A. P. (2002). Memory enhancement training for older adults with mild cognitive impairment: A preliminary study. *Aging and Mental Health, 6,* 5–11.

Rapport, L. J., Farchione, T. J., Dutra, R. L., Webster, J. S., & Charter, R. A. (1996). Measures of hemi-inattention on the Rey Figure copy for the Lezak-Osterrieth scoring method. *The Clinical Neuropsychologist, 10,* 450–454.

Raskin, S. A., & Sohlberg, M. M. (1996). The efficacy of prospective memory training in two adults with brain injury. *Journal of Head Trauma Rehabilitation, 11,* 32–51.

Rath, J. F., Langebahn, D. M., Simon, D., Sherr, R., Fletcher, J., & Diller, L. (2004). The construct of problem solving in higher level neuropsychological assessment and rehabilitation. *Archives of Clinical Neuropsychology, 19,* 613–635.

Rath, J. F., Simon, D., Langenbahn, D. M., Sherr, R. L., & Diller, L. (2003). Group treatment of problem-solving deficits in outpatients with traumatic brain injury: A randomized outcome study. *Neuropsychological Rehabilitation, 13,* 461–488.

Rathore, S. S., Hinn, A. R., Cooper, L. S., Tyroler, H. A., & Rosamond, W. D. (2002). Characterization of incident stroke signs and symptoms: Findings from the atherosclerosis risk in communities study. *Stroke, 33,* 2718–2721.

Rausch, R. (1985). Differences in cognitive function with left and right temporal lobe dysfunction. In D. F. Benson & E. Zaidel (Eds.), *The dual brain: Hemispheric specialization in humans* (pp. 247–261). New York: Guilford Press.

Rausch, R., Serafetinides, E. A., & Crandall, P. H. (1977). Olfactory memory in patients with anterior temporal lobectomy. *Cortex, 13,* 445–453.

Raven, J. C. (1998). *Raven's Progressive Matrices.* San Antonio, TX: Psychological Corporation.

Raymer, A. M., & Rothi, L. J. G. (2001). Cognitive approaches to impairments of word comprehension and production. In R. Chapey (Ed.), *Language intervention strategies in adult aphasia* (4th ed., pp. 524–550). New York: Lippincott, Williams & Wilkins.

Raymer, A. M., Thompson, C. K., Jacobs, B., Le Grand, H. R. (1993). Phonological treatment of naming deficits in aphasia: Model-based generalization analysis. *Aphasiology, 7,* 27–53.

Rayner, H., & Marshall, J. (2003). Training volunteers as conversation partners for people with aphasia. *International Journal of Language and Communication Disorders, 38,* 149–164.

Razani, J., Boone, K. B., Miller, B. L., Lee, A., & Sherman, D. (2001). Neuropsychological performance of right- and left-frontotemporal dementia compared to Alzheimer's disease. *Journal of the Neuropsychological Society, 7,* 468–480.

Records, N. L. (1994). A measure of the contribution of a gesture to the perception of speech in listeners with aphasia. *Journal of Speech and Hearing Research, 37,* 1086–1099.

Records, N. L., Tomblin, J. B., & Freese, P. R. (1992). The quality of life of young adults with histories of specific language impairment. *American Journal of Speech-Language Pathology, 1,* 44–53.

Reilly, S. (2004a). The challenges in making speech pathology evidence based. *Advances in Speech-Language Pathology, 6,* 113–124.

Reilly, S. (2004b). Introducing evidence-based practice. In S. Reilly, J. M. Douglas, & J. Oates (Eds.), *Evidence-based practice in speech pathology.* London: Whurr Publishers.

Reinmuth, O. M. (1997). Stroke: Mechanisms and effects. *Special Interest Division 2: Neurophysiology and Neurogenic Speech and Language Disorders Newsletter, 7,* 16–19.

Reitan, R. M. (1981). *Aphasia Screening Test* (2nd ed.). Tucson, AZ: Reitan Neuropsychology Laboratory.

Reitan, R. M., & Wolfson, D. (1985). *The Halstead-Reitan Neuropsychology Test Battery.* Tucson, AZ: Neuropsychology Press.

Reitan, R. M., & Wolfson, D. (1993). *The Halstead-Reitan Neuropsychological Test Battery* (2nd ed.). Tucson, AZ: Neuropsychology Press.

Rende, B. (2000). Cognitive flexibility: Theory, assessment and treatment. *Seminars in Speech and Language, 21,* 121–134.

Rey, G. J., Sivan, A. B., & Benton, A. L. (1991). *Multilingual Aphasia Examination-Spanish Version.* Lutz, FL: Psychological Assessment Resources.

Reynolds, C. R. (2002). *Comprehensive Trail-Making Test.* Lutz, FL: Psychological Assessment Resources.

Richards, K., Singletary F., Gonzalez-Rothi, L. J., Koehler, S., & Crosson, B. (2002). Activation of intentional mechanisms through utilization of nonsymbolic movements in aphasia rehabilitation. *Journal of Rehabilitation Research and Development, 39,* 445–454.

Richards, K., Wierenga, C., Singletary, F., Fuller, R., Rodriguez, A., Kendall, D., et al. (2003*). Comparison of intention and attention treatments in nonfluent aphasia.* Poster presentation at the annual International Neuropsychology Society conference, Waikiki, HI.

Richardson, J. T., & Barry, C. (1985). The effects of minor closed head injury upon human memory: Further evidence on the role of mental imagery. *Cognitive Neuropsychology, 2,* 149–168.

Richeson, N. E. (2003). Effects of animal-assisted therapy on agitated behaviors and social interactions of older adults with dementia. *American Journal of Alzheimer's Disease and Other Dementias, 18,* 353–358.

Rinne, J. O., Portin, R., Ruottinen, H., Nurmi, I., Bergman, J., Haaparanta, M., & et al. (2000). Cognitive impairment and the brain dopaminergic system in Parkinson's disease. *Archives of Neurology, 57,* 470–475.

Rios, M., Perianez, J. A., & Munoz-Cespedes, J. M. (2004). Attentional control and slowness of information processing after severe traumatic brain injury. *Brain Injury, 18,* 257–272.

Ripich, D. N. (1996). *Alzheimer's disease communication code: The FOCUSED program for caregivers.* Austin, TX: The Psychological Corporation.

Ritchie, K., & Lovestone, S. (2002). The dementias. *The Lancet, 360,* 179–1766.

Rizzo, M., Reinach, S., McGehee, D. V., & Dawson, J. (1997). Simulated car crashes and crash predictors in drivers with Alzheimer disease. *Archives of Neurology, 54,* 545–553.

Robertson, I. H. (1991). Use of left versus right hand in responding to lateralized stimuli in unilateral neglect. *Neuropsychologia, 29,* 1129–1135.

Robertson, I. H. (1996). *Goal Management Training: A clinical manual.* Cambridge, UK: Psy-Consult.

Robertson, I. H., & Halligan, P. W. (1999). *Spatial neglect: A clinical handbook for diagnosis and treatment.* Hove, East Sussex. UK: Psychology Press.

Robertson, I. H., Hogg, K., & McMillan, T. M. (1998). Rehabilitation of unilateral neglect: Improving function by contralesional limb activation. *Neuropsychological Rehabilitation, 8,* 19–29.

Robertson, I. H., & Murre, J. M. (1999). Rehabilitation of brain damage: Brain plasticity and principles of guided recovery. *Psychological Bulletin, 25,* 544–575.

Robertson, I. H., North, N., & Geggie, C. (1992). Spatio-motor cueing in unilateral neglect: Three single case studies of its therapeutic effectiveness. *Journal of Neurology, Neurosurgery, and Psychiatry, 55,* 799–805.

Robertson, I. H., Ward, T., Ridgeway, V., & Nimmo-Smith, I. (1994). *The Test of Everyday Attention.* Gaylord, MI: Northern Speech Services.

Robertson, I. H., Ward, T., Ridgeway, V., & Nimmo-Smith, I. (1996). The structure of normal human attention: The Test of Everyday Attention. *Journal of the International Neuropsychological Society, 2,* 525–534.

Robey, R. (1994). The efficacy of treatment for aphasic persons: A meta-analysis. *Brain and Language, 47,* 582–608.

Robey, R. R. (2004). A five-phase model for clinical-outcome research. *Journal of Communication Disorders, 37,* 401–411.

Robey, R. R., & Schultz, M. C. (1998). A model for conducting clinical-outcome research: An adaptation of the standard protocol for use in aphasiology. *Aphasiology, 12,* 787–810.

Robin, D. A., & Scheinberg, S. (1990). Subcortical lesions and aphasia. *Journal of Speech and Hearing Disorders, 55,* 90–100.

Robin, D. A., Tranel, D., & Damasio, H. (1990). Auditory perception of temporal and spectral events in patients with focal left and right cerebral lesions. *Brain and Language, 39,* 539–555.

Robson, J., Marshall, J., Chiat, S., & Pring, T. (2001). Enhancing communication in jargon aphasia: A small group study of writing therapy. *International Journal of Language and Communication Disorders, 36,* 471–488.

Robson, J., Marshall, J., Pring, T., & Chiat, S. (1998a). Phonological naming therapy in jargon aphasia: Positive but paradoxical effects. *Journal of the International Neuropsychological Society, 4,* 675–686.

Robson, J., Pring, T., Marshall, J., Morrison, S., & Chiat, S. (1998b). Written communication in undifferentiated jargon aphasia: A therapy study. *International Journal of Language and Communication Disorders, 33*, 305–328.

Rochon, E., & Reichman, S. (2003). A modular treatment for sentence processing impairment in aphasia: Sentence production. *Journal of Speech-Language Pathology and Audiology, 27*, 202–210.

Rochon, E., & Reichman, S. (2004). A modular treatment for sentence processing impairment in aphasia: Sentence comprehension. *Journal of Speech-Language Pathology and Audiology, 28*, 25–33.

Rode, G., Tiliket, C., Charlopain, P., & Boisson, D. (1998). Postural asymmetry reduction by vestibular caloric stimulation in left hemiparetic patients. *Scandinavian Journal of Rehabilitation Medicine, 30*, 9–14.

Rogers, H. B., Schroeder, T., Secher, N. H., & Mitchell, J. (1990). Cerebral blood flow during static exercise in humans. *Journal of Applied Physiology, 68*, 2358–2361.

Rosenbek, J. C., LaPointe, L. L., & Wertz, R. T. (1989). *Aphasia: A clinical approach*. Austin, TX: Pro-Ed.

Rosenbek, J. C., McCullough, G. H., & Wertz, R. T. (2004). Is the information about a test important? Applying the methods of evidence-based medicine to the clinical examination of swallowing. *Journal of Communication Disorders, 37*, 437–450.

Rosenthal, W. S. (2004). Group therapy is better than individual therapy: With special attention to stuttering. *Special Interest Division 2: Neurophysiology and Neurogenic Speech and Language Disorders Newsletter, 14*, 3–8.

Rosetta Stone Language Learning Programs [computer software]. (2001). Harrisonburg, VA: Fairfield Language Technologies.

Ross, D. (1986). *Ross Information Processing Assessment*. Austin, TX: Pro-Ed.

Ross, E. (1984). Right hemisphere's role in language, affective behavior and emotion. *Trends in Neuroscience, 7*, 342–346.

Ross, K. B., & Wertz, R. T. (1999). Comparison of impairment and disability measures for assessing severity of, and improvement in, aphasia. *Aphasiology, 13*, 113–124.

Ross, K. B., & Wertz, R. T. (2001). Possible demographic influences on differentiating normal from aphasic performance. *Journal of Communication Disorders, 34*, 115–130.

Ross, K. B., & Wertz, R. T. (2002). Relationships between language-based disability and quality of life in chronically aphasic adults. *Aphasiology, 16*, 791–800.

Ross, K. B., & Wertz, R. T. (2003). Discriminative validity of selected measures for differentiating normal from aphasic performance. *American Journal of Speech-Language Pathology, 12*, 312–319.

Ross, K. B., & Wertz, R. T. (2004). Accuracy of formal tests for diagnosing mild aphasia: An application of evidence-based medicine. *Aphasiology, 18*, 337–355.

Ross-Swain, D. (1996). *Ross Information Processing Assessment* (2nd ed.). Austin, TX: Pro-Ed.

Ross-Swain, D., & Fogle, P. (1996). *Ross Information Processing Assessment-Geriatric*. Austin, TX: Pro-Ed.

Rossetti, Y., Rode, G., Pisella, L., Farne, A., Li, L., Boisson, D., et al. (1998). Prism adaptation to a rightward optical deviation rehabilitates left hemispatial neglect. *Nature, 395*, 166–169.

Rossor, M. N. (2001). Pick's disease: A clinical overview. *Neurology, 56 (Suppl. 4)*, S3–S5.

Roth, E. J., & Lovell, L. (2003). Seven-year trends in stroke rehabilitation: Patient characteristics, medical complications, and functional outcomes. *Topics in Stroke Rehabilitation, 9,* 1–9.

Roth, H., & Heilman, K. M. (2000). Aphasia: A historical perspective. In S. Nadeau, L. J. Gonzales Rothi, & B. Crosson (Eds.), *Aphasia and language: Theory to practice* (pp. 3–28). New York: Guilford Press.

Rothi, L. J. G., & Moss, S. (1992). Alexia without agraphia: Potential for model assisted therapy. *Clinics in Communication Disorders, 2,* 11–18.

Rothi, L. J. G., Raymer, A. M., & Heilman, K. M. (1997). Limb praxis assessment. In L. J. G. Rothi & K. M. Heilman (Eds.), *Apraxia: The neuropsychology of action* (pp. 61–73). Hove, East Sussex, UK: Psychology Press.

Rothi, L. J. G., Raymer, A. M., Maher, L., Greenwald, M., & Morris, M. (1991). Assessment of naming failures in neurological communication disorders. *Clinics in Communication Disorders, 1,* 7–20.

Roux, F. E., Lubrano, V., Lauwers-Cances, V., Tremoulet, M., Mascott, C. R., & Demonet, J. F. (2004). Intra-operative mapping of cortical areas involved in reading in mono- and bilingual patients. *Brain, 127,* 1796–1810.

Royall, D. R., Cordes, J. A., & Polk, M. (1998). CLOX: An executive clock drawing task. *Journal of Neurology, Neurosurgery, and Psychiatry, 64,* 588–594.

Royall, D. R., Espino, D. V., Polk, M. J., Verdeja, R., Vale, S., Gonzales, H., et al. (2003). Validation of a Spanish translation of the CLOX for use in Hispanic samples: The Hispanic EPESE study. *International Journal of Geriatric Psychiatry, 18,* 135–141.

Royall, D. R., Mahurin, R. K., Cornell, J., & Gray, K. F. (1993). Bedside assessment of dementia type using the Qualitative Evaluation of Dementia (QED). *Neuropsychiatry, Neuropsychology, and Behavioral Neurology, 6,* 235–244.

Royall, D. R., Mahurin, R. K., & Gray, K. F. (1992). Bedside assessment of executive dyscontrol: The Executive Interview (EXIT). *Journal of the American Geriatrics Society, 40,* 1221–1226.

Ruff, R. (1996). *Ruff Figural Fluency Test.* Lutz, FL: Psychological Assessment Resources.

Ruff, R. M., Nieman, H., Allen, C. C., Farrow, C. E., & Wylie, T. (1992). The Ruff 2 and 7 Selective Attention Test: A neuropsychological application. *Perceptual and Motor Skills, 75,* 1311–1319.

Ruiz, A. (2000). Aphasia treatment. On drugs, machines, and therapies: What will the future be? *Brain and Language, 71,* 200–203.

Ryalls, R., Joanette, Y., & Feldman, L. (1987). An acoustic comparison of normal and right-hemisphere-damaged speech prosody. *Cortex, 23,* 685–694.

Ryan, L. M., & Warden, D. L. (2003). Post concussion syndrome. *International Review of Psychiatry, 15,* 310–316.

Ryff, C. D. (1989). Happiness is everything, or is it? Explorations on the meaning of psychological well-being. *Journal of Personality and Social Psychology, 57,* 1069–1081.

Rymer, S., Salloway, S., Norton, L., Malloy, P., Correia, S., & Monast, D. (2002). Impaired awareness, behavior disturbance, and caregiver burden in Alzheimer disease. *Alzheimer Disease and Associated Disorders, 16,* 248–253.

Sabe, L., Leiguarda, R., & Starkstein, S. E. (1992). An open-label trial of bromocriptine in nonfluent aphasia. *Neurology, 42,* 1637–1638.

Sackett, D. L., Richardson, W. S., Rosenberg, W., & Haynes, R. B. (1997). *Evidence-based medicine: How to practice and teach EBM.* London: Churchill Livingstone.

Sackett, D. L., Rosenberg, W. M., Gray, J. A., Haynes, B., & Richardson, W. S. (1996). Evidence based medicine: What it is and what it isn't. *British Medical Journal 312*, 71–72

Sackett, D. L., Strauss, S. E., Richardson, W. S., Rosenberg, W., & Haynes, R. B. (2000). *Evidence-based medicine: How to practice and teach EBM* (2nd ed.). London: Churchill Livingstone.

Sacktor, N. (2002). The epidemiology of human immunodeficiency virus-associated neurological disease in the era of highly active antiretroviral therapy. *Journal of Neurovirology, 8*, 115–121.

Saffran, E. M., Berndt, R. S., & Schwartz, M. F. (1989). The quantitative analysis of agrammatic production: Procedure and data. *Brain and Language, 37*, 440–479.

Sakai, C. S., & Mateer, C. A. (1984). Otological and audiological sequelae of closed head trauma. *Seminars in Hearing, 5*, 157–174.

Samsa, G. P., & Matchar, D. B. (2004). How strong is the relationship between functional status and quality of life among persons with stroke. *Journal of Rehabilitation Research and Development, 41*, 279–282.

Samuel, C., Louis-Dreyfus, A., Kaschel, R., Makiela, E., Troubat, M., Anselmi, N., et al. (2000). Rehabilitation of very severe unilateral neglect by visuospatiomotor cueing: Two single case studies. *Neuropsychological Rehabilitation, 10*, 385–399.

Sands, E. S., Sarno, M. T., & Shankweiler, D. P. (1969). Long-term assessment of language function in aphasia due to stroke. *Archives of Physical Medicine, 50*, 202–207.

Saniova, B., Drobny, M., Kneslova, L., & Minarik, M. (2004). The outcome of patients with severe head injuries treated with amantadine sulphate. *Journal of Neural Transmission, 111*, 511–514.

Santo Pietro, M. J., & Boczko, F. (1998). The Breakfast Club: Results of a study examining the effectiveness of a multi-modality group communication treatment. *American Journal of Alzheimer's Disease, 13*, 146–158.

Sargeant, R., Webster, G., Salzman, T., White, S., & McGrath, J. (2000). Enriching the environment of patients undergoing long-term rehabilitation through group discussion of the news. *The Journal of Cognitive Rehabilitation, 18*, 20–23.

Sarno, J, E., Sarno, M. T., & Levita, E. (1973). The functional life scale. *Archives of Physical and Medical Rehabilitation, 54*, 214–220.

Sarno, M. T. (1969). *The functional communication profile.* New York: NYU Medical Center Monograph Department.

Sarno, M. T., Buonaguro, A., & Levin, E. (1986). Characteristics of verbal impairment in closed head injured patients. *Archives of Physical Medicine and Rehabilitation, 67*, 400–405.

Sarno, M. T., Silverman, M. G., & Sands, E. S. (1970). Speech therapy and language recovery in severe aphasia. *Journal of Speech and Hearing Research, 13*, 607–23.

Saxton, J., Swihart, A. A., & Boller, F. (1993). *Severe Impairment Battery.* Bury St. Edmunds, Suffolk, England: Thames Valley Test Company.

Saygin, A. P., Dick, F., Wilson, S. M., Dronkers, N. F., & Bates, E. (2003). Neural resources for processing language and environmental sounds: Evidence from aphasia. *Brain, 126*, 928–945.

Sbordone, R. J. (1996). Ecological validity: Some critical issues for the neuro-psychologist. In R. J. Sbordone & C. J. Long (Ed.), *Ecological validity of neuropsychological testing* (pp. 15–41). Delray Beach, FL: St. Lucie Press.

Sbordone, R. J., Seyranian, G. D., & Ruff, R. M. (1998). Are the subjective complaints of traumatically brain injured patients reliable? *Brain Injury, 12*, 505–515.

Schacter, D. L. (1992). Understanding implicit memory. *American Psychologist, 47,* 559–569.

Schatz, J., Hale, S., & Myerson, J. (1998). Cerebellar contribution to linguistic processing efficiency revealed by focal damage. *Journal of the International Neuropsychological Society, 4,* 491–501.

Scherder, J., Bouma, A., & Steen, L. (1992). Influence of transcutaneous electrical nerve stimulation on memory in dementia of the Alzheimer's type. *Journal of Clinical and Experimental Neuropsychology, 14,* 951–960.

Scherder, J., Bouma, A., & Steen, L. (1995). Effects of short-term transcutaneous electrical nerve stimulation on memory and affective behavior in patients with probable Alzheimer's disease. *Behavioral Brain Research, 67,* 211–219.

Schindler, I., Kerkhoff, G., Karnath, H. O., Keller, I., & Goldenberg, G. (2002). Neck muscle vibration induces lasting recovery in spatial neglect. *Journal of Neurology, Neurosurgery, and Psychiatry, 73,* 412–419.

Schlund, M. W. (1999). Self awareness: Effects of feedback and review on verbal self reports and remembering following brain injury. *Brain Injury, 13,* 375–380.

Schmitter-Edgecombe, M., & Wright, M. J. (2004). Event-based prospective memory following severe closed head injury. *Neuropsychology, 18,* 353–361.

Schneider, S. L., Thompson, C. K., & Luring, B. (1996). Effects of verbal plus gestural matrix training on sentence production in a patient with primary progressive aphasia. *Aphasiology, 10,* 297–317.

Schretlen, D. (1997). *Brief Test of Attention.* Lutz, FL: Psychological Assessment Resources.

Schuell, H. (1965a). *Differential diagnosis of aphasia with the Minnesota Test.* Minneapolis, MN: University of Minnesota Press.

Schuell, H. (1965b). *The Minnesota Test for Differential Diagnosis of Aphasia.* Minneapolis, MN: University of Minnesota Press.

Schuell, H., & Jenkins, J. J. (1959). The nature of language deficit in aphasia. *Psychological Review, 66,* 45–67.

Schuell, H., Jenkins, J. J., & Jimenese-Pabon, E. (1964). *Aphasia in adults.* New York: Harper and Row.

Schultheis, M. T., Caplan, B., Ricker, J. H., & Woessner, R. (2000). Fractioning the Hooper: A multiple-choice response format. *Clinical Neuropsychologist, 14,* 196–201.

Schwartz, M. F., Buxbaum, L. J., Veramonti, T., Ferraro, M., & Segal, M. (2002). *Naturalistic Action Test.* Bury St. Edmunds, Suffolk, England: Thames Valley Test Company.

Schwartz, M. F., Saffran, E. M., Fink, R. B., Myers, J. L., & Martin, N. (1994). Mapping therapy: A treatment programme for agrammatism. *Aphasiology, 8,* 19–54.

Schwartz, R. (1989). Early rehabilitation in trauma centers: Have speech-language pathology services progressed? *American Speech-Language-Hearing Association, 31,* 91–94.

Searle, J. (1969). *Speech acts.* London: Cambridge University Press.

Seashore, C., Lewis, D., & Saetveit, J. (1960). *Seashore measures of musical talents.* New York: The Psychological Corporation.

Shadden, B. (1998). Obtaining the discourse sample. In L. R. Cherney, B. Shadden, & C. A. Coelho (Eds.). *Analyzing discourse in communicatively impaired adults.* Gaithersburg, MD: Aspen.

Shadden, B. B., Burnette, R. B., Eikenberry, B. R., & DiBrezzo, R. (1991). All discourse tasks are not created equal. *Clinical Aphasiology, 20,* 327–342.

Shallice, T. (1982). Specific impairments of planning. *Philosophical Transactions of the Royal Society of London, 298,* 199–209.

Shallice, T. (1988). *From neuropsychology to mental structure.* Cambridge, MA: Cambridge University Press.

Shankar, K. K., & Orrell, M. W. (2000). Detecting and managing depression and anxiety in people with dementia. *Current Opinion in Psychiatry, 13,* 55–59.

Shankar, K. K., Walker, M., Frost, D., & Orrell, M. W. (1999). The development of a valid and reliable scale for rating anxiety in dementia. *Aging and Mental Health, 3,* 39–49.

Shapiro, L. P. (1997). Tutorial: An introduction to syntax. *Journal of Speech, Language, and Hearing Research, 40,* 254–272.

Shatz, R. S. (1998). Behavioral neurology. In A. F. Johnson & B. H. Jacobson (Eds.). *Medical speech-language pathology: A practitioner's guide* (pp. 243–284). New York: Thieme.

Shaw, D., & May, H. (2001). Sharing knowledge with nursing home staff: An objective investigation. *International Journal of Language and Communication, 33,* 200–205.

Shelton, J. R., Weinrich, M., McCall, D., & Cox, D. M. (1996). Differentiating globally aphasic patients: Data from in-depth language assessments and production training using C-VIC. *Aphasiology, 10,* 319–342.

Sherer, M., Bergloff, P., Levin, E., High, W. M., Oden, K. E., & Nick, T. G. (1998). Impaired awareness and employment outcome after traumatic brain injury. *Journal of Head Trauma Rehabilitation, 13,* 52–61.

Sherratt, S. M., & Penn, C. (1990). Discourse in a right-hemisphere brain-damaged subject. *Aphasiology, 4,* 539–560.

Shewan, C. M., & Kertesz, A. (1980). Reliability and validity characteristics of the Western Aphasia Battery. *Journal of Speech and Hearing Disorders, 45,* 308–324.

Shewan, C. M., & Kertesz, A. (1984). Effects of speech and language treatment on recovery from aphasia. *Brain and Language, 23,* 272–299.

Shiel, A., Wilson, B. A., McLellan, D. L., Horn, S., & Watson, M. (2000). *Wessex Head Injury Matrix.* Bury St. Edmunds, Suffolk, England: Thames Valley Test Company.

Shum, D. H. K., Harris, D., & O'Gorman, J. G. (2000). Effects of severe traumatic brain injury on visual memory. *Journal of Clinical and Experimental Neuropsychology, 22,* 25–39.

Shuster, L. I. (2004). Resource theory and aphasia reconsidered: Why alternative theories can better guide our research. *Aphasiology, 18,* 811–830.

Sieroff, E., Piquard, A., Auclair, L., Lacomblez, L., Derouesne, C., & Laberge, D. (2004). Deficit of preparatory attention in frontotemporal dementia. *Brain and Cognition, 55,* 444–451.

Silkes, J. P. (2003). Cerebral vascular imaging: Methods, applications, and considerations. *Special Interest Division 2: Neurophysiology and Neurogenic Speech and Language Disorders Newsletter, 13,* 10–17.

Simard, M., van Reekum, R., & Myran, D. (2003). Visuospatial impairment in dementia with Lewy bodies and Alzhiemer's disease: A process analysis. *International Journal of Geriatric Psychiatry, 18,* 387–391.

Simmons-Mackie, N. (2001). Social approaches to aphasia intervention. In R. Chapey (Ed.), *Language intervention strategies in aphasia and related neurogenic communication disorders* (4th ed., pp. 246–268). Philadelphia: Lippincott, Williams & Wilkins.

Simmons-Mackie, N., & Kagan, A. (1999). Communication strategies used by "good" versus "poor" speaking partners of individuals with aphasia. *Aphasiology, 13,* 807–820.

Simmons-Mackie, N. N., & Damico, J. S. (1996). Accounting for handicaps in aphasia: Communicative assessment from an authentic social perspective. *Disability and Rehabilitation, 18,* 540–549.

Simon, H. A. (1975). The functional equivalence of problem solving skill. *Cognitive Psychology, 7,* 268–288.

Singer, B. D., & Bashir, A. S. (1999). What are executive functions and self-regulation and what do they have to do with language-learning disorders? *Language, Speech, and Hearing Services in Schools, 30,* 265–273.

Sinotte, M. P., Nicholas, M., & Helm-Estabrooks, N. (2003). *Cognitive skills predict response to alternative communication aphasia treatment.* Poster presentation at the annual International Neuropsychology Society conference, Waikiki, HI.

Sivan, A. B. (1991). *Benton Visual Retention Test.* San Antonio, TX: The Psychological Corporation.

Skelly, M. (1979). *Amer-Ind gestural code based on universal American Indian hand talk.* New York: Elsevier.

Sklar, M. (1983). *Sklar Aphasia Scale.* Los Angeles, CA: Western Psychological Services.

Slachevsky, A., Villalpando, J. M., Sarazin, M., Hahn-Barma, V., Pillon, B., & Dubois, B. (2004). Frontal assessment battery and differential diagnosis of frontotemporal dementia and Alzheimer disease. *Archives of Neurology, 61,* 1104–1107.

Slosson, R. L., Nicholson, C. L., & Larson, S. (1990). *Slosson Oral Reading Test-Revised 3.* East Aurora, NY: Slosson Educational Publications.

Small, J. A., Geldart, K., & Gutman, G. (2000). Communication between individuals with Alzheimer's disease and their caregivers during activities of daily living. *American Journal of Alzheimer's Disease, 15,* 291–302.

Small, J. A., Geldart, K., Gutman, G., & Clarke Scott, M. (1998). The discourse of self in dementia. *Ageing and Society, 18,* 291–316.

Small, J. A., & Gutman, G. (2002). Recommended and reported use of communication strategies in Alzheimer caregiving. *Alzheimer Disease and Associated Disorders, 16,* 270–278.

Small, S. L. (2002). Biological approaches to the treatment of aphasia. In A. E. Hillis (Ed.), *The handbook of adult language disorders: Integrating cognitive neuropsychology, neurology, and rehabilitation* (pp. 392–411). New York: Psychology Press.

Smith, A. (1971). Objective indices of severity of chronic aphasia in stroke patients. *Journal of Speech and Hearing Disorders, 36,* 167–207.

Smith, E. E., & Jonides, J. (1998). Neuroimaging analyses of human working memory. *Proceedings of the National Academy of Science, 95,* 12061–12068.

Smith Doody, R. (2003). Update on Alzheimer drugs (donepezil). *The Neurologist, 9,* 225–229.

Smollan, T., & Penn, C. (1997). The measurement of emotional reaction and depression in a South African stroke population. *Disability and Rehabilitation, 19,* 56–63.

Snow, P. C., & Douglas, J. M. (2000). Conceptual and methodological challenges in discourse assessment with TBI speakers: Towards an understanding. *Brain Injury, 14,* 397–415.

Sohlberg, M. M. (1992). *The Profile of Executive Control System.* Gaylord, MI: Northern Rehabilitation Services.

Sohlberg, M. M. (2000). Assessing and managing unawareness of self. *Seminars in Speech and Language, 21,* 135–152.

Sohlberg, M. M., Avery, J., Kennedy, M., Ylvisaker, M., Coelho, C., Turkstra, L., et al. (2003). Practice guidelines for direct attention training. *Journal of Medical Speech-Language Pathology, 11,* xix-xxxix.

Sohlberg, M. M., Johnson, L., Paule, L., Raskin, S. A., & Mateer, C. A. (2001). *Attention Process Training-II: A program to address attentional deficits for persons with mild cognitive dysfunction* (2nd ed.). Wake Forest, NC: Lash & Associates.

Sohlberg, M. M., & Mateer, C. A. (1986). *Attention Process Training (APT).* Puyallup, WA: Association for Neuropsychological Research and Development.

Sohlberg, M. M., & Mateer, C. A. (2001). *APT Test-Revised.* Wake Forest, NC: Lash & Associates.

Sohlberg, M. M., & Mateer, C. A. (2001a). *Cognitive rehabilitation: An integrative neuropsychological approach.* New York: Guilford Press.

Sohlberg, M. M., & Mateer, C. A. (2001b). *Prospective Memory Screening/Training (PROMS/T).* Wake Forest, NC: Lash & Associates.

Sohlberg, M. M., McLaughlin, K., Pavese, A., Heidrich, A., & Posner, M. I. (2000). Evaluation of attention process training and brain injury education in persons with acquired brain injury. *Journal of Clinical and Experimental Neuropsychology, 22,* 656–676.

Sohlberg, M. M., & Raskin, S. A. (1996). Principles of generalization applied to attention and memory interventions. *Journal of Head Trauma Rehabilitation, 11,* 65–78.

Sohlberg, M. M., Sprunk, H., & Metzelaar, K. (1988). Efficacy of an external cuing system in an individual with severe frontal lobe damage. *Cognitive Rehabilitation, 6,* 36–41.

Sohlberg, M. M., White, O., Evans, E., & Mateer, C. A. (1992). Background and initial case studies into the effects of prospective memory training. *Brain Injury, 6,* 129–138.

Solomon, P. R. (2002). *Alzheimer's Disease Caregiver's Questionnaire.* Lutz, FL: Psychological Assessment Resources.

Sorin-Peters, R. (2004). The evaluation of a learner-centred training programme for spouses of adults with chronic aphasia using qualitative case study methodology. *Aphasiology, 18,* 951–975.

Sparks, R. (2001). Melodic Intonation Therapy. In R. Chapey (Ed.), *Language intervention strategies in aphasia and related neurogenic communication disorders, 4th ed.* (pp. 703–717). New York: Lippincott, Williams & Wilkins.

Sparks, R., Helm, N., & Albert, M. (1974). Aphasia rehabilitation resulting from Melodic Intonation Therapy. *Cortex, 10,* 303–316.

Speech, T. J., Rao, S. M., Osmon, D. C., & Sperry, L. T. (1993). A double-blind controlled study of methylphenidate treatment in closed head injury. *Brain Injury, 7,* 333–338.

Spencer, K. A., Tompkins, C. A., & Schulz, R. (1997). Assessment of depression in patients with brain pathology: The case of stroke. *Psychological Bulletin, 122,* 132–152.

Spreen, O., & Benton, A. L. (1977). *Neurosensory Center Comprehensive Examination for Aphasia* (rev. ed.). Victoria, BC: University of Victoria, Neuropsychology Laboratory.

Spreen, O., & Strauss, E. (1998). *A compendium of neuropsychological tests* (2nd ed.). New York: Oxford University Press.

Square, P. A., Martin, R. E., & Bose, A. (2001). Nature and treatment of neuromotor speech disorders in aphasia. In R. Chapey (Ed.), *Language intervention strategies in aphasia and related neurogenic communication disorders* (4th ed., pp. 847–884). Philadelphia: Lippincott, Williams & Wilkins.

Squire, L. R. (1987). *Memory and brain.* New York: Oxford University Press.

Squires, E. J., Hunkin, N. M., & Parkin, A. J. (1996). Memory notebook training in a case of severe amnesia: Generalizing from paired associate learning to real life. *Neuropsychological Rehabilitation, 6,* 55–65.

Stanczak, D. E., Lynch, M. D., McNeil, C. K., & Brown, B. (1998). The Expanded Trail Making Test: Rationale, development, and psychometric properties. *Archives of Clinical Neuropsychology, 13*, 473–487.

State University of New York at Buffalo Research Foundation. (1993) *Guide for the use of the uniform data set for medical rehabilitation: Functional independence measure.* Buffalo: State University of New York.

Stein, N. L., & Glenn, C. G. (1979). An analysis of story comprehension in elementary school children. In R. O. Freedle (Ed.), *New directions in discourse processing* (pp. 53–120). Norwood, NJ: Ablex.

Stein, R. A., & Strickland, T. L. (1998). A review of the neuropsychological effects of commonly used prescription medications. *Archives of Clinical Neuropsychology, 13*, 259–284.

Stern, R. A. (1998). *Visual Analog Mood Scales.* Odessa, FL: Psychological Assessment Resources.

Stern, R. A. (1999). Assessment of mood states in aphasia. *Seminars in Speech and Language, 20*, 33–50.

Stern, R. A., Javorsky, D. J., Singer, E. A., Singer Harris, N. G., Somerville, J. A., Duke, L. M., et al. (1999). *The Boston Qualitative Scoring System for the Rey-Osterrieth Complex Figure.* Lutz, FL: Psychological Assessment Resources.

Stern, R. A., & White, T. (2003). *Neuropsychological Assessment Battery.* Lutz, FL: Psychological Assessment Resources.

Stern, Y., Albert, M., Brandt, J., Jacobs, D. M., Tang, M. X. M., Marder K., et al. (1994). Utility of extrapyramidal signs and psychotic symptoms as predictors of cognitive and functional decline, nursing home admission, and death in Alzheimer's disease: Prospective analyses from the predictors study. *Neurology, 44*, 2300–2307.

Stierwalt, J., & Murray, L. L. (2002). Attention impairment in traumatic brain injury. *Seminars in Speech and Language, 23*, 129–138.

Stone, S. P., Patel, P., Greenwood, R. J., & Halligan, P. W. (1992). Measuring visual neglect in acute stroke and predicting its recovery: The visual neglect recovery index. *Journal of Neurology, Neurosurgery, and Psychiatry, 55*, 431–436.

Stout, J. C., & Murray, L. L. (2001). Assessment of memory in neurogenic communication disorders. *Seminars in Speech and Language, 22*, 137–145.

Stringer, A. Y. (1996). Treatment of motor aprosodia with pitch biofeedback and expression modeling. *Brain Injury, 10*, 583–590.

Sturm, W., Willmes, K., Orgass, B., & Hartje, W. (1997). Do specific attention deficits need specific training? *Neuropsychological Rehabilitation, 7*, 81–103.

Stuss, D. (1991). Disturbances of self-awareness after frontal system damage. In G. P. Prigatano & D. L. Schacter (Eds.), *Awareness of deficit after brain injury: Clinical and theoretical issues* (pp. 63–83). New York: Oxford University Press.

Stuss, D. T., & Levine, B. (2002). Adult clinical neuropsychology: Lessons from studies of the frontal lobes. *Annual Review of Psychology, 53*, 401–433.

Suarez, J. I. (2000). Acute ischemic stroke: Current treatment and future direction. *Special Interest Division 2: Neurophysiology and Neurogenic Speech and Language Disorders Newsletter, 10*, 5–10.

Suhr, J. S., Anderson, S., & Tranel, D. (1999). Progressive muscle relaxation in the management of behavioral disturbance in Alzheimer's disease. *Neuropsychological Rehabilitation, 9*, 31–44.

Sunderland, T., Alterman, I. S., Yount, D., Hill, J. L., Tariot, P. N., Newhouse, P. A., et al. (1988). A new scale for assessment of depressed mood in demented patients. *American Journal of Psychiatry, 145,* 955–959.

Sundin, K., Jansson, L., & Norberg, A. (2000). Communicating with people with stroke and aphasia: Understanding through sensation without words. *Journal of Clinical Nursing, 9,* 481–488.

Surian, L., & Siegal M. (2001). Sources of performance on theory of mind tasks in right hemisphere-damaged patients. *Brain and Language, 78,* 224–232.

Sutcliffe, L. M., & Lincoln, N. B. (1998). The assessment of depression in aphasic stroke patients: The development of the Stroke Aphasic Depression Questionnaire. *Clinical Rehabilitation, 12,* 506–513.

Sutton-Brown, M., & Suchowersky, O. (2003). Clinical and research advances in Huntington's disease. *Canadian Journal of Neurological Sciences, 30,* S45–S52.

Swartz, R., Miller, B. L., Darby, A., & Schuman, S. (1997). Frontotemporal dementia: Treatment response to serotonin selective reuptake inhibitors. *Journal of Clinical Psychiatry, 58,* 212–216.

Swigert, N. B. (1997). *The source for dysarthria.* East Moline, IL: Linguisystems.

Syder, D., Body, R., Parker, M., & Boddy, M. (1993). *Sheffield Screening Test for Acquired Language Disorders.* Manual: NferNelson.

Talland, G. A. (1965). *Deranged memory.* New York: Academic Press.

Tanaka, Y., & Albert, M. L. (2003). *Selective serotonin re-uptake inhibition as a treatment for depression and language disturbance in aphasia.* Paper presented at the annual International Neuropsychology Society Meeting, Waikiki, HI.

Tanaka, Y., & Bachman, D. L. (2000). Pharmacotherapy of aphasia. In L. T. Connor & L. K. Obler (Eds.), *Neurobehavior of language and cognition* (pp. 159–176). Boston, MA: Kluwer Academic Publishers.

Tanaka, Y., Miyazaki, M., & Albert, M. L. (1997). Effects of increased cholinergic activity on naming in aphasia. *The Lancet, 350,* 116–117.

Tanaka, Y., Nakano, I., & Obayashi, T. (2002). Environmental sound recognition after unilateral subcortical lesions. *Cortex, 38,* 69–76.

Tanner, D. C., & Culbertson, W. (1999a). *Caregiver-Administered Communication Inventory.* Oceanside, CA: Academic Communication Associates.

Tanner, D. C., & Culbertson, W. (1999b). *Quick Assessment for Aphasia.* Oceanside, CA: Academic Communication Associates.

Tanner, D. C., & Culbertson, W. (1999c). *Quick Assessment for Apraxia of Speech.* Oceanside, CA: Academic Communication Associates.

Tanner, D. C., & Culbertson, W. (1999d). *Quick Assessment for Dysarthria.* Oceanside, CA: Academic Communication Associates.

Tate, R. L. (1997). Beyond one-bun, two-shoe: Recent advances in the psychological rehabilitation of memory disorders after acquired brain injury. *Brain Injury, 11,* 907–918.

Tatemichi, T. K., Desmond, D. W., Stern, Y., Paik, M., Sano, M., & Bagiella, E. (1994). Cognitive impairment after stroke: Frequency, patterns, and relationship to functional abilities. *Journal of Neurology, Neurosurgery, and Psychiatry, 57,* 202–207.

Teasdale, G., & Jennett, B. (1976). Assessment and prognosis of coma after head injury. *Acta Neurochirurgica, 34,* 45–55.

Teng, E. L., & Chui, H. C. (1987). The Modified Mini-Mental State (3MS) Examination. *Journal of Clinical Psychiatry, 48,* 314–318.

Teri, L., Borson, S., Kiyak, H. A., & Yamagishi, M. (1989). Behavioral disturbance, cognitive dysfunction and functional skill: Prevalence and relationship in Alzheimer's disease. *Journal of the American Geriatrics Society, 37,* 109–116.

Terrell, B., & Ripich, D. (1989). Discourse competence as a variable in intervention. *Seminars in Speech and Language, 10,* 282–297.

Tham, K., & Tegner, R. (1997). Video feedback in the rehabilitation of patients with unilateral neglect. *Archives of Physical Medicine and Rehabilitation, 78,* 410–413.

Theodoros, D. G., Murdoch, B. E., & Goozee, J. V. (2001). Dysarthria following traumatic brain injury: Incidence, recovery and perceptual features. In B. E. Murdoch & D. G. Theodoros (Eds.), *Traumatic brain injury: Associated speech, language, and swallowing disorders* (pp. 27–51). Clifton Park, NY: Singular Thomson Delmar Learning.

Thompson, C. K. (2001). Treatment of underlying forms: A linguistic specific approach for sentence production deficits in agrammatic aphasia. In R. Chapey (Ed.), *Language intervention strategies in adult aphasia* (4th ed., pp. 605–628). New York: Lippincott, Williams & Wilkins.

Thompson, C. K., Ballard, K. J., & Shapiro, L. P. (1998). The role of syntactic complexity in training wh-movement structures in agrammatic aphasia: Optimal order for promoting generalization. *Journal of the International Neuropsychological Society, 4,* 661–674.

Thompson, C. K., Shapiro, L. P., Kiran, S., & Sobecks, J. (2003). The role of syntactic complexity in treatment of sentence deficits in agrammatic aphasia: The complexity account of treatment efficacy (CATE). *Journal of Speech, Language, and Hearing Research, 46,* 591–607.

Thompson, C. K., Shapiro, L. P., Tait, M. E., Jacobs, B. J., Schneider, S. L., & Ballard, K. J. (1995). A system for the linguistic analysis of agrammatic language production. *Brain and Language, 51,* 124–129.

Thomsen, I. V. (1984). Late outcome of very severe blunt head trauma: A 10-15-year second follow-up. *Journal of Neurology, Neurosurgery, and Psychiatry, 47,* 260–268.

Thurman, D., Alverson, C., Dunn, K., Guerrero, J., & Sniezek, J. (1999). Traumatic brain injury in the United States: A public health perspective. *Journal of Head Trauma and Rehabilitation, 14,* 602–15.

Thurstone, L. L., & Thurstone, T. G. (1962). *Primary mental abilities* (rev. ed.). Chicago: Science Research Associates.

Tiberti, C., Sabe, L., Jason, L., Leiguarda, R., & Starkstein, S. (1998). A randomized, double-blind, placebo-controlled study of methylphenidate in patients with organic amnesia. *European Journal of Neurology, 5,* 297–299.

Tingley, S. J., Kyte, C. S., Johnson, C. J., & Beitchman, J. H. (2003). Single-word and conversational measures of word-finding proficiency. *American Journal of Speech-Language Pathology, 12,* 359–368.

Togher, L. (2001). Discourse sampling in the 21st century. *Journal of Communication Disorders, 34,* 131–150.

Toglia, J. P. (1993). *Contextual Memory Test.* San Antonio, TX: The Psychological Corporation.

Tombaugh, T. N., & Hubley, A. M. (1997). The 60-item Boston Naming Test: Norms for cognitively intact adults aged 25 to 88 years. *Journal of Clinical and Experimental Neuropsychology, 19,* 922–932.

Tombaugh, T. N., & McIntyre, N. J. (1992). The Mini-Mental State Examination: A comprehensive review. *Journal of the American Geriatrics Society, 40,* 922–935.

Tomer, R., Levin, B. E., & Weiner, W. J. (1993). Side of onset of motor symptoms influences cognition in Parkinson's disease. *Annals of Neurology, 34,* 579–584.

Tomlin, K. J. (2002). *Workbook of activities for language and cognition-2.* East Moline, IL: Linguisystems.

Tompkins, C. A. (1995). *Right hemisphere communication disorders: Theory and management.* Clifton Park, NY: Singular Thomson Delmar Learning.

Tompkins, C. A., Bloise, C. G. R., Timko, M. L., & Baumgaertner, A. (1994). Working memory and inference revision in brain-damaged and normally aging adults. *Journal of Speech and Hearing Research, 37,* 896–912.

Tompkins, C. A., & Flowers, C. R. (1985). Perception of emotional intonation by brain-damaged adults: The influence of task processing levels. *Journal of Speech and Hearing Research, 28,* 527–538.

Tompkins, C. A., Jackson, S., & Shulz, R. (1990). On prognostic research in adult neurologic disorders. *Journal of Speech and Hearing Research, 33,* 398–401.

Tompkins, C. A., & Lehman, M. T. (1997). Outcomes measurement in cognitive communication disorders. Section 2: Right-hemisphere brain damage. In C. M. Frattali (Ed.), *Measuring outcomes in speech-language pathology* (pp. 281–292). New York: Thieme.

Tompkins, C. A., Lehman Blake, M., Baumgaertner, A., & Fassbinder, W. (2001). Mechanisms of discourse comprehension impairment after right hemisphere brain damage: Suppression in inferential ambiguity resolution. *Journal of Speech, Language and Hearing Research, 44,* 400–415.

Tompkins, C. A., & Lustig, A. P. (2001). Research principles for the clinician. In R. Chapey (Ed.), *Language intervention strategies in aphasia and related neurogenic communication disorders* (4th ed., pp. 129–147). Baltimore: Lippincott, Williams & Wilkins.

Tonkonogy, J. M. (1986). *Vascular aphasia.* Cambridge, MA: MIT Press.

Torgesen, J. K., Wagner, R., & Rashotte, C. (1999). *Test of Word Reading Efficiency.* Austin, TX: Pro-Ed.

Torti, F. M., Gwyther, L., Reed, S. D., Friedman, J., & Schulman, K. (2004). A multinational review of recent trends and reports in dementia caregiver burden. *Alzheimer Disease and Associated Disorders, 18,* 99–109.

Trahan, D. E., & Larrabee, G. J. (1988). *Continuous Visual Memory Test.* Lutz, FL: Psychological Assessment Resources.

Trenerry, M. R., Crosson, B., DeBoe, J., & Leber, W. R. (1989). *Stroop Neuropsychological Screening Test.* Lutz, FL: Psychological Assessment Resources.

Trenerry, M. R., Crosson, B., DeBoe, J., & Leber, W. R. (1990). *Visual Search and Attention Test.* Lutz, FL: Psychological Assessment Resources.

Turkstra, L. S. (1999). Language testing in adolescents with brain injury: A consideration of the CELF-3. *Language, Speech and Hearing Services in Schools, 30,* 132–140.

Turkstra, L. S. (2001). Treating memory problems in adults with neurogenic communication disorders. *Seminars in Speech and Language, 22,* 149–156.

Turkstra, L. S., & Flora, T. (2002). Compensation for executive function impairments after TBI: A single case study of functional intervention. *Journal of Communication Disorders, 35,* 167–182.

Turkstra, L. S., & Holland, A. L. (1998). Assessment of syntax after adolescent brain injury: Effects of memory on test performance. *Journal of Speech, Language and Hearing, 41,* 137–149.

Ulatowska, H. K., Chapman, S. B., & Johnson, J. K. (1995). Processing of proverbs in aphasics and old-elderly. *Clinical Aphasiology, 23,* 179–193.

Ulatowska, H. K., Doyel, A. W., Freedman-Stern, R. F., Macaluso-Hayes, S., & North, A. J. (1983). Production of procedural discourse in aphasia. *Brain and Language, 18,* 315–341.

Ulatowska, H. K., Olness, G. S., Hill, C. L., Roberts, J. A., & Keebler, M. W. (2000). Repetition in narratives of African Americans: The effects of aphasia. *Discourse Processes, 30,* 265–283.

Ulatowska, H. R., & Richardson, S. M. (1974). A longitudinal study of an adult with aphasia: Considerations for research and therapy. *Brain and Language, 1,* 151–166.

Vakil, E., Biederman, Y., Liran, G., Groswaser, Z., & Aberbuch, S. (1994). Head-injured patients and control group: Implicit versus explicit measures of frequency of occurrence. *Journal of Clinical and Experimental Neuropsychology, 16,* 539–546.

Vallar, G., Rusconi, M. L., & Bernardini, B. (1996). Modulation of neglect hemianesthesia by transcutaneous electrical stimulation. *Journal of the International Neuropsychology Society, 2,* 452–459.

Vallino-Napoli, L. D., & Reilly, S. (2004). Evidence-based health care: A survey of speech pathology practice. *Advances in Speech-Language Pathology, 6,* 107–112.

Van der Linden, M., Meulemans, T., & Lorrain, D. (1994). Acquisition of new concepts by two amnesic patients. *Cortex, 30,* 305–317.

Vanderploeg, R. D., Axelrod, B. N., Sherer, M., Scott, J. G, & Adams, R. L. (1997). The importance of demographic adjustments on neuropsychological test performance: A response to Reitan and Wolfson (1995). *The Clinical Neuropsychologist, 11,* 210–217.

van de Sandt-Koenderman, M. W. M. (2004). High-tech AAC and aphasia: Widening horizons? *Aphasiology, 18,* 245–263.

van De Weg, F. B., Kuik, D. J., & Lankhorst, G. J. (1999). Post-stroke depression and functional outcome: A cohort study investigating the influence of depression on functional recovery from stroke. *Clinical Rehabilitation, 13,* 268–272.

van Harskamp, F., & Visch-Brink, E. (1991). Goal recognition in aphasia therapy. *Aphasiology, 5,* 529–539.

Van Mourik, M., Verschaeve, M., Boon, P., Paquier, P., & Van Harskamp, F. (1992). Cognition in global aphasia: Indicators for therapy. *Aphasiology, 6,* 491–499.

Van Zomeren, A. H., & Brouwer, W. H. (1994). *Clinical neuropsychology of attention.* New York: Oxford University Press.

Varney, N. R. (1982). Pantomime recognition defect in aphasia: Implications for the concept of asymbolia. *Brain and Language, 15,* 32–39.

Varney, N. R. (1998). Neuropsychological assessment of aphasia. In G. Goldstein, P. D. Nussbaum, & S. R. Beers (Eds.), *Neuropsychology* (pp. 357–378). New York: Plenum Press.

Verdolini, K. (1994) Voice disorders. In J. B. Tomblin, H. L. Morris, & D. C. Spriestersbach (Eds.) *Diagnosis in speech-language pathology* (pp 247–297). Clifton Park, NY: Singular Thomson Delmar Learning.

Vickers, C. (2004). Communicating in groups: One stop on the road to improved participation for persons with aphasia. *Perspectives on Neurophysiology and Neurogenic Speech and Language Disorders, 14,* 16–20.

Vignolo, L. A. (1964). Evolution of aphasia and language rehabilitation: A retrospective exploratory study. *Cortex, 1,* 344–67.

Vignolo, L. A. (2003). Music agnosia and auditory agnosia: Dissociations in stroke patients. *Annals of the New York Academy of Sciences, 999,* 50–57.

Vignolo, L. A., Boccardi, E., & Caverni, L. (1986). Unexpected CT-scan findings in global aphasia. *Cortex, 22,* 55–69.

Visser-Keizer, A. C., Meyboom-de Jong, B., Deelman, B. G., Berg, I J., & Gerritsen, M. J. J. (2002). Subjective changes in emotion, cognition, and behavior after stroke: Factors affecting the perception of patients and partners. *Journal of Clinical and Experimental Neuropsychology, 24,* 1032–1045.

Vogel, D., & Cannito, M. P. (2001). *Treating disordered speech motor control.* Austin, TX: Pro-Ed.

Vogel, D., Carter, J. E., & Carter, P. B. (2000). *The effects of drugs on communication disorders.* Clifton Park, NY: Singular Thomson Delmar Learning.

Wagner, A. K., Sasser, H. C., Hammond, F. M., Wierciseiwski, D., & Alexander, J. (2000). Intentional traumatic brain injury: Epidemiology, risk factors, and associations with injury severity and mortality. *The Journal of Trauma Injury, Infection, and Critical Care, 49,* 404–410.

Walker, R., Young, A. W., & Lincoln, N. B. (1996). Eye patching and rehabilitation in unilateral neglect. *Neuropsychological Rehabilitation, 6,* 219–231.

Walker-Batson, D., Curtis, S., Natarajan, R., Ford, J., Dronkers, N., Salmeron, E., et al. (2001). A double-blind, placebo-controlled study of the use of amphetamine in the treatment of aphasia. *Stroke, 32,* 2093–2098.

Walker-Batson, D., Curtis, S., Wolf, T., & Porch, B. (1996). Amphetamine treatment accelerates recovery from aphasia. *Brain and Language, 55,* 27–29.

Walker-Batson, D., Smith, P., Curtis, S., Unwin, H., & Greenlee, R. G. (1995). Amphetamine paired with physical therapy accelerates recovery from stroke: Further evidence. *Stroke, 26,* 2254–2259.

Walker-Batson, D., Unwin, H., Curtis, S., Allen, E., Wood, M., Smith, P., et al. (1992). Use of amphetamine in the treatment of aphasia. *Restorative Neurology and Neuroscience, 4,* 47–50.

Wallace, G., & Hammill, D. D. (2002). *Comprehensive Receptive and Expressive Vocabulary Test* (2nd ed.). Austin, TX: Pro-Ed.

Wambaugh, J. L. (2003). A comparison of the relative effects of phonologic and semantic cueing treatments. *Aphasiology, 17,* 433–441.

Wambaugh, J. L., Doyle, P. J., Martinez, A. L., & Kalinyak-Fliszar, M. (2002). Effects of two lexical retrieval cueing treatments on action naming in aphasia. *Journal of Rehabilitation Research and Development, 39,* 455–466.

Wambaugh, J. L., Linebaugh, C. W., Doyle, P. J, Martinez, A. L., Kalinyak-Fliszar, M., & Spencer, K. A. (2001). Effects of two cueing treatments on lexical retrieval in aphasic speakers with different levels of deficit. *Aphasiology, 15,* 933–950.

Wambaugh, J. L., & Martinez, A. L. (2000). Effects of modified response elaboration training with apraxia and aphasic speakers. *Aphasiology, 14,* 603–617.

Wambaugh, J. L., Martinez, A. L., & Alegre, M. N. (2001). Qualitative changes following application of modified response elaboration training with apraxic-aphasic speakers. *Aphasiology, 15,* 965–976.

Ward, H., Shum, D., Dick, B., McKinlay, L., & Baker-Tweney, S. (2004). Interview study of the effects of paediatric traumatic brain injury on memory. *Brain Injury, 18,* 471–495.

Ward-Lonergan, J., & Nicholas, M. (1995). Drawing to communicate: A case report of an adult with global aphasia. *European Journal of Disorders of Communication, 30,* 475–491.

Warner, T. T., & Schapira, A. H. V. (2003). Genetic and environmental factors in the cause of Parkinson's disease. *Annals of Neurology, 53,* S16–S25.

Warren, R. L. (1992). Functional outcome: An introduction. *Clinical Aphasiology, 21,* 59–65.

Warrington, E. K. (1999). *Recognition Memory Test.* Lutz, FL: Psychological Assessment Resources.

Warrington, E. K., & James, M. (1991). *Visual Object and Space Perception Battery.* Gaylord, MI: National Rehabilitation Services.

Watanabe, Y., & Taki, K. (2000). An evaluation of neurobehavioral problems as perceived by family members and levels of family stress 1–3 years following traumatic brain injury in Japan. *Clinical Rehabilitation, 14,* 172–177.

Watt, S., Shores, S. E., & Kinoshita, S. (1999). Effects of reducing attentional resources on implicit and explicit memory after severe traumatic brain injury. *Neuropsychology, 13,* 338–349.

Webster, J. S., McFarland, P. T., Rapport, L. J., Morrill, B., Roades, L. A., & Abadee, P. S. (2001). Computer-assisted training for improving wheelchair mobility in unilateral neglect patients. *Archives of Physical Medicine and Rehabilitation, 82,* 769–775.

Wechsler, D. (1981). *Wechsler Adult Intelligence Scales-Revised.* San Antonio, TX: The Psychological Corporation.

Wechsler, D. (1987). *Wechsler Memory Scale-R.* San Antonio, TX: The Psychological Corporation.

Wechsler, D. (1991). *Wechsler Intelligence Scales for Children-III.* San Antonio, TX: The Psychological Corporation.

Wechsler, D. (1997a). *Wechsler Adult Intelligence Scales-III.* San Antonio, TX: The Psychological Corporation.

Wechsler, D. (1997b). *Wechsler Memory Scale-III.* San Antonio, TX: The Psychological Corporation.

Wechsler, D. (1999). *Wechsler Abbreviated Scale of Intelligence.* San Antonio, TX: The Psychological Corporation.

Wechsler, D. (2001). *Wechsler Test of Adult Reading.* San Antonio, TX: The Psychological Corporation.

Wee, J., & Menard, M. R. (1999). "Pure word deafness": Implications for assessment and management in communication disorder—a report of two cases. *Archives of Physical Medicine and Rehabilitation, 80,* 1106–1109.

Weidner, W. E., & Lasky, E. Z. (1976). The interaction of rate and complexity of stimulus on the performance of adult aphasic subjects. *Brain and Language, 3,* 34–40.

Weigl, E. (1981). *Neuropsychology and neurolinguistics: Selected papers.* New York: Mouton.

Weindling, F. H. (2000). Speech-language pathology: A home care viewpoint. *American Journal of Speech-Language Pathology, 9,* 99–106.

Weintraub, S., & Mesulam, M. M. (1985). *Verbal and Nonverbal Cancellation Test.* Philadelphia: F. A. Davis.

Weintraub, S., Mesulam, M. M., & Kramer, L. (1981). Disturbances in prosody: A right-hemisphere contribution to language. *Archives of Neurology, 38,* 742–744.

Weintraub, S., Rubin, N. P., & Mesulam, M. M. (1990). Primary progressive aphasia. Longitudinal course, neuropsychological profile, and language features. *Archives of Neurology, 47,* 1329–335.

Welch, L. W., Doineau, D., Johnson, S., & King, D. (1996). Education and gender normative data for the Boston Naming Test in a group of older adults. *Brain and Language, 53,* 260–266.

Welden, S., & Yesavage, J. (1982). Behavioral improvement with relaxation training in senile dementia. *Clinical Gerontologist, 1,* 43–49.

Welland, R. J., Lubinski, R., & Higginbotham, D. J. (2002). Discourse comprehension test performance of elders with dementia of the Alzheimer's type. *Journal of Speech, Language and Hearing Research, 45,* 1175–1187.

Wen, P. Y., Fine, H. A., Black, P. M., Shrieve, D. C., Alexander, E., & Loeffler, J. S. (1995). High-grade astrocytomas. *Neurologic Clinics, 13,* 875–900.

Wertz, R. T. (1998). *Treatment studies in communication disorders: Nosology, phase I–V outcomes, levels of evidence, interpretation, and who's who.* Nashville, TN: 1998 Treatment Efficacy Conference at Vanderbilt University School of Medicine.

Wertz, R. T., Deal, J. L., & Robinson, A. J. (1984). Classifying the aphasias: A comparison of the Boston Diagnostic Aphasia Examination and the Western Aphasia Battery. *Clinical Aphasiology, 14,* 40–47.

Wertz, R. T., & Irwin, W. H. (2001). Darley and the efficacy of language rehabilitation in aphasia. *Aphasiology, 15,* 231–247.

Wertz, R. T., & Katz, R. C. (2004). Outcomes of computer-provided treatment for aphasia. *Aphasiology, 18,* 229–244.

West, J., Sands, E., & Ross-Swain, D. (1998). *Bedside Evaluation Screening Test of Aphasia.* (2nd ed.). Austin, TX: Pro-Ed.

Wetherell, J. L. (1998). Treatment of anxiety in older adults. *Psychotherapy, 35,* 444–458.

Whiteneck, G. G., Charlifue, S. W., Gerhart, K. A., Overholser, J. D., & Richardson, G. N. (1992). Quantifying handicap: A new measure of long-term rehabilitation outcomes. *Archives of Physical and Medical Rehabilitation, 73,* 519–526.

Whitworth, A., Perkins, L., & Lesser, R. (1997). *Conversation Analysis Profile for People with Aphasia.* Philadelphia: Taylor & Francis.

Whurr, M., & Lorch, M. (1991). The use of a prosthesis to facilitate writing in aphasia and right hemiplegia. *Aphasiology, 5,* 411–418.

Whurr, R. (1997). *The Aphasia Screening Test* (2nd ed.). Philadelphia: Taylor & Francis.

Whyte, J., Hart, T., Schuster, K., Fleming, M., Polansky, M., & Coslett, H. B. (1997). Effects of methylphenidate on attentional function after traumatic brain injury: A randomized, placebo-controlled trial. *American Journal of Physical Medicine and Rehabilitation, 76,* 440–450.

Wiederholt, J. L., & Blalock, G. (2001). *Gray Silent Reading Test.* Austin, TX: Pro-Ed.

Wiederholt, J. L., & Bryant, B. R. (2002). *Gray Oral Reading Tests* (4th ed.). Austin, TX: Pro-Ed.

Wierenga, C. E., Richards, K. S., Singletary, F., Rodriguez, A., Kendall, D., Leon, S., et al. (2003). *Intention and attention treatments of high functioning nonfluent aphasia.* Poster presentation at the annual International Neuropsychology Society conference, Waikiki, HI.

Wiig, E. H., Nielsen, N. P., Minthon, L., & Warkentin, S. (2002). *Alzheimer's Quick Test: Assessment of Parietal Function.* San Antonio, TX: The Psychological Corporation.

Wiig, E. H., & Secord, W. (1989). *Test of Language Competence-Expanded Edition.* San Antonio, TX: The Psychological Corporation.

Wiig, E. H., & Secord, W. A. (1992). *Test of Word Knowledge.* San Antonio, TX: The Psychological Corporation.

Wilkinson, G. S. (1993). *Wide Range Achievement Test* (3rd ed.). Wilmington, DE: Wide Range.

Wilkinson, R., Bryan, K., Lock, S., Bayley, K., Maxim, J., Bruce, C., et al. (1998). Therapy using conversation analysis: Helping couples adapt to aphasia in conversation. *International Journal of Language and Communication Disorders, 33,* 144–149.

Willer, B., Rosenthal, M., Kreutzer, J. S., Gordon, W.A., & Rempel, R. (1993). Assessment of community integration following rehabilitation for traumatic brain injury. *Journal of Head Trauma Rehabilitation. 8,* 75–87.

Williams, J. M. (1987). *Cognitive Behavior Rating Scales.* Lutz, FL: Psychological Assessment Resources.

Williams, L. S., Weinberger, M., Harris, L. E., Clark, D. O., & Biller, H. (1999). Development of a stroke-specific quality of life scale. *Stroke, 30,* 1362–1369.

Williams, M. (1990). *Test of Auditory Perception.* Woodsboro, MD: Cool Spring Software.

Williams, M. (1994a). *Criterion-Oriented Test of Attention.* Marlton, NJ: Brainmetric Software.

Williams, M. (1994b). *Test of Visual Field Attention.* Marlton, NJ: Brainmetric Software.

Williams, M. (1994c). *The Category Test.* Marlton, NJ: Brainmetric Software.

Williams, M. (1994d). *Williams Inhibition Test.* Marlton, NJ: Brainmetric Software.

Williams, M. (1996*). The Naming Test.* Marlton, NJ: Brainmetric Software.

Wilson, B. (1982). Success and failure in memory training following a cerebral vascular accident. *Cortex, 18,* 581–594.

Wilson, B. A. (1996). *Wilson reading system.* Milbury, MA: Wilson Language Training Corporation.

Wilson, B. A., Alderman, N., Burgess, P., Emslie, H., & Evans, J. J. (1996). *Behavioral Assessment of the Dysexecutive Syndrome.* Bury St. Edmunds, Suffolk, England: Thames Valley Test Company.

Wilson, B. A., Baddeley, A. D., Evans, E., & Shiel, A. (1994). Errorless learning in the rehabilitation of memory impaired people. *Neuropsychological Rehabilitation, 4,* 307–326.

Wilson, B. A., Clare, L., Baddeley, A., Cockburn, J., Watson, P., & Tate, R. (1998). *The Rivermead Behavioral Memory Test-Extended Version.* Bury St. Edmunds, Suffolk, England: Thames Valley Test Company.

Wilson, B. A., Cockburn, J., & Baddeley, A. (1985). *The Rivermead Behavioral Memory Test.* Bury St. Edmunds, Suffolk, England: Thames Valley Test Company.

Wilson, B. A., Cockburn, J., & Baddeley, A. (2003). *The Rivermead Behavioral Memory Test* (2nd ed.). Bury St. Edmunds, Suffolk, England: Thames Valley Test Company.

Wilson, B. A., Cockburn, J., Baddeley, A. D., & Hiorns, R. (1989). The development and validation of a test battery for detecting and monitoring everyday memory problems. *Journal of Clinical and Experimental Neuropsychology, 11,* 855–870.

Wilson, B. A., Cockburn, J., & Halligan, P. (1987). *The Behavioral Inattention Test.* Bury St. Edmunds, Suffolk, England: Thames Valley Test Company.

Wilson, B. A., Emslie, H. C., Quirk, K., & Evans, J. J. (2001). Reducing everyday memory and planning problems by means of a paging system: A randomized control crossover study. *Journal of Neurology, Neurosurgery, and Psychiatry, 70,* 477–482.

Wilson, B. A., & Evans, E. (1996). Error-free learning in the rehabilitation of people with memory impairments. *Journal of Head Trauma Rehabilitation, 11,* 54–64.

Wilson, B. A., Evans, J. J., Emslie, H., & Malinek, V. (1997). Evaluation of NeuroPage: A new memory aid. *Journal of Neurology, Neurosurgery and Psychiatry, 63,* 113–115.

Wilson, B. A., Shiel, A., Foley, J., Emslie, H., Groot, Y., Hawkins, K., et al. (2005). *Cambridge Test of Prospective Memory.* Bury St. Edmunds, Suffolk, England: Thames Valley Test Company.

Wilson, B. A., Watson, P. C., Baddeley, A. D., Emslie, H., & Evans, J. J. (2000). Improvement or simply practice? The effects of twenty repeated assessments on people with and without brain injury. *Journal of the International Neuropsychological Society, 6,* 469–479.

Wilson, C., & Manly, T. (2003). Sustained attention training and errorless learning facilitates self-care functioning in chronic ipsilesional neglect following severe traumatic brain injury. *Neuropsychological Rehabilitation, 13,* 537–549.

Wilson, C., & Robertson, I. H. (1992). A home-based intervention for attentional slips during reading following head injury: A single case study. *Neuropsychological Rehabilitation, 2,* 193–205.

Wilson, R. S., Rosenbaum, G., & Brown, B. (1979). The problem of premorbid intelligence in neuropsychological assessment. *Journal of Clinical Neuropsychology, 1,* 49–53.

Wilson, S. L., Powell, G. E., Elliot, K., & Thwaites, H. (1993). Evaluation of sensory stimulation as a treatment for prolonged coma: Seven single experimental case studies. *Neuropsychological Rehabilitation, 3,* 191–201.

Winograd, P., & Hare, V. C. (1988). Direct instruction of reading comprehension strategies: The nature of teacher explanation. In C. Weinstein, E. Goetz & P. Alexander (Eds.), *Learning and study strategies: Issues in assessment, instruction and evaluation* (pp. 121–138.). New York: Academic Press.

Wiseman-Hakes, C., Stewart, M. L., Wasserman, R., & Schuller, R. (1998). Peer group training of pragmatic skills in adolescents with acquired brain injury. *Journal of Head Trauma Rehabilitation, 13,* 23–28.

Witol, A. D., Kreutzer, J. S., & Sander, A. M. (1999). Emotional, behavioral and personality assessment after traumatic brain injury. In M. Rosenthal, E. R. Griffith, J. S. Kreutzer, & B. Pentland (Eds.), *Rehabilitation of the adult and child with traumatic brain injury* (3rd ed., pp. 167–182). Philadelphia: F. A. Davis.

Wolman, R. L., Cornall, C., Flucher, K. R., & Greenwood, R. (1994). Aerobic training in brain-injured patients. *Clinical Rehabilitation, 8,* 253–257.

World Health Organization (1980). *International classification of impairments, disabilities, and handicaps: A manual relating to the consequences of disease.* Geneva, Switzerland: Author.

World Health Organization (2001). *ICF: International classification of functioning, disability, and health.* Geneva, Switzerland: Author.

Wressle, E., Eeg-Olofsson, A., Marcusson, J., & Henriksson, C. (2002). Improved client participation in the rehabilitation process using a client-centred goal formulation structure. *Journal of Rehabilitation Medicine, 34,* 5–11.

Wright, H. H., & Newhoff, M. (2005). Pragmatics. In L. L. La Pointe (Ed.), *Aphasia and related neurogenic language disorders* (3rd ed., pp. 237–248). New York: Thieme.

Wright, P., Rogers, N., Hall, C., Wilson, B., Evans, J., Emslie, H., et al. (2001). Comparison of pocket-computer memory aids for people with brain injury. *Brain Injury, 15,* 787–800.

Wymer, J. H., Lindman, L. S., & Booksh, R. L. (2002). A neuropsychological perspective of aprosody: Features, function, assessment and treatment. *Applied Neuropsychology, 9,* 37–47.

Yamadera, H., Ito, T., Suzuki, H., Asayama, K., Ito, R., & Endo, S. (2000). Effects of bright light on cognitive and sleep-wake (circadian) rhythm disturbances in Alzheimer-type dementia. *Psychiatry and Clinical Neurosciences, 54,* 352–354.

Yampolsky, S., & Waters, G. (2002). Treatment of single word oral reading in an individual with deep dyslexia. *Aphasiology, 16,* 455–471.

Yasuda, K., Misu, T., Beckman, B., Watanabe, O., Ozawa, Y., & Nakamura, T. (2002). Use of an IC Recorder as a voice output memory aid for patients with prospective memory impairment. *Neuropsychological Rehabilitation, 12,* 155–166.

Yasuda, K., Nakamura, T., & Beckman, B. (2000). Comprehension and storage of four serially presented radio news stories by mild aphasic subjects. *Brain and Language, 75,* 399–415.

Yesavage, J. A., Brink, T. L., Rose, T. L., Lum, O., Huang, V., Adey, M., et al. (1983). Development and validation of a geriatric depression screening scale: A preliminary report. *Journal of Psychiatric Research, 17,* 37–49.

Ylvisaker, M., & Feeney, T. (1998). A Vygotskyan approach to rehabilitation after TBI: A case illustration. *Special Interest Division 2: Neurophysiology and Neurogenic Speech and Language Disorders Newsletter, 8,* 14–18.

Ylvisaker, M., Szekeres, S. F., & Feeney, T. J. (1998). Cognitive rehabilitation: Executive functions. In M. Ylvisaker (Ed.), *Traumatic brain injury rehabilitation: Children and adolescents* (2nd ed., pp. 221–269). Boston, MA: Butterworth-Heinemann.

Yoo, E., Park, E., & Chung, B. (2001). Mental practice effect on line-tracing accuracy in persons with hemiparetic stroke: A preliminary study. *Archives of Physical Medicine and Rehabilitation, 82,* 1213–1218.

Yorkston, K., & Beukelman, D. (1980). An analysis of connected speech samples of aphasic and normal speakers. *Journal of Speech and Hearing Disorders, 45,* 27–36.

Yorkston, K. M., Beukelman, D. R., Strand, E. A., & Bell, K. R. (1999). *Management of motor speech disorders in children and adults* (2nd ed.). Austin, TX: Pro-Ed.

Yorkston, K. M., Beukelman, D. R., & Traynor, C. (1984). *Assessment of Intelligibility of Dysarthric Speech.* Austin, TX: Pro-Ed.

Young, A., Perrett, D., Calder, A., Sprengelmeyer, R., & Elkman, P. (2002). *Facial Expression Stimuli and Test.* Bury St. Edmunds, Suffolk, England: Thames Valley Test Company.

Zafonte, R., Hammond, F., & Peterson, J. (1996). Predicting outcome in the slow to respond traumatically brain injured patient: Acute and subacute parameters. *NeuroRehabilitation, 6,* 19–24.

Zafonte, R. D., Elovic, E., Mysiw, W. J., O'Dell, M., & Watanabe, T. (1999). Pharmacology in traumatic brain injury: Fundamentals and treatment strategies. In M. Rosenthal, J. S. Kreutzer, E. R. Griffith, & Pentland, B. (Eds.), *Rehabilitation of the adult and child with traumatic brain injury* (3rd ed., pp. 536–555). Philadelphia: F. A. Davis.

Zangwill, O. L. (1967). Speech and the minor hemisphere. *Acta Neurologica et Psychiatrica Belgica, 67,* 1013–1020.

Zeman, A. (1997). Persistent vegetative state. *The Lancet, 350,* 795–799.

Zgaljardic, D. J., Borod, J. C., Foldi, N. S., & Mattis, P. (2003). A review of the cognitive and behavioral sequelae of Parkinson's disease: Relationship to frontostriatal circuitry. *Cognitive and Behavioral Neurology, 16,* 193–210.

Zhang, Z. (1989). Efficacy of acupuncture in the treatment of post-stroke aphasia. *Journal of Traditional Chinese Medicine, 9,* 87–89.

Zhang, Z., & Zhao, C. (1990). Comparative observations on the curative results of the treatment of central aphasia by puncturing the yumen point versus conventional acupuncture methods. *Journal of Traditional Chinese Medicine, 10,* 260–263.

Ziegler, W. (2002). Psycholinguistic and motor theories of apraxia of speech. *Seminars in Speech and Language, 23,* 231–244.

Ziegler, W., Kerkhoff, G., Cate, D., Artinger, F., & Zierdt, A. (2001). Spatial processing of spoken words in aphasia and in neglect. *Cortex, 37,* 754–756.

Zingeser, L. B., & Berndt, R. S. (1990). Retrieval of nouns and verbs in agrammatism and anomia. *Brain and Language, 39,* 14–32.

Zollman, C., & Vickers, A. (1999). Users and practitioners of complementary medicine. *BMJ, 399,* 836–838.

Index